The Path

Book II: Mind and Body

Dedicated to Mihoko Kobayashi
who has always been there
and has the purest heart
I have ever known.
domo, Michan
Araiguma
ag

The Path:
A Book of Potential
by
Eric A. Smith
copyright 2012

BOOK II: MIND AND BODY

Cover art: Parc de Marly Cathedral Trees,
Margot van der Heijden 2011. Used with permission.

Long ago, it's said, a Cherokee elder told his grandson,
"There is a battle between two wolves inside each of us.
One is Evil: anger, jealousy, regret, greed,
arrogance, self-pity, guilt, resentment, & lies.
The other is Good: joy, peace, love, hope, serenity,
humility, empathy, generosity, truth, compassion and faith."

Said the child, "Which wolf wins?"
To which the elder replied, "The one you feed."

– John Bisagno, 1965

Foreword

Dear Reader:

Welcome back!

In Book I, you learned of the incredible power and astounding complexity of your brain, genetic heritage, endocrine and nervous systems, and of how to use this knowledge to initiate profound, lasting changes in your life.

Here, you'll learn how to unleash the awe-inspiring capacities that lie dormant within you, and how to harness your body for astonishing strength, robust health and longevity. You'll discover how you can boost your IQ, maximize your learning, and shatter the limits of memory, of how to maximize your influence, and the true secrets of happiness.

You're going to learn about the truly awesome power you possess in your body, how it converts food into its energy and building blocks, nutrients to heal you and supercharge your health, and how to feed and otherwise maintain your body for superb, lifelong health and youth.

Discover superfoods under research now by the US government that reverse the effects of Alzheimer's, and about revolutionary technology that's about to enable you to live well past the century mark. You'll study the roots of human attraction and learn magnetic social skills taught nowhere else.

Volume I was all about teaching you how to reach your potential. Now you're going to learn how to become superhuman.

Whenever you're ready, let's continue.

Contents

BOOK II: MIND AND BODY

Part IV: Connecting

Deadly

"Men, for the sake of getting a living, forget to live."
- Margaret Fuller, The Dial Magazine, 1843

Every single day you encounter it. It's your worst enemy, and you probably aren't even aware of its silent, unremitting assault, causing premature aging, lowering your defenses against disease, making you fat, irritable and tired, sapping your energy, destroying your libido, concentration and appetite, and shortening your life. The culprit is *stress*, and it's deadly. Fortunately, there are ways to fight it and its devastating effects.

Stress is a term first coined by American biologist Hans Selye in the 1930s. It refers to when a living creature – human or animal – feels fear, anger or related negative emotions because of a threat. These threats don't even have to be real; imaginary threats can also cause stress.

Dr. Selye said there are two kinds of stress – *eustress* (positive stress, which leads to improvement) and *distress* (negative stress, which leads to physical and mental disease). He says that positive stress comes from people's work, and is necessary to a healthy life. On the other hand, *distress* is insidious and deadly.

What A Baboon Can Teach You About Stress

Since 1978, Stanford University's Dr. Robert Sapolsky has been studying the effects of stress on the bodies of baboons in the Masai Mara wild game reserve in Kenya, Africa:

> *You live in a place like this, you're a baboon, and you only have to spend about three hours a day getting your calories. And if you only have to work three hours a day, you've got nine hours of free time every day to devote to making somebody else just miserable.*

> *They're not being stressed by lions chasing them all the time, they're being stressed by each other. They're being stressed by social and psychological tumult invented by their own species. They're a perfect model for westernized stress-related disease.*

By anaesthetizing baboons with a blow gun, Dr. Sapolsky is able to subdue them without adding anticipatory stress, and can measure stress hormone levels in blood samples. He says two hormones are the primary *workhorses* of the stress response – epinephrine and glucocorticoids, both released by the adrenal glands in response to stress.

In the wild, stress is primarily about only thing: eat or be eaten. Because of this, when the adrenal glands release stress hormones, the body prepares for three minutes of "kill or be killed" level activity, causing you to hyperventilate and your heart rate and blood pressure to increase, pumping huge amounts of oxygen into your bloodstream so your muscles can respond instantly, and turning off all nonessential processes, such as digestion, waste elimination, tissue growth and repair, and immune and reproductive functions.

In the wild, once it's no longer needed, the stress response immediately shuts down. Unfortunately, in humans, our ability to worry and ruminate means we artificially and continuously stimulate this life or death emergency system, and it often just stays activated, with deadly cumulative effects, making us, as *National Geographic* science writer John Heminway puts it, "...wallow in a corrosive bath of hormones." The effects are deadly, resulting in:

- *atherosclerosis* – damage to artery walls, with pits and scarring that provide sites for a deadly buildup of plaques that can lead to heart attacks and strokes;

- *neural atrophy and die-off*, particularly in the hippocampus, critical to memory and learning;

- *abdominal adipose tissue accumulation*, better known as belly fat, the most dangerous type of all, slowing the metabolism and greatly increasing the risks of obesity, heart attacks and diabetes;

- *lower dopamine levels*, meaning life is less fulfilling for the stressed;

- *Suppression of the immune system*, leading to an increase in bacteria responsible for *peptic ulcers* – sores caused by bacteria eating at the lining of the stomach. Simultaneously, this slows metabolic rate, so your body is less effective at repairing such damage

Dr. Sapolsky's 30 years of study have demonstrated a direct link between social status, stress hormone levels and poor health and longevity among baboons. Social rank, he says, directly correlates with stress hormone levels in each creature's system. Alpha baboons are the least affected, enjoying lives of relative comfort, ease and robust health, while beta baboons are subject to torment, and suffer ill health, shorter life spans, increased heart rates, higher blood pressure, elevated stress hormone levels, depressed immune responses and even poorer reproductive function. "And all that stuff," says Dr. Sapolsky, "those are not predictors of a hale and hearty old age."

Sapolsky's results align completely with one of the largest, most highly controlled studies in human history – the four-decade *Whitehall Study* that has been tracking the health of over 28,000 British citizens. London University College professor Sir Michael Marmot named his study after Whitehall, the British civil service headquarters, where occupations are ranked according to a very precise hierarchy, the perfect opportunity to see if there's a similar link between social ranking and stress in humans. The subjects are in stable office jobs with no hazardous exposures, and in the British civil service system, everyone has the same universal health care. In other words, their environment is just as stable and predictable as that of baboons in the wild.

According to Sir Marmot, the results are the same: the lower you are in the human hierarchy, the worse are the effects upon your health and longevity. Longevity and the risks of heart attacks and other life-threatening illnesses directly correspond with employment ranking. The Whitehall findings and those of his own studies, agrees Dr. Sapolsky, are "virtually identical".

Stress And Your Body

Your body has two adrenal glands above your kidneys. These help control blood sugar, *metabolism* (the rate of chemical breakdown, synthesis and energy consumption) heartbeat and respiration.

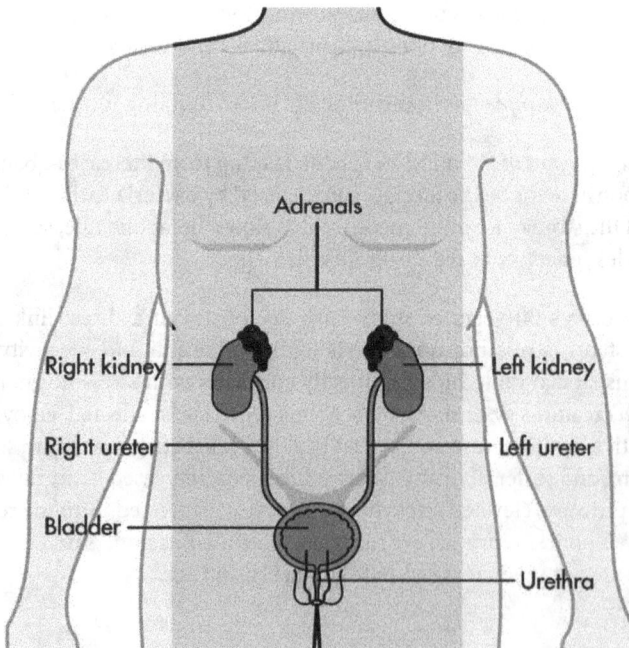

Position of the Adrenal Glands, MacMillan Cancer Support, 2011

Here's how your brain reacts when stress makes you angry, anxious, nervous, or upset:

Your hypothalamus receives a message that you're in danger. It sends emergency signals to your pituitary gland, which releases hormones prompting your adrenal glands to release cortisol into your bloodstream, leading to a sudden flood release of sugar. This sugar is the super-energy your body can use to fight or run in response to danger. In ancient times, this allowed your ancestors to, for example, have the energy to run for shelter from a predator or to fight a rival tribesman.

However, in modern society, such dangers are no longer part of your everyday life. Still, your primitive subcortical brain, particularly the limbic system, can't tell the difference between stress from being late for work in the morning or from the presence of a predator. So the emergency rush of sugar into your bloodstream that gives you super-energy for fighting or running from danger stays unused in your body and gets stored, primarily as adipose tissue around your midsection – better known as belly fat. This can lead to major, potentially fatal health problems such as diabetes and heart disease.

Constantly overtaxing your adrenal glands with stress also leads to a condition called *adrenal burnout*, where your adrenal gland function is severely impaired or even stops.

Boss Monkey - Flunky Monkey

In *Why Zebras Don't Get Ulcers,* Dr. Sapolsky says that when animals are exposed to pathological amounts of stress, it creates behavioral changes "strikingly similar" to human depression. He says that repeated stress, combined with total absence of control, quickly leads to depression. When it comes to stress, "...a lack of predictability and control are at the top of the list of things you want to avoid," he notes.

At Rockefeller University, Dr. Sapolsky and his mentor, Dr. Bruce McEwen, found chronic stress leads to dramatically shrunken brain cells, with sparse dendrite growth, the effects primarily concentrated in the hippocampus, seat of learning and memory.

Wake Forest University neuroscientist Dr. Carol Shively has been studying the effects of stress on monkeys, and says that dopamine levels are significantly affected by social hierarchy: "What we see is that the brains of dominant monkeys light up bright with lots of dopamine binding in this area that's so important to reward and feeling pleasure about life."

Comparatively, "...the brains of the subordinate monkeys are very, very dull because there's much less receptor binding going on in this area...."

When you have less dopamine, everything around you that you would normally take pleasure in is less pleasurable, so the sun doesn't shine so bright, the grass is not so green, food doesn't taste as good. It's because of the way your brain is functioning that you're doing that, and your brain is functioning that way because you're low on the social status hierarchy.

Long-Term Stress

A 2009 University of Toronto study of more than 1,000 Americans aged 18 and older found that time pressures, economic hardship and workplace conflicts were the leading stressors, increasing anger, particularly among younger people, parents and the least-educated. The study found those with higher education levels experienced less stress-related anger and had better coping skills.

Your immediate physical responses to stress include epinephrine and cortisol release, resulting in elevated heartbeat. But severe, long-term stress can eventually cause a complete breakdown of your mental and/or physical health. Joe Dispenza, author of *Evolve Your Brain – The Science of Changing Your Mind*, says stress may even be responsible for as much as 90% of physical illnesses. According to the nonprofit organization Helpguide, symptoms of stress include:

- poor judgment
- irritability
- negativity
- fidgeting
- excessive worrying
- moodiness, withdrawal
- an inability to relax
- loneliness or depression
- bodily aches and pains
- dizziness

- nausea
- chest pain
- rapid heartbeat
- appetite change
- over- or under-sleeping
- neglect of responsibilities
- increased alcohol/drug use
- nervous habits like aimless pacing or nail-biting
- diarrhea or constipation.

Sources of stress can include pain, bright light, loud noises, overcrowding, a lack of control over the environment, unmet homeostatic needs (food, housing, health, freedom, or mobility), or social conflict. Social stressors include struggles with others, social defeat, relationship conflicts, deception, break ups, and major events such as births, deaths, marriage, and divorce.

Life situations such as poverty, unemployment, alcoholism, or a lack of sleep can also cause stress. Students and workers may feel stress from exams, deadlines or problems with coworkers or bosses. Constant exposure to crowded areas and loud noise also compound the problem, adding quiet, chronic stress. According to the organization Helpguide, here are the top 10 causes of stress, in order of severity:

1. Death of a partner

2. Divorce

3. Separation from a partner

4. Imprisonment

5. Death of a close family member

6. Personal illness or injury

7. Marriage

8. Dismissal from work

9. Job change

10. Retirement

If you continue to experience stress, your mind and body try to find ways to resist the source. But the energy required to do this will eventually wear your body down to exhaustion. If the source of stress isn't removed or lessened, it will eventually create chronic anxiety or withdrawal into the state called depression.

At this point, your body's coping resources have been so depleted you can no longer function normally. If the situation continues, there may be permanent damage to your adrenal glands, your immune system will cease functioning, and it becomes very easy to contract illnesses, and very difficult to recover.

Long-term stress effects can include mental illness, memory loss, ulcers, depression, diabetes, digestive trouble and even heart attacks and strokes. In homes with alcoholism, child abuse or serious marital problems, chronic stress can even impede the physical growth of a child by lowering hormone production.

Chronic Stress And Your Brain

Normally, your prefrontal cortex controls emotional impulses generated by your amygdala, but you're constantly under stress, the neural circuitry centered on your amygdalae potentiates – becomes more sensitive and likely to activate, thus giving it greater influence over your thoughts, emotions and behavioral responses.

This can worsen existing mental disorders like anxiety, OCD and worry. In other words, chronic stress will physically alter your nervous and endocrine systems over time, particularly if you're already emotionally sensitive to begin with. Experiments have shown that within a matter of only one week of repeated stress (in the form of mild shocks), laboratory animals will begin to have seizures, and from that moment forward, these seizures will occur spontaneously, with little to no provocation.

Neuroscientist Philip Gold calls this progressive stress hypersensitivity *"kindling"*, a cascade of chemical reactions that, particularly in the young, permanently alters gene expression in the brain and establishes lifelong alterations to neural function.

Your brain's lobes and the association areas that integrate their processing into a unified sensory experience (*consciousness*) converge into the hippocampal region. Here, your hippocampus and connecting structures consolidate your outer- and inner-world experiences (experiences, thoughts and emotions) into *memories*.

Your hippocampus and related structures like the amygdala process and integrate stimuli, provide input to your hypothalamus and autonomic nervous system (ANS). This means just the memory of a traumatic event can trigger the stress responses of your ANS, before logic or evaluative thought processes can even begin to occur in your cortex.

> *Reversing the signals* – *Dr. Jaideep Bains of the University of Calgary has discovered that stress causes the hypothalamus (which governs stress responses) to read neurochemical "off" messages (inhibition signals) as "on" messages (excitatory signals). This is analogous to a car's brakes causing the vehicle to speed up instead of slowing down.*
>
> *These neural "brakes" (GABA inhibitory signals) only function if low chloride ion levels are maintained by a protein called KCC2. Stress impairs KCC2 function, so GABA signal inhibition is impeded. This loss of the brain's ability to moderate signalling may underlie the health damage of stress.*

Stress Kills Your Memory

Extensive animal and human research has shown that the hippocampus is not only crucially involved in memory formation, but is also highly sensitive to stress. The University of Washington's Dr. Jeansok Kim has demonstrated that stress slows your brain's firing as well as its ability to connect neurons to form memories, memories that also participate in higher cognitive functions such as decision-making.

Several independent studies have shown that stress impairs memory in a number of species. It also impairs long-term potentiation (LTP) in the hippocampus, the key brain structure for forming declarative memories. Instead, stress enhances long-term depression (LTD) in the hippocampus.

High levels of stress-response hormones called *glucocorticoids* are released under severe stress or trauma (in life-or-death situations), and, says Daniel Goleman, they are "…neurotoxic to the hippocampi". This potential damage to the hippocampi may be the reason neurons *atrophy* (wither) in long-term depressives. This atrophy has been proven to *result* from depression (a form of stress) rather than causing it. What's more, the longer depression lasts, the greater the hippocampus cell atrophy and the worse memory problems become.

Too Much Of A Good Thing

The effects of stress on memory formation are complex. As any good teacher knows, a small amount of tension helps firmly fix a lesson in a student's memory – speaking in front of the class, and being mildly anxious about a test can heighten retention. But too much stress leads to memory decline, and is believed to be a major factor in age-related memory loss.

Dr. Joyce Yau of Edinburgh's University's Centre of Cardiovascular Science believes she knows why: she's found two receptors react very differently to cortisol, the stress hormone linked to age-related memory decline. At low levels, cortisol activates one type of receptor (*high-affinity mineralocorticoid receptors* – MRs) which enhance memory. At high levels, however, cortisol activates a second type of receptor (*low-affinity glucocorticoid receptors* – GRs) which leads to memory impairment.

Using mice in maze-navigation experiments, Dr. Yau's team found that, while low levels of stress hormone enhanced their memory, high levels impeded their ability to remember how to navigate through the maze. When the GR receptor was blocked, however, their recall returned to normal. The study helps to explain how excessive, chronic stress interferes with the normal processing of memories, and is leading to the development of drugs to help maintain memory in the face of stress- and age-related decline.

Stress Injures Your Body

Wake Forest University's Dr. Carol Shively says stress hormones trigger intense negative cardiovascular responses, elevating heart rate and increasing blood pressure. Over time, this damages arterial walls, making them ideal sites for plaque deposits, which can build and narrow the channels through which blood flows. These effects also directly correlate with social status, so beta members of a group tend to have significant *atherosclerosis* – plaque deposits in their arteries – while alpha members have none.

Because of this partial blockage, says Dr. Shively:

> *...now when you feel threatened, your arteries don't expand and your heart muscle doesn't get more blood and that can lead to a heart attack. This is not an abstract concept, it's not something that maybe someday you should do something about. You need to attend to it today because it's affecting the way your body functions, and stress today will affect your health tomorrow and for years to come.*

Maryland cardiologist Dr. Jeffrey Ritterman says you can also draw direct links between health, longevity and stress, seen in the correlation between neighborhoods and life expectancy; among poor neighborhoods, people are more vigilant and live more stressful lives. The high stress hormones this produces have a very clear effect.

Sir Michael Marmot's Whitehall study also found a correlation between stress, social status and weight, as well as the distribution of excess weight: fat tends to accumulate around the abdomen in relation to your position in the socioeconomic hierarchy.

The same phenomenon can be seen in monkeys, says Dr. Shively, as they also organize themselves into a social hierarchy. Subordinate monkeys tend to grow fatter in their abdomens than do dominant monkeys - and this abdominal fat is much worse for health than fat elsewhere in the body, producing different hormones.

Stress Disrupts Your Genes

Stress also exerts profound epigenetic effects. Dutch geneticist Dr. Tessa Roseboom has been studying the effects of a 1944 famine called the "Dutch Hunger Winter" upon families under the Nazi regime. In testing over 2,400 people carried within their mothers' wombs during that brutal winter, she found the stress of that famine during fetal life still had profound effects six decades later.

Now in their sixties, these survivors have an increased risk of cardiovascular disease, are more sensitive to stress, and are in poorer general health than those conceived after or born before the famine. She believes maternal stress hormones triggered changes in the nervous systems of these fetuses.

Dr. Sapolsky observes that this profoundly affected their brain chemistry, impairing their learning, capacity to cope with stress, and making them vulnerable to psychiatric illnesses such as depression: "An adverse, stressful environment can leave imprints, can leave scars lasting a whole lifetime."

Stress Significantly Shortens Your Life

Stress exerts major influence upon your genes in another disturbing manner: *telomeres* are caps at the ends of your chromosomes, which appear to protect your nuclear DNA strands from unravelling. As you grow older, your telomeres wear down and shorten. And stress, says Dr. Sapolsky, accelerates this shortening. Thus, for low-ranking members of society under significant stress, telomeres will be shorter, and you simply won't live as long.

Dr. Elizabeth Blackburn was corecipient of a 2009 Nobel for co-discovering *telomerase*, an enzyme which repairs telomeres, which may be the key to significant life extension. Says Dr. Blackburn "We have 46 chromosomes and they're capped off at each end by telomeres.... What we found was the length of the telomeres directly relates to the amount of stress somebody is under and the number of years that they've been under the stress."

Dr. Sapolsky estimates that every year of extreme stress correlates to roughly six years' of aging. Adds Dr. Blackburn: "This is real. This is not just somebody whining. This is real, medically serious aging going on, and we can see that it's actually caused by the chronic stress."

Stress, Fertility and Libido

Dr. Mark Wilson, chief of Psychobiology at Emory University, says chronic stress can lead to several behavioral changes and health problems such as anxiety, depression and even infertility. Using laboratory animals, his team found that *corticotrophin releasing factor* (CRF) is a key neurohormone in stress.

CRF is found throughout the brain, where it primarily aids you in adapting to everyday stressors and maintaining your emotional and physical health. CRF levels rise in response to stress, and decrease when stressors disappear. But in the case of chronic stress, the duration and levels of CRF increase in brain regions that process emotions like fear, including in your amygdala. This increase in CRF is believed to lead to health-related stress

11

problems which include depression, anxiety and infertility. Persistent CRF release affects a number of body systems, leading to anxious and depressive behavior, disrupting ovarian cycles and decreasing libido, changes common in women under severe daily stress.

Crippling Children For Life

In adolescents, chronic stress may even lead to mood disorders in adulthood, according to a 2010 study conducted at Concordia University. Dr. Mark Ellenbogen, who led the study, believes the current surge in depression rates is linked to increases in stress from modern daily life. He has been focusing on links between early stress-filled environments, hormones, and mood disorders like depression or bipolar disorder. Major depression is "one of the most pressing health issues in both developing and developed countries," he says.

> What is especially alarming is that depression in young people is increasing in successive generations. People are suffering from depression earlier in life and more people are getting it. We want to know why and how. We believe that stress is a major contributor.

His research team measured cortisol levels of children living with a parent suffering from a mood disorder. Studies have previously shown kids from at-risk families are more likely to develop a mental disorder at some point in their lives. According to Ellenbogen, these children aren't just inheriting the traits, but are being raised in stressful, chaotic, unstructured environments.

His team discovered that adolescent children from these homes have higher levels of cortisol in their saliva than children from more families whose parents don't suffer from mental disorders. These elevated cortisol levels persist into young adulthood.

There may be a number of causes for the increased cortisol levels, including exposure to family stress and disruptive parenting. And while the subsequent development of adult mood disorders is still unproven, at this point, high adolescent levels of cortisol appear to double the risk of developing a serious mood disorder in young adulthood.

Social Stress And Neurodegenerative Disease

Texas A & M University researchers have shown that social stress affects your immune system, presumably through stress-triggered increases of *cytokines*, proteins which regulate immune and inflammatory functions and influence the onset of diseases such as MS. Chronic stress intensifies *inflammation* (tissue swelling), increasing the risk of CNS infections and neurodegenerative diseases like *multiple sclerosis* (MS) and others, according to 2007 research presented at the American Psychological Association convention.

Stress increases and sustains high levels of infection-fighting *interleukin-6 (IL-6) cytokines*, proteins which respond to viral infections by triggering inflammation. But excessive inflammation interferes with the immune response to infections.

This in turn leads to increased viral levels, prolonged infections, increased CNS inflammation, and worsening of chronic autoimmune diseases. In this way, excessive cytokines inhibit your immune system's ability to fight off infections and make inflammation spiral out of control, increasing vulnerability to neurodegenerative viruses like MS.

Mice exposed to social stress show elevated IL-6 levels in the CNS and PNS, which can increase the severity of CNS diseases. And just like mice exposed to repeated social defeat, people exposed to chronic social stressors suffer high levels of stress leading to immune system dysfunction, increasing their vulnerability to diseases. The health effects might be preventable or reversible by blocking cytokine increases. Evidence suggests that some anti-inflammatory drugs, exercise, antidepressants, omega-3 fatty acids, and mindfulness meditation can help, but the evidence is still sparse.

Your Attitude Matters

How you view your life's difficulties directly alters your body's neurochemical states, according to 2011 research conducted at the University of Pittsburgh. People who respond to stress with high levels of anger or anxiety show increased inflammation compared with those who maintain calm, according to Dr. Judith Carroll, who led the study. Dr. Carroll believes this may be one of the reasons highly stressed people suffer from chronic illnesses.

The study indicates people who get angry or stressed in the face of minor life challenges are more likely to suffer increased inflammation, an immune system defense and repair response which can eventually make them prone to health problems such as cardiovascular disease. This study is part of a relatively new and growing field of neurobiology called *Psychoneuroimmunology*, which explores the links between mental processes and health.

A Whole Host Of Problems

Inglewood California veterinarian Dr. Richard Palmquist recommends "tuning in to your biology" to naturally reduce stress. He points out that the body is extremely sensitive to biochemical changes; for example, minute quantities of hormones released by your thyroid can trigger major changes in your body's tissue growth. Additionally, minor fluctuations in blood sugar alter function of your pancreas, which secretes insulin to regulate sugar usage by your body. The tiniest of electrical signals can trigger immune system responses, alter heartbeat, respiration and more. All this, of course, creates significant changes to your inner chemistry, affecting your digestion, cardiovascular function, sugar and fat metabolism, immune function and neurochemistry. Says Dr. Palmquist, being aware of this means you can start to see how your emotions can work for you or against you, optimizing your health or triggering disease:

> Chronic fear, grief, anger and stress makes our immune cells less effective. When a body is stressed it releases cortisone. This hormone assists the body initially by increasing sugar levels and allowing the body to live under difficult circumstances.

> If the stress lasts too long then the cortisone suppresses the immune system, damages the gastrointestinal lining, makes the body less responsive to other hormones like insulin, and blocks the body from being able to cycle through its normal fluctuations of acid and gel phases. A stressed body cannot heal optimally. It cannot repair properly. Such a body ages prematurely, but if we diminish the stress, reduce the fear, increase our understanding, improve the communication and take other steps toward addressing the correct cause of the stress, then the body can begin to manifest its normal care, control and repair systems.

Stress can even make your hair fall out, among a host of other superficial problems. Raising cortisol levels can lead to alopecia (bald spots), in both men and women. This is, fortunately, temporary if the stressors are removed, but grey hairs can grow in where the bald spots appeared. In addition, cortisol triggers increases in sebum (oil) production, which can contribute to acne.

On a much more serious level, chronic stress and depression can disrupt the balance of microorganisms in your intestines, resulting in an increase of harmful bacteria and a decrease of beneficial bacteria. Such changes have "profound implications for physiological function", primarily weakening your immune function, according to 20 separate studies conducted at Texas Tech University. Healthy intestinal bacteria help your body fight a number of illnesses, not the least of which includes cancer.

Stress and depression also appear to affect *VEGF protein* production. VEGF stimulates tumor growth and shortens cancer survival. A 2011 study at Fox Chase Cancer Center revealed that a patient's reported stress and depression levels coincided with high levels of the protein VEGF, which is regulated by stress hormones, and promotes tumor growth in a variety of cancers.

Passing It On

You don't live in a social vacuum, and your moods, for better or for worse, have a profound effect upon everyone around you, particularly those closest to you. Your emotions are the outward reflection of your inner states, and your pets are particularly sensitive to this. As a pet owner, your animals see you as the "alpha member of their pack", and will mirror your emotional states: if you're happy and content, your animals will also be well-adjusted; but if you're constantly on edge with worry, your pets will be tense and unhappy too.

Neglecting management of your own stress transmits stress – and illness – to your pets, which mirror both your behavior and your emotional states. By extension, of course, you affect all your loved ones in exactly the same way. If someone cares about you, your unhappiness adds stress to their lives. In neglecting your own "emotional hygiene" (self-care), you're not only worsening your own health and shortening your own life, you're doing the same to those who care about you the most. Their very affection for you is what makes them vulnerable.

Crash And Burn

Chronic stress and feeling unappreciated at work are major sources of *burnout syndrome*. Being over-burdened by work, monotony or a perceived lack of recognition can all trigger burnout. The condition "…poses a serious problem to society because of the economic losses it causes and its consequences for health," according to Jesús Montero-Marín, senior researcher at the Aragon Institute of Health Sciences in Spain and lead author of a 2011 study on the disease. Using questionnaires, his team surveyed employees throughout the University of Zaragoza system, including administrative, services, teaching and research staff and interns.

The study examines the underlying sociodemographic and employment factors linked to three sub-types of burnout– *frenetic, under-challenged* and *worn out*.

"The 'frenetic' profile is associated with the number of hours worked," explains Dr. Montero-Marín; people holding down multiple jobs, and people on temporary contracts end up with frenetic burnout syndrome.

Frenetic employees are typically ambitious, heavily invested in their positions, and have a serious work overload. Spending over 40 hours a week at work is six times more likely to lead to this kind of burnout than working less than 35.

Workers who perform monotonous tasks tend to get bored, and lack personal development opportunities are at a greater risk of developing the "under-challenged" profile. Administrative and services staff had three times the likelihood of falling within this group than the teaching and research staff, and the profile applies primarily to men. "While men tend to distance themselves from the company's objectives, women are more likely to develop emotional exhaustion," according to Dr. Montero-Marín.

Meanwhile, the "worn out" profile generally appears among employees who have been in the same job the longest, who end up ignoring their responsibilities because they feel unappreciated. Workers with over 16 years of service at the same workplace are five times more likely to develop this type of burnout than workers with service records of under four years.

Emotional exhaustion, cynicism or poor work ability are indications of burnout. Experts consider burnout to be present if someone has at least one of these characteristics. Your type of employment contract also impacts whether or not you will develop burnout. Temporary employees are at risk of developing a "frenetic" profile when they work hard to secure more stable positions. This is also a possibility among half-day workers who often hold down multiple jobs.

As well as the factors which lead to burnout, your social environment can counterbalance stress, preventing burnout before it develops. "Having a family, partner or children can act as a protective 'cushion', because when people finish their day at work they leave their workplace worries behind them and focus on other kinds of tasks," Dr. Montero-Marín explains.

Academic level also contributes to risk. Those at the opposite ends of the academic scale are most likely to suffer from burnout – those with the least training and those with the most. This is believed to be because those with little education usually work at jobs which have fewer qualifications, and for which they can receive little recognition, while PhDs with long work histories can "...feel they are investing more in the job than they get in return," according to Dr. Montero-Marín.

Autonomy Protects

Sir Michael Marmot says massive combined studies show the social conditions in which you live and work are "absolutely vital" for your health. He says the studies show the amount of control you have in your environments is intimately linked to your place in the hierarchy; generally, as people report their life conditions have worsened, and work-related stress has increased, illness rates increase. And when they report greater control and fair treatment, illness rates decrease. He says providing greater involvement, greater individual empowerment, and better rewards for individual effort create both a healthier and more productive workplace.

A stress experiment by Rockefeller University's Dr. Jay Weiss demonstrates the underlying principle – how a perceived lack of control worsens stress.

In the laboratory, two groups of rats received electric shocks to their tails. One group labelled "Control," could turn off the shocks by turning a wheel; the other group, labelled "No Control," had no way of shutting off the shocks.

Over time, the animals that couldn't control whether or not they received shocks developed stomach ulcers and had significantly higher levels of stress hormones in their blood, while those able to stop the shocks did not. Dr. Weiss says this experiment clearly demonstrates how unpredictability and a lack of control affect health.

Traumatic life events can vary in their effects, depending upon how well you cope with them, but this psychological safety mechanism seems to function as a buffer against the adverse effects of stress. According to Cambridge Professor of Cognitive Neuroscience Dr. Trevor W. Robbins, having control over a stressful situation reduces its negative consequences in both your mind and body.

It's thought that the ventral medial prefrontal cortex gauges the amount of control you have over a stressful situation and the region exercises control over the raphé nucleus – knowing you have control over a stressor allows your vmPFC to inhibit excessive serotonin and norepinephrine release. Your raphé nucleus is the primary source of serotonin output to your neocortex, striatum, and amygdala. Stressors elevate raphe nucleus serotonin release. When you judge stressors to be out of your control, serotonin release increases, impairing cortical, striatal and limbic function. This potentially leads to serotonin depletion, depression and other disorders.

The Healing Gift Of Connections

A number of studies are beginning to point to compassion as a major antidote to chronic stress. Being connected, kind, caring, and sharing close social ties with others seems to exert a powerful influence upon stress.

Twenty years ago, when tuberculosis wiped out half the male population of the first baboon troop Dr. Sapolsky had been studying, he noticed an amazing thing: every single alpha male had died, leaving only the gentler males and females:

> *If you were aggressive and if you were not particularly socially connected, socially affiliative, you didn't spend your time grooming and hanging out, if you were that kind of male, you died. And what you were left with was twice as many females as males, and the males who were remaining were, you know, just to use scientific jargon, they were good guys. They were not aggressive jerks. They were nice to the females. They were very socially affiliative. It completely transformed the atmosphere in the troop.*

The social transformations have remained in the baboon troop for two decades; it now has very low aggression levels and very high social affiliation levels; blood measurements show these kinder, gentler baboons have none of the health problems – elevated blood pressure, brain deterioration or stress hormones – of the past. With the bullies out of the picture, the creatures are free to live in harmony and significantly improved health.

The same effects are found in humans, although we tend to belong to multiple rather than single social hierarchies. According to Dr. Sapolsky, if you've got some measure of control, predictability and status in at least one of your social groups, these psychological controls are enough to help you cope with your life stress. In other words, social ties matter. Friendships matter. Family matters.

Dr. Sapolsky summarizes his lifelong research into primate socialization and stress by refuting the maxim that "nice guys finish last":

> *Don't bite somebody because you're having a bad day. Don't displace on them in any sort of matter. Social affiliation is a remarkably powerful thing.... Those things are real important and one of the greatest forms of sociality is giving rather than receiving, and all those things make for a better world. Another one of the things that baboons teach us is if they're able to, in one generation, transform what are supposed to be textbook social systems sort of engraved in stone, we don't have an excuse when we say there's certain inevitabilities about human social systems.*

Are You An Adrenaline Junkie?

The classical adrenaline junkie you see in movies is a thrill seeker who loves to do dangerous or exciting things. While these people certainly exist, more typical in everyday life is the sort of person who overschedules her days, waits until the last minute and then rushes things, has a life full of drama and crises, takes on more work than she can easily manage, and is often looking to help out "charity case" people.

There are obviously people with troubled lives or genuine problems, but if you persistently have these behavior patterns, it's quite possible you're addicted to the rush of sensations that come from the release of adrenaline (epinephrine) in your body. Psychologist Elizabeth Scott says the habit of seeking adrenaline stimulation in your life can become a problem if you're always "…unwittingly creating crises for yourself or becoming needlessly engulfed in stressful situations".

Over time, this can lead to burnout, where stress begins to impair or even break down your body's normal healthy functions. She suggests cutting activities which cause you unnecessary stress and using relaxation techniques to reduce stress's effects on your body when things get out of hand.

Self-Test: How Much Stress Do You Have?

You've seen the major physical and mental health problems that stress can cause. So how much are you dealing with?

The first signs you're suffering from too much stress are brief flashes of panic or anxiety with no immediate cause. Please consider it an alarm. You must identify the sources of your stress and take steps to eliminate or at least reduce it. The following quiz will help you recognize stress, even in its earliest stages. Please answer Yes or No.

1. Do you always see the negative side in everything you do?

2. Do you often feel overwhelmed by small incidents or tasks?

3. Do you often have sudden, uncontrollable mood changes?

4. Are you compelled to eat constantly, even when you're not hungry, or are you repulsed by food?

5. Do you find there is nothing that motivates you to get out of bed in the morning?

6. When you awaken, are you mentally or physically unable to function until you have caffeine?

7. Do you have back, neck or joint pain with no physical reason?

8. Do you often catch colds or flus from which you don't recover quickly?

9. Do you find sex no longer interests you?

10. Do you often have stomach problems such as gas, bloating, a lack of appetite or uncontrollable appetite?

11. Have you recently developed high or low blood pressure?

12. Does fat accumulate around your waist while your hands, legs, neck and face remain thin?

13. Do you ever have sudden lower back pain?

14. Is there a large amount of cholesterol in your blood?

15. Do you have an impulse to quit everything and just run away?

16. Do you completely cut yourself off from those who care for you, and prefer to live in isolation?

17. Have you thought of suicide as an escape?

18. Are you often forgetful?

19. Do you feel guilty about things that go wrong around you, even when they're not your fault?

20. Are you at times unable to think clearly about a favourite topic or situation?

21. Does life at times seem surreal?

If you answered 'Yes' to only 2-5 questions, you are leading a very balanced, healthy life.

If you answered 'Yes' to 6-12 questions, you are showing some signs of stress, which can lead to health problems if you don't take steps to reduce the negative stress in your life.

If you answered 'Yes' to 13 or more questions, you have a seriously large amount of negative stress. You need to carefully examine your life and take immediate steps to reduce your negative stress. Remember that a great number of health problems are caused by negative stress – it's critical that you get a handle on your own, or it will almost certainly be very detrimental to your health.

Additional, specific symptoms of stress include:

Physical – chest tightness, chest pain, palpitations, indigestion, breathlessness, nausea, muscle twitches, aches and pains, headaches, skin conditions, recurrence of previous illnesses and/or allergies, constipation or diarrhea, weight loss or gain, changes in menstrual cycles, insomnia or fatigue

Emotional – mood swings, anxiety, tension, anger, guilt, shame, lack of enthusiasm, cynicism, feelings of a lack of control or helplessness, decrease in confidence or self-esteem, poor concentration

Behavioral – drop in work performance, becoming accident-prone, increased drinking and/or smoking, overeating or loss of appetite, change in sleeping patterns, poor time management, no time to relax, withdrawal from family and friends, loss of interest in sex, poor judgment, inability to express feelings, overreacting

Psychological – Negative thought processes such as "I am a failure", "I should be able to cope; why can't I?", "why is everyone picking on me?", "no one understands me", "I don't know what to do", "I can't cope", "what's the point?", "I don't seem to be able to get on top of things", "I keep forgetting where I put things", loss of judgment

If you have 10 or more of these symptoms, you need to take immediate action to reduce your stress. Professional therapy is recommended – you need someone to help you unburden.

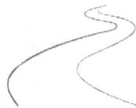

Negative Affective Responses to a Speech Task Predict Changes in Interleukin (IL)-6, Judith E. Carroll, Carissa A. Low, Aric A. Prather, Sheldon Cohen, Jacqueline M. Fury, Diana C. Ross, Anna L. Marsland. 2011, Brain, Behavior, and Immunity; 25 (2): 232 DOI: 10.1016/j.bbi.2010.09.024; http://www.psy.cmu.edu/~scohen/Carroll_etal_BBI_2011.pdf

Researchers Create Animal Model Of Chronic Stress, Emory University (2008, September 4),

Stress: Portrait of a Killer, 2008, John Heminway, Stanford University and National Geographic

Does Adolescent Stress Lead to Mood Disorders in Adulthood? press release, Sylvain-Jacques Desjardins, 2010, Concordia University; http://www.concordia.ca/now/media-relations/press-releases/20101109/does-adolescent-stress-lead-to-mood-disorders-in-adulthood.php

High Cortisol Levels in the Offspring of Parents with Bipolar Disorder During Two Weeks of Daily Sampling, Mark A Ellenbogen, Jonathan B Santo, Anne-Marie Linnen, Claire-Dominique Walker, Sheilagh Hodgins, 2010, Bipolar Disorders, DOI: 10.1111/j.1399-5618.2009.00770.x;

The Stressed Hippocampus, Synaptic Plasticity and Lost Memories, Jeansok J. Kim and David M. Diamond, Nature Reviews Neuroscience 3, 453-462 (June 2002) | doi:10.1038/nrn849;

11 -Hydroxysteroid Dehydrogenase Type 1 Deficiency Prevents Memory Deficits with Aging by Switching from Glucocorticoid Receptor to Mineralocorticoid Receptor-Mediated Cognitive Control, J. L. W. Yau, J. Noble, J. R. Seckl. , Journal of Neuroscience, 2011; 31 (11): 4188 DOI: 10.1523/JNEUROSCI.6145-10.2011; http://www.jneurosci.org/content/31/11/4188.short

Severe or Traumatic Stress and Inflammation in Multiple Sclerosis, presentation, Dr. Mary W. Meagher, Texas A&M University, 2007, Symposium: Traumatic Stress, Cardiovascular Disease, Metabolic Syndrome, and Neurodegenerative Disease

How Chronic Stress Worsens Neurodegenerative Disease Course, American Psychological Association (2007, August 20).

Perceived Stress and Depressive Symptoms Are Associated with Biomarkers Indicative of Shorter Disease-Free Survival in Head and Neck Cancer Patients, Fox Chase Cancer Center press release, 2011; http://www.fccc.edu/news/2011/2011-04-28-fang.html

Exposure to a Social Stressor Alters the Structure of the Intestinal Microbiota: Implications for Stressor-Induced Immunomodulation?, Michael T. Bailey, Scot E. Dowd, Jeffrey D. Galley, Amy R. Hufnagle, Rebecca G. Allen and Mark Lytee, 2011, Brain, Behavior, and Immunity; 25 (3): 397 DOI: 0.06/j.bbi.200.0.023

New And Unexpected Mechanism Identified How The Brain Responds To Stress, University of Calgary (2009, March 4), ScienceDaily. Retrieved May 11, 2011, from http://www.science-daily.com /releases/2009/03/090302133226.htm

Microbial Translocation Augments the Function of Adoptively Transferred Self/Tumor-Specific CD8+ T cells Via TLR4 Signalling, Chrystal M. Paulos, Claudia Wrzesinski, Andrew Kaiser, Christian S. Hinrichs, Marcello Chieppa, Lydie Cassard, Douglas C. Palmer, Andrea Boni, Pawel Muranski, Zhiya Yu, Luca Gattinoni, Paul A. Antony, Steven A. Rosenberg and Nicholas P. Restifo, 2007, Journal of Clinical Investigation, 2007; 117(8):2197–2204. doi: 10.1172/JCI32205;

Sociodemographic and Occupational Risk Factors Associated With the Development of Different Burnout Types: the Cross-Sectional University of Zaragoza Study, Jesús Montero-Marín, Javier García-Campayo, Marta Fajó-Pascual, José Carrasco, Santiago Gascón, Margarita Gili, Fermín Mayoral-Cleries, BMC Psychiatry, 2011; 11 (1): 49 DOI: 10.1186/1471-244X-11-49

What Is An Adrenaline Junkie? What Can You Do If You Are One? Are YOU Subconsciously Hooked On Adrenaline? Elizabeth Scott, M.S., 2007, About.com

Solutions

I am your constant companion. I am your greatest helper or heaviest burden. I will push you onward or drag you down to failure. I am completely at your command. Half of the things you do you might as well turn over to me and I will do them – quickly and correctly.

I am easily managed – you must be firm with me. Show me exactly how you want something done and after a few lessons, I will do it automatically. I am the servant of great people, and alas, of all failures as well. Those who are great, I have made great. Those who are failures, I have made failures.

I am not a machine, though I work with the precision of a machine plus the intelligence of a person. You may run me for profit or run me for ruin – it makes no difference to me. Take me, train me, be firm with me, and I will place the world at your feet. Be easy with me and I will destroy you.

Who am I?

I am Habit.

– John Di Lemme, Champions Are Born, Losers Are Made! 2007

The Role Of Perspective

Whether a stressful situation affects you negatively or positively depends very much upon how you judge the situation and your ability to cope with it. If you see the situation as threatening, harmful or causing a loss, and believe you have no way of escaping or fixing the situation, it will have a harmful effect. Conversely, if you see such a situation as a "healthy challenge", it has the potential to help you. In other words, the neurochemicals and hormones your brain and body release in response to stressful events can be altered, depending upon your mental perspective – interpreting a situation as a threat triggers a completely different neurochemical release in your brain than viewing the same situation as an "interesting challenge".

The Role Of Diet And Exercise

To reduce wear on your adrenal system, you need to exercise, and either find solutions to the situations giving you stress, or remove yourself from these situations to restore calm to your life and boost your sense of well-being. You can lessen the effects of stress significantly by eating and resting properly. Seven or more hours of sleep every night will help in restoring your adrenal gland health. Conversely, night after night of less than this amount will gradually and steadily deplete your adrenal function.

Proper eating entails not just what, but also how you eat. You need to eat steadily all day. Skipping meals wreaks havoc on your system – dropping your blood sugar, stressing your adrenal glands and pancreas, and triggering dizziness, cravings, anxiety and tiredness. In fact, skipping meals, particularly breakfast, is one the best method to ensure you get fat and wear down your body.

A 2008 Swedish study of over 3,600 seniors showed that skipping meals and other irregular eating habits greatly increases the risk of developing metabolic syndrome, a condition in which the body is at extreme risk for heart attacks and other dangers, increasing abdominal fat, glucose intolerance and the chance of contracting diabetes. To avoid this, make sure you eat a healthy, substantial, protein-rich breakfast, and then eat small amounts regularly throughout the day, every two to three hours. This will keep your energy levels high and your metabolism revved up.

What Not To Eat for Stress

You don't want to be eating an excess of sugar, and alcohol should only be consumed in moderation, if at all. Fruit juices are also chemically little better for you than sugary drinks. Dieticians also recommend avoiding starchy carbohydrates like white breads, pasta and rice, which are little different from simple sugars, as you'll see in a later chapter. Potassium-rich fruits also worsen *adrenal fatigue* – if you're stressed, you might want to limit or avoid eating bananas, melons, raisins, dates, figs, oranges and grapefruit.

Caffeine will give you a temporary energy lift, but too much depletes your body's B vitamins and stresses your adrenal glands. Artificial sweeteners and preservatives like MSG are likewise not the best nutritive choices.

The Science Of Comfort Foods

Food, sex, and other pleasurable activities don't just cause sensations of pleasure; according to 2010 findings at the University of Cincinnati, they reduce your stress – helping calm your sympathetic nervous system. The reduction in SNS response can last up to a week or more. This explains such things as the motivation to eat "comfort foods" and similar behaviours after stressful events, according to Drs. Yvonne Ulrich-Lai and James Herman. Even small portions of pleasure-inducing foods can trigger stress-reduction, they add.

By feeding rats a sugar solution twice daily for two weeks and testing their stress responses, the team found that rats which ate sugar had reduced heart rates and stress hormone levels compared with non-sugar-eating rats when placed in stressful conditions. Artificial sweeteners and sex also had the same calming effects, but, when sucrose was fed directly into their stomachs, there was no reduction in stress responses, suggesting that it was the pleasure of *consumption* itself – the *tastes* and *sensations* of foods, rather than the caloric content, which was triggering the reduction in stress responses. Enjoyment reduces stress. Thus, when you're stressed, you want to eat junk foods.

Unfortunately, you pay for the short-term comfort later: when you eat sugary, fatty or oily foods for a quick energy or mood boost, breaking down the fat and sugar molecules saps your body of essential nutrients which help you manage stress levels, such as vitamins B and C. Thus, fast foods give you a short-term energy high, but you end up irritable, tired, and unable to concentrate. Chronic habits such as reaching for donuts when you're tired will also lead to permanent weight gain and metabolic slowdown.

Supplements and Stress

The following supplements help repair adrenal damage:

- Vitamins B5, B6, niacin, C, and E

- Ginseng

- Magnesium

- Trace minerals: zinc, manganese, selenium, chromium, molybdenum, copper and iodine.

To counter stress, instead of junk foods, you need to consume a diet rich in vitamins B and C, *essential fatty acids* (deep-sea fish oils), and green leafy vegetables. Specifically recommended foods for burnout recovery include brewer's yeast, brown rice, flax, olive and safflower oils, beans, nuts, seeds, wheat germ, and whole grains.

In addition, the trace element germanium has been shown to boost the immune system, and it can be found in garlic, pearl barley, sauerkraut, tomatoes, onions, broccoli, celery, milk, rhubarb, aloe vera, ginseng, and shitake mushrooms.

Stressbusters

If you're under a lot of stress, you need to take steps to reduce it – work, family, monetary, and relationship stresses must be reduced or eliminated whenever and wherever possible. If that's unmanageable on your own, a counsellor can help you develop stress-coping skills.

Exercise and meditation also reduce stress tremendously, strengthening your body and mind and making you more capable of coping with external events. Spending time with loved ones and pets is very important, as it increases feelings of security. The touch of a loved one has also been shown to release the "feel-good" and "bonding" hormone *oxytocin* in addition to dopamine, soothing you and increasing happiness.

Making warm personal connections is mentally and physically essential, and helps your body fight stress by increasing oxytocin, decreasing cortisol and improving your sense of general wellbeing. Make friends with coworkers and acquaintances. Cultivate kindness toward everyone you encounter, throughout daily life.

Enjoying at least one fun, novel and interesting experience every day will likewise enrich your life and reduce your stress. Looking forward each day to something positive, such as an approaching vacation, a concert, or a crafts project takes your energy away from worry. Regularly try new, small things. A little bit of novelty in your life will keep your mind flexible, so you're better equipped to handle situations which bring you stress. Try a new hobby or go along a different route to work and/or school.

Joe Robinson, author of *Work to Live* and *Don't Miss Your Life* has additional insight. It's his contention that modern-day life has conditioned us to be too goal-oriented; we've come to believe that if something isn't practical and profitable it's a waste of time. Wage slavery, he contends, kills. To be happy and fulfilled, you need to experience your passions fully, set loose your inner child, and fully engage in carefree play.

Thus, if you love hiking, that's exactly what you need to be doing, regardless of the negative notions that you should be spending time more productively. If baking is your kick, immerse yourself in it, and your life will begin to light up more fully. Letting loose and occasionally doing what you damned well please is a vital stress buster, energy and immunity booster – and it's essential to reaching self-actualization.

Moments in which you are fully engaged in what you're doing are the peak of human experience, and when you're doing what you really love, regardless of the value judgments of others around you, you're truly living. So have a snowball fight. Or a pillow fight. Shoot some hoops. Dance the worm. Roll down that hill. Sing during your commute (just not on a crowded train).

Robinson also suggests that watching screens endlessly, day in and day out, robs you of authentic life experiences – you're reduced to watching others experience life moments while yours passes you by.

Here are some additional powerful strategies for lessening stress:

- Spend time with people who are uplifting, and don't try to exploit others for your personal benefit – as a famous song's lyrics suggest, it's important to love people and use things – not the opposite.

- Encourage your body's own natural, biological healing mechanisms through consistent exercise, good nutrition, adequate rest, and a healthy emotional environment.

- Cultivate awareness of your own emotional state and be aware that you can choose to deliberately change it in habit-forming ways.

- If you're anxious, find out more about what's giving you stress and how you can change it.

- Close your eyes and relax, using deep breathing to induce alpha wave activity in your brain and activate your parasympathetic nervous system response.

- Be aware that you're not your job, goals or possessions. Learn to recognize your strengths and take pride in them, and treat areas you need to improve gently.

- Take time to connect with others, cultivating authentic human moments, sharing pleasures and disappointments with real caring and trust. The strength of your relationships can sustain you in the darkest of times.

- Stop perfectionist habits – have realistic expectations for yourself and others.

- Avoid stretching yourself too thin – don't schedule more than you can handle, and drop activities if you feel overloaded.

- Be sure to always sleep regularly to maintain proper neurochemical and endocrine balance.

- Schedule "me time" into your day when you can properly unwind.

Please take a moment to consider the areas in your life that are causing you stress, and how to reduce or eliminate them.

Worrybusters

1. If you're bothered by constant worry, psychologists suggest putting a notepad beside your bed, making a list of the worries and then putting them aside until a time you've put aside as your designated *daily worry time*; for example at 10 am the following day.

2. Rate your worries from 1 to 10, with 10 being a complete, life-destroying disaster. It's likely they're not as serious as you believe when they're put into proper perspective the next time you see them.

3. Finding a way to solve what's causing you worry, or otherwise changing the situation or your perspective on it in a way you can accept is the key – for example, learning to set limits or to say no to demands from bosses or family members.

4. Avoiding the situation that causes the stress, if possible, is another method. My personal preference is to seek quiet and solitude in nature, but any hobby that brings significant enjoyment can reduce your stress.

5. Make relaxation a daily part of your life, and learn to be in control of your mind and body, and you will instinctively know how to manage your stressful situations. In the next chapter, you'll be learning the deeply powerful "Oasis" meditation, where you go inside your mind to find your personal source of healing.

"TLC" – Your Ticket To Health And Happiness

A few simple changes to your lifestyle, like adding a little daily exercise, enjoying natural surroundings or volunteering to help those less fortunate than you is now believed to be just as effective as medication or counselling in treating a wide range of mental illness, according to a 2011 study by the American Psychological Association. Dr. Roger Walsh, who led the study, says positive lifestyle changes can be used to treat anxiety and depression just as well as they improve conditions like diabetes and obesity. *"TLCs"* or *"therapeutic lifestyle changes"* include:

- positive social relationships

- exercise

- nutrition

- recreation

- relaxation

- stress management

- spending time in nature

- religious or spiritual involvement

- service to others

TLCs, says Dr. Walsh, are inexpensive, powerful and have fewer complications or side effects than medicines. On the other hand, the worst lifestyle behavior, he says, include insufficient outdoor activity, social isolation, and excessive sitting and watching television or computer monitors.

Take Time To Smell The Rosemary... And Lavender – *Although inhaling certain plants has been a folk remedy for fighting depression, inflammation, insomnia and stress since at least the ancient Egyptian era, solid scientific evidence has only recently emerged.*

In 2009, Dr. Akio Nakamura and others at the University of Tokyo School of Agricultural and Life Science demonstrated that inhaling certain scents like jasmine, lavender, lemon, mango, mint, cinnamon and other fragrant plants can reduce stress by significantly altering blood chemistry, and even alter gene expression of 115 specific genes.

Linalool, an oil found in over 200 plant species, is one of the most popular substances for soothing stress. Dr. Nakamura and his team had laboratory rats inhale linalool while restrained – restraint being a proven method of artificially inducing stress. Vital immune response cells (neutrophils and lymphocytes) decline under stress, but are restored to near-normal levels after inhaling linalool. Linalool inhalation also reduced activity in 109 genes which overexpress in response to stress, and 6 which underexpress. At present, the team is testing a variety of fragrances for their stress-relieving effects.

Japanese researchers have also recently found that breathing the scent of lavender or rosemary for five minutes lowers cortisol as much as 24%, increasing the body's cleansing of free radicals (oxygen ions that leach electrons, distroying cell intergrity, causing aging and disease). Bergamot and rose are also said to promote calm, though this has not yet been substantiated by clinical research. Essential oils made with these ingredients are inexpensive and easy to find.

Bluesbusters

Four-time NY Times bestselling author Dr. Mark Hyman is a heavyweight of the relatively new field of functional medicine. He coauthored and introduced the *Take Back Your Health Act* of 2009 in the United States Senate, to provide reimbursement for lifestyle treatment of chronic disease. He is also chairman of the Institute for Functional Medicine and recipient of the 2009 Books for a Better Life and Linus Pauling Awards for Leadership in Functional Medicine.

Dr. Hyman recommends the following steps for treating depression without resorting to drugs:

1. Switch to an anti-inflammatory diet which eliminates food allergens – food allergies and the inflammation they cause, he says, have been linked to depression and other mood disorders.

2. If you're feeling depressed, have your thyroid examined for *hypothyroidism*, which he says is a leading cause of depression.

3. Supplement with 1,000 to 2,000 mg of purified fish oil every day. Omega-3 fatty acids are vital for your brain, which is composed of such fatty tissue. Deficiencies can result in a number of serious health problems.

4. Supplement with 1,000 mcg (micrograms) of B12, 800 mcg of folic acid, and 25 mg (milligrams) of vitamin B6 every day. These three essential vitamins are necessary for your body to use *homocysteine*, a factor in depression. You needn't worry about toxicity in this case; B and C vitamins are *water soluble*, which, as you'll see later, means any excess is eliminated from your body without a possibility of toxic buildup.

5. Have a medical exam for mercury. *Heavy metal toxicity* has been linked to depression and other serious mood and neurological disorders.

6. Exercise strenuously for at least 30 minutes, five days a week at a minimum. This will increases BDNF (brain-derived neurotrophic factor), essential for proper brain function.

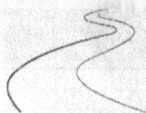

Understanding Stress: Signs, Symptoms, Causes, and Effects, Melinda Smith, M.A., Ellen Jaffe–Gill, and Jeanne Segal, Ph.D., helpguide.org, 2010 http://helpguide.org/mental/stress_signs.htm;

Don't Miss Your Life, Joe Robinson, 2010;

Evolve Your Brain – The Science of Changing Your Mind, Joe Dispenza, 2007;

Stress and the Brain: from Adaptation to Disease, E. Ron de Kloet, M. Joels, F. Holsboer, 2005, Nature Reviews Neuroscience;

Smelling Lavender and Rosemary Increases Free Radical Scavenging Activity and Decreases Cortisol Level in Saliva, T. Atsumi and K. Tonosaki, Psychiatry Research, 2007 Feb 28;

Prescription for Nutritional Healing, 4th Edition, Phyllis A. Balch, CNC, 2004;

Eating Meals Irregularly: A Novel Environmental Risk Factor for the Metabolic Syndrome; Justo Sierra-Johnson, Anna-Lena Undén, Madeleine Linestrand, Magdalena Rosell, Per Sjogren, Maria Kolak, Ulf De Faire, Rachel M. Fisher and Mai-Lis Hellénius, 2008, Obesity 16 (6): 1302 DOI http://www.nature.com/oby/journal/v16/n6/full/oby2008203a.html

Pleasurable Behaviours Reduce Stress Via Brain Reward Pathways, Y. M. Ulrich-Lai, A. M. Christiansen, M. M. Ostrander, A. A. Jones, K. R. Jones, D. C. Choi, E. G. Krause, N. K. Evanson, A. R. Furay, J. F. Davis, M. B. Solomon, A. D. de Kloet, K. L. Tamashiro, R. R. Sakai, R. J. Seeley, S. C. Woods, J. P. Herman, 2009, Proceedings of the National Academy of Sciences, 2010; DOI: 10.1073/pnas.1007740107; http://www.pnas.org/content/107/47/20529

Stop and Smell the Flowers – the Scent Really can Soothe Stress, press release, Michael Woods, 2009, American Chemical Society; http://www.eurekalert.org/pub_releases/2009-07/acs-sas072209.php

Stress Repression in Restrained Rats by (R)-(-)-Linalool Inhalation and Gene Expression Profiling of Their Whole Blood Cells, Akio Nakamura, Satoshi Fujiwara, Ichiro Matsumoto and Keiko Abe, Journal of Agricultural and Food Chemistry, 2009, 57 (12), pp 5480–5485 DOI: 10.1021/jf900420g; http://pubs.acs.org/doi/pdf/10.1021/jf900420g

Stress Management: Tapping Into Your Biology to Reduce Stress, Dr. Richard Palmquist, November 9, 2010 The Huffington Post; http://www.huffingtonpost.com/richard-palmquist-dvm/stress-disease-and-the-he_b_770293.html

Revolutionary Act No. 2: Want to Reduce Stress? Eliminate Annoyances, Pilar Gereasimo, February 6, 2011, The Huffington Post; http://www.huffingtonpost.com/pilar-gerasimo/energy-drainers_b_816671.html

Free

"To lick your wounds, to smack your lips over grievances long past, to roll your tongue over the prospect of bitter confrontations still to come, to savor to the last toothsome morsel both the pain you are given and the pain you are giving back—in many ways it is a feast fit for a king. The chief drawback is that what you are wolfing down is yourself. The skeleton at the feast is you."—Frederick Buechner

"Forgiving is not forgetting. Forgiving is anchoring a wrong in its own time, letting it recede into the past as we live and move toward the future."
– Greta Crosby, Tree and Jubilee, p. 54

"The people who hurt us the most, and whom we either need to forgive or be forgiven by, are also the people we love the most. Love is at the root of hatred and anger."
– Minister Barbara Wells ten Hove

"To forgive is not just to be altruistic. It is the best form of self-interest. It is also a process that does not exclude hatred and anger. These emotions are all part of being human. You should never hate yourself for hating others who do terrible things: the depth of your love is shown by the extent of your anger. However, when I talk of forgiveness I mean the belief that you can come out the other side a better person. A better person than the one being consumed by anger and hatred. Remaining in that state locks you in a state of victimhood, making you almost dependent on the perpetrator. If you can find it in yourself to forgive then you are no longer chained to the perpetrator. You can move on, and you can even help the perpetrator to become a better person too." —Desmond Tutu, No Future Without Forgiveness

"Living well is the best revenge"—George Herbert

Hanging onto hate and anger is toxic. Chronic, unused epinephrine, norepinephrine and cortisol tear down your body and mind, bringing you to an early, unhappy grave. But there are means of coping.

Dr. Edward Hallowell is a Massachusetts psychiatrist and author of *Dare to Forgive: The Power of Letting Go and Moving On*. In the best-seller, he points out that forgiveness, rather than a sign of weakness or "giving in", is an act of courage which is liberating, healing, and contagious. It's also, he contends, essential to living a healthy, happy life.

Dr. Hallowell shows how even the most gravely wronged have found courage to forgive – a mother able to forgive her daughter's murderer, business people falsely accused forgiving those who had framed them, even incest and rape survivors forgiving their attackers. This act of forgiveness set them upon the path to healing and freedom from the prison of reliving past hurts.

Says Hallowell, the word forgiveness:

> *...goes back to the Greek root word that means 'to set free,' as in freeing a slave. Ironically, when we forgive, the slave we free is ourselves. We free ourselves from being slaves to our own hatred....*
>
> *Forgiveness is much stronger, not to mention much wiser, than vengeance or retribution, and it begets the best kind of justice... Vengeance lets hatred rule you. Forgiveness overrules hatred ... Forgiveness takes intelligence, discipline, imagination and persistence, as well as a special psychological strength, something athletes call mental toughness and warriors call courage.*

Hallowell outlines four steps to the process of forgiving:

1. ***Admit you've been hurt*** – Don't try to deny your pain, or carry a chip on your shoulder while pretending nothing happened. Says Hallowell, admission of your pain will bring a flood of very hurtful emotions that will "rip great holes in your sense of well-being". He advises that this can be a very traumatic period, so avoiding the instinct to withdraw, instead staying connected to and talking with two or three people you trust deeply, are vital at this time. He also advises immersing yourself in activities you love.

2. ***Revisit the events and reflect on them*** – As you mentally relive the painful events, your instincts will be to exact revenge, to never trust again, or to withdraw, but instead you need to override your instincts with logic and ask where you want this pain to lead, look down the possible paths it could lead to, and search your deep beliefs and core values about life and people to guide you.

   Anger is a defense mechanism masking sadness or fear of a loss, so you need to search within deeper than the anger and grieve over your loss of hope, trust or opportunity. You need to discover the main reason the issue bothers you and why you're unable to let go of your anger. Hallowell calls this reason a "hook", like a fishhook buried in your guts, keeping you from being free. He suggests asking yourself "why does this bother me so much?" followed by "is it possible I'm acting like a fool?"

   Anger's also often a defense mechanism used when you feel threatened or out of control, providing (often illusory) feelings of power and control. If you're still afraid after this period of reflection, Dr. Hallowell suggests taking steps such as getting an apology, a restraining order or having the person responsible arrested, so that you're able to regain your feelings of control and security.

Finally, Hallowell teaches his patients to empathize with the person or people who hurt them – to try to understand their point of view in the situation. He points out that, while this is very difficult, shutting down this capability in yourself is very damaging and self-limiting. Losing human empathy to the forces of hatred, bitterness and cynicism is a tragic loss of human potential and joy.

3. *Work Through it* – Struggle within yourself to get rid of the "hook" – the reason for not forgiving. Perhaps, he points out, it's pride or jealousy; think, pray or meditate deeply upon the situation; feel gratitude for the things you have; remind yourself of your own need for forgiveness from others, and that both you and the world will be better if you forgive; if you must, indulge briefly in fantasies of vengeance and then put them away; finally, focus on living well in the future.

4. *Assess and Move On* – Disown and reject your anger and resentment, and keep repeating these four steps until the anger and resentment are gone. Dr. Hallowell suggests envisioning these feelings as ugly troll-like creatures that, when the reappear, you should practice addressing with "Go away you ugly things; I don't need or want you". Finally, he suggests letting the act of forgiveness heal you and help you grow, and then go on to teach others what you've learned from it.

Mental Jiu Jitsu – Defeating Your Anger

Anger can range from fleeting irritation to a full-fledged rage. Feeling angry is a signal that something is troubling you, and, rather than giving in to the immediate impulse to vent, it's an alert that's telling you to look within and find the root causes, so you can fix them and move on.

While it's a normal human emotion, anger tends to build because you're stifling or not communicating a deeper, underlying issue: blocked feelings of powerlessness, frustration, resentment, pain, fear, or disappointment. It's possible to vent anger and feel better for a time, or to distract yourself, but until these core feelings which underlie it are addressed and resolved, it will continue to build and come back again and again. Eventually, mounting anger can slip out of your control, with destructive consequences, damaging your relationships at home, with friends, or at work, and seriously degrading the quality of your life. At its extreme, it can lead to violence, with tragic results.

Anger can be triggered by not just external, but also internal, events. You might be worrying, remembering traumatic events or brooding about personal problems, all of which can lead to anger. External events like traffic jams or flight delays, and specific people like coworkers or supervisors may be bothering you, and your natural instincts are to respond with aggression.

34

Contrary to popular opinion, when it comes to anger, "letting it all out" is destructive to your environment, relationships and health. Just "expressing yourself", like "just kidding" is all too frequently a mask used by people who enjoy aggressing at others, humiliating or hurting their feelings. Angry outbursts actually compound the neural and endocrine rage state, escalating aggression and inevitably resulting in damage of one sort or another. It's far more constructive to uncover the specific causes and triggers of your anger, and to develop skills for how to handle those specific triggers.

Giving in to your aggressive impulses causes neurological, hormonal and even genetic changes in your brain and body, which not only increase your likelihood of acting violent or destructive in the future, but actually serve to profoundly compromise your cardiovascular, endocrine, and immune systems. As with every emotion, anger is accompanied by biological changes; increases in heart rate and blood pressure, and higher circulation of the action-promoting hormones epinephrine and norepinephrine.

There are three main strategies for handling anger: expressing, suppressing, or calming. When all three strategies fail, trouble is guaranteed to follow.

1. ***Expressing*** your anger assertively is the healthiest method. This means you make your needs clear, and determine how you can meet them, without hurting anyone else. Assertiveness differs from aggressiveness in that it involves respect for both yourself and others, instead of being pushy or demanding.

2. ***Suppressing*** your anger means holding it in, then changing your focus to something more positive. Here you attempt to convert your negative energy into more constructive behaviours. However, with this strategy, the likelihood is that if you don't eventually express your anger, you'll turn it upon yourself. This self-directed anger can lead to high blood pressure and eventually depression.

   It can also lead to problems such as pathological (unhealthy) expression, such as a cynical, sarcastic, negative and even hostile personality. People who constantly criticize, put others down, or make snide remarks have never developed the social skills to express their anger in healthy ways. This can lead to problems in all their relationships.

   Another pathological means of suppressing anger is *passive-aggression* – doing things to get back at someone else indirectly without telling them why, instead of directly saying what's bothering you.

3. *Calming* is a third strategy, in which you deliberately choose to engage your parasympathetic nervous system, slowing your heart-beat and respiration, calming yourself, and letting your feelings pass. Again, this doesn't permanently address any underlying emotional or situational concerns which are not being addressed.

The Hotheads: Low Frustration Tolerance

Anger management aims to reduce both your mental and physiological responses that result from anger. Sometimes, your control of people or events which bother you is limited, and you can't avoid, eliminate or change them, so it's more practical to learn to control your own responses to these triggers.

Dr. Jerry Deffenbacher specializes in anger management, and says that some people are naturally more anger-prone than others; it's easier for them to lose their tempers, and they react much more intensely than the average person. Some of these anger-prone people may not show intense or overt anger, but instead seem constantly irritable. They may not curse or throw things, but instead choose to withdraw, sulk, and even get physically ill.

If you're easily angered, it typically means you have *low frustration tolerance,* meaning you feel *entitled* to not have to deal with annoyance, being inconvenienced or frustrated. You can't easily accept things as they are, and when something you see as "unfair" occurs, it can enrage you.

The causes of low frustration tolerance can be genetic or physiological: some children are genetically predisposed to being cranky, fussy, and easily angered, signs which are present from early on. Environment also plays a major role – Broken or disruptive, chaotic homes teach poor communication skills. Or if you've been raised to believe it's acceptable to express worry, sadness, and other feelings, but not anger, you may not have learned how to manage and express it. Tests can determine how anger-prone you are, the intensity of your anger, and how effective you are at handling it.

Temperbusters

Relaxation – Close your eyes, use deep, slow breathing from your diaphragm (not your chest) and picture yourself in your perfect scene of serene nature; slowly repeat calming phrases such as "It's all okay", or "relax". Slow stretching or even yoga exercises will drain tension from your muscles and calm you.

This will activate your parasympathetic nervous system and put you into an alpha brain wave state. From there, you can effectively use some very powerful techniques for visualization and health enhancement you'll learn in the next chapter. Practice these relaxation techniques daily, so they become habitual, and you can fall back upon them automatically when you feel tense.

Cognitive Restructuring – Change the way you think about situations. When you're angry, you may be mentally cursing, or speaking to yourself in overly dramatic terms; try replacing these words with more rational thoughts: instead of thinking, "It's all over – everything's completely ruined!" you might say to yourself, "this is frustrating, and I'm naturally upset, but the world isn't coming to an end and my anger won't help things anyway."

Avoid using the words *never* or *always* when talking about yourself or someone else: "There's *never* an empty parking spot available!" or, "You're *always* late!" are almost certainly not true, and allow you to feel justified in your anger, and to believe that there's no solution. Such absolutes also humiliate and alienate others who might otherwise be willing to help you fix the problem.

Remember that getting angry won't fix a situation, but will almost always worsen it and make you feel worse than before. Anger tends to become irrational, even when you have a good reason for it. This is why logic is helpful. Don't think of things as the world trying to "get you", but instead, whenever you get angry, try to realize that life is full of ups and downs for everyone.

Anger Is Demanding

When you're angry, you tend to have expectations that you demand others meet. You expect people to act more fairly, appreciative, or agreeable toward you, or to do things the way you want them done. While everybody hopes to have these things, and becomes disappointed when they're unable to get them, people who are angry expect them, and when things don't live up to their expectations, disappointment turns into what Dr. Panksepp calls *frustration rage*.

When changing how you think, it's important to first recognize if you have a demanding nature, and then learn to transform your demands into wishes. It's much more constructive to say "I would like that" than "It had better be that way or else!" or "I *demand* it!".

As a result of changing your thinking, when you can't get what you want, you'll begin to have more reasonable reactions, such as disappointment or frustration, but not anger. Anger might be your way of preventing yourself from being hurt, but the hurt won't simply vanish – you'll still have to deal with the underlying issues.

Problem Solving – Your anger or frustrations may be the result of some very concrete problems; sometimes anger is a justified, healthy response to setbacks. While we're raised to believe there's a solution to every problem, there are some circumstances you'll simply be unable to change, which can cause you frustration. In cases like these, when it's apparent there's no solution, it's more constructive to think of how you might better cope with the problem.

Devise a plan, and monitor your progress. Make up your mind to do the best you can, but don't mentally "beat yourself up" if you can't improve things immediately. Tackling the situation with your greatest effort will decrease the likelihood of your losing patience, or falling into *all-or-nothing* thought patterns, even when your problem can't be immediately solved.

Better Communication – Anger tends to make people jump to conclusions and instantly act upon these assumptions, even though they can often be quite inaccurate. When you're in a situation which has the potential to trigger your anger – such as an argument – the best action is to slow down and carefully consider how you'll respond. Avoid blurting out the first thing which pops into your mind, instead pausing to carefully consider what it is you need to say. Especially when situations are tense, learn to listen carefully to what the other person says, and take a little time before you answer.

Search within yourself to find out what's motivating your anger. For example, you may want more personal space or freedom, and your partner may be asking for a closer connection. If your partner's complaining about your actions, don't attack them with accusations, claiming they're prison wardens or the like.

People naturally tend to become defensive in response to criticism, but you need to avoid fighting back. A much more effective strategy is to listen for what's *behind* the words in a verbal attack: your partner may be feeling unloved or neglected. Getting to the heart of the matter may require a great deal of patient probing, and both of you may need time and "breathing space", but keep yours and your partner's anger from letting the conversation spiral out of control. Keep cool, to avoid worsening the situation.

Change Your Environment – At times, your surroundings are the source of your irritation and anger. Responsibilities or difficulties can press upon you, making you angry at having fallen into a "trap", including people and things you consider part of that trap. Take a break, and be sure to have "me time" scheduled into your day at times you know tend to be stressful.

An example might be the working housewife whose rule is that when she gets back home, she has 15 minutes in which nobody talks to her unless there's a disaster. After her brief stress break, she's better equipped to deal with demands from the family without losing her temper.

Look for alternatives. If your daily commute makes you enraged and frustrated, find or plan an alternative route that's less crowded and perhaps even more scenic. There may even be alternative transportation, like a bus, bicycle or commuter train.

Counselling – If your anger is out of your control, damaging your relationships or other critical aspects of your life, a trained therapist may be able to help you learn to cope with things more constructively. A counsellor or psychologist can help you to develop a wider range of strategies for dealing with your thoughts and behavior. Psychologists say counselling can move a highly angry person into a midrange of anger in about two months, depending upon the individual and the techniques which are employed.

Anger can't and shouldn't be completely eliminated – it's actually necessary for your survival and well-being. No matter what you do, life will be full of events and people that frustrate, disappoint and hurt you. This is something you can't change, but you can change how you respond, resulting in a longer and more satisfying life for you.

Amen's Ants

Dr. Daniel G. Amen is a psychiatrist with some particularly excellent recommendations. In particular, he suggests you begin to treat food like medicine, concentrating on lean proteins, complex carbohydrates, *phytochemicals* (plant-based nutrients) and omega fatty acids. We'll look at nutrition and how your body uses it in detail later, but Dr. Amen also highlights the very real and substantial physical effects your thoughts have upon your health:

Every time you have a thought, your brain releases chemicals. Negative thoughts – anger, fear, worry, hatred, loneliness, sadness, boredom, stress – release chemicals which physically alter your brain and body in destructive ways. Chronic exposure to stress hormones in particular is toxic to cells in the hippocampus, and there are now very clear indications that stress triggers epigenetic changes which age you and make you ill, even helping to give you cancer.

Positive thoughts, on the other hand – love, kindness, joy, excitement, interest, cooperation – release chemicals which physically change your brain and body in positive ways. We've already looked at the specific processes, and the clinical proof of how they activate your endocrine and autonomic nervous systems. But every thought you have holds the potential to profoundly affect every single cell in your body. Thoughts are based on memories and complex chemical reactions. Many are automatic, but they're also very often erroneous, so it's important to question thoughts which hold you back.

Dr. Amen teaches a special children's program on "How to Think". It's very easy to remember using his mnemonic device, which describe *ANTs* – Automatic Negative Thoughts – and how to overcome them:

Ant Species (negative thought processes) can be consistently overcome by establishing a habitual response: when you feel recurring anger, cynicism, complaints, hatred, irritation, sadness or worry, you need to stop, identify the emotion, write it down, and then logically decide if it's true or not.

The three most dangerous ants are:

Mind-reading – Thinking you can clearly read someone else's thoughts, even if they haven't told you what they're thinking. Even experts in human behavior can't tell what most people are thinking, most of the time. But you can be certain that, whatever someone else is thinking, it's almost never about you. They're almost certainly thinking about something much more important – themselves! An irritated glance from a stranger may be nothing more than stomach gas; there's no possible way for you to tell.

Fortune-telling (catastrophizing) – Assuming the worst will happen, without any evidence for your predictions. This can even lead to panic attacks. In such cases, rather than fleeing the site of your stress, feel your internal sensations, slow your breathing, write down your thoughts and then logically determine whether they're true or not, and how you can regain control over the situation.

Guilt – Guilt is an important teacher to avoid repeating behaviours that harm others, but when guilt takes over your life, it's time to let things go. It's also a bad idea to use guilt to try and control others; it may work in the short term, but eventually those you've manipulated will resent you.

Here are the most common A.N.T. species Dr. Amen speaks of:

- *Thinking in Absolutes:* using phrases like *always, never, no one, everyone, every time,* and *everything*;

- *Negative thinking*: focusing only on negative aspects of a situation;

- *Thinking with your emotions*: automatically believing negative emotions without questioning them;

- *Guilt*: using the words *should, must, ought,* or *have to*;

- *Labelling*: negatively labelling yourself or someone else;

- *Personalizing*: thinking there is personal meaning in events completely unconnected to you;

- *Blaming:* Believing others have caused your problems

Here are some typical ANT phrases you need to stomp out or your life:

- *"You're always late because you don't care about anyone but yourself."* STOMP!

- *"It's all your fault!"* STOMP!

- *"You never listen to what I have to say!"* STOMP!

- *"One successful year is nothing. I know things will get much worse."* STOMP!

- *"You don't care about me."* STOMP!

- *"Things may be good now, but I'm sure it's only temporary. I just know something bad is about to happen."* STOMP!

- *"They all hate me."* STOMP!

- *"I should have done better. I'm a loser."* STOMP!

- *"You think you're so superior."* STOMP!

Exterminating Your Ants

Accept that your thoughts are okay to have, but then notice how your body reacts to your thoughts. When you lie, you'll typically sweat, and your heart rate will increase, and you may even blush.

Notice the physical effects specifically negative thoughts have on your body. Whenever you think an angry, sad, or unkind thought, your brain releases neurochemicals and hormones which affect your mood, body sensations and health. For example, the last time you were sad, you probably felt drained of energy, tight in the chest and a little powerless. This is your body reacting to your negative thoughts.

Over time, the impact on your health will be profound. Start to consider bad thoughts as pollutants. Thoughts are extremely potent, able to make your mind and your body feel good or bad. This has profound effects throughout your body, even upon your immune system, which is why emotional upset can be followed by physical symptoms like headaches, stomachaches, and even illness. There are even studies that show a correlation between negativity and cancer. Conversely, if you think positively, you'll feel better.

Notice the physical effects specifically positive thoughts have on your body. Whenever you think a happy, hopeful or kind thought, your brain releases neurochemicals and hormones which also affect your mood, body sensations and health. For example, the last time you were happy, you probably felt energized, relaxed, and your breath and heartbeat were slow. Over time, this state also has a profound impact on your health.

Realize that your pet Automatic Negative Thoughts aren't always true. Unless you actually reflect upon what you're thinking, your ANTs will just automatically march in and start feasting. But they're not necessarily true, or completely true. At times they are even 180 degrees incorrect. Dr. Amen gives one example of a college student who believed he scored poorly on tests, but was surprised when tests showed he had a near-genius level IQ.

Evaluate your thoughts to determine whether they're helping or harming you. If you never challenge your ANTs, you will simply go on believing them, even when they're completely untrue.

Tame your ANTs. You have the choice of lazily allowing your negative thought patterns to fester, take deep root, control your life, and make you feel perpetually miserable, or of establishing habits that will train your thought processes, making you more optimistic.

One path to taming your negative thoughts is to increase your self-awareness of them, and then to talk back to them. If you simply accept a negative thought without challenging it, your brain will accept and process it as truth, with negative consequences for your life and health. But by saying, "Wait a minute. Is that really what's going on?" you can render these negative thoughts harmless.

Stomp out your ANTs. If you envision your negative thoughts as ants disturbing your picnic, a single negative idea, like an ant, is only a minor annoyance. But as the numbers grow, and the ants start to swarm, the situation becomes intolerable. That's why, when you first notice such automatic negative thought patterns, you want to stomp them out of existence before they can rob you of your self-confidence, healthy relationships, and personal power.

Learn to crush them by writing them down as they occur, and then talking back to them. So if you hear yourself thinking, "My boyfriend never pays attention to me," write it down, then write down a more reasoned response to the thought, such as, "He didn't listen to me on the telephone tonight, but maybe he has stress at work; actually, most of the time, he gives me a lot of affectionate attention."

Writing down negative thoughts and talking back to them robs them of power and makes you feel better.

Some people may believe talking back to their negative thoughts is difficult, as it feels like being dishonest, but your own thoughts can be mistaken. If your negative thoughts are having a strong effect on your life, you owe it to yourself to confirm whether or not they're real, or if you're just mistaken.

Your ANTs can make you feel depressed and hopeless. Thoughts like "People don't like me" set you up for failure. You can cause these negative events to happen by consistently thinking this way – what psychologists call a self-fulfilling prophecy: for example, if you believe you're doomed to fail at something, you don't expend maximal effort, and you subconsciously create the failure.

Likewise, the suffering you cause yourself by thinking gloomy thoughts can drive you to act in disturbing manners that alienate those around you, pushing you into isolation. However, positive thinking and a sunny outlook projects a sense of well-being and self-management that makes you more approachable and attractive to others. Positive thinking also makes you more effective in everything you do. In this manner, the thought processes you carry around in your head throughout the day largely determine whether you succeed or fail in life.

Training your mind requires learning to choose healthy, positive thought patterns from moment to moment. As you've seen, habit physically alters your brain, your basal ganglia gradually making habits automatic and powerful. This also permanently affects how your limbic system operates.

Polygraph machines (better know as lie detectors) – like other "biofeedback machines" – measure deviations from your normal body state in terms of sweat, blood pressure, and heart rate. During a polygraph test, the subject is strapped to equipment which measures such metrics as body temperature, heart rate, blood pressure, breathing, muscle tension, and galvanic response (changes in electrical conductivity from sweating).

The tester establishes a base level by asking neutral questions such as a person's daily routine, and then moves on to the important phase, with such questions as "Did you rob the bank?" In most cases, the subject will experience stress if he did rob the bank or knows about it. His blood pressure will rise, his heartbeat will quicken, he will sweat ever so slightly more, and his muscles will tighten.

These reactions are almost immediate, even without a response. This is the limbic system triggering the sympathetic nervous system response, translating your emotional state into physical responses – muscle activation, and, in this case tension. In the same way, your body reacts to every one of your thoughts – positive or negative – every moment of your life.

Lifelong Mental Habits

Try to learn new and different things. You have to learn NOVEL things to keep using energy; things you're already good at have *potentiated* the neural circuits in your brain, which thereafter require minimal energy to activate. To keep your brain healthy, you need to be doing things which provide you with a challenge, subjects in which you're not so skilled or knowledgeable.

Social ties are vital for your mental health, and social cutoffs are like poison – let your grudges go – learn to forgive. Start to look for the good in people. Drop thinking about what you don't like, and focus on what you do like.

Clearing Your Clutter – Inside And Out

If you're constantly tired, drained by your daily existence, it's time to examine little things in your life which are adding up to major extra stress. Thomas Leonard, founder of the life-coaching industry, coined the term *tolerations* to mean endless small sources of irritation in daily life which add up to a huge amount of unnecessary extra stress. Distractions and minor annoyances you simply put up with sap your energy and hinder your progress in life, without your awareness.

Leonard suggested tolerations are a mirror of what's going on inside you, reflecting the unconscious choices you've made about what you deserve in life and how you choose to live. You may be tolerating hundreds of minor energy-drainers, from tiny inconveniences to major sources of frustration you've simply given up on doing anything about. But you carry the combined burden of all these tolerations everywhere you go, it colors your moods, self-image, health and social interactions. Accepting these annoyances holds you back; like swimming in a winter coat, it can be done, but why not do it the easy way?

Allowing pesky little irritations to continue draining your energy when you could make them vanish is settling for less than comfort in your life. Suppressing the irritation of all these little annoyances takes serious energy. For example, if you wake up in the morning, and the alarm clock is stuck, the shower head leaking, the window cracked, and your coffee machine a little hinky, you'll gradually get into a progressively darker mood. By the time you get to work, the slightest thing may be enough to get you fuming.

As we've seen, the neurohormones produced by anger make it erupt quickly and dissipate slowly, so minor annoyances like this simply build up the emotion until your body is in fight or flight mode, and stress hormones are coursing through it, lingering throughout the day and gradually poisoning you. Is saving a chipped cup or a scorched pot really worth losing health and possibly even shaving months off of your life? By identifying and eliminating these irritations, you'll free up more energy and time to devote to the things which matter most to you.

Psychologist Rich Broderick says taking time to repair, replace and organize tiny things that drive you nuts will go a long way towards eliminating your life stress. He recommends making a list of all the situations, people, places, things and feelings that bother you, no matter how tiny, and then working to fix them, one by one.

Are These On Your Fix-It List?

- nosy or noisy coworkers

- broken coffee machine

- dripping faucet

- dried up pens

- a constantly ringing phone

- keys you always lose

- a relationship which gives you stress and anxiety

- hurrying to and from work

You need to start saying goodbye to the things doing you more harm than good. Throw out things you don't need and never use, which clutter your shelves and closets. Say goodbye to toxic relationships. Establish behavioral and conversation boundaries – things you will and will not tolerate. Clearing away the clutter in your life and mind will start to bring you inner peace and mental clarity. And for each step you take, it becomes easier to eliminate ever more burdensome tolerances. This will have a huge impact on your life.

However, be aware that unless you're doing this as a positive step, the clutter in your life will eventually return. But every step forward helps – repair or throw away what's broken, and clear your shelves, closets and kitchen. It will start to transform your life, boosting your energy and mood significantly.

A Few Nevers

"Never dare to judge till you've heard the other side," – Euripides, 415 BC

"Never continue in a job you don't enjoy. If you don't like it, stop doing it."–
Johnny Carson 1976, commencement address at Norfolk High School, Nebraska

"Never feel self-pity, the most destructive emotion there is."
– Congresswoman Millicent Fenwick

"Never let the odds keep you from pursuing what you know in your heart you were
meant to do." – Leroy "Satchel" Paige, baseball's oldest rookie, age 42

"Never lose a chance of saying a kind word." –
William Makepeace Thackeray, Vanity Fair, 1847

Bouncing Back From Adversity – Lessons In Resilience

One of the fundamental secrets of patience is a simple realization: Things
are going to get better. They always do. But the corollary to positivity is that
pollyannaism – blind, unfounded optimism – is limiting, because things are
also going to get worse. They always do.

The overwhelmingly good news is that, if you're fortunate enough to be
educated and bright enough to read and use this book, you've got a distinct
socioeconomic advantage over at least 75% of the world. The ability to speak
and read fluently means you've enjoyed an educational advantage much of
the world will never have, and you live a kingly life in comparison to the
average Afghani or Congolese.

Think you've got it tough? You don't know tough: consider the average Con-
golese, who lives on the equivalent of $300 US per year; or their wealthy neigh-
bors in Somalia, living the high life on $600 per year. The average Somalian
can expect to live 50 years, contending with constant war, slavery, drought,
starvation, rampant AIDS, hepatitis, malaria, typhoid, dengue, Rift Valley
fever, and even rabies. Just over one in three is able to read and write, and three
years' of schooling is the most the average Somalian can ever hope to receive.

If the horrible circumstances you've just read about have moved you, rather
than simply feeling smug about your great good fortune, why not find out what
you can do to help? UNICEF, The Red Cross, CARE, Doctors Without Borders,
Save the Children, The World Food Program, OXFAM International, The
International Medical Corps and many more organizations are desperately
working to save lives as you're reading this. You can find out more at this link:
http://www.msnbc.msn.com/id/43841708/ns/nightly_news/t/famine-horn-
africa-how-help/#.Tnx2VNRipB

46

The point is, whoever you are, if you're in any position to read these words, Lady Luck's dealt you a blackjack, and no matter how bad you think your situation may be, it's guaranteed SOMEBODY is in a significantly tougher situation than you. Bearing that in mind, your dizzyingly great fortune to be born in an era and place where you can enjoy unprecedented access to health, wealth, nutrition, education, longevity and happiness is good reason to be optimistic.

Bushido: Legacy Of The Samurai Spirit

The samurai were Japan's Renaissance-era elite warriors, prizing honour, loyalty and duty above even life itself. The code they were taught to live and die by was known as Bushido, literally, "The Knight's Path". Many Japanese today still practice the principles of Bushido in their lives.

The Bushido code is perhaps the height of the remarkable hardiness of the Japanese. Deeply ingrained into Japanese culture is the concept of 我慢強さ – *gamman-zuyo-sa* – tough, enduring patience; the Japanese have historically been as tough as nails.

This island race (which, for better or for worse, belongs to its own distinct genomic *haplotype* (distinct genetic family) because of strictly-enforced closed borders) has endured earthquakes, fires, floods, invasions and multiple civil wars, and very quickly bounced back, at various times dominating the eastern world militarily, technologically and economically. During the 2011 earthquake, that historical toughness and resilience was once again evident, as people adjusted to the disaster and its aftermath in a very short timespan. Such resilience, in particular, is a mental skill that is invaluable for longevity, achievement and health.

Dr. Barbara Fredrickson is a leading researcher on positivity. She has recently determined that the core of such resilience is positivity – the ability to hold onto and even ramp up positive emotions when everything around seems to be falling to pieces. Some years back, Fredrickson and her colleagues found a "tipping-point" for positivity – a 3:1 ratio of three positive emotions for every negative one. People above this tipping point are resilient, with the psychological resources for change, growth, and the capacity to rebound from adversity. People below this tipping point languish and descend into a downward spiral.

In her best-seller *Positivity*, Dr. Fredrickson lists 10 positive emotions which contribute to resiliency: amusement, awe, gratitude, hope, inspiration, interest, joy, love, pride, and serenity. These emotions are inspired by triumph over adversity, and supply the positive energy that spurs hope: a belief that better times lie ahead, and that you have the strength to persevere until you arrive.

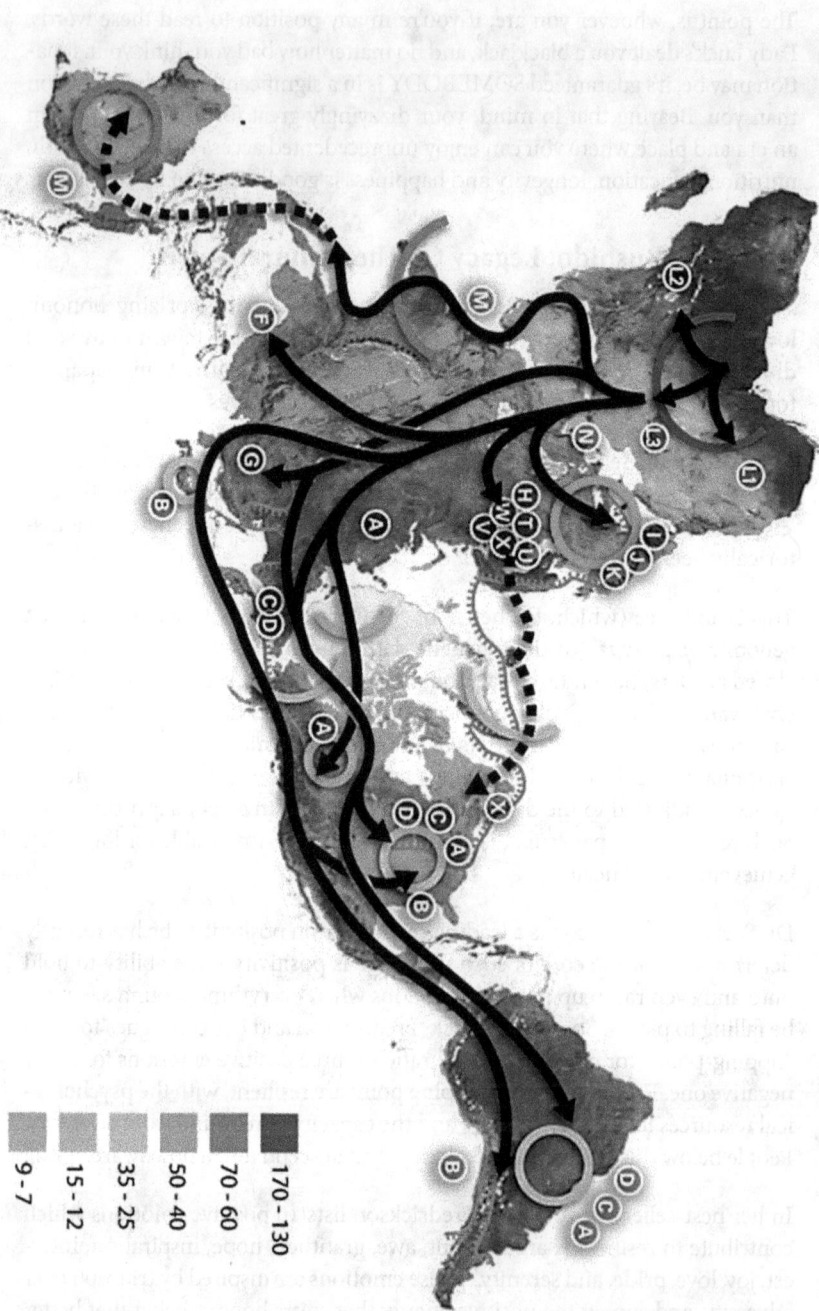

Illustration: Human migrations across the world, North Pole in center. These migrations can be tracked by shared DNA patterns. Africa, being the birthplace of the human species, is the origin of the migrations (top left), and South America is the far right. The numbers in the index indicate thousands of years before the present day. The thin blue line surrounds areas covered with ice or tundra within the most recent ice age (Wikipedia, 2011).

The letters represent DNA haplogroups (pure lineages). Haplogroups define genetic populations and primarily correspond to geographical locations. The following are common haplogroups:

- *African: L, L1, L2, L3*

- *Near Eastern: J, N*

- *Southern European: J, K*

- *General European: H, V*

- *Northern European: T, U, X*

- *Asian: A, B, C, D, E, F, G (note: M is made up of C, D, E, and G)*

- *Native American: A, B, C, D, and sometimes X*

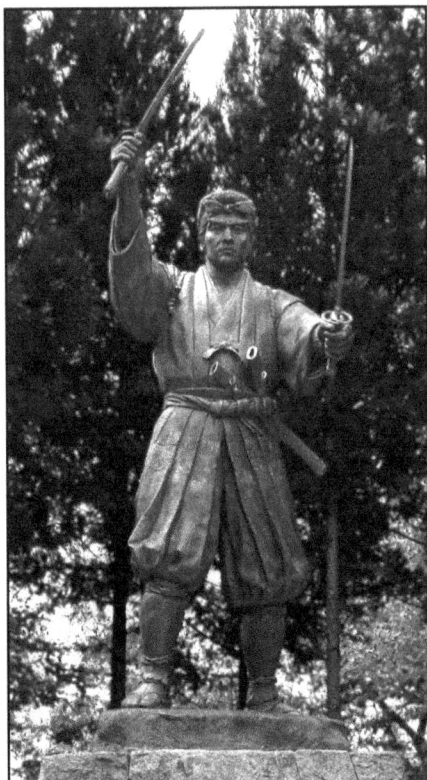

Hachidai Shrine, Kyoto, Japan. Miyamoto Musashi (1584-1645), said to be one of the greatest fighters who ever lived, defeated a samurai headmaster, then ambushed and defeated dozens of samurai who had come to punish him for the duel. His strategies are immortalized in The Book of Five Rings.

Japanese Secrets To Resilience

Dr. Margaret Moore, also known as "Coach Meg", points out that having hope for the future is particularly critical for optimism and well-being. If you can envision better times to come, it becomes possible for you to weather the worst of fate's storms.

Seeing courage and altruism in others can also inspire and spread. The response to the Fukushima earthquake in particular inspired Dr. Moore to pen the column *Japanese Secrets to Resilience*:

> *Crises often bring us to our knees and help us appreciate how our relationships with others are truly the backbone of our lives, to survive and, beyond that, to thrive. Taking time to help another, even ahead of one's own needs, is nourishing for both giver and receiver. There is also a global wave of love and support from far-away onlookers, earnest in their prayers and contributions, and hoping to help even a little.*

> *Another common response to crisis is a sense of deep gratitude and appreciation for one's life -- that we and others are alive, having survived a serious crisis. The value of material possessions slips away as we come to appreciate the gift of waking up every morning to a new day, new possibilities and new learning. We may even feel awe for the amazing talents of humans to adapt and respond beautifully to enormous loss and suffering. Some feel awe for the power and force of Mother Nature -- even when she unleashes massive destruction in natural disasters.*

> *Faced with adversity, resilient people are interested, open and curious, hunting for silver linings and ways to foster positive emotions as the fuel for putting one foot in front of the other in order to rebuild lives and communities. Developing a sense of profound meaning and purpose is a rich vein of positivity: "How can I make a difference? How can I use my strengths to help others recover and rebuild? How can I make lemonade out of lemons -- noticing, amplifying and harvesting the many lessons that emerge from a huge setback?"*

Moore says that making a difference in the community and lives of others teaches patience, and instills a sense of pride in your accomplishments. This in turn provides the impetus you need to keep moving forward, even in the darkest of times.

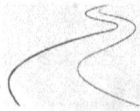

Dare to Forgive: The Power of Letting Go and Moving On, Dr. Edward Hallowell, 2004

Emotional Intelligence, Dr. Daniel Goleman, 1996

Change Your Brain, Change Your Life, Dr. Daniel G. Amen, 1999

The Portable Coach: 28 Sure-fire Strategies for Business and Personal Success, Thomas J. Leonard, 1999

Revolutionary Act 2: Want to Reduce Stress? Eliminate Annoyances, Pilar Gerasimo, February 6, 2011, The Huffington Post

World Factbook, Central Intelligence Agency, 2011

Succeed: How We Can Reach Our Goals, Dr. Heidi Grant Halvorson, 2011

Japanese Secrets to Resilience, Maragaret Moore, March 20, 2011, The Huffington Post

Haplogroup, Wikipedia, 2011

Miyamoto Musashi, Wikipedia, 2012

Positivity: Groundbreaking Research Reveals How to Embrace the Hidden Strength of Positive Emotions, Overcome Negativity, and Thrive, Dr. Barabara Frederickson, 2009

Laugh

"Laughter is an instant vacation." – Milton Berle

"Laughter is the shortest distance between two people." – Victor Borge

"If I can get you to laugh with me, you like me better, which makes you more open to my ideas. And if I can persuade you to laugh at the particular point I make, by laughing at it you acknowledge its truth." – John Cleese

*"I don't think so; therefore, I'm probably not."
– Rene DesCartes' confused younger brother Claude*

*"You don't stop laughing because you grow older.
You grow older because you stop laughing." – Maurice Chevalier*

*"We used to laugh at Grandpa when he'd head off and go fishing.
But we wouldn't be laughing that evening when he'd come back with
some whore he picked up in town." – Jack Handy, Saturday Night Live*

Laughter is an interesting behavior humans share with several other animal species. Behavioral psychologists say it's a bonding signal, signifying agreement, mutual understanding and group membership. It also signifies acceptance, approval and a positive mutual relationship.

Research also shows laughter is incredibly good for your health. Among the amazing things it does for your body:

- boosts immunity

- reduces pain, anxiety and fear

- improves overall mood and sense of well-being

- increases emotional resilience

- improves circulation

- protects the heart

- lowers adrenaline, cortisol, and blood sugar levels

- relieves muscular tension and mental stress for up to 45 minutes

- reduces hostility

- strengthens social bonds

The ways in which these physical changes occur were precisely mapped out in 2002 by American Dr. Lee Berk, who measured biochemical changes in subjects laughing at comedy videos. What he discovered was that laughing:

- increased well-being and joy by raising endorphin levels 27% on average

- tremendously enhanced immunity, increasing human growth hormone an average of 87%. This increases antibody-producing cells and enhances T cell effectiveness.

- dramatically lowered stress by reducing the dopamine byproduct-DOPAC by 38%, and the stress hormones cortisol and adrenaline by an average of 39% and 70%, respectively.

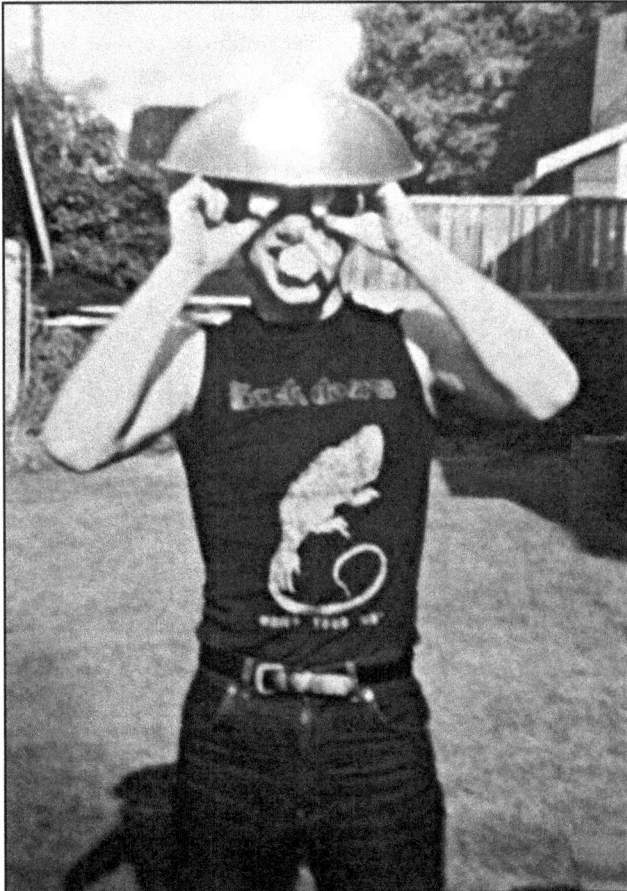

The author playing with his food Photo: Marcus Brunt, circa 1984.

Worldwide Prescription For Laughter

Around the globe, the therapeutic power of laughter is well-recognized. In Korea, for example, Dr. Lee Im-Seon is currently a "laughter therapist" for Seoul National University Hospital. He says "the hormones secreted when people laugh are known to alleviate pain 200-300 times better than morphine."

In Norway, A 2001-2006 study of 54,000 Norwegian patients found patients with a strong sense of humor had on average a 35% greater chance of survival – and up to 70% greater chance of survival if they'd been diagnosed with cancer but retained their senses of humor.

Doctors have recognized a link between humor and health as far back as the Middle Ages, when French surgeon Henri de Mondeville would request that hospital visitors tell jokes to his patients. Scientists first began to research the specific mechanisms behind the laughter healing process in 1964, however, when *New York Post* editor Norman Cousins was the recipient of what seemed a scientific miracle: having been diagnosed with a fatal, incurable, and deeply painful form of spinal arthritis, Cousins began a "pain-reduction regimen", throwing out his painkiller medicine, and watching a marathon of comedies:

> I made the joyous discovery that ten minutes of genuine belly laugh-
> ter had an anaesthetic effect and would give me at least two hours
> of pain-free sleep," he reported. "When the pain-killing effect of the
> laughter wore off, we would switch on the motion picture projector
> again and not infrequently, it would lead to another pain-free inter-
> val.

Not only did Cousins survive, he went on to live for another 26 years, inspiring the new field of *integrative medicine*. He wrote about the experience in 1979, in the best-seller *Anatomy of an Illness as Perceived by the Patient*.

Homework: *Watch the movies Mrs. Doubtfire, Clerks, Mystery Men, Ground-hog Day, Brain Donors, Monty Python and the Holy Grail, and the television series Fawlty Towers.*

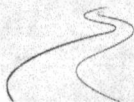

Mirthful Laughter, As Adjunct Therapy in Diabetic Care, Increases HDL Cholesterol and Attenuates Inflammatory Cytokines and hs-CRP and Possible CVD Risk, Dr. Lee Berk, pH, MPH, and Dr. Stanley Tan, MD, PhD, 122nd Annual Meeting of the American Physiological Society, April, 2009;

Modulation of Neuroimmune Parameters During the Eustress of Humor-Associated Mirthful Laughter, Dr. Lee Berk, pH, MPH, and Dr. Stanley Tan, MD, PhD, et al. Alternative Therapies in Health and Medicine, March 2001;

A Healthy Laugh, Charmaine Liebertz, September 21, 2005, Scientific American Mind 16;

A Seven-Year Prospective Study of Sense of Humor and Mortality in an Adult County Population: The HUNT-2 study, Sven Svebak, Solfrid Romundstad, PhD, and Professor Jostein Holmen, 2010, International Journal of Psychiatry in Medicine, 40, 125-146

Will

"To assert your willpower is simply to make up your mind that you want something, and then refuse to be put off. In short, think about what you want and hold to that thought. Believe in it as a reality, regardless of what may appear to be true. This is willpower in action, and anyone can do it."
– Phillip Cooper, Secrets of Creative Visualization, 1999

"It is fatal to enter any war without the will to win it."
– General Douglas MacArthur, Republican national convention, 1952

"Your own mind is a sacred enclosure into which nothing harmful can enter except by your promotion." – Ralph Waldo Emerson, The Essential Writings, 2000

"It is not the mountain we conquer but ourselves." Sir Edmund Hillary

Impulsivity can be controlled, and you can train to improve it, with measurable physical changes to your cortex, according to a 2010 Queen's University study.

Professor Cella Olmstead, the study's leader, says the neural mechanism controlling impulsivity is at the heart of addiction, obsessive compulsive disorder and gambling. Her team has trained rats to control their impulses until a signal is presented – like the dog that has learned not to eat a biscuit balanced on its nose until its owner gives a command.

The medial prefrontal cortex (mPFC) controls impulsivity by sending inhibitory signals which dampen neural activity in the limbic and basal ganglia systems. Dr. Olmsted's team found that training in impulse control increases conductivity and receptor growth within this mPFC-striatum circuit – after training, the synaptic connections and signals grew stronger in her laboratory test animals.

Similarly, in 2011, researchers at Ireland's Trinity College compared fMRI scans of former and current smokers to nonsmokers, as volunteers engaged in impulse control, self-monitoring and focusing attention, all cognitive skills necessary for quitting smoking, The scientists found that, while performing such cognitive tasks, current smokers showed reduced PFC activity, related to behavior and impulse control, and increased activation of the nucleus accumbens, the part of the dopamine reward pathways which responds to nicotine.

In direct contrast, smokers who had quit showed increased PFC and reduced nucleus accumbens activity; in fact, PFC activity among former smokers was at "super-normal" levels, compared with those among a control group which had never smoked. This demonstrates how neural circuits responsible for willpower become measurably more active in ex-smokers, implying that the mental skills used in resisting impulses can be trained and strengthened with use, resulting in neurological, functional changes.

Willpower involves decision-making – choosing between short-term gains (positive sensations) and long-term rewards (also positive sensations, but derived from different rewards). When willpower fails, it's because your brain's "autopilot" – your striatal-limbic circuitry – is at work. This autopilot controls your mundane daily activity, your daily commute and washing, allowing you to concentrate on other things.

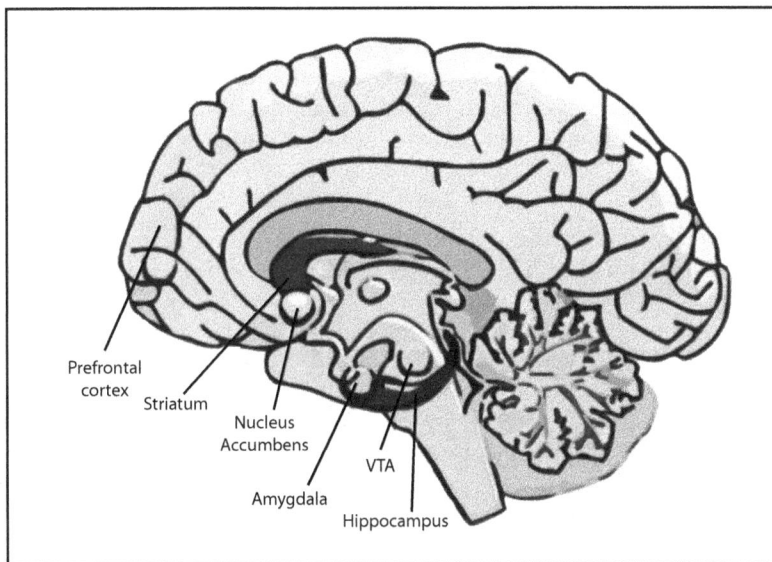

The Mesolimbic reward pathway, 2012 Polyglot Studios

But if your daily habits include such unhealthy behaviours as buying a box of donuts on the way to work, this habit-forming striatal-limbic circuitry has begun to work against you. Guilty pleasures like late-night snacking, smoking, or impulsive shopping represent a choice between short-term and long-term rewards, and here, you've allowed short-term gains to win, and strengthened the neural circuitry driving you to act in the unhealthy way.

University of Texas professor Russell Poldrack says:

The autopilot mechanism can be very powerful when an unhealthy habit – like lighting a cigarette with your morning coffee – is already ingrained in your daily routine. The immediate gratification of deliciousness and comfort that comes along with indulgences like eating a cupcake or taking a drag off a cigarette can trigger an overwhelming 'let's do it again' message in the brain. This overwhelming feeling can override a person's goal to prevent cancer or lose weight.

Self Control And Attention

Deciding whether or not you'll eat a healthy dinner – wild salmon and cauliflower vs. fried chicken and cola – is a complex mental process, but, says a team of neuroscientists at the California Institute of Technology, this decision can be swayed by simply shifting your attention toward the healthier aspects of things.

This same shift in attention can help you make healthier choices everywhere in your life, from diet to leisure activities to toxic behaviours like addictions. When choosing what you'll eat, your brain performs a complex cost-benefit analysis, calculating taste, health benefits, size and even packaging, then deciding the relative importance of each of these factors nearly instantaneously.

Drs. Antonio Rangel of Caltech and Todd Hare of the University of Zurich in Switzerland have been studying this evaluative process for many years, specifically focusing upon what makes some people more capable of exercising self-control than others.

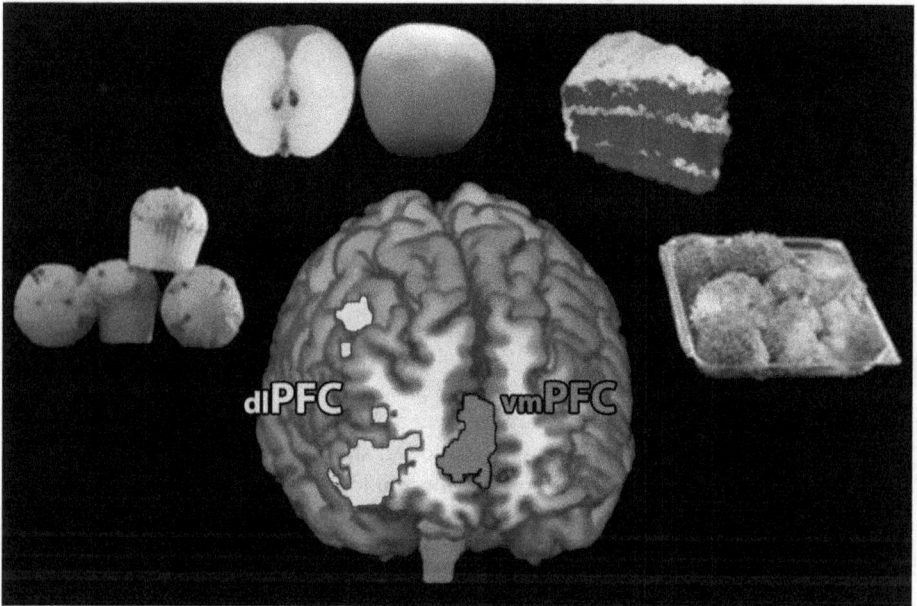

Regions of the prefrontal cortex responsible for self-control. 2011 studies at Caltech show the vmPFC (ventromedial prefrontal cortex) compares relative benefits of actions (such as what kind of food to eat), while the dlPFC (dorsolateral prefrontal cortex) is the main center for self-control – exercising willpower over destructive impulses. Todd A. Hare, 2011, Caltech. Used with permission.

They have discovered that everyone uses the same brain region – the vmPFC (ventral medial prefrontal cortex) – when making value-laden choices such as what to eat, but a second brain region – the dlPFC (dorsolateral prefrontal cortex) activates when exercising self-control in these decisions.

When the dlPFC engages, it lets the vmPFC consider health benefits in addition to taste when assigning relative values to a food item. In a new study, they've discovered how you can trigger your own dlPFC's engagement in decision-making, using external cues to shift your attention in a positive direction and allow greater self-control than normal.

Drs. Rangel and Hare ran fMRI scans upon 33 adult volunteers, none of whom were following a specific diet or trying to lose weight. Each volunteer was shown images through a set of video goggles of 180 a range of healthy and unhealthy food items – from chips and candy bars to apples and broccoli – while in a functional magnetic resonance imaging (fMRI) machine.

The volunteers were all asked to fast for three hours before the experiment, so they were in a state of hunger when they arrived. They were each given up to three seconds to respond to each food image, deciding and stating whether or not they'd be willing to eat that food after the experiment. Responses included "strong no," "no," "yes," or "strong yes."

Instructions would appear onscreen for five seconds before every 10 food items, instructing the volunteers to consider healthiness, tastiness, or simply "make decisions naturally." Out of 180 decisions, subjects made 60 based on each of three considerations. This was designed to shift the participants' attention and, potentially, their decision-making. After every image had been displayed, one food item was randomly chosen, and if the subject had responded with a "yes" or "strong yes" to that food, it was served to him or her after exiting the scanner.

Participants next rated the food in terms of tastiness (very untasty, untasty, tasty, and very tasty) and healthiness (very unhealthy, unhealthy, healthy, very healthy). In this manner, the research team could link subject choices with their assessments of food attributes, for example, showing a volunteer that chose broccoli when instructed to "consider the healthiness" part of the experiment might still consider it untasty. The research team then organized the foods for each volunteer based upon that volunteer's assessments: unhealthy-untasty, healthy-untasty, unhealthy-tasty, and healthy-tasty. The subjects generally chose foods which they considered both healthy and tasty no matter what they had been focused upon during the scans.

Among the remaining three categories, however, they discovered:

- While considering health, volunteers were unlikely to choose unhealthy foods, even if they found them tasty, choosing instead the healthy-untasty foods.

- Being instructed to consider healthiness led volunteers to refuse foods more frequently than when asked to naturally choose.

- Food choices during the "consider the tastiness" and "make decisions naturally" segments of the study were the same. In other words, the default basis of human dietary choices appears to be primarily based upon considerations of taste.

Upon examining the results of the fMRI scans, the research team discovered that the vmPFC was, "more responsive to the healthiness of food in the presence of health cues," as was expected, according to Dr. Rangel. The strength of that neural response, however, was influenced by the dlPFC, the region responsible for self-control. The dlPFC was significantly quieter as volunteers considered taste or personal preferences than when asked to consider healthiness. According to Dr. Hare, "This increased influence of the health signals on the vmPFC results in an overall value for the food that is based more on its health properties than is the case when the subject's attention is not focused on healthiness". The results are almost certainly applicable to other decisions unrelated to food, according to Dr. Hare:

"Our findings are also relevant to the current changes to cigarette warnings many governments have started to make.... These changes include adding graphical images of the health risks of smoking. It remains to be seen whether these images will be more effective in drawing attention to the unhealthiness of smoking than the text warnings. If the graphical warnings do increase attention to health, then our results suggest that they could decrease the desire to smoke."

The Number One Secret to Life:
Breaking Bad Habits – And Forming Good Ones

"First we make our habits; then our habits make us."
– Charles C. Noble, Faith for the Future, 1950

We've all got them – our pet vices. Perhaps you smoke a pack-and-a-half a day, or can't put down the potato chips. Maybe you procrastinate or stay up too late texting friends. Whatever your bad habits may be, the reason they're so hard to break is that they get naturally hard-wired into your brain. The latest research, worldwide, across several scientific disciplines and spanning decades, shows conclusively that your habits – dietary, exercise, behavioral, thinking and even emotional– significantly alter your brain and body chemistry and functionality, and ultimately shape your destiny. In 1931, Sigmund Freud wrote "anatomy is destiny".

I would strongly disagree. Habit is destiny. Master your habits and you *will* master your destiny.

Behaviours, beliefs and attitudes are habitual – acting evil is indeed a slippery slope, and the more you lie or engage in morally weak or criminal behaviours, the easier it becomes to do them, and the harder to act in a more responsible or morally upstanding manner:

When you lie, the physical stress (raised cortisol levels, accelerated heartbeat, raised blood pressure, etc.) that naturally follows acting dishonest begins to lessen, and changes within your brain and body make it progressively easier and more likely that you'll choose to lie in the future.

Giving in to cravings and overeating fatty or sweet food blunts your brain's response to dopamine over time, so you need to eat ever greater amounts to receive the same biological "rewards". Get fatter, and it becomes progressively harder to resist bad eating habits. Get lazier, and it becomes progressively harder to be active. Get sloppier, and your tolerance for clutter grows (even while it creates toxins in your body from stress and environmental pollutants). And laziness begets laziness.

Conversely, discipline can also become habitual. You can become addicted to the neuro- and endocrine chemistry of sociability, happiness, human kindness and exercise (dopamine, serotonin, human growth hormone and oxytocin, endorphins, etc.) These chemical changes will not only make you feel good – they'll make you live longer, be healthier, more effective in life and more attractive to those around you.

Want more energy? Paradoxically, using energy, by getting up and getting busy – through exercise, straightening up around the house, socializing, working and studying – will boost your mood, energy and concentration. Using energy brings you more. What's even more amazing is that you can "infect" all those you contact – human and animal – with your attitudes, beliefs and behaviours, giving the gifts of health, happiness, longevity and success, or selfishly worsening and shortening the lives of every person and animal you meet, functioning as a toxic element in their lives. The choice is entirely yours, from moment to moment, but be careful, as one path or the other becomes ever increasingly easy for you to tread.

Your frontal cortex is your brain's decision-making center. The first time you try a behavior (e.g. drinking coffee), you have to consciously choose to take the actions, using your frontal cortex to do it.

If you judge the experience to be pleasant, the portion of your brain called your *striatum* releases the neurochemical dopamine into your brain. Because dopamine release feels good (and boosts brain function and creativity), you want to repeat the action that led to the dopamine release.

Dopamine is enormously important as the driving force that makes living creatures, for example, eat and drink, or even move. In short, it's the vital key to all motivation. Knowing how it functions is therefore the key to training yourself to do anything and everything you want. Or stopping what you don't want.

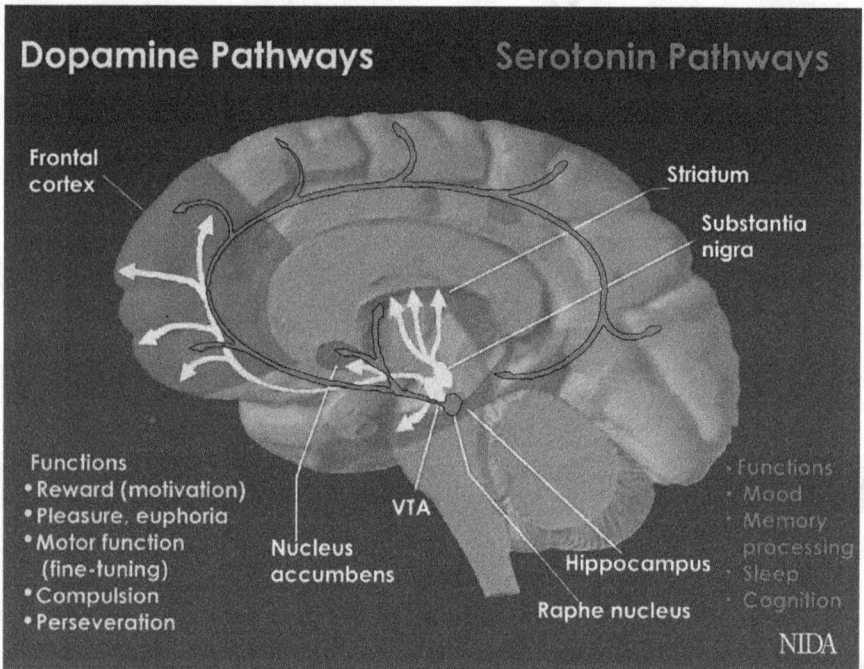

Dopamine and Serotonin Pathways, NIH, 2009, public domain

As you repeat an action over and over, you no longer need to use your frontal cortex as much to logically think about and choose making decisions, and the actions become gradually more automatic each time you're in the same situation or environment. Eventually your brain will begin to associate the circumstances (e.g. chatting with friends in a cafe) with the pleasurable release of dopamine, and a habit will take root. So how can you put this knowledge to use in breaking bad habits and forming good ones?

There are six keys to the process of forming (or breaking) a habit:

- developing patience

- repetition

- consistent timing

- controlling exposure to triggering situations

- controlling exposure to stress

- rewarding yourself

The Willpower Key: Delaying Gratification

Dr. Nora Volkow, director of the US National Institute on Drug Abuse, is the perhaps world's foremost authority on the brain's reward pathways. As she puts it, people prefer immediate rewards over something in the future. That's why it's easier to eat ice cream at midnight than to stick to a diet for a week, because the reward comes sooner.

But developing the willpower to delay this gratification is perhaps the single key to mastering anything in life – if you can just persevere, you can eventually do anything. Remember your visualization exercises? One of the reasons you want to visualize yourself succeeding and enjoying the rewards of your hard work is that you will give yourself an immediate dopamine release and your brain will begin to make the association between images of you performing those actions and pleasurable rewards.

Constant repetition will also disengage your frontal cortex, and you will continue to be rewarded with dopamine for the actions. After you've formed the habit, the situation changes; now if you *don't* perform the activity, your brain will crave the dopamine it's used to, and you will feel anxious or "not quite right". But to really program a habit, you want to repeat the action *at the same time every day*.

It will take from 14 to 60 days, depending upon the difficulty and complexity of the behavior, but you will eventually reach the point where a habitual behavior is a natural part of your identity. In fact, practicing by referring to yourself mentally or verbally as a "non-smoker" or an "exercise buff" will also speed up the behavior. Visualizing an action can release the motivational dopamine as well as actually performing it. In addition to dopamine, exercise also releases the feel-good chemical endorphins, so if you keep with a routine, you can addict yourself to health.

Another way to give yourself a hit of dopamine is to reward yourself with things you like when you've achieved a goal. A new outfit or a movie – whatever makes you happy and feel good. Tell yourself "I've earned it" to associate the reward with the new habit you're trying to form. Learn to substitute a positive ritual for your negative one – go for a brisk walk or a short jog in the sunshine instead of reaching for a cigarette, for example.

Be very careful when something stressful happens or you're in an unpleasant environment, because your desire for comfort (a dopamine hit) to relieve the unpleasant feelings of stress will make you want to perform your bad habit. Ruthlessly cut out *rituals* (repeated behavior sequences) linked to your bad habits, such as lighting up after a meal. Immediately do something else, like taking a walk or brushing your teeth.

The key to avoiding giving in to guilty pleasures is to change your environment. Because willpower can be weaker than you realize, you need to avoid situations that make you confront your bad habits; for example, ridding the kitchen of all junk food, and even taking a different route to and from work to avoid fast food restaurants.

The Success Formula

Why are some people more successful at achieving their goals than others? According to *Harvard Business Review*, it's because they approach goals differently. Dr. Heidi Grant Halvorson, a motivational psychologist and author of *Succeed: How We Can Reach Our Goals*, outlines the nine strategies that separate the successful – and make the difference between "trying" and "succeeding":

1. *Be Specific* – Expressing a goal in very specific, measurable terms creates a much clearer end result. Clearly defining your goal and the steps necessary to reach it keeps you motivated and on track. For example, "I'm going to save 5000 dollars this year" is a very clear target as opposed to the vague "I plan to save more money".

2. *Use the Time on Hand* – It's likely that you tell yourself things like "I'd love to exercise, but just can't seem to find the time!" In all likelihood, the time is there, and you're just avoiding taking action. Once you've defined your goals, set a specific time and day and you'll increase your chances of success by about 300%.

3. *Monitor Your Progress* – Keeping honest, up-to-date track of your progress will keep your eye on the goal.

4. ***Be realistically optimistic*** – While setting goals, you need to believe in your ability to achieve them, but be careful not to underestimate the difficulty of reaching them.

    Worthwhile goals require planning, effort, time and persistence – believing things will come to you easily is setting yourself up for disappointment. Be aware of, and realistic about, the investment involved in achieving what you want.

5. ***Focus on the journey, not the destination*** – Real change doesn't happen overnight. To achieve something important, if you focus on improving rather than excelling, you can be fully "present" and engage your focus and energy better than if you're distracted by visions of results. Slowly, over the long term, you will improve if you stay focused.

6. ***Stick to your guns*** – If self-improvement were easy, we would all be perfect. But improvement inevitably means times of extreme difficulty, when your patience will be tested. The Japanese in particular are masters of this process, employing what they call "gamman zuyoi" – powerful patience.

    Perseverance is one of the most powerful mental skills you can develop; studies show that those with the greatest patience earn better grades and salaries, and make better athletes.

7. ***Strengthen your willpower*** – Perhaps the one central, overriding theme of this book is that the principle of "use it or lose it" is the most profound principle not just of physical exercise, but also cognition. Remember, you heard it here: habit is destiny. If you never try to build your willpower, it will remain weak. Conversely, every time you use it, it will strengthen.

    Dr. Halvorson recommends doing something you find unpleasant as a first step toward building up your willpower:

Give up high-fat snacks, do 100 sit-ups a day, stand up straight when you catch yourself slouching, try to learn a new skill. When you find yourself wanting to give in, give up, or just not bother — don't. Start with just one activity, and make a plan for how you will deal with troubles when they occur ("If I have a craving for a snack, I will eat one piece of fresh or three pieces of dried fruit.") It will be hard in the beginning, but it will get easier, and that's the whole point. As your strength grows, you can take on more challenges and step-up your self-control workout.

This progressive training works in exactly the same way as strength training with weights – gradually increase the difficulty and your ability will grow.

8. **Don't press your luck** – Studies have found that, particularly when it comes to addictions, people overestimate their willpower. Tackling multiple bad habits at the same time, or putting yourself deliberately in situations where your willpower is tested will slowly drain your (finite) resistance.

9. **Focus on the positive** – As we learned earlier, one of the most effective ways to improve is to replace bad habits with good ones. Trying to suppress negative thoughts and behaviours only brings them back with a vengeance (don't think of a white elephant!); instead put some other thought or activity in its place.

For example, instead of lighting up when the urge to smoke grips you, decide to take a brisk walk around the block or climb the stairs to your office/class. In this way, you'll eventually wear your bad habits down to nothing.

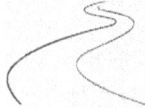

Lifestyle and Mental Health, Roger Walsh. 2011, American Psychologist, 2011; DOI: 10.1037/a0021769

Focusing Attention on the Health Aspects of Foods Changes Value Signals in vmPFC and Improves Dietary Choice, Todd A. Hare, Jonathan Malmaud, and Antonio Rangel, 2011, Journal of Neuroscience; 31 (30): 11077 DOI: 10.1523/JNEUROSCI.6383-10.2011; http://www.jneurosci.org/content/31/30/11077

Tobacco Addiction, 2010, National Institute on Drug Abuse; http://drugabuse.gov/PDF/TobaccoRRS_v16.pdf

Questions About Smoking, Tobacco, and Health, What in Cigarette Smoke is Harmful? American Cancer Society, 2010, http://www.cancer.org/Cancer/CancerCauses/TobaccoCancer/QuestionsaboutSmokingTobaccoandHealth/questions-about-smoking-tobacco-and-health-intro-and-background;

Reduced Thickness in Medial Orbitofrontal Cortex in Smokers, Kühn, S.; et al., 2010, Biological Psychiatry, volume 68, number 11;

Immediate Consequences of Cigarette Smoking: Rapid Formation of Polycyclic Aromatic Hydrocarbon Diol Epoxides, Zhong Y. et al., Chemical Research in Toxicology, Dec 27 http://pubs.acs.org/stoken/presspac/presspac/full/10.1021/tx100345x;

Dicarbonyl Enolates: A New Class of Neuroprotectants, Dr. Richard M. LoPachin, et al, Journal of Neurochemistry, 2011 Jan;

Nicotine Patch Plus Lozenge Best for Quitting Smoking, Amanda Gardner, Nov. 02, 2009 BusinessWeek, http://www.businessweek.com/lifestyle/content/healthday/632704.html

Healthy Minds: Neuroplasticity, Dr. Jeffrey Borenstein, 2011 WNET, New York Public Media; http://www.wliw.org/productions/local/healthy-minds/video-neurogenesis/171/

The World's Technological Capacity to Store, Communicate, and Compute Information, Martin Hilbert, Priscila López, 2011, Science Magazine, DOI: 10.1126/science.1200970; http://www.sciencemag.org/content/early/2011/02/09/science.1200970.abstract

The Innate Genius of Baby Brains, Jane G. Goldberg, Ph.D., 2011, Huffington Post; http://www.huffingtonpost.com/jane-g-goldberg-phd/your-baby-is-a-genius_b_824857.html

Astrocytes Impose Postburst Depression of Release Probability at Hippocampal Glutamate Synapses, M. Andersson, E. Hanse, 2010, Journal of Neuroscience; 30 (16): 5776 DOI: 10.1523/JNEUROSCI.3957-09.2010

How the Brain Works, Dr. Mark Wm. Dubin, 2002

Emotional Intelligence, Daniel Goleman, 2002

Variants of "Umami" Taste Receptor Contribute to Our Individualized Flavor Worlds, Qing-Ying Chen et al, 2009, Monell Chemical Senses Center;

The Greatest Map of All, Douglas Fox, Feb. 7, 2011, New Scientist

Muscles Remember Past Glory, Tina Hesman Saey, 2010, Science News

Sleep Improves Memory of Movements Even Without Practice, PNAS doi: 10.1073_pnas.0901320106

Stress Impairs Prefrontal Cortical Function, Amy F.T. Arnsten, 1988

Empathy Is Moderated by Genetic Background in Mice, Qi Liang Chen, Jules B. Panksepp, Garet P. Lahvis, 2009, Public Library of Science ONE 4(2): e4387. doi:10.1371/journal.pone.0004387

Affective Neuroscience: the Foundations of Human and Animal Emotions, Jaak Panksepp, 2004, Oxford University Press, ISBN: 019517805X

Controlling Anger Before it Controls You, author unattributed, 2011, American Psychological Association; http://www.apa.org/topics/anger/control.aspx

Change Your Brain, Change Your Life, Daniel G. Amen, M.D., 1998 eISBN: 978-0-307-45333-4

Dare to Forgive: The Power of Letting Go and Moving On, Dr. Edward M. Hallowell, 2006

No Future Without Forgiveness, Barbara W. ten Hove, 2007; http://www.pbuuc.org/worship/sermons/sermons0708/Forgiveness.pdf

National Psychological Association for Psychoanalysis: Ninth Annual Oscar Sternbach Award Ceremony, Dr. Jaak Panksepp, Oct 15, 2009.

The Trouble with Testosterone and Other Essays on the Biology of the Human Predicament, Robert M. Sapolsky, 1997;

Supranormal Stimulation of D1 Dopamine Receptors in the Rodent Cortex Impairs Spatial Working Memory Performance, Zahrt et al., 1997, Arnsten

Eliminating Clutter Will Set You Free, Rich Broderick, The Huffington Post, April 2010

Japanese Secrets to Resilience, Margaret Moore, 05/20/11 The Huffington Post

Neverisms: 11 Things You Should Never Do, Never Say, Never Forget, article, Dr. Mardy Grothe, March 11, 2011, The Huffington Post; http://www.huffingtonpost.com/dr-mardy-grothe/neverisms-things-you-should-never_b_860133.html#s277067&title=Never_dull_your

Thomas Edison, Wikipedia; http://en.wikipedia.org/wiki/Thomas_Edison

Growing the Distance: Timeless Principles for Personal, Career, and Family Success, Jim Clemmer; http://www.clemmer.net

From Telegraph to Light Bulb with Thomas Edison, Deborah Hedstrom, 2007 p. 22

Why Do Some People Learn Faster, Jonah Lehrer, October 4, 2011, Wired Magazine

Mindset, Dr. Carol Dweck, 2006; http://www.mindsetonline.com/abouttheauthor/index.html

How Not to Talk to Your Kids: The Inverse Power of Praise, Po Bronson, Feb 11, 2007

The Talent Myth - Are smart people overrated? July 22, 2002, The New Yorker

Focusing Attention on the Health Aspects of Foods Changes Value Signals in the vmPFC and Improves Dietary Choice, Dr. Antonio Rangel, Todd Hare, and Jonathan Malmaud, 2011, Journal of Neuroscience;

Nine Things Successful People Do Differently, Heidi Grant Halvorson, Ph.D., 2011, Harvard Business Review; http://blogs.hbr.org/cs/2011/02/nine_things_successful_people.html

Within

"All that we are is the result of what we have thought. If a man speaks or acts with an evil thought, pain follows him. If a man speaks or acts with a pure thought, happiness follows him, like a shadow that never leaves him."
– Siddhartha Gautama Buddha, circa 500 BC

Your Incredible Inner Power

Want to add years to your life, supercharge your brain, shed stress and boost memory, concentration and decision-making, while significantly improving your health?

Three separate 2010 studies show that just 20 minutes of mindfulness meditation over five days improves attention, concentration, memory, decision-making skills and focus (as much as ten times!). Researchers also believe that, over time, the enhanced enzyme and blood flow may even result in permanent, positive, ongoing physical changes to the brain. Subjects of studies also showed improved mood, with lower anxiety, depression, anger and fatigue.

Mindfulness meditation involves fully and nonjudgmentally focusing on the present, concentrating upon sensations like your breathing, without allowing your mind to wander.

MRI scans show practiced meditators can significantly reduce amygdala activity; this translates into heightened emotional mastery and self-control, a reduction in pain sensitivity, and assists in a wide range of positive effects from addiction and depression recovery to weight loss.

As for the physical benefits, meditation also significantly reduces stress and cortisol levels, lowers blood pressure as much as prescription drugs but without the side effects, dramatically offsets memory-loss effects of Alzheimer's disease through improved blood flow, and creates a significant increase in production of *telomerase,* which protects against cellular aging, all very compelling reasons to be sure to have your daily "quiet time".

Lest you dismiss the benefits of meditation as "New Age superstition", consider this: in 2009, the US Army awarded a $2 million grant to Dr. Amishi P. Jha of the University of Pennsylvania to test the effects of meditation upon marines being deployed into combat. Her research team found 12 minutes of daily mindfulness meditation improved mood and bolstered memory among marines who participated, improving their emotional control and problem-solving skills critical to crisis situations.

According to Dr. Jha, the same benefits can be applied to everyday stressful situations, such as planning a wedding, having a baby, entering surgery, or undergoing a career change. She likens mindfulness training to exercise, advising that you can improve with practice.

Finding Your Answers Deep Within

If you've never practiced visualization before, what follows are some powerful techniques that will radically transform your physical, emotional and cognitive health very quickly. You're going to start the bulk of your program with a meditation of power – the power to change your life forever. Please read through and practice this exercise at least once before attempting it with your eyes closed.

First, you want to arrange yourself comfortably, with your hands loosely resting on your knees. Gently close your eyes, and slowly take a deep, full breath through your nostrils. Really expand your chest with air, to the bottom of your belly, fully expanding your chest and stomach as much as possible. Hold it for a count of five. Let your breath slowly out, under control, through your mouth.

Do it again: a big, full breath in through the nose, and hold it. Slowly let it out through the mouth, and feel your belly and lungs empty, your shoulders fall. With your eyes remaining closed, keep breathing deep, full, greedy breaths of air, and, as you're doing so, focus on the sensations of your feet. Clench them hard, as hard as you can, and then let them relax. Keep breathing. Do it again, and relax.

Work up to your lower legs and calves. Really tighten them, hold, and release, breathing deeply, fully and slowly. Again: Tighten; hold; release. Your upper legs: Clench hard – hold, and release. Again: clench, hold and release. Feel the tension draining as you release, relaxing your body. Keep breathing in this manner – deep, full inhalations, five second breath-holding followed by slow, full exhalations.

Move to your buttocks and pelvis – clench hard, hold and release. Again: Clench, hold, and release. Keep breathing deeply, fully, slowly, relaxing deeper and deeper into your chair. Progress to tightening your belly and mid-back. Tighten – hold and release. Tighten, hold, and release. Feel the tension draining away…

Move up to your upper back and shoulders. Clench – hold, and release. Clench, hold and release. Feel the tension melting slowly away from your body as you relax deeper and deeper into your thoughts. Clench your hands into tight fists – hold it – and relax. Again, clench, hold and release. Tense the muscles in the back of your neck and around your face; really grimace hard – hold it, and relax. Once again, Clench, hold, and release.

Keep breathing slowly, deeply, fully. Your body should feel fully relaxed, and your eyes remain gently closed. With practice, you'll learn to reach a theta brainwave state which is extremely powerful for visualization.

Begin by picturing yourself in your room, sitting with your eyes closed, breathing slowly. See the things and people around you clearly in your mind's eye. Picture up in the clouds high above your head, a great, shimmering, golden column of light shooting down from the sun, bathing you in its light. You're surrounded by this golden energy. Clearly picture it and feel the sensations of it bathing you in golden light. *Shoot* that light out all around you in a blast of golden energy, filling the room, bathing everything and everyone in it. See the coruscating light energy, like rippling golden water, washing over everyone and everything in the room. Watch this golden light soak into your skin, into their skin, and feel its energy, like rippling electricity within you, a great, beautiful power. Stay with it for as long as you wish, and, when you're ready, open your eyes.

Enlightenment

Light is a metaphor for personal energy. In the morning when you awaken, as an experiment, clearly visualize a great, golden bolt of sunlight shooting down from the heavens upon you, and like a beacon, imagine that light beaming out from your solar plexus, making a shining path, lighting the way before you as you go about your day. Watch how your day progresses as a result.

The 2500-year-old *Upanishads* – a collection of books that form the central core of Indian philosophy – teach of a higher state of being called *enlightenment* – the root word *light* indicating that the light of knowledge has shone upon someone. These ancient scriptures say the entire universe is one great pool of connected spiritual energy – out of this pool of energy, your spirit came, and into it you'll return. That energy, it's believed, is within everything in the universe.

In its entirety, the universe is, they say, *Brahma* or God, and you and every grain of dust in the universe are a part of that great pool of energy, a Cosmic Consciousness. Across the globe and throughout human history, the most widely-revered ancient spiritual texts – the *Tao Te Ching, Bhagavad Gita, Buddhist Avatmsaka Sutras*, Hebrew and Christian *Bibles* and even Native American shamans – all speak of a Universal Consciousness in which all living and nonliving things are constituent elements. Perhaps there is a logical argument in favor of the idea:

In the realm of science, the *Law of Conservation of Energy* says that energy (and matter) are neither created nor destroyed – they simply change form.

For example, if you burn a piece of wood, it doesn't disappear. The energy you release – the light, heat and sound of a fire – is the chemical energy stored in the molecular bonds that make *starch*, plant sugar. That chemical energy is stored sunlight energy, converted and trapped in chemical bonds through *photosynthesis* – the use of sunlight for energy storage in the force of plant starch. So in the act of burning wood, you're freeing stored sunlight energy.

When the molecules of carbon, hydrogen, oxygen and nitrogen are sufficiently excited through heat of a flame, the bonds rupture, releasing heat and light – the stored sunlight energy which the plant used to drive its growth. The heat burns the wood, leaving ash, and releasing steam, carbon dioxide and trace gases into the air.

In this and myriad other chemical reactions, both energy and matter are constantly recirculating in an endless cycle. Neither is ever created nor destroyed. And if it's possible such a thing as a spiritual energy exists, it seems reasonable to suppose it follows the same principles – a Law of Conservation of spiritual Energy, if you will.

It's not our purpose to explore metaphysics or religion, but there are both spiritualists and scientists who teach that the universe is connected by an energy present in all things, from the life energy within you to the much quieter energy of the stones beneath your feet, to the comet 10,000 light-years away. *Pilot Wave Theory* (see book one) seems to support this.

I'm personally convinced there's more to the universe than what our five senses report, but you're welcome to be skeptical regarding such matters, as they are, at this point, unfalsifiable. The tremendous physical and psychological benefits of meditation, however, have been scientifically proven.

Life Transformation Through Visualization

You want to begin in a deeply relaxed state. Designate an area to be your "quiet space", where you can spend 20 minutes without distractions or interruptions. Unplug the telephone and turn off your cellphone's ringer. Arrange yourself comfortably. You can be sitting in a chair, lying down, or in a cross-legged meditation pose – the choice is yours. Make sure your spine is straight, and gently close your eyes.

Begin deep breathing and relaxing in the manner you practiced earlier, tensing and relaxing all your muscle groups. When you're fully relaxed, as you breathe out deeply, imagine you are breathing out stress, daily tension, worries, and pollutants. As you breathe in, imagine you're taking in purity and goodness.

Keep deep breathing, and, as you exhale, start counting down backwards from ten to one, gradually sinking into an ever greater state of relaxation and peace. When you've reached "one", gently ride with the peaceful calm of your body and experience the sensation for a few moments.

When you feel ready to proceed, continue to keep your eyes closed and breathe in a deep, easy, natural rhythm, then proceed with one of the visualization exercises below. Start with the elementary and then work your way up to more advanced (and powerful) visualizations.

Don't struggle; visualization can be initially challenging, but you don't want the process to be something you have to try too hard to achieve. As leadership coach Adam Chalker suggests, "...visualizing is like holding a bird: hold it too loose and you lose it; hold it too tightly and you crush it. Keep your concentration as if you're holding the bird."

Focus gently away from distractions. As you focus, negative thoughts may encroach upon you. It's okay; allow them to remain. Just acknowledge them without trying to fight them, as they're also a part of your inner self. Gently return your focus back to your chosen meditation theme. The most effective meditation work focuses on manifesting your highest aspirations, your "authentic self".

I. Beginner Level – Breathing And Focus

Deep Breathing – Inhale through your nose, pushing your stomach forward until your belly is tight, lifting your chest and collarbone as you breathe in,

Exhale through your mouth, simply relaxing your collarbone, chest and ribs; this will automatically push out the air in your lungs. When you feel like all the air is out, pull your stomach muscles in to push out the remaining air.

Focus

1) Aim for maintaining a mental picture of these shapes for about two to three minutes each:

- Yellow triangle

- Red circle

- Blue star

2) Visualize numbers, starting with a single digit, then two digits, then three, four, five, six, etc. Maintain focus on the largest number you can "see" entirely.

3) Visualize your favourite food, making it as real as possible. In your mind, you want to smell and taste it. Feel yourself savoring it as fully as possible; make it real.

Health

Picture a golden ball of warmth, energy and light in the center of your chest. As you inhale, imagine it expanding and brightening. With every breath, feel this golden warmth spreading and expanding throughout your body, and then radiating out into the world.

Serenity

1) The Silent Temple – When you have reached a state of complete calm and feel you're ready, begin by imagining you're in a bustling city. Walk through it, into a quieter neighborhood that gives way to countryside, and gradually more natural surroundings. As you proceed, the surroundings become ever more sylvan. Presently, you're walking through dense, lush, untouched forest (or jungle, if you prefer). After a while, you arrive at the scene of an ancient, utterly silent temple.

In this temple, the silence has been sacred since the dawn of humanity, and not a single word has ever been spoken here. As you enter, look around in awe at the magnificence of this temple of solitude. Seat yourself in its throne, in the heart of silence. Drink in the details all around you. This is your quiet place. Feel free to linger, relaxing in peace.

When you wish, stand, carrying the inner peace within you, like a glowing, silent ball of serenity. Exit the temple, returning along the path you came by, through the forest, through the countryside, through the neighborhood, carrying the serenity within you, back to the town. Finish your visualization when you feel ready.

2) Your Place of Power – When you've reached a state of complete calm and feel you're ready, begin imaging that you're walking through natural surroundings until you arrive at your favourite scene – any natural environment you wish. Look around; feel, hear, see, smell, touch and taste it in vivid detail. Are there buildings or is it all natural? What are the colors, sights, sounds and scents? What does the air taste like? How does it feel on your skin? Is it warm or cool? Linger here and rest, until you feel fully refreshed and ready to return to your waking life.

As you stand to leave, give thanks for the blessing of your own personal sanctuary, and leave knowing it is always here, right where you left it, whenever you wish to return.

II. Intermediate Level – Guidance and Purpose

1. Communing With Your Inner Guide – When you've reached a state of complete calm and feel you're ready, begin: Start by visiting your inner sanctuary and resting there. After a time, picture a radiance approaching you, materializing into a figure – your personal guide. Imagine your guide as vividly as possible. What does he (or she, or even it) look like? How is its voice? What sort of "air" does it emanate?

Express thanks to your inner guide for coming to you and ask it whatever questions you wish. If it cannot answer, have faith that these answers will come at a later date. (As a cautionary note, if this figure is more like a critic, turn it away gently with gratitude, instructing it to send your true inner guide.

When you've finished communing, send your guide back to where it came from with your thanks, watching as it retreats into the distance, the radiation fading. Feel free to linger and rest at your leisure. When you feel completely ready, leave your inner sanctuary and return to your waking world.

2. Meeting Your Future Self – When you've reached a state of complete calm and feel you're ready, begin:

Imagine a great ray of light entering your room, surrounding you. Step into the ray; it raises you into the air, and the ceiling and roof dissolve as you continue to rise, higher and higher. You can see the ground retreating ever further, buildings, streets, then your neighborhood, your city, your province and country....

You keep rising, until you're in the upper atmosphere and beyond, above the clouds, looking at the blue-green curve of the Earth from space. From above the Earth, suspended, floating in space, there is a great quietude. Relax and enjoy the serenity.

Time passes differently here. Here, only minutes have passed, but down below, on Earth, years are passing with every minute you linger. When you feel ready, follow the ray of light below you back down, down, seeing the earth, and then your country, your province, your neighborhood growing.

ADVANCED VISUALIZATION: KUNDALINI AWAKENING

From a purely rational standpoint, concentrating on mentally creating the complex shapes and feelings associated with each spiritual center in your mind is incredibly powerful for increasing inward focus.

CROWN CHAKRA

"Sahasrara", the 1000-petalled lotus (all colors fuse into white), top of the head. *Meaning:* when the chakra awakens you have accessed pure consciousness. Being and matter no longer exist in this state of mind, and you have fused spiritually with the universe.

BROW CHAKRA

"Ajna" the two-petaled violet/deep-blue lotus. The "third eye" chakra. *Meaning:* when this chakra awakens, gender disappears, you are simply a living entity, and your spiritual and mental self are in harmony with your physical self. This is when you have full access to your intuition and inner guidance.

THROAT CHAKRA

"Vishuddha" is surrounded by 16 pale blue/turquoise petals. *Meaning:* When this chakra awakens, thinking becomes smooth and fluid; it also grants rich communication, mature growth, emotional independence and expressiveness.

HEART CHAKRA

"Anahata" is depicted as a circular flower with twelve green petals. Within are two intersecting triangles which depict the coming together of the male and female through love, forming a star of David shape. *Meaning:* complex emotions including unconditional love, devotion, balance, compassion, love of the self and others, well-being. It also governs circulation (appropriate, as the heart and thymus are here.

SOLAR PLEXUS CHAKRA

"Manipura" is yellow, envisioned as a triangle pointing downward, surrounded by ten petals. *Meaning:* This chakra controls life energy through metabolism and digestion, as this is where the stomach is found. Also located here are the pancreas (which controls blood sugar levels) and the adrenal glands. It is also where the diaphragm controls breath, and the center of "ki" energy in martial arts. Meaning: Physical energy, growth and personal power. Also governs the ability to transform base emotions into more productive ones (fear into courage. anxiety into mental focus, etc.)

SACRUM CHAKRA

"Swadhisthana" is located in the "sacrum" (pelvic region). It's envisioned as a a crescent moon in a white lotus surrounded by six orange petals. *Meaning:* Physical pleasures, both positive and negative (including addictions and satisfying basic emotional needs). Also destructive impulses such as violence. Reproduction, joy and enthusiasm.

ROOT CHAKRA

"Muladhara" is depicted as a square within four red petals. This is related to the most basic impulses - instincts, survival, security, lust. It's located in the area known as the "perineum", between the genitals and the anus. This region is where the muscles contract during orgasm, which is the basis of human reproduction.

This is thought of as where the "genetic code" of human life originates (through sperm and the ovaries), and mentally envisioned as the coiled, dormant spiritual serpent called the "kundalini".

Tantric yoga is a practice devoted to awakening spiritual power through sexual discipline, and involves delaying orgasm - allowing hours-long, continuous orgasms - for both men and women. I will attest (through years of arduous and extensive field research) to the truth that the perenium is indeed an orgasmic "hot button". Further research is certainly in order.

Sources: http://www.kundaliniyoga.org/ http://en.wikipedia.org/wiki/Chakra Image: Polyglot Studios, 2011

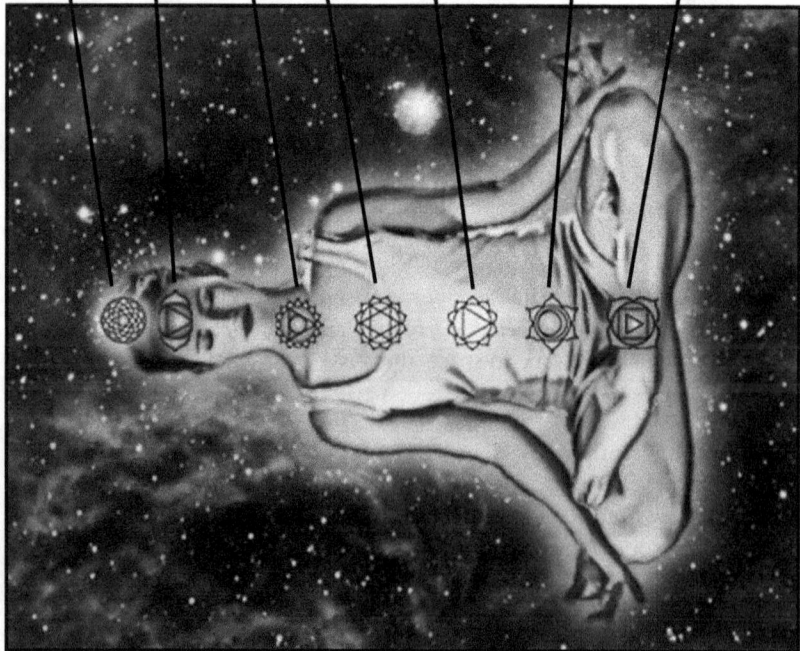

Please note: I absolutely do not advocate any religion or cult; I'm interested purely in furthering the cause of self-empowerment, through any path of wisdom available, be it science, religion art, mathematics or philosphy. Therefore, I'm just as comfortable recommending the parables of Jesus Christ as the lyrics of Bob Dylan, the prose of Herman Melville as the principles of Aristotelian logic. If I've offended anyone by recommending unfamiliar teachings, please take it as a gentle suggestion that you might want to examine your inner, self-imposed limitations.

Finally levitate gently down into your room, where the figure of you from 10 to 50 years older stands. It's the "you" of the future, here to meet with you. The future you is full of great wisdom and joy. Ask "future you" anything you want. When you're finished, "future you" gives you a gift – what's your gift?

When you've finished communing, thank "future you", and step back into the ray of light, then rise back above your home, your neighborhood, your city, your province, your country, the Earth, back into space. Relax in the calm of space until you're ready to return, back down the ray of light, to your present-day world.

3. Discovering Your Life Purpose – When you have reached a state of complete calm and feel you're ready, begin: Picture yourself walking through natural surroundings, when a path appears before you. You see people and things on the sides of the path, all trying to distract you, but no matter what they do they're unable to step onto your path.

As you proceed along your pathway, you can feel their influence pulling at you, but you continue, unfazed. Eventually, you come to the end of your path and see an image or symbol. What is it? Walk up to it and examine it in detail. Take time to reflect upon it, and to ask it whatever questions are within you. Listen carefully to its teachings. When you have finished, give thanks, return to the waking world, and write down everything you have learned.

III. Advanced Level – Awareness, Courage, Health, Love And Wisdom

Eastern Kundalini Yoga teaches how to maximize health by awakening energy centers in your body called chakras. Your spine is a conduit for channelling this energy and connecting with the power of the Universe.

The energy channeled through your spine works its way upward, awakening each of the chakras in turn. This energy is envisioned as a glowing blue serpent of light, like a cobra, rising through your spinal column. Each of the energy centers is pictured as opening like a beautiful flower of light, and each in turn awakens a gradually higher level of spiritual attunement ("enlightenment"), starting from the base (physical), through the sexual, emotional, mental and finally the spiritual, in the "crown" of your head, which is said to connect you with the spiritual energy flowing throughout the Universe.

The chakras are said to be absorbing this prana (universal life force) and distributing it throughout your body. There is said to be a huge amount of energy locked in your root chakra, the energy center at the base of your spine, which can be unlocked and released, to travel up your spine, through all your chakras, finally opening your crown chakra, allowing you to experience higher wisdom and spiritual awareness.

The idea is to contemplate each of your chakras opening in turn, as kundalini energy rises slowly up from the root at the base of your spine through each of these energy centers. Each of the seven chakras has an associated color and power, and if you want to find out more, the information is freely available on a number of websites. You don't have to accept the mystic aspects of this to benefit from the exercise, but it's been practiced by billions of people for thousands of years, and that is usually a good indication that there is some form of benefit to the practice.

Personally, I find it interesting that each of the chakras corresponds to key anatomical points:

- Your *crown* is centered upon your cerebral cortex;

- Your pineal gland is in the third eye position; it produces melatonin, which is responsible for sleeping (and, by extension, dreaming);

- Your *larynx* (voice box) is in your throat, allowing you to "connect" with others through speech; so is your thyroid, which controls energy use and your body's sensitivity to hormones;

- Your heart is, of course, vital to all life;

- Your *solar plexus* is where your diaphragm controls breath. It's also the seat of what eastern health and martial arts practitioners call your *chi power*, of which you will learn more presently; this is also where your adrenal glands and major spinal stability muscles are, giving you "courage" or "backbone";

- Your sexual organs are where you "connect" with others physically;

- The base of your spine – your *coccyx* – is where your spine connects you to your lower limbs, and thus the earth; it's also connected to the muscles responsible for evacuating bodily waste.

Based on all we've seen so far, it seems clear that what this practice has been teaching people to do for thousands of years is to use the hypothalamus to activate the parasympathetic nervous system and control endocrine functions; and based on the latest scientific research, mental effects upon the endocrine system are indisputably powerful.

Please note: I'm not advocating any religion or cult, merely practices which can help you achieve your goals in life. Even if you accept the spiritual aspects on a purely metaphoric, utilitarian basis, the principles will still help you.

Interestingly, yoga is becoming much more mainstream: in 2009, Austrian video game publisher JoWooD Productions began marketing Yoga for Nintendo Wii; with a balance board, you can receive direct feedback on your actions.

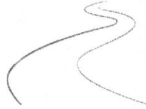

Examining the Protective Effects of Mindfulness Training on Working Memory Capacity and Affective Experience, Elizabeth A. Stanley and Amishi P. Jha, et al, Emotion Journal, 10.1 2010: 54-64;

Mind Fitness: Improving Operational Effectiveness and Building Warrior Resilience, Elizabeth A. Stanley and Amishi P. Jha, Joint Force Quarterly, 55.4, 2009: 144-151;

Mindfulness Meditation Improves Cognition: Evidence of Brief Mental Training, Fadel Zeidan, Susan K. Johnson, Zhanna David, Paula Goolkasian, and Bruce J. Diamond, Consciousness and Cognition, 2010, 19 (2):597-605;

Chinese Meditation, Yi-Yuan Tang, Michael I. Posner, Qilin Lu, Xiujuan Geng, Elliot A. Stein, Yihong Yang;

IBMT Found to Boost Brain Connectivity, 2010, http://www.yi-yuan.net/english/pdf/2010/Media%20Relations.pdf;

Neural Correlates of Focused Attention and Cognitive Monitoring in Meditation, Manna A, Raffone A, Perrucci MG, Nardo D, Ferretti A, Tartaro A, Londei A, Del Gratta C, Belardinelli MO, Romani GL, Brain Research Bulletin, 2010 Apr 29;82(1-2):46-56.;

Neural Correlates of Attentional Expertise in Long-Term Meditation Practitioners, Brefczynski-Lewis J. A., Lutz, A., Schaefer, H. S., Levinson, D. B. & Davidson, R. J., Proceedings of the National Academy of Sciences, 2007 104(27) 11483-11488.;

Does Meditation Training Lead to Enduring Changes in the Anticipation and Experience of Pain? Jason Buhleemail, Tor D. Wager, Journal of the International Association for the Study of Pain, 2010;

Blood Pressure Response to Transcendental Meditation: A Meta-Analysis, James W. Anderson, Chunxu Liu and Richard J. Kryscio, American Journal of Hypertension, 2008;

Effect of Compassion Meditation on Neuroendocrine, Innate Immune and Behavioral Responses to Psychosocial Stress, Pace, T. W. W., Negi, L. T., Adame, D. D., Cole, S. P., Sivilli, T. I., Brown, T. D., Issa, M. J., & Raison, C.L., Psychoneuroendocrinology, 2009, 34, 87-98;

Meditation Effects on Cognitive Function and Cerebral Blood Flow In Subjects with Memory Loss: A Preliminary Study, Andrew Newberg, MD, et al., Journal of Alzheimer's Disease, Volume 20:2, April 2010;

Intensive Meditation Training, Immune Cell Telomerase Activity, and Psychological Mediators, Tonya L. Jacobs, Elissa S. Epel, Jue Lin, Elizabeth Blackburn, Owen M. Wolkowitz, David A. Bridwell, Anthony P. Zanesco, Stephen R. Aichele, Baljinder K. Sahdra, Katherine A. MacLean, Brandon G. King, Phillip R.Shaver, Erika L. Rosenberg, Emilio Ferrer, B. Alan Wallace, Clifford D. Saron, Psychoneuroendocrinology, 2010

Guided meditation exercise as originally taught by Asst. Prof. Kelly Ann Charlton, UNCP, 1999.

Best Personal Growth Resources, Adam Chalker, 2009, http://www.best-personal-growth-resources.com/about-me.html

Addicted

"Use it once, it might let you go; use it twice, and it owns your soul."
– Popular prisoner's aphorism about methamphetamine

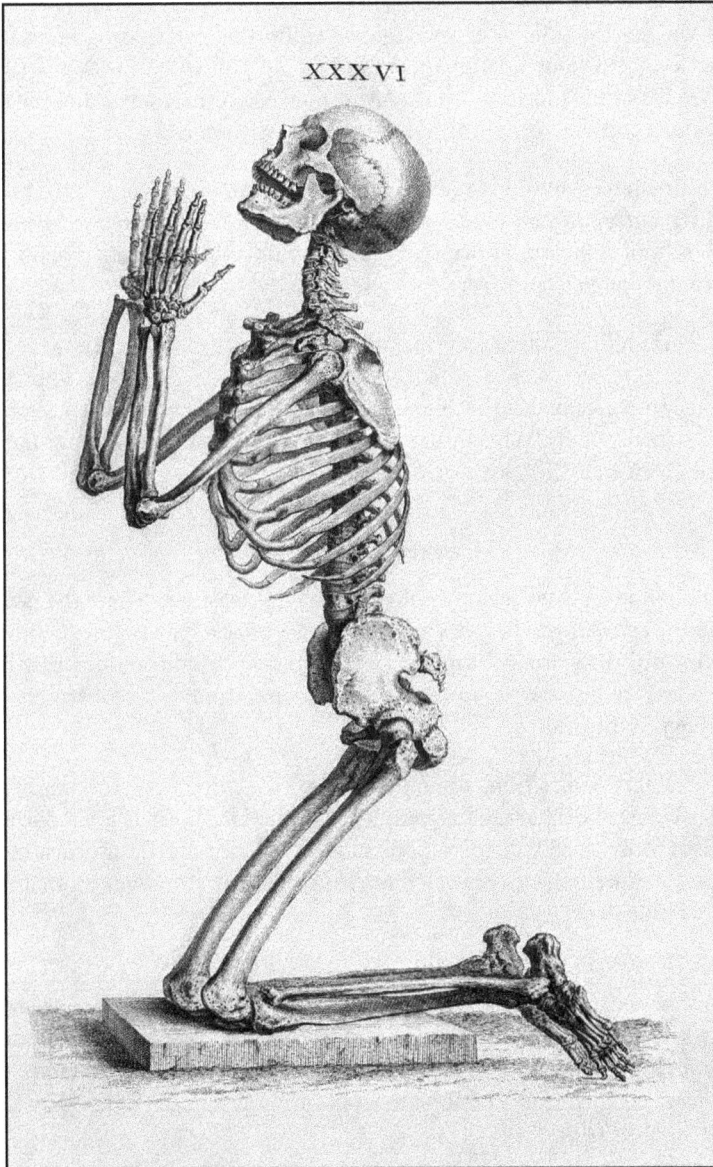

Osteographia or the Anatomy of the Bones. William Cheselden, 1733,
US National Library of Medicine, public domain

America's Horrific Modern Epidemic

If you're so inclined, for 60 dollars and about an hour of your time, you can "shake and bake" a week's supply of methamphetamine from common household products, which include battery acid, lighter fluid, drain cleaner and other deadly, shiver-inducing chemicals. The mixture is highly caustic, and will eat the skin from your fingers while you're preparing it. Usually completely untrained, anonymous, functionally illiterate locals mix it in plastic containers in their homes. And then, of course, an addict buys it, and snorts, smokes or injects it into his bloodstream. Nice.

An estimated 1.2 million (one out of every 260) Americans have tried meth, and it's currently considered the country's worst drug problem. Among high school students, who are particularly vulnerable, the rate is about 1.5 percent – one in a hundred.

These are chilling statistics, if you know a little about meth's effects: after two to three short weeks of use, meth addicts' personalities have been known to change so radically that they'll murder best friends or even family members over a small supply. Why on Earth would anybody willingly engage in this sort of behavior?

Causes And Effects

Addiction is, in essence, a pathological form of learning, where the neural circuits that train you to adapt and survive are hijacked by synthetic sources of pleasure. Your brain learns by building synaptic connections that link two ideas or sensations, so that whenever one occurs, it will trigger the memory of the other.

Vulnerability comes from a number of factors – living in high crime areas, where drugs or dealers are frequently present and the lifestyle is glamorized. Poverty is likewise a factor – poor kids have higher levels of fearfulness, anxiety and depression, putting them at greater risk than their more finan-cially stable peers.

Says Dr. Daniel Goleman, addicts (as opposed to casual users), tend to use drugs for self-medicating, attempting to soothe anger, depression or anxi-ety with a chemical hit. Studies have shown, he says, the most emotionally distraught have the highest rates of substance abuse. The inner distress that has plagued them for a lifetime is often instantly quietened the first time they try alcohol or drugs.

Director of the Center for Education and Drug Abuse Research, Dr. Ralph Tarter, says this *predisposition*, a vulnerability to addiction, means the first time such people take a particular drug or drink, the effect is profound – they often report feeling "normal" for the first time in their lives.

The biological predisposition for addiction can be hereditary, characterized by low levels of the neurotransmitter GABA, which helps regulate anxiety. When these individuals drink alcohol or take sedatives, their GABA levels rise and their anxiety drops – their brain chemistry temporarily "normalizes". Unfortunately, over time, seeking calm from alcohol or sedatives leads to a dangerous dependency, which results in all sorts of very well-known and incredibly destructive circumstances.

Impaired frontal lobe function is also often a factor, resulting in reduced working memory capacity and impulse control – so short-term comfort is chosen as a quick-fix response to anxiety. The addictive substance becomes the easiest way to kill emotional pain, to self-medicate and reduce anxiety.

People who are predisposed to restlessness, boredom, and impulsiveness – kids who are restless, fidgety, and so-called "troublemakers", are susceptible to falling in with companions on the fringes of society – criminals and drug addicts. Usually these questionable individuals are male, with a predisposition for seeking risk and excitement. It's believed, says Goleman, that such risk-taking behavior is linked to deficiencies in serotonin and *MAO*s.

Serotonin promotes calm and well-being and reduces aggression, while MAOs (monoamine oxidases) are enzymes which inactivate and break down several neurotransmitters – dopamine, epinephrine, melatonin, norepinephrine and serotonin. MAO deficiency can result in abnormally high levels of central nervous system-stimulating catecholamines – dopamine, epinephrine, and norepinephrine.

For depressives, low serotonin puts them at risk for dependency on stimulants like cocaine, and for those predisposed to rage and other hyperactive states, opioids like heroin are the drugs which give them peace. But repeated drug use changes the way their brains react to pleasant stimuli. After long periods of drug abuse, their mesolimbic pathways require the drug just to function at normal levels. Thus, addiction is the state in which a drug is needed to feel normal or happy.

Born Vulnerable

Drug addiction has been repeatedly linked to inheritable genetic susceptibility, and epigenetics appear to alter gene expression in ways that pass susceptibility down through several generations; for example, children of alcoholics have a 400% greater risk of alcohol addiction than others.

According to Dr. Kenneth Blum, a pioneer in the study of alcoholism, substance abuse is largely driven by genetics, which make some of us more easily addicted than others. One commonly-inherited trait results in dopamine reductions, leading to *reward deficiency syndrome*; people with these inherited characteristics crave artificially-increased dopamine stimulation just to feel "normal".

Drs. Kenneth Blum and Ernest P. Noble found a region of DNA associated with severe alcoholism they dubbed the *reward gene*, which produces dopamine D2 receptors. Carriers of a variant gene (*DRD2 A1 polymorphism*) have about 30-40 percent fewer D2 receptors than most people. If they have two copies of the polymorphism – one from each parent – the number of receptors is even lower.

This results in reward deficiency syndrome – a general state of anxiety, stress, pain, discomfort and agitation that sufferers learn to relieve with addictive behaviours. Dr. Blum says extensive studies link alcoholism to a wide range of disorders, including cocaine addiction, smoking, carbohydrate binging, pathological gambling, Tourette's Syndrome, PTSD, ADHD, internet gaming, compulsive lying, obesity and sexual addiction, all of which appear to emerge due to faulty D2 receptor genes in the mesolimbic pathway.

Dopamine receptor gene D4 is also thought to play a role in addictions, encoding receptors, the tiny lumps of specialized proteins on neural surfaces to which neurochemicals bind. Just like turning on a light switch, dopamine triggers a sequence of chemical chain events whenever it binds to one of its five known receptors. Genetic differences that reduce the number of these synaptic receptors are thought to diminish the ability to experience pleasure, and predispose someone to using drugs which elevate their naturally subdued mental states.

Since 1990, additional dopamine and other genes have been tentatively linked to a susceptibility to alcoholism and other addictions. Inherited variations among these genes change the efficiency of dopamine function; for example, a superefficient dopamine-transporter gene which is too adept at clearing dopamine from the synapses can predispose one to alcoholism and other addictions, it's believed, keeping the synapses perpetually low in dopamine.

Conversely, knocking out this dopamine-transporter gene creates mice so well-equipped with dopamine that they are immune to addictions, lending weight to the theory that dopamine underlies it all.

Researchers have begun honing in on additional genes tied to virtually all drug addictions. In 2009, Dr. Ming Li, professor of psychiatry and neurobehavioral sciences at the UVA School of Medicine, and Dr. Margit Burmeister, professor of psychiatry and human genetics at the University of Michigan, presented a paper showing several genes linked to multiple addictions. They pointed out specific gene clusters on 11 chromosomes linked to alcohol, cannabis, cocaine, heroin, nicotine and opioid addictions.

Cravings

Motivation is controlled by two opposing drives — *appetitive* and *aversive* motivation. Appetitive motivation directs you toward goals which bring satisfaction: eating, sex, companionship, etc. Aversive motivation prompts you to escape unpleasant stimuli: pain, cold, stress, etc. Appetitive motivation is driven by your brain's mesolimbic reward system, a chemical cascade that frees you from stress and returns your body to homeostasis, giving you feelings of general well-being and comfort.

The neurohormone CRF (corticotropin-releasing-factor) plays a major role in drug addiction withdrawal and relapse. When an addict is deprived of his drug, his amygdala secretes high levels of CRF, which activates the adrenal cortex. This elevated CRF secretion increases anxiety and decreases interest in normally rewarding activities – both symptoms of drug withdrawal.

Stress creates cravings – your brain saying it wants more dopamine. By activating D2 receptors in the nucleus accumbens, this craving is satisfied. Several neurotransmitters work in harmony to produce feelings of well-being: serotonin, dopamine, norepinephrine, GABA and endorphins – when levels of these chemicals decline or the receptors are blocked, stress, pain, discomfort and agitation result.

Those suffering from Reward Deficiency Syndrome are unable to produce an adequate feeling of well-being and consequently often self-medicate with substances that help raise the levels of pleasurable chemicals in their system – if only temporarily. This relieves stress, anxiety and emotional pain, allowing them to function. Such substances needn't be illegal drugs; the list also includes junk foods, sugars, chocolate, alcohol, nicotine or other stimulants. Unfortunately, self-medication only provides temporary relief, while bringing with it the possibility of worse long-term consequences, weight gain, addictions, and health problems.

Nowhere To Turn – Stigmatized For A Disease

Dr. Nora Volkow, director of the US National Institute on Drug Abuse, has revolutionized modern understanding of addictions. She says society stigmatizes addicts for what is actually a mental illness. Drug addictions, she explains, are a brain disease which wipes out your ability to exert control – destroying circuits that allow you to exercise what's commonly called free will: disrupting the neural pathways which allow you control of your behavior makes it so that, even if you know your habit is destructive, you cannot stop.

Volkow was set onto her career path by seeing her favourite uncle, an alcoholic, rejected by everyone around him, for the brain disease disrupting control of his self-destructive behavior. Her grandfather also committed suicide after struggling with alcoholism. Fear of the social stigma attached to drug addiction, she says, makes it impossible for people like them to seek help, with tragic consequences.

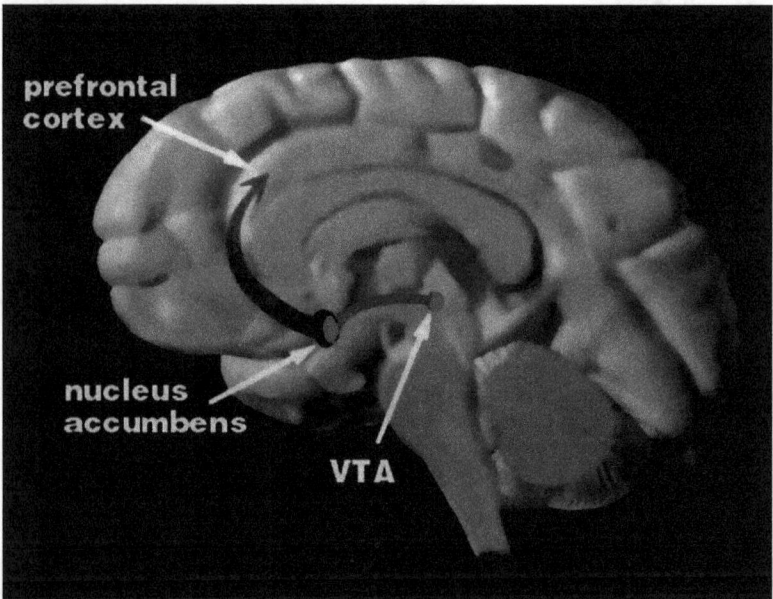

Drug "rewards" are the rushes of pleasure that come from a heightened dopamine neurotransmission in the mesolimbic pathway, originating from the ventral tegmental area (VTA) and terminating in the nucleus accumbens (NAcc), and onward to the prefrontal cortex, which processes the experience. National Institutes of Health, 2004, Public domain.

Hijacking The Hedonic Highway

Your brain's mesolimbic pathway, called the *hedonic highway* because of its relation to pleasure-seeking, directs you toward goals which promote your sur-

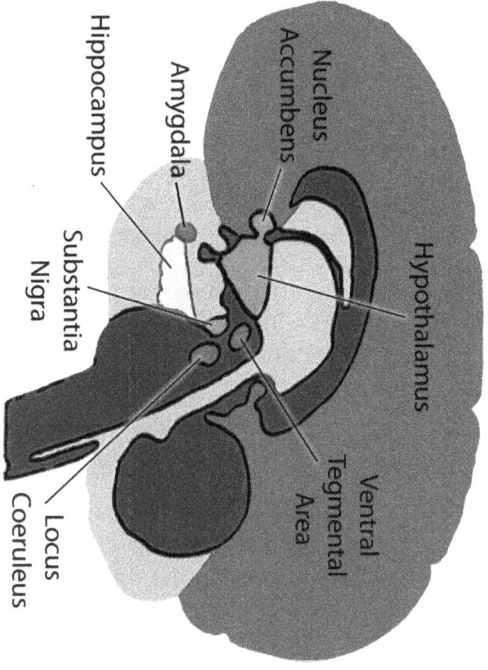

Schematic of the Reward Cascade

adapted from *Perspectives on Brain Functioning: The Addictive Brain,* by Jay M. Holder, DC and Kenneth Blum, PhD, 1990

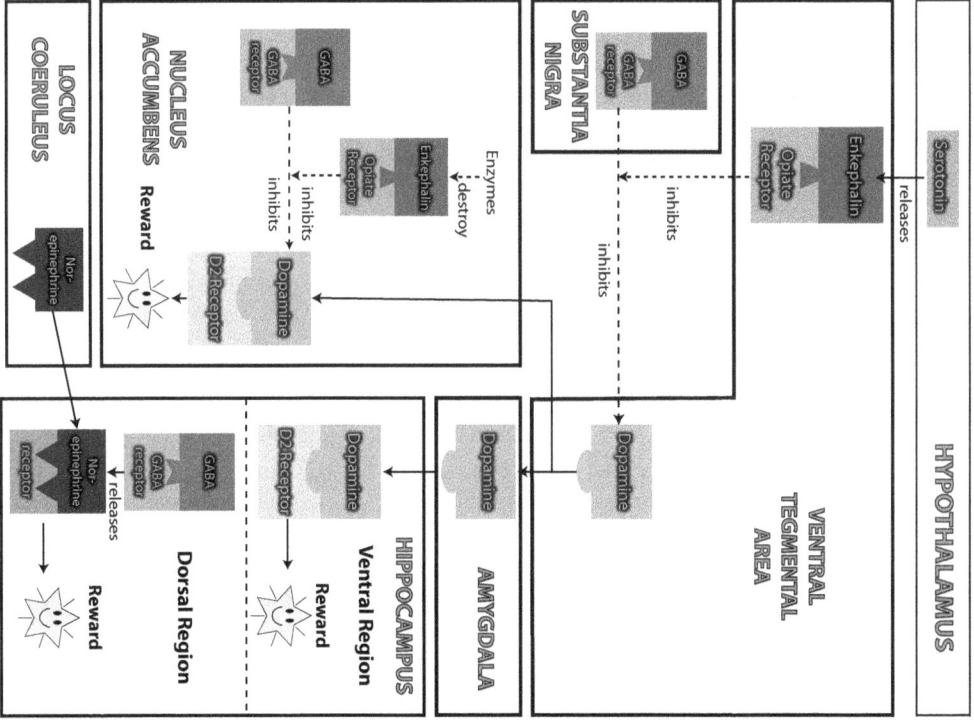

Hippocampus

Amygdala

Nucleus Accumbens

Substantia Nigra

Hypothalamus

Ventral Tegmental Area

Locus Coeruleus

HYPOTHALAMUS

Serotonin — releases

Enkephalin — Opiate Receptor

SUBSTANTIA NIGRA

GABA — GABA receptor

inhibits

VENTRAL TEGMENTAL AREA

Dopamine

inhibits

NUCLEUS ACCUMBENS

GABA — GABA receptor

Enkephalin — Opiate Receptor

Enzymes destroy

inhibits   inhibits

Dopamine — D2 Receptor   Reward

AMYGDALA

Dopamine

HIPPOCAMPUS

Ventral Region

Dopamine — D2 Receptor   Reward

Dorsal Region

GABA — GABA receptor

Nor-epinephrine

releases

LOCUS COERULEUS

Nor-epinephrine — Nor-epinephrine receptor

Reward

vival: food, water, sex and nurturing. When your hypothalamus signals a need, you seek out things you have learned will satisfy these needs. The process which teaches you how to meet these needs is triggered when your Ventral Tegmental Area transmits dopamine to your nucleus accumbens. Dopaminergic neurons from the VTA project into the nucleus accumbens and then onward to your frontal cortex, the seat of conscious thought and willpower.

Dopamine exercises tremendous power over attention, learning and memory. It promotes brain function, and in high concentrations causes feelings of elation. On a chemical level, every pleasurable experience you know – winning a card game, looking into the face of a loved one, enjoying tasty food, hearing praise from a classmate – feels good because of the release of dopamine in the mesolimbic pathway of your brain.

The neural pathways that are modulated by dopamine reach throughout your brain, including into your limbic system, which generates your emotions, and hippocampus, which generates your long-term memories. Dopamine focuses neurotransmission, so that only the strongest, coordinated signals from other neurotransmitters are communicated. This regulates your attention and working memory, and enhances overall CNS function. The end result is that a dopamine surge makes you feel alive, energized, engaged, excited, powerful and capable. Insufficient dopamine stimulation, on the other hand, results in diffuse, unfocused information. When you try something and get a positive result (for example, eating a favourite food), your cortex signals your ventral tegmental area. This region triggers the "reward cascade", a flood of dopamine. This reduces your stress and makes you feel focused, energized, alert and powerful, and conveys a general sense of wellbeing.

Normal dopamine levels create pleasure from healthy daily activities, and these feelings of comfort and pleasure calm and soothe stress. Psychologists believe that every time a reward is better than anticipated however, dopamine-releasing neurons increase their output – raising the salience of that stimulus for memory encoding; decrease their output when the result is worse, and maintain a steady firing rate when the result is just as expected.

The reward cascade is your brain's behavior-encouraging payoff for satisfying survival drives for food, mating, and safety, giving feelings of comfort and satisfaction. Your brain encodes memories of such pleasure and seeks to repeat it. The first time you get a specific reward, the reward itself triggers dopamine release, but from that point, sensory cues which indicate presence of the reward trigger dopamine release.

The Reward Cascade

Dopamine release is not as simple as it seems at first glance; when dopamine is released into the nucleus accumbens in the striatum of your basal ganglia, it binds to receptors and enhances neurotransmission, an exceedingly pleasurable state. Activating one type of dopamine receptors (D1) stimulates neurotransmission, but also leaves your nervous system in a "jittery" state, while the second type (D2) has a calming, pleasurable effect.

Serotonin begins the reward cascade, a domino effect of chemical processes that operate like water cascading down a waterfall... It's released into the hypothalamus, which triggers the release of opioids (enkephalins). These bind to opiate receptors in the substantia nigra, inhibiting GABA transmission. GABA is a regulator, inhibiting dopamine release into the nucleus accumbens.

This reward cascade is the basis of every action you take, and is responsible for motivation and learning. At the most basic level, this neurochemical circuit underlies the "drive to survive" in humans and other living creatures. Thus, dopamine is the main chemical behind virtually everything you do, from getting up out of bed in the morning to eating, to sex. If you remove the dopamine circuit or suppress its function, everything from fruit flies to mice to human beings is reduced to a lazy, listless existence, generally hunkering down in a corner without the will to pursue any behavior whatsoever.

Genetic variations called *polymorphisms* can alter protein production, in some cases underproducing receptors in the reward cascade. As we've seen, a lack of D2 receptors in particular results in a predisposition for addictions – there is a lack of receptors with which dopamine can bind, and the predisposed person has higher natural stress. But receptor-producing genes for *every* neurochemical in the reward cascade have to be properly encoded for the process to function properly. Genetic anomalies in any step of the process can result in inefficient function, and reward deficiency syndrome can result. It's extremely common, it's estimated about a third of Americans have the condition.

Genetic defects can lead to deficiencies and imbalances in neurotransmitters, an excess or underproduction of the enzymes that "mop them up" or of the receptors to which they bind. Such a deficiency or imbalance can alter the reward cascade, resulting in disturbing emotions or cravings for substances which mask or relieve such disturbing emotions.

The Artificial Rush

Stimulants, opiates, nicotine and alcohol all hijack your VTA-NA mesolimbic dopamine pathway through various chemical pathways. In other words, for addicts, drugs have taken over control of the brain's chemical reward system which underlies all motivation. Drugs like cocaine, heroin, amphetamines and nicotine trigger the same dopamine release as natural pleasures like food and sex, but in concentrated spikes of up to 200 to 1000 percent. While each drug uses a different chemical mechanism, the result is the same: increased dopamine in synapses of the mesolimbic pathway.

Regardless of how they are administered, the active ingredients from "recreational drugs" like alcohol, nicotine, cocaine, heroin, amphetamines and marijuana are sent to your brain via your bloodstream, and the more quickly the drug affects your brain, the stronger the association between the action (administering the drug) and the result (dopamine surge), and thus the greater its potential for addiction.

The dopamine "hit" from nicotine and crack cocaine is almost instantaneous, making the brain's link between the behavior and the pleasurable feelings stronger than normal, and the risk of addiction significantly higher. This is thought to be why these two drugs in particular are so quickly habit-forming, and difficult to stop using. Heroin, cocaine and methamphetamine addicts often say nicotine is the hardest drug of all to quit.

Feeling No Pain

Endogenous opiates – endorphins – bind to opioid receptors throughout your body, inhibiting transmission of:

- pain-signaling substance P – producing analgesia

- catecholamines such as epinephrine and norepinephrine – reducing anxiety

- GABA – disinhibiting (allowing) dopamine release and causing euphoria, a feeling of blissful joy.

The VTA seems to be where endogenous and *exogenous* (created outside the body) opiates, such as heroin and morphine, activate dopamine release. What this means is that addicts don't crave specifically amphetamines, cocaine, heroin or nicotine, they crave unnaturally massive amounts of dopamine produced by the drugs.

90

Drugs alter interneural transmission at the synapses, the control point of neural communication, targeting either the postsynaptic receptors (like nicotine and marijuana) or presynaptic reuptake mechanisms (like cocaine). By altering synapses, drugs change your brain's functions, and can profoundly alter your behavior, mood, cognition, memory, judgment, learning, movement and sensory perception. These effects can be beneficial – when treating disease – or detrimental – when drugs are abused.

Once dopamine binds to appropriate receptors, triggering an impulse, it either gets reabsorbed into the presynaptic terminals from which it was released, or it's broken down by an enzyme. Addictive drugs affect dopamine in the synapse in different ways: amphetamines stimulate the production of higher levels of dopamine, cocaine prevents dopamine re-absorption back into the presynaptic cells which produced it; and alcohol, heroin and nicotine trigger a series of neurochemical activities which result in higher synaptic dopamine levels.

Cocaine In Your Synapses

By mimicking natural neurotransmitters, drugs like cocaine disrupt the system. Cocaine blocks molecules which reuptake dopamine, noradrenaline and serotonin. An increase in the three neurotransmitters results in increased euphoria (dopamine), confidence (serotonin) and energy (noradrenaline). To produce a "high", cocaine needs to occupy just under half of these sites, although the preferred results for addicts occur when 60% – 80% of the reuptake sites are blocked, preventing reabsorption of dopamine and allowing it to remain in circulation within the synapses.

This makes the pleasurable effects outlast natural behavioral rewards. The pleasurable effects of addictive substances can be much stronger and longer lasting in your brain, compelling you to repeat the behavior and ignore less stimulating, normal behaviours, forgetting to eat, groom, neglecting social relationships and virtually everything that matters in a non-addict's life.

Drugs like cocaine create associations when paired with environmental stimuli, which serve as "cues" to trigger craving. You become *conditioned* by subconsciously linking environments, situations and people with addictive substances, so whenever you encounter the same environments, situations and people, you're overwhelmed by the desire to start using again. It's the same principles of *operant conditioning* at work with Pavlov's dogs (see book I), below the level of your conscious thought or control.

The Trap Is Sprung

Nora Volkow is one of the world's foremost authorities on addiction, and has led the field of research, using PET scans on the brains of alcoholics, cocaine addicts and smokers. Volkow's studies in the 1980s showed a consistent pattern of reduced dopamine receptors in patients addicted to cocaine, primarily in the striatum of the basal ganglia.

The mesolimbic pathway responds to salient stimuli – noteworthy things in your environment that are pleasurable, surprising, novel, off-putting, or otherwise worth paying attention to. In other words, says Dr. Volkow, dopamine shouts, "pay attention to this—it's important! Dopamine signals salience."

The point at which rewards from normal behavior lose their ability to direct your behavior – called *motivational toxicity* – is when addictive drugs like cocaine and heroin rapidly begin to seize control of your life. Things that normally motivate you lose their attraction, as drug addiction makes you neglect formerly potent rewards such as your job, friends, family and sex, and you focus more and more upon obtaining and using your drug of choice. Motivational toxicity is thus the point at which salience shifts from mundane pleasures of food, sex and companionship onto the drug of choice. Your brain has learned it can get a massive dopamine surge with which everyday pleasures simply cannot compete.

When neurons are exposed to a neurotransmitter for an extended period, they gradually lose sensitivity, the ability to respond with their original intensity. This is *habituation*, the result of the cell producing fewer receptors for that specific neurotransmitter. Your brain has reacted to the massive flood of dopamine by protecting itself from dangerous overstimulation, a form of neuroadaptation called *downregulating*, killing off dopamine receptors, thus reducing the number of sites onto which dopamine can bind. The end result is that your neurons no longer efficiently receive and transmit dopamine when you're not using.

So when you take a drug (like cocaine) which acts as a neuromodulator, it causes abnormally excessive neurotransmitter levels to remain in your synapses for extended periods. This initially creates a pleasurable "rush", but leads to a reduction in receptors; to protect themselves from dying due to overstimulation, your neurons begin to reduce dopamine receptors. The next time, you need a larger dose to feel the same euphoric effects as the first time. With repeated use, your nervous system builds up a "tolerance" – and progressively stronger amounts are required to receive the same high.

Over time, the decline in your dopamine sensitivity leads to *dysphoria* – unpleasant sensations, irritableness, poor mental function, a loss of motivation and an inability to feel pleasure, even to the point of complete apathy. Antisocial behavior and depression often result. To relieve the symptoms, you use again.

Via this destructive cycle, eventually all life's pleasures – from food to the company of friends and loved ones – become dulled. Your brain gradually becomes desensitized to everything good in life, and, apart from the ever-diminishing pleasure of taking your chosen drug, all of life becomes a grey, pointless, meaningless passage of time. At this point, you come to need the drug just to feel "normal" again. It's a downward spiral, in which the shift in salience – meaningfulness – narrows your world until nothing matters but the drug you crave.

How To Get Hooked In Eight Easy Steps

1. You encounter a pleasurable experience. It triggers your VTA, and dopamine is released into your nucleus accumbens.

2. This signals your amygdala, which marks the stimulus as highly salient and your hippocampus creates a strong memory.

3. By continuing to seek that pleasure, your brain rewires its neural pathways, strengthening the memory of the pleasure.

4. When angry, bored, in pain, lonely, stressed or tired, your limbic system prompts a search for memories of strategies to restore positive feelings (neurochemical homeostasis).

5. In time, the limbic system raises the salience (importance) of the addictive behavior to the level of a survival behavior. Because it's closely tied to your autonomic nervous system, which controls such deep-level functions as breathing, heartbeat and more, your addiction has tremendous hold over your physical state.

6. To escape stress or other negative feelings, you indulge

7. Over time, neural impulse control systems in the PFC and elsewhere degrade, reducing your ability to resist your addiction.

8. Dopamine transmission to your nucleus accumbens decreases, and your pituitary releases the stress hormone CRF, targeting the amygdala, causing anxiety, irritability, and other withdrawal symptoms, and increasing the synaptic strength of special inhibitory circuits. This triggers unpleasant sensations of withdrawal. For some addictions, withdrawal can lead to fatal biological shock and shutdown.

But addiction is a "double whammy": first your brain's reward system – driven by the feel-good neurotransmitter dopamine – craves ever more of an addictive drug, while at the same time the prefrontal cortex regions responsible for resisting temptation (inhibitory control) suffer crippling incapacitation.

An additional effect of addiction is altered levels of glutamate, the primary neurotransmitter responsible for the formation of memory traces – learning. When glutamate levels are altered through drug abuse, your hypothalamus attempts to re-establish chemical homeostasis, with the potential for severe damage to cognitive function. In the brains of recovering cocaine addicts, researchers have also discovered a significant impairment in the ability to process glucose, the brain's main energy source. This impairment lasts up to three and a half months after withdrawal, and is strongest in the PFC, the region responsible for controlling impulses and suppressing inappropriate behavior.

And just as strokes and injuries in the PFC destroy the mental network allowing people to gauge and suppress inappropriate behaviours, addictions can lead to inappropriate acts, according to Dr. Antonio Damasio. Dopamine supplied to your frontal cortex normally allows you to control the impulses, emotions and reactions of your primitive subcortical brain; but in addicts, at the same time the PFC becomes gradually less effective at control of these subcortical regions, the compulsion-triggering subcortical neural pathways are being used more frequently and strengthening. Your ability and likelihood of resorting to impulsive, emotional, instinctive desires strengthens, while your powers of self-control, logic, reason and empathy, and such moral considerations as justice and fairness progressively weaken.

Thus, as excessive dopamine release alters your PFC, it also alters not just your control over your addiction, but also other aspects of your personality such as your judgment, morality, willpower, foresight, learning capacity, ability to recognize cause and effect, what you care about, and your general temperament.

In this manner, addictions don't just take deep root, they fundamentally change who you are. You become a different person. Overstimulating dopamine receptors in your PFC impedes neurotransmission. The end result is a loss of self-control, focus, concentration, reasoning and working memory function. You feel muddled, confused, weakened, tired, drained, unmotivated and unable to function.

The insidious trap has been sprung – you begin to find the drug has become necessary just for you to feel functionally normal. This is the point at which you've become addicted. At this point, your sensitivity to all but the largest of dopamine hits has declined. This severely disrupts the motivational system of everyday life. All the things that once gave you pleasure seem dull, drab, and grey, and you feel worse and worse without chasing the ever-diminishing dopamine rush your addiction provides.

The Highway To Hell

In recent studies of laboratory animals addicted to amphetamines, switching off the insula shuts off drug cravings, and re-activating it restarts the cravings. In humans, the insula, the body's inner "discomfort reporter", informs the prefrontal cortex of homeostatic needs, relaying sensations of physical and emotional discomfort such as pain and cravings. When the insula reports you need a fix, it triggers anxiety and irritation.

At this point, your brain and body switch from a state of tolerance to one of dependency. You no longer seek out the drug to feel pleasure; at this point it's needed to keep you from entering *withdrawal* – severe mental and physical distress, including seizures, nausea, chills and a flu-like state, chattering teeth, irritability, diarrhea and hypersensitivity. Abrupt withdrawal from severe alcohol addiction can even lead to death.

By this point, the need to find your next fix becomes the only thing that matters, no matter how destructive that quest has become. Choice, self-control and anything that once mattered to you have all vanished – the drug has become your entire world.

Habit Is Destiny

The central theme throughout this book is that repeated behavior strengthens neural circuits that encode the behavior and its reward, so the pattern becomes much easier and more natural to repeat: habit is destiny. But in the case of addictions, it's not merely a matter of neural reinforcement, but also of irreversible destruction. Your cerebral cortex is responsible for inhibitory control – your conscious ability to master your emotions, thoughts and behaviours. Such abilities weaken as addiction progresses; in essence, the primitive animal regions of the brain hold sway over the minds of addicts, and controlling their impulses becomes increasingly harder to do.

Compounding the problem is that most drug abusers have multiple addictions – to nicotine, alcohol, cocaine and more, in many cases. Depending upon the drug, sudden physical withdrawal can causes severe painful physical effects, such as seizures, vomiting, diarrhea, chills, severe anxiety and other problems. Aside from these physical side effects, one of the reasons it's so difficult to stop abusing addictive substances is that so much of the brain is modulated by dopamine pathways – the hypothalamus, amygdala, thalamus and prefrontal cortex.

Dopamine itself acts like a valve – a primary modulator of information flow throughout the entire brain, directly affecting mood, memory, decision making, perception and logical thought, among other brain functions. It also allows prefrontal control of the limbic system, and as you've seen, the limbic system controls autonomic functions throughout the body and is critical to memory formation and learning in general.

In addition to the VTA, the substantia nigra releases dopamine into your striatum, an area critical to social behaviours, error correcting, motor control and learning in general. In fact, there are eight dopaminergic pathways in your brain, circulating dopamine throughout your CNS. Dopamine's effects are all-powerful.

Your Brain's Weak Link:
Permanent Destruction Of Control Centers

The mesolimbic circuit, your *Go circuit,* can be inhibited by your PFC, but the link inhibiting both dopamine-releasing VTA neurons and serotonin releasing raphe nucleus neurons is a very frail one: in 1992, UCLA neuroscientist Dr. Gaylord Ellison discovered this vulnerability in a twin bundle of axons only a few hundred thick called the *fasciculus retroflexus* (FR). Your FR relays vital control signals between your frontal lobes, midbrain and brain stem, but it's thin and highly sensitive.

These axons run from the *habenula* (a tiny neural cluster between your pineal gland and the rear of your thalamus), to dopaminergic cells in your VTA, which governs motivation and reward-based learning; your substantia nigra, which, if you recall, governs initiation and cessation of movement; and your brainstem's raphe nuclei, the source of your brain's serotonin, used to control arousal states and mediate neurotransmission throughout your CNS.

The *lateral* (outer edge of the) habenula inhibits VTA dopamine release, and it's believed the organ sends messages indicating "negative rewards" in this way. Recent studies also link the region to helping control arousal states and chronic stress responses. In other words, it's a tiny organ, but with a huge influence.

Your habenula has the ability to inhibit dopamine and serotonin output, and is therefore involved in all your behavior, playing a central role in learning, memory, and attention. Since dopamine and serotonin are the two primary neuromodulators controlling neurotransmission, your prefrontal cortex uses this function to inhibit unwanted behaviors. If you think of the nucleus accumbens as your brain's behavioral "go switch", the prefrontal cortex is its "stop switch", and the Fasciculus Retroflexus is the neural path down which these stop signals travel. This allows your judgment center to control your cravings, impulses and drives. Damage to this slender neural pathway results in compulsive behaviors and addiction.

The bundle of nerves called the fasciculus retroflexus connects your cortex – your thought and decision centers – to your midbrain – where impulses and cravings originate. The pathway affects emotional control, sexual arousal, and REM sleep. When these neurons function properly, you're able to control your urges, cravings, temper and impulses, but when they're not, your cravings and impulses control you.

These very slender nerve bundles (only a few hundred cells thick) are extremely sensitive to dopamine. After high exposure to dopamine from addictive drugs like nicotine, cocaine, methamphetamine, etc., they die. Says UCLA neuroscientist Dr. Gaylord Ellison, the fasciculus retroflexus is the brain's "weak link for stimulant addictive drugs. This tract is affected more by chronic drug use than any other tract in the brain."

In over two decades of study, Dr. Ellison's team has demonstrated how addictive drugs like amphetamines, cocaine and ecstasy damage one half of the fasciculus retroflexus. In 2000, the team discovered that nicotine damages the other half. The effects are rapid – after administering high doses of nicotine to rats for just five days, the pathway was almost completely destroyed. And the larger the dosage, the greater the damage to the region.

For those genetically more sensitive to dopamine, the pathway's destruction can occur quite quickly – after a short time or even a single major binge. In this way, the control circuitry of the brain loses its power over the motivation system, and control from the cortex is effectively shut down – permanently.

> For some drugs, such as cocaine, this is virtually the only degeneration induced in the brain. Continuous nicotine also selectively induces degeneration in the FR, but in the other half of the tract.... the finding that these descending control pathways are compromised following simulated drug binges has implications for theories of drug addiction but also psychosis in general.

97

The Most Dangerous Drug In The World

Alcohol erodes these same FR control-signal axons, but at a comparatively slower pace – it's estimated that alcohol takes several months to a year or more to destroy the FR to the point where self-control is obliterated. But cocaine can accomplish the job in a few short weeks, and methamphetamine, which *National Geographic* calls "the most dangerous drug in the world", can destroy this vital self-control link after a single night, resulting in addiction – and the addict never even feels the change.

Meth travels through the bloodstream to the nucleus accumbens, the primary receptive center for dopamine, the "chemical key to human pleasure". Methamphetamine forces an unnaturally large dopamine release. One hit can trigger the release of 1200 units of dopamine, a "rush" of pleasure three and a half times that triggered by cocaine, and about six times the human body's natural amount. A meth high can also last up to 12 hours; much longer effects than those provided by other drugs.

Most people have heard of tolerance, where ever higher doses are necessary to achieve a buzz, so it's easy to assume this must be true of all addictions. But in the early stages of meth addiction, *sensitization* occurs, the opposite of tolerance, and the CNS becomes more sensitive to methamphetamine; so that each dose produces a stronger effect than before.

Because each high seems better than before, and requires less meth to experience, so you'll likely assume you're not addicted. Early on, after you come down, you'll feel a little blue, a mild depression which is far less intense than an alcohol hangover. But the more you use, the worse the crashes will get, the longer they'll last and the worse you'll feel. Eventually, these horrible episodes will own you.

You'll soon find you've begun using meth regularly, and have a compulsion – intense desires and behavior you can no longer control. You've already gotten hooked, and never even saw it coming. What's worse is you won't be able to stop without help, no matter how strong you may believe yourself to be.

Statistically, after you first try meth, there is a 75% chance you'll take it again in a week, a 90% chance you'll take it again within a month, and a 98% chance you'll take it again within a year. Very soon however, you'll start to realize your "choice" to take it has become an illusion. It's no longer a desire you can control. You've long since killed the cells which once allowed you to suppress and control that desire.

You can never regain these dead brain cells – they don't regenerate. The best you can hope for is that, after one or two years without using, your brain will slowly remold itself to compensate. But drug rehabilitation, just like rehabilitation from a stroke or major head injury, is hard work.

After a period of a year or two, if you can manage to refrain from taking the drug to which you've become addicted, your brain may slowly begin to reroute normal functions to alternative pathways, generating some semblance of your former powers of self-control.

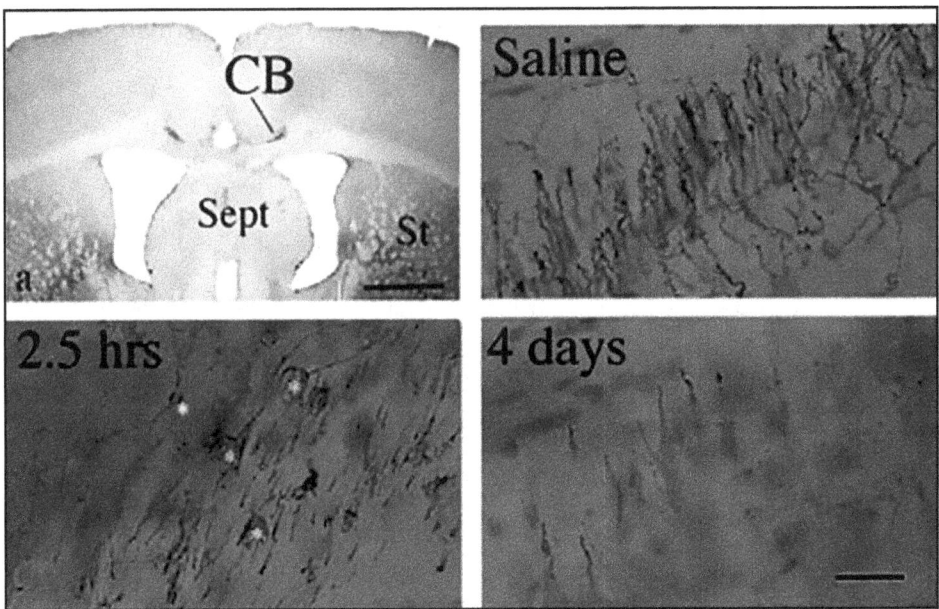

A Micrograph of a rat's fasciculus retroflexus cells. The slide reading saline shows approximately 125 healthy cells. 2.5 hours after a single administration of methamphetamine, these cells swell, rupture and die. Within four days of this single methamphetamine dose, only about 6 cells remain. Source: Mothers Against Methamphetamine, Dr. Mary Holly, 2010. Used with permission.

The Anti-Reward Pathway

Your FR bundle projects out from the tiny structure on your thalamus called the habenula. The habenula (Latin for *reins*) is a group of neurons at the stalk of your pineal gland. It receives input directly from your frontal cortex and preoptic area, as well as your basal ganglia and extensive regions of your limbic system. It strongly inhibits several midbrain areas involved in releasing neuromodulators like dopamine, norepinephrine, and serotonin, including the VTA, SN and raphe nuclei.

In this way, your habenula is centrally involved in the reward pathways, and in pain processing, sexual behavior, nutrition, sleep-wake cycles, stress responses, and learning. fMRI scans have closely linked the region with *negative feedback* – encoding negative rewards. It's thought this negative reward processor works hand-in-hand with the positive reward system in your basal ganglia, using dopamine and serotonin to signal errors in reward-prediction.

Several dopamine-boosting addictive drugs have neurotoxic effects which destroy the fragile fasciculus retroflexus axons, connecting the habenula to targets of its control – midbrain cells in the SN, VTA, and raphe nuclei.

Destruction of these FR neurons is linked to impaired motor control, emotional, social, and cognitive functions, cortical control of which appear to be supported by the habenula. Dysfunctions of the habenula have also been linked to schizophrenia, psychosis and depression.

In laboratory animals, depression markedly increases the habenula's consumption of glucose, more than in any other brain region. And as depression worsens, hyperactivation of the habenula and the serotonin-producing raphe nuclei rapidly depletes the brain of tryptophan – the precursor of the mood-stabilizer serotonin.

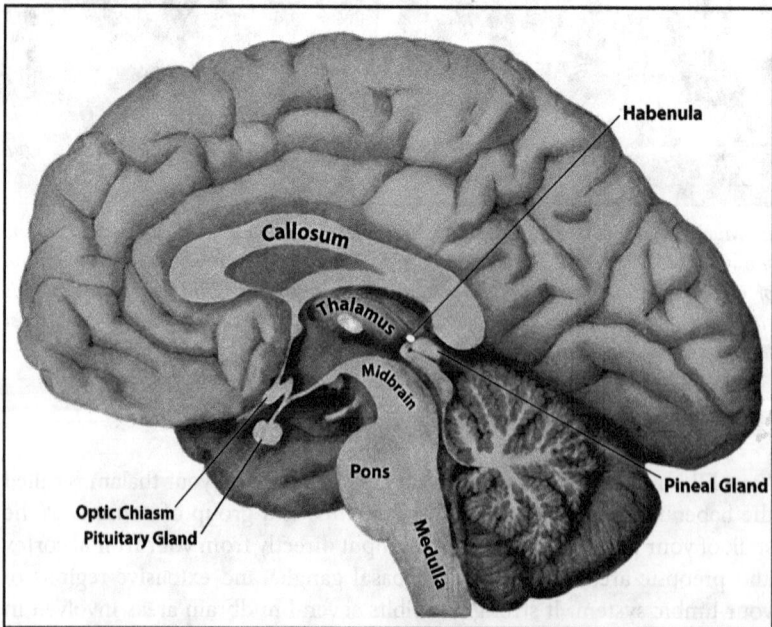

Habenula and Midbrain. Adapted from Gray's Anatomy, public domain

Input from most of your limbic system, preoptic area, dopamine from your VTA, norepinephrine from your locus coeruleus, serotonin from your raphe nuclei and direct projections from your cerebral cortex run through the slender FR bundle. Your *outer* (lateral) habenula strongly inhibits dopamine production from the VTA and SN, and serotonin from the raphe nuclei, as well as regions of the hypothalamus.

Your *central* (medial) habenula outputs transmits acetylcholine and substance P to your brain stem and pineal gland. This central habenula region seems to participate in endocrine stress responses, helping regulate salt and water balance by coregulating the adrenal cortex and inhibiting the thyroid gland. Stressors such as defeat, courtship or involuntary restraint increase medial habenula activity, resulting in a strong increase in immune cell release, possibly one source of stress-induced inflammation.

The habenula is *well-conserved* in all vertebrates (it's existed throughout millions of years of evolution across a wide range of species), so it almost certainly performs vital functions, although these functions are only just beginning to be understood. Among its apparent functions are:

1) Negative reward signals – In experiments, habenula neurons are *excited* by signs of no reward, and *inhibited* by signs of a reward – the opposite pattern from dopamine neurons in the mesolimbic reward pathway. Thus, neurons in the lateral habenula are *reward-negative* – activated by unpleasant events such as punishment or the absence of a reward, especially when the unpleasant event was not predicted. This reward information is fed to the habenula by the striatum.

Reward prediction error signals are used for training – guiding motor behavior to maximize rewards. These signals also encode unexpected and novel events to help guide motor behavior. When volunteers perform motion predicting tasks, negative feedback from the insula and elsewhere activates the ACC, insula, and habenula, and memory traces are formed which encode the error.

The region also strongly inhibits VTA and SN dopamine neurons, thus suppressing motor responses to stimuli which don't hold rewards: dopaminergic neurons are believed to modulate cortical feedback to the striatum, so when the habenula inhibits dopaminergic activity, it may suppress body movements when no reward is expected. The basal ganglia, if you recall, control body movements through direct connections to the brain stem motor networks, or through indirect connections to the motor cortices via the thalamus.

2) Influence of behaviours related to aversive stimuli (pain, stress and anxiety) – The lateral habenula appears to be involved in behaviours linked to negative emotions, particularly sensitivity to pain and anxiety, and in conditioned avoidance to aversive stimulation like electrical shocks.

3) Inhibitory control of dopamine release – A major inhibitory target of the lateral habenula is the dopamine-rich midbrain – the VTA and SN via GABAergic interneurons. This region is itself also under dopaminergic control, receiving looping input back from the VTA. This means the habenula plays a possibly central role in the midbrain circuits which govern learning and controlling body movements.

4) Circadian influence of behavior – Circadian rhythms (sleep-wake and metabolic cycles), controlled mainly by the *suprachiasmatic nucleus* of the hypothalamus, may also be partly governed by the habenula; the habenula is closely connected to your pineal gland, which excretes melatonin to trigger sleep, and it appears to regulate activity patterns according to a circadian timetable set by the suprachiasmatic nucleus, which is photosensitive, responding to natural changes in light.

5) Inhibitory movement control – Injury of the habenula in rats increases exploratory behavior, heightening responses to novelty and environmental stimuli.

6) Maternal and female sexual instincts – The region appears to participate in maternal behaviours, as well as female sexual behaviours such as *lordosis* – arching upward of the rump to present the pelvis for mounting.

7) Social and Emotional Influence – Social and emotional behaviours are thought to be mediated by serotonin from the raphe nuclei, one of the main targets of the lateral habenula. This connection is thought to suppress serotonergic release to the basal ganglia (serotonin here helping regulate movement and behavior response choices).

8) Cognitive functions – Involved in spatial cognition (navigating through mazes), as well as motor task control through dopamine suppression, and influencing the memory-forming hippocampus through multiple pathways.

Consequences

Addicts chase their addictions even knowing full well how destructive their habits are. The pattern is the same for any kind of addiction, from shooting heroin to gorging on unhealthy food. So while it's easy to make resolutions to quit, the hardest part is overcoming major physical changes which have fundamentally rewired your brain.

The cumulative, heartbreaking effect of addiction – as anyone knows who has a family member or friend who's fallen victim to the downward spiral – is always destructive. Eventually, the addict's brain has been so radically altered it instinctively "needs the drug to survive", and every other consideration is sacrificed in the pursuit of getting another fix. Marriages, jobs, personal possessions – none of it matters in the feverish pursuit for the next fix. Addicts under the spell of heroin or cocaine will quite literally sell their own children for another fix. In other words, addictions can persist despite someone's strength of character and in spite of their good intentions. The endless pursuit of the next fix holds greater sway over the nervous and endocrine systems of an addict than even essential needs such as food, water and the need for human attachments.

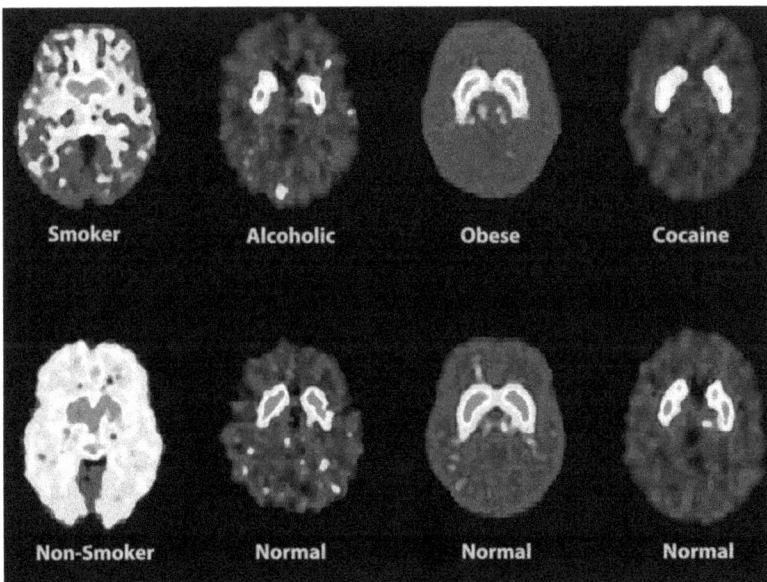

Repeated drug exposure changes brain function. Positron emission tomography (PET) scans show dopamine activity for addicts (top row) vs. non-addicts (bottom row). Regions of greatest dopamine receptor activity are indicated with a color scale starting from red (most active), descending through yellow and green to blue and purple (least active). Note the extreme lack of dopamine activity in the top row images. National Institutes of Health 2006, public domain.

Teenagers At Risk

Adolescents in particular are particularly vulnerable to addictions. Because the PFC doesn't fully mature until about 20 years, impulse control hasn't yet developed in teens, and drug effects last longer than in adults. Additionally, the mental associations between drugs and cues appear to be stronger among adolescents, who assign greater salience to drug-linked cues than do adults.

Dopamine D1 receptors are thought to play a role in this increased salience attribution – adolescents have elevated D1 expression compared with juveniles and adults, suggesting that D1 receptor expression may create a window of vulnerability to drug addictions during adolescence.

A Rogue's Gallery: The Most Addictive Drugs

Vicodin – Not every abused drug is bought from a street-corner pusher, as recovering oxytocin addict and right wing demagogue Rush Limbaugh can attest. Vicodin is one of the most commonly abused prescription drugs, preferred because of it's active ingredient, the narcotic *hydrocodone*.

Hydrocodone binds to opioid receptors, but its effects are much weaker than those of morphine. However, vicodin addiction can develop within a week, and has been a challenge for pop stars Courtney Love and Eminem, and actor Matthew Perry. Overdosing is easy, and often kills.

Cocaine – This a stimulant purified by German chemists in the mid-1800s from a shrub native to the Andes area of South America, which natives have chewed for some 2,000 years when they wanted an energy boost. Many physicians initially considered cocaine a miracle drug, prescribing it for all sorts of physical and mental ailments; it was even added to soft drinks. Today US law forbids the importation, manufacture, and use of cocaine for nonmedical purposes, and medical use is highly restricted.

Cocaine acts by binding to reuptake transporters in the synapses, blocking natural reabsorption of dopamine, serotonin and norepinephrine, resulting in high levels of the three neurotransmitters, which remain circulating in the synapses.

Alcohol and tranquillizers – both drugs slow neural activity by triggering inhibitory GABA release. When animals consume alcohol, it produces two *psychoactive* (brain altering) substances called *THP* (tetrahydropapaveroline) and *TIQ* (tetrahydroisoquinoline salsolinol). These substances are also derived from opium poppies, the source of heroin and morphine. Stress can motivate drinking if someone naturally lacks production or activation of endorphins, the body's natural opioids. So when alcoholics feel stressed, they want to drink, because it triggers their underactive opioid receptors.

Heroin and morphine – These synthetic opioids bind to VTA receptors which normally respond to the body's endorphins, triggering dopamine release in the mesolimbic reward pathway. Opioids also block pain signals transmitted by substance P from the body through the spinal cord, and deactivate the anterior cingulate cortex (ACC), which concentrates attention upon unpleasant (aversive) inner stimuli. These twin effects dull pain.

Withdrawal from opioids, however, is associated with a sharp rise in stress hormones, which act upon the hypothalamus to trigger cravings, and withdrawal can be excruciatingly painful, lasting about a week after stopping. Sudden heroin withdrawal can even be fatal, if an addict is in extremely poor health, but heroin withdrawal isn't as directly dangerous as alcohol withdrawal. The much more prevalent dangers are from overdosing – street purity is unpredictable – and from contracting highly infectious diseases such as AIDS, hepatitis and other blood-borne viruses.

Tobacco – According to the World Health Organization, tobacco use kills over five million people worldwide every year. Why anyone would inhale toxic fumes to the point at which it destroyed their health may seem perplexing to a nonsmoker. But heroin and cocaine addicts often remark that the toughest addiction to overcome is nicotine addiction. I can believe it; I started at age 11 and smoked over a pack and a half every day for 16 years, even as I saw lung cancer and emphysema kill both my grandparents and my great-aunt. A combination of running and the patch enabled me to finally overcome my own deadly addiction.

Nicotine imitates acetylcholine in your brain, binding to *cholinergic* receptors, giving a surge of focus and artificial energy, and triggering a dopamine release in the mesolimbic pathway. It also indirectly results in the release of glutamate and endorphins. This powerful, combined chemical rush of euphoria and alertness is something you're soon compelled to repeat throughout the day.

Acetylcholine is normally used by your brain to trigger muscle contraction, but it also helps control your energy levels, heart rate and breathing, and helps regulate neurotransmission throughout your brain and nervous system. It's also at the center of memory formation.

Nicotine mimics acetylcholine, binding to its receptors and simultaneously triggering a burst of receptor activity throughout several brain regions. This stimulation:

- heightens attention and sharpens focus and timing, the energizing and focus boost that smokers experience

- triggers dopamine release in the mesolimbic reward pathways, giving pleasurable, calm, happy feelings that reinforce the habit

- triggers the release of glutamate, central to forming the neural connections that make up memories. In this case, neural reinforcement builds up memories of the pleasures from inhaling cigarette smoke and further drive the addiction.

- increases endorphins, the neurotransmitters that act as your body's natural pain blockers (morphine and heroin hijack the effects of endorphins). This artificially creates the "endorphin rush" of pleasure that long-distance runners often experience.

The Gene Which Hooks You AND Makes You Susceptible To Cancer – Your vulnerability to nicotine addiction seems to be largely based upon genetics. Your habenula plays a key role in the process, according to Dr. Inés Ibañez-Tallon of Germany's Max Delbrück Center for Molecular Medicine (MDC). Interestingly, studies showed that variations in a single gene cluster control risk factors for both nicotine dependence and for lung cancer. Her team, in cooperation with researchers from the Pasteur Institute in Paris, France and the Russian Academy of Sciences in Moscow, has illuminated the process at work in generating this addiction.

A receptor for the neurotransmitter acetylcholine, activated by nicotine in smokers, is encoded by three genes in a cluster. This gene cluster is in the DNA of every cell in your body, but the receptor is only actually expressed in a few restricted brain regions, such as the habenula. One of the three genes in this cluster is alpha5. A single mutation in this gene – present in a majority of smokers – makes them both more vulnerable to nicotine addiction and to developing lung cancer.

Hooked After Your First

A 2007 study published in the Archives of Pediatric and Adolescent Medicine says that 10 percent of adolescents become addicted within two days of first smoking, and 25 percent get addicted within a month. Researchers observed 1,246 sixth-grade students over a period of four years in six Massachusetts communities. Half of the addicted students reported strong withdrawal symptoms after smoking just seven cigarettes a month.

According to Dr. Joseph R. DiFranza, of the University of Massachusetts Medical School and leader of the research team, "Nobody expects to get addicted from smoking one cigarette", however, "…experiments confirm that nicotine alters the structure and function of the brain within a day of the very first dose. In humans, nicotine-induced alterations in the brain can trigger addiction with the first cigarette." He says these changes to the brain are permanent, remaining decades after a smoker has quit; this explains why a single cigarette can trigger immediate relapse in ex-smokers.

Nicotine addiction can emerge when adolescents smoke just a single cigarette per month. Initially, only one cigarette is needed to relieve the craving of nicotine withdrawal for weeks, but as nicotine tolerance builds, smokers find they have to smoke increasingly more to suppress withdrawal. The cravings are so powerful that some smokers try unsuccessfully to quit smoking their entire lives.

In addition to the young, 2008 research at the University of Western Ontario has shown that some people are extremely vulnerable to nicotine addiction in particular, and can even become hooked after only smoking a single cigarette. Dr. Steven Laviolette of the Schulich School of Medicine & Dentistry says there are two types of initial reactions to nicotine: most find their first cigarette to be extremely unpleasant, but some find it immediately highly rewarding, and they quickly develop a dependency.

Individual susceptibility to addiction appears to depend chiefly upon genetics rather than personal willpower; dopamine receptors control the brain's initial sensitivity to nicotine's rewarding and addictive properties. But Dr. Laviolette and his team were able to successfully manipulate these receptors to control whether nicotine is processed as rewarding or aversive. Dopaminergic receptors D1 and D2 in the nucleus accumbens "switch" how the mesolimbic system processes the first exposure to nicotine – determining whether the first exposure feels good or bad, and regulating individual sensitivity to these reactions.

As addiction progresses, these dopaminergic receptors trigger feelings of pleasure when the brain receives nicotine, and unpleasant feelings of anxiety when the brain is deprived of nicotine, usually within 30 to 50 minutes. Your sensitivity to these twin motivations for continued nicotine is controlled by your DA receptors. How you react the first time you try smoking is also linked to variations in the *CHRNA5 gene*, which encodes special (*"nicotinic"*) acetylcholine receptors that also respond to nicotine.

Butt Out!

Emphysema from lifelong smoking killed my aunt, grandfather and grandmother, which is one of the reasons I chose to quit after almost two decades of smoking a pack and a half a day. I'm lucky: smoking is now the number one preventable cause of death. Worldwide, smoking kills one in 10 (four million) adults every year through heart disease, strokes, lung disease or cancer of the lungs, larynx, esophagus, mouth, bladder, cervix, pancreas, and kidneys. Currently nearly one in five U.S. adults smokes. Globally, it's one in three adults.

It's estimated that 440,000 Americans a year die from smoking – more than from AIDS, car accidents, drug and alcohol abuse, suicides and murders combined. The National Institutes of Health estimates that as many as 6.4 million children who are living today will die prematurely as adults because they began to smoke cigarettes during adolescence.

Nicotine, the major addictive substance in tobacco, has only one known practical use – as an insecticide. And in addition to the poisonous gases carbon monoxide and nitrogen oxide, cigarette smoke contains "tar", a chemical compound with more than 4,000 toxic and 60 carcinogenic chemicals, among the worst of which are:

- Cyanide (one of the world's deadliest poisons – a mining chemical that dissolves ores and metals)

- Formaldehyde (a preservative for corpses)

- Arsenic (another of the deadliest poisons known)

- Benzene (poisonous gas found in gasoline fumes which causes leukemia – blood or bone marrow cancer)

- Cadmium (major carcinogenic component in car batteries)

- Toluene (industrial cleaning solution)

- Methanol (wood alcohol)

- Butane (lighter fluid)

- Ethanol (major component of anti-freeze)

- Acetylene (welding torch fuel)

- Methanol (rocket fuel)

- Ammonia (cleaning product)

- Acetone (paint stripper)

- Polonium 210 (radioactive substance that comes from the soil the leaves are grown in)

If smoking doesn't give you cancer, a stroke, heart attack, emphysema, or chronic asthma, it's certainly going to impair your memory, concentration, cognitive function, energy levels, sleep cycles, immune system, and wound healing – and pipes, cigars and chewing tobacco are equally as dangerous.

How about brain decay? Smokers have been shown to have thinner orbito-frontal cortices, the part of the brain linked to addictions, decision-making, and controlling impulses and compulsive behaviours. This brain decay is also progressive – it grows the longer you smoke.

If brain-rot isn't enough to cure you of smoking, how about this?

The very latest studies show that chemicals in tobacco smoke called PHAs cause DNA damage that can lead to cellular mutation and cancer within only 15 minutes to half an hour after smoking a single cigarette. And once the mutation has occurred, the damage is done and it's permanent. Finally, in 2010, type-2 alkenes, the chemicals found in cigarette smoke and car exhaust, have also been found to damage brain nerve endings and are believed to be the cause of Alzheimer's disease. (As an aside, the same chemicals have been found in French fries, so you might want to rethink indulging in that fast food fix).

The truth is most people have heard similar scary stories about tobacco. So the perplexing question for nonsmokers is "Why the Hell do people insist on doing this to themselves?"

Well, according to the American Lung Association, half of American smokers try to quit every year, but less than 5 percent manage to succeed. The truth is it's very, very difficult – in fact, heroin users and other drug addicts say tobacco is by far the hardest drug to quit. So what's going on internally to compel someone to want to continue doing this to himself?

When a smoker lights up, nicotine causes an adrenaline release that speeds up the heart rate, giving a feeling of alertness. This is followed by a release of dopamine, along with several other feel-good chemicals called endogenous opioids that heighten pleasurable feelings and dull negative ones. This causes feelings of relaxation and comfort. Neurons in the brain (and other parts of the body) sprout additional receptors, which multiply with prolonged use, so that every time a smoker gets a hit of nicotine, she receives a dopamine release and feels pleasurable emotions and sensations.

So when the addict tries to quit, numerous receptors aren't being supplied the customary level of dopamine and other mood-enhancing chemicals, and the negative effects of withdrawal are felt, which include:

- irritability

- impatience

- hostility

- headaches

- anxiety

- depression

- difficulty concentrating

- restlessness

- decreased heart rate

- increased appetite

- weight gain

When I first quit, I would have episodes similar to panic attacks if I didn't have a cigarette every 20 minutes. It took me about ten attempts before I finally succeeded in quitting. But even now, nearly twenty years later, I still have minor cravings and occasionally dream of smoking. The addiction is that powerful.

The other addictive element of smoking is environmental cues, which your brain associates with the action of smoking. If you're used to smoking in the car or after dinner, these events trigger your brain to expect a dopamine release. If you're trying to quit, these are the danger spots you need to look out for. Fortunately, although cigarette smoking is an incredibly powerful drug addiction, there are a number of resources and tools to help you overcome it, among them free telephone counselling , behavioral modification therapy, hypnosis, acupuncture, and at least five types of nicotine replacement therapy including:

- nicotine patches

- nicotine gum

- nasal sprays

- inhalers

- lozenges

Although a study last year concluded that a combination of the patch and lozenges is the most effective way to stop, the patch and a running program got me over my addiction, and the "hump period" was about two weeks. If you can endure the withdrawal symptoms beyond that point, you've essentially freed yourself from the slavery of addiction. If you need help quitting, why not call the American Cancer Society for free counselling? *1-800-ACS-2345*

Your Brain On Junk Food – Eating Your Way Into A Grave

During the Society for Neuroscience's 2009 and 2010 annual meetings, a number of respected scientists presented startling and sobering findings: in addition to ruining your health and shortening your life, eating unhealthy food alters your brain chemistry and functionality in ways that make it progressively harder to stop. Fat, sugar and salt all activate mesolimbic dopamine pathways, but these pathways become progressively desensitized in rats fed a high-fat, high-calorie diet. These neurological changes mirror those of cocaine- or heroin- addicted rats. After these changes, rats become less likely to eat nutritious food, even when it's all that is available.

What's even scarier is that these neuroadaptations appear to be progressive, permanent and irreversible. Mice and rats fed sugary, fatty diets (with unlimited access to foods like bacon, sausage, cheesecake, and chocolate) showed significant destructive changes in their dopamine and opioid pathways after as little as six weeks, lowering their ability to derive pleasure from food, leading to lifelong, compulsive overeating and a lifelong preference for unhealthy foods.

Lest you're thinking these findings may not apply to humans, in 2009, Dr. Eric Stice at the Oregon Research Institute used fMRI scans to show people can also be genetically predisposed to impaired dopamine function. Genetically predisposed subjects show the greatest one-year weight gains, leading Dr. Stice to conclude that this lower level of mental rewards from eating leads them to overeat to achieve typical levels of eating pleasure.

According to Dr. Gene-Jack Wang, chairman of the US Department of Energy's Brookhaven National Laboratory medical department, when you see your favourite foods, your orbital prefrontal cortex (your decision-making center) triggers a flood of dopamine, just as if you were a cocaine addict shown a bag of white powder. But if you're obese, the pleasure you receive from eating these foods begins to dull with continued consumption: obese subjects consistently show fewer dopamine receptors in their striata than their leaner counterparts. These neuroadaptations are "virtually identical" to those found in heroin and cocaine addictions, according to the Scripps Research Institute and University of Pennsylvania.

In The Mouths Of Babes

Junk food preferences are also hereditary; a pregnant mother's diet can exert epigenetic changes which manifest in the DNA encoding the same biological systems in her children. In turn, these same children, even if they ate healthy diets, still pass the genetic traits on to their own offspring, leading to increased risk of obesity and diabetes through multiple generations. Nursing appears to be the critical window in determining infant dietary habits and future health, according to 2010 studies presented at the Society for the Study of Ingestive Behavior, which linked a high-fat diet in nursing mothers with infant obesity and pre-diabetes.

These neuroadaptations can lead to dangerous habits, including chronic food consumption beyond metabolic need. A number of hereditary gene mutations can also alter hypothalamic function, which controls appetite and energy expenditure. A 2010 Yale study found there's an additional factor making it progressively harder to reverse weight gain: obese people tend to lose sensitivity to their bodies' hunger mechanisms. In 2011, a team at the University of Texas Southwestern Medical Center also found that being overweight leads to the brain being progressively unable to receive messages of satiety (fullness).

Adipose (fat) cells release a hormone called leptin, which alerts your hypothalamus that you've eaten enough. Your hypothalamus, which regulates and balances your body's chemical, biological and temperature balances, uses leptin signals to make you feel full and stop eating. The sights or smells of your favourite foods act as cues which stimulate your hypothalamus, which controls your desires, and builds your anticipation. If you're slender, after having eaten a sufficient amount, leptin causes your hypothalamus to shut down your desire to eat, but if you're obese, this desire remains switched on.

Over time, an excess of dietary and body fat floods your bloodstream with leptin, and your hypothalamus loses its ability to recognize the presence of leptin when you've eaten enough. As a result, you'll continue to feel hungry, craving high-calorie foods like candy and pastries, and to store the excess calories as body fat – leading to an ever-increasing, spiralling loss of sensitivity and metabolic slowdown. So the next time you're about to reach for a doughnut, think twice about the long-term consequences for you and even your future generations.

Considering

Recall the food choice experiment from the previous chapter: to examine how well people's good intentions align with what they actually eat, in 2009, a group of Caltech neurobiologists took fMRI scans of the brains of dieters as they chose, weighing taste vs. healthiness among the foods. The scans focused on two areas in the prefrontal cortex believed to be key to decision-making. A number of those who had planned to eat healthily wound up choosing junk food against their better intentions, a lack of self-control the scientists were able to monitor in real-time.

Prior to the experiment, volunteers rated 50 foods on taste and health. They were then separated into two groups – those who reported they had little self-control, and those who reported high levels of it. Those who had high self-control would, it was assumed, base their food choices on taste and healthiness, whereas those with low self-control would choose based solely upon taste.

Researchers believed consciously evaluating each food item would take place in the ventromedial prefrontal cortex (vmPFC). They surmised that evaluations and choices would be modulated – the signals amplified or attenuated – by the dorsolateral prefrontal cortex (dlPFC), associated with self-control. fMRI scans supported their theory, showing that, while both groups had similar activity in the evaluative portions of their PFCs, those with greater self-control, who chose foods based upon nutritive value, showed greater dlPFC activity. Based on their findings, the researchers suggest these regions evolved to serve different purposes – the vmPFC evolved early to predict short-term rewards, and later, the DLPFC emerged to enable suppression of short-term desires in favor of long-term rewards.

Understanding these mechanisms of self-control has important implications for humanity, in finding treatments for addiction, marketing, and even determining in courts of law whether someone can be legally held responsible for a given decision. It also lends weight to the principle that you can exercise self-control and other mental capabilities like a muscle, thereby gaining mastery over your decisions and ultimate destiny.

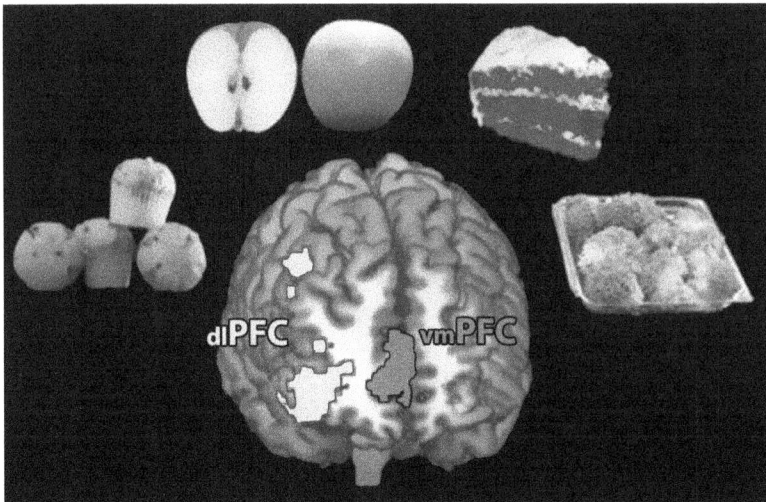

3-D projection of a transparent brain shows the regions of activation: the ventral medial prefrontal cortex (vmPFC) is in red, and the dorsolateral prefrontal cortex (DLPFC) is in yellow. Caltech, Todd Hare, 2010, used with permission

The Allure Of Gambling

Why gamble if you know the odds are against you and the house always wins in the long run? University of Cambridge researchers say it's the near-misses, where you almost hit the jackpot, that drive gambling addiction. Close calls, such as when a slot machine stops one turn away from a payoff, drives compulsive gamblers are driven to continue. These near-misses activate brain regions which normally process winning.

The 2009 study scanned 15 volunteers as they used a computerized slot machine which periodically gave 50 pence wins. These wins activated the mesolimbic pathway. But near-misses – for example, two liberty bells and a cherry – also triggered the mesolimbic pathway. A follow-up experiment outside the scanner had participants rate their experiences. While they reported they found near-misses to be unpleasant, their combined responses showed their desire to continue playing rose after such near-misses. Similar studies have demonstrated that gamblers will play at slot machines that give near-misses longer than those set up to produce no such near-misses. The team found neural responses to near-misses were centered in the striatum and insula, the same regions found to drive drug addictions. The study's authors believe insula function changes with the onset of gambling addiction.

Compulsive gamblers experience cravings and the compulsion to bet progressively larger amounts of money, a pathology which mirrors the symptoms of drug addiction. This study showed volunteers with the highest near-miss insula responses agreed most strongly with statements endorsed by compulsive gamblers, such as "Losses when gambling are bound to be followed by a series of wins". Dr. Luke Clark, who led the research, said:

> Gamblers often interpret near-misses as special events, which encourage them to continue to gamble. Our findings show that the brain responds to near-misses as if a win has been delivered, even though the result is technically a loss. On games where there is some skill involved, like target practice, it makes sense to pay attention to near-misses. However, on gambling games where the wins are random, like slot machines or roulette, near-misses do not signal your future success. Importantly, our volunteers in this study were not regular or problem gamblers, and so these findings suggest that the brain may naturally respond to near-misses in this way.

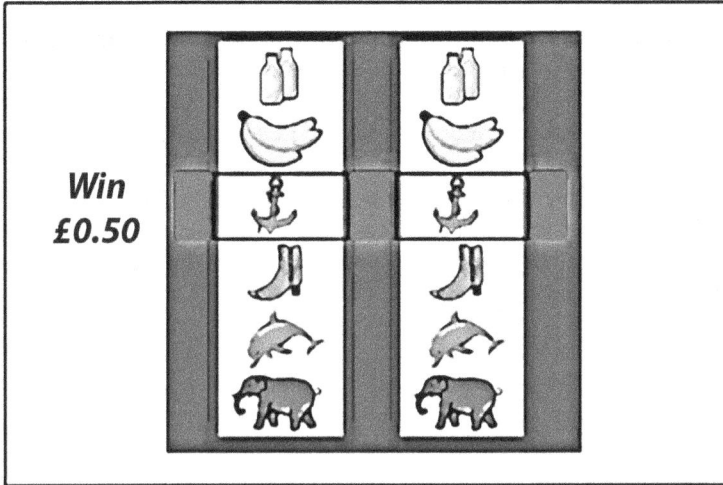

The slot machine task. Chase and Clark, 2010. Used with permission

The mesolimbic pathways of compulsive gamblers react more intensely to near misses than casual players, which is thought to be why they continue, according to a 2010 follow-up study. Dr. Clark and colleague Dr. Henry Chase now believe the severity of gambling addiction corresponds to sensitivity to near-misses.

These findings are exciting because they suggest that near-miss outcomes may elicit a dopamine response in the more severe gamblers, despite the fact that no actual reward is delivered," Clark said. "If these bursts of dopamine are driving addictive behavior, this may help to explain why problem gamblers find it so difficult to quit." The team found strong activity in the midbrain, which is dense with dopaminergic neurons. Near misses were also linked to increased activation of the ventral striatum and anterior insula, which are at the heart of reward-based learning.

Research has shown people that gamble on games of pure chance (like lotteries or slot machines) often mistakenly think skill is involved in the process. This illusionary belief of control drives them to continue playing. Increased dopamine resulting from witnessing near misses may be what drives compulsive gambling and the mistaken belief that such games of luck involve skill on the part of the players. Compulsive gambling is currently estimated to be a problem for over two million U.S. adults.

Slave To The Shopping Mall

Advertisers spend a great deal of money and time studying human motivation and behavior. One of the most useful principles, they've discovered, is that low self-esteem drives reckless spending and credit card use. If you're feeling down on yourself, you're more likely to rack up bills you can't afford. This human weakness drives several very profitable industries. In particular, people tend to engage in compensatory consumption, purchasing goods perceived as "high-status" when depressed, and are more likely to make such high-priced purchases on credit, according to 2010 research conducted at London Business School and Cornell University.

When your confidence is low from feeling powerless, or having been judged negatively, studies show you're likely to try and repair your sense of self-worth by buying luxury items. What's more, say researchers Niro Sivanathan and Nathan Pettit, because parting with cash specifically triggers psychological "pain" and regret in your insula, when you're down, you're more likely to use a credit card – it seems less "real" of a loss than spending money.

In the experiment, volunteers took a meaningless computer test. Afterward, half were told their "spatial reasoning" and "logic abilities" were "in the 12th percentile" (geekspeak for "you're a dumbass"). The other half were told they had scored in the 88th percentile. After, when asked how they would pay for a purchase they'd been planning on making, those who had undergone the ego bashing were about 60% more likely to answer that they planned to use credit. In a follow-up, 150 volunteers were asked to consider buying jeans. Half were asked to think about a pair of high-status exclusive designer jeans, and the others were asked to consider normally-priced jeans. After taking the same computer test and being told the same results, threats to their self-esteem made the "low-scoring" volunteers willing to pay about 30% more for designer jeans, and over 60% more likely to purchase them on credit.

Sivanathan and Pettit believe that people tend to believe luxury items confer high status, reassuring us of our self-worth, and we believe these items will increase our status in the eyes of others, serving as "identity signals". This tendency to seek comfort in luxury items means you're most vulnerable to overspending and overextending credit when you're feeling low. A similar study at Harvard has shown that sadness is a trigger of compensatory consumption, leading to eating more unhealthy food, and to a willingness to pay higher prices for new goods.

Such effects of sadness are generally beneath your awareness, and therefore out of your control. You carry over your emotions from one situation to another, and this colors your behavior in unrelated tasks, influencing your judgment, decisions, risk-taking, information processing, choices, and financial transactions.

Emotions strongly influence unrelated behavior. Sadness, rather than leading to negative evaluations of consumer goods, along with negative evaluations of the world, brings positive evaluations of new products, and a willingness to pay more for them. The sadder you are, studies indicate, the more you'll be willing to spend on these consumer goods. This "carry-over effect" of sadness also drives consumption in terms of eating, particularly preferences for fatty junk foods (so-called comfort foods), and for choosing high-risk/high-reward options. Regret often follows the overspending or overeating, leading to a repetitive cycle of negativity, reinforcing the original sadness.

Sadness is believed to be a response to loss or helplessness, a state from which you consciously or unconsciously attempt to repair the situation and your mood. In modern societies, we tend to purchase material goods to compensate for feelings of insecurity, overspending to obtain status-related items – a potentially disastrous coping strategy for psychological threats like feelings of powerlessness.

Training The Addicted Mind To Think Ahead

So why do some choose destructive behaviours like drug abuse, even when they're fully aware of the unpleasant and even disastrous consequences? And why does understanding those consequences protect some people but not others?

Researchers have found that people susceptible to addiction focus upon immediate pleasure, placing lesser value on future consequences, a process called *delay discounting*. It's an evaluation that occurs in your frontal cortex, using short-term working memory for temporary storage, much like a piece of scrap paper is used to jot down temporary notes while you make a decision.

Dr. John Krystal, Editor of the *Journal of Biological Psychiatry,* says,

> *The legal punishments and medical damages associated with the consumption of drugs of abuse may be meaningless to the addict in the moment when they have to choose whether or not to take their drug. Their mind is filled with the imagination of the pleasure to follow. We now see evidence that this myopic view of immediate pleasures and delayed punishments is not a fixed feature of addiction.*

In fact, it is possible to exercise and strengthen working memory, and thus improve impulse control. Center for Addiction Research Director Dr. Warren Bickel and colleagues at Little Rock, Arkansas teach substance abusers working memory-strengthening exercises, which help train them to better compare the consequences of short-term vs. long-term rewards. Strengthening working memory reduces the tendency to devalue future rewards, allowing substance abusers to see the value in resisting their impulses to use.

Nearly every spiritual teacher throughout history has taught that the key to mastering anything is learning to delay gratification. It's said (and experiments seem to support it) that if you can just have the self-control to put off things you want, you can master your brain's reward center and have ultimate control over your entire life.

Slave To The Past – Emotional Addictions

Dr. Daniel Goleman writes that emotionally-charged memories from your past can re-emerge, and your limbic system will experience them as if the events were occurring in the present. Thus, if you were beaten as a child, when you see someone scowling, having learned as a child to associate that facial expression with fear, hatred and retaliatory anger, you can be overwhelmed by the same emotions as an adult, without knowing the source.

When a sudden rush of negative emotion appears, to a degree disproportionate to the situation, it's likely to stem from such long-buried, early childhood memories. The key to not being driven by these overwhelming emotions is to stop and logically examine them when they arise, and question whether or not the response is appropriate or helpful at the time.

Deep-seated emotional maladaptations can be almost overwhelmingly powerful, and the temptation is to give in and respond to them in the same old familiar way – to run in panic, burst into tears, start swinging, shout yourself hoarse, shut down and refuse to communicate, or collapse into a quivering ball of worry and anxiety. But you have a choice, alternatives to these "default behaviours". While any and all of your thoughts are "okay" to have, how you respond to them is definitely a matter of choice, and the more often you choose healthy alternatives, the greater your self-control and wider your range of options will become.

Habit is destiny: through repeated use, your thought patterns and behaviours will build and strengthen synaptic connections, and through reuse, they will require less energy to activate in the future, therefore becoming easier to access at those times when you need them most.

Developing healthy alternatives – self-confidence, effective social skills, optimism, persistence in spite of failures, an easygoing attitude and the ability to quickly bounce back from frustrations – is the key to managing your emotional environment. Be aware that, just as with substance addictions, emotions trigger substantial neurochemical and hormonal releases, and, to your CNS, one addiction – to a favourite junk food, a syringe full of heroin, or a familiar, comfortable, destructive emotional surge – is essentially the same as any other.

The Long Road Home

While effective treatments are widely available, the constant danger of relapse into addiction is the greatest challenge in treatment; aside from destroying cortical impulse control, long-term drug abuse also builds powerful habits through deep, unconscious memory associations. These memory traces formed during addiction link people, places and circumstances to the addictive substance, so anytime these cues are encountered, overwhelming cravings overtake the addict, even many years after quitting.

Triggers such as stress, depression or trauma can severely test a recovering addict's resources, driving the instinctive desire to achieve homeostasis – relief from stress – in the most powerful and direct way the addict knows. Because dopamine is the brain's natural "anti-stress" drug, highly-stressful situations can trigger strong cravings and the danger of relapse. But the most powerful trigger for addictive relapses appears to be social interactions – hanging out with former drug-abusing friends.

Physically, it can take a former addict anywhere from several months to four years to recover from downregulation – the dopamine receptor die-off that accompanies addiction. Unfortunately, the potential for relapse seems to last indefinitely –acute cravings may fade after weeks or months, but they never quite completely disappear, a fact friends and family of addicts need to always remember.

How Anger Fuels Relapse

In *It Will Never Happen to Me,* addiction and recovery specialist Dr. Claudia Black talks about the role of anger in driving addictions. Addiction, she says, may be fueled by anger in several ways:

- Intense anger moves activity and control from the prefrontal cortex to the limbic system, so energy needed for logical thinking and impulse control is diverted to emotional responses; the results are poor decisions, and "giving in" to destructive impulses.

- Feeling angry and victimized leads to feelings of entitlement – a feeling of justification in doing something aggressive toward someone else, such as cheating on a husband or wife, verbally or physically abusing someone, invading privacy, and inflicting pain by indulging addictive impulses.

- Anger acts as an emotional barrier, preventing intimacy. This in turn leads to loneliness and the desire to self-medicate.

- Fear of another's anger and a desire to avoid conflict drive a desire to escape; as long as the conflict remains unresolved, an addict is apt to fall back into the destructive behavior pattern.

- Fear of expressing anger can lead to self-medicating to avoid so-called "unacceptable" feelings.

- A passive-aggressive way of "getting back" at someone with whom the addict is angry, but doesn't wish to directly confront

- Buried anger at parents, a spouse, or an abuser

- Suppressing anger builds up guilt and shame, and wanting to stop these unpleasant feelings fuels addiction.

To combat the role of anger in the cycle of addiction, it's critical to fully, openly and honestly address the underlying reasons for anger – and the fears that are driving it.

The aim of Alcoholics Anonymous and other recovery programs is to teach people how to regain control over their emotions without resorting to addictive drugs for self-medication. Learning healthy ways to soothe inner anxiety, quieten anger and lift depression are the targets of their 12-Step Recovery system. Once those emotional self-management skills are in place, the need for artificial control begins to diminish, although the addiction remains dormant for life, with the chance of relapse always near.

Taming The Beast

A very promising 2010 experiment in Chile may point the way to more powerful future treatments: researchers at the Pontifical Catholic University of Chile found that blocking the insula appears to stop amphetamine cravings. The insula, if you recall, is your brain's deep inner "reporter", part of your somatosensory system which informs your prefrontal cortex of your body's negative physical states and needs. When your insula reports that you "need a hit", it triggers anxiety and irritation.

Experiments on animals show that inhibiting insular activity stops drug cravings, and re-activating it restarts cravings. Suppressing signals from the region also seems to turn off the ability to feel stomach aches. According to Dr. Fernando Torrealba, the study's lead researcher, the insula reports cravings to your conscious mind, so shutting its messages down means, if you're an addict, you're no longer consciously aware of your body's "need" for drugs.

If you or somebody you know is struggling with a dependency issue, you can find out where to get help online here:

http://www.drugfreeworld.org

http://www.ncadd.org

or toll-free here:

24-hour HOPE Line: 800 NCA CALL (800-622-2255)

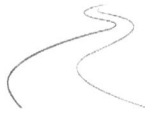

American Underworld, Mark Allen Johnson, Sept. 19, 2011, Discovery Communications, Ltd.; http://dsc.discovery.com/videos/american-underworld-sneak-peak-videos/

Methamphetamine, 2009, National Institute on Drug Abuse; http://www.nida.nih.gov/drug-pages/methamphetamine.html

The Owner's Manual for the Brain: Everyday Applications from Mind-Brain Research, 3rd ed. 2006. Austin: Bard Press. ISBN 1885167644

Pleasure: The Politics and the Reality, D.M. Warburton, 1994, New York: John Wiley & Sons;

Nora Volkow, interview, Tony Cenicola, July 13, 2011, NY Times; http://video.nytimes.com/video/2011/06/13/science/100000000862646/nora-volkow.html

The Pleasure Seekers, Helen Phillips, 11 October 2003, New Scientist Magazine

The Three-Pound Universe, Judith Hooper and Dick Teresi, 1991

New Insights into the Genetics of Addiction, Ming D. Li & Margit Burmeister, Nature Reviews Genetics, 2009; DOI: 10.1038/nrg2536

Research Reveals Why Some Smokers Become Addicted With Their First Cigarette, press release, Jeff Renaud, 2008, The University of Western Ontario; http://communications.uwo.ca/com/media_newsroom/media_newsroom_stories/research_reveals_why_some_smokers_become_addicted_with_their_first_cigarette__20080805442566/

Aversion to Nicotine Is Regulated by the Balanced Activity of b4 and a5 Nicotinic Receptor Subunits in the Medial Habenula, Silke Frahm et al, Neuron, May,12, 2011, Vol. 70, Issue 3, pp: 522-535 DOI: 10.1016/j.neuron.2011.04.013

A User's Guide to the Brain, Dr. John J. Ratey, 2002

Extended Amygdala and Emotional Salience: A PET Activation Study of Positive and Negative Affect, Israel Liberzon, K Luan Phan, Laura R Decker and Stephan F Taylor, 2003, Neuropsychopharmacology 28, 726–733. doi:10.1038/sj.npp.1300113; http://www.nature.com/%3Ffile%3D/npp/journal/v28/n4/full/1300113a.html

Dopamine Signalling through D1-Like versus D2-Like Receptors in the Nucleus Accumbens Core versus Shell Differentially Modulates Nicotine Reward Sensitivity, Steven R. Laviolette, Nicole M. Lauzon, Stephanie F. Bishop, Ninglei Sun, and Huibing Tan, 2008, The Journal of Neuroscience, 28(32): 8025-8033; doi: 10.1523/?JNEUROSCI.1371-08.2008 http://www.jneurosci.org/content/28/32/8025.full.pdf+html

NMDA Receptor Hypofunction in the Prelimbic Cortex Increases Sensitivity to the Rewarding Properties of Opiates via Dopaminergic and Amygdalar Substrates, Stephanie F. Bishop, Nicole M. Lauzon, Melanie Bechard, Shervin Gholizadeh and Steven R. Laviolette

Cerebral Cortex (2011) 21 (1): 68-80. doi: 10.1093/cercor/bhq060; http://cercor.oxfordjournals.org/content/21/1/68.full

The Role of Dopamine in the Prelimbic Cortex and the Dorsomedial Striatum in Instrumental Conditioning, Bjoern Lex and Wolfgang Hauber

Lower Quit Rates Among African American and Latino Menthol Cigarette Smokers at a Tobacco Treatment Clinic, Gandhi et al. , 2009, International Journal of Clinical Practice, 2009; DOI: 10.1111/j.1742-1241.2008.01969.x

The Fasciculus Retroflexus Controls the Integrity of REM Sleep by Supporting the Generation of Hippocampal Theta Rhythm and Rapid Eye Movements in Rats, Valjakka A, Vartiainen J, Tuomisto L, Tuomisto JT, Olkkonen H, Airaksinen MM, Brain Research Bulletin, 1998 Sep 15;47(2):171-84; http://www.ncbi.nlm.nih.gov/pubmed/9820735

Neural Degeneration Following Chronic Stimulant Abuse Reveals a Weak Link in Brain, Fasciculus Retroflexus, Implying the Loss of Forebrain Control Circuitry, Gaylord Ellison, 2002 European Neuropsychopharmacology 2002 Aug;12(4):287-97; http://www.europeanneuropsychopharmacology.com/article/S0924-977X%2802%2900020-2/fulltext

Perspectives on Brain Functioning: The Addictive Brain, by Jay M. Holder, D.C. and Kenneth Blum, PhD, 1990

Mothers Against Methamphetamine, Dr. Mary Holly, 2010; http://mamasite.net

Think What You Eat: Studies Point to Cellular Factors Linking Diet and Behavior, Kat Snodgrass and Sarah Bates, 2009, Society for Neuroscience; http://www.sfn.org/SiteObjects/published/0000BDF20016F63800FD712C30FA42DD/8A9303AF1029933F739A98FF4817335E/file/Think%20What%20You%20Eat%20News%20Release.pdf

Brain Dopamine and Obesity, Gene-Jack Wang, et al, 2001, The Lancet, Volume 357, Issue 9253, Pages 354-357; http://linkinghub.elsevier.com/retrieve/pii/S0140673600036436

Maternal High-Fat Diet Alters Methylation and Gene Expression of Dopamine and Opioid-Related Genes, Zivjena Vucetic, Jessica Kimmel, Kathy Totoki, Emily Hollenbeck and Teresa M. Reyes, 2010, Endocrinology Vol. 151, No. 10 4756-4764; http://endo.endojournals.org/cgi/content/short/151/10/4756

Relation of Obesity to Consummatory and Anticipatory Food Reward, Eric Stice, Sonja Spoor, Janet Ng, and David H. Zald, 2009, Journal of Physiological Behavior, July 14; 97(5): 551–560; http://www.ncbi.nlm.nih.gov/pmc/articles/PMC2734415/

Gambling Severity Predicts Midbrain Response to Near-Miss Outcomes, Henry W. Chase, Luke Clark, Journal of Neuroscience, 2010; 30 (18): 6180 DOI: 10.1523/JNEUROSCI.5758-09.2010

A High Fat Diet Alters Crucial Aspects of Brain Dopamine Signalling, Jackson J. Cone, J.D. Roitman and M.F. Roitman, 2010, Society for the Study of Ingestive Behavior; http://www.ssib.org/web/index.php?page=press&release=2010-8

Greater Obesity in Offspring of Nursing Mothers Consuming a High-Fat Diet, Bo Sun et al, 2010, Society for the Study of Ingestive Behavior; http://www.ssib.org/web/index.php?page=press&release=2010-5

Brain Responses of Obese Individuals are More Weakly Linked to Feelings of Hunger, Francois Chouinard-Decorte, 2010, Society for the Study of Ingestive Behavior; http://www.ssib.org/web/index.php?page=press&release=2010-6

Signalling Path in Brain May Prevent That 'I'm full' Message, UT Southwestern Scientists Discover, Kristen Holland Shear, 2011, Southwestern Medical Center; http://www.utsouthwestern.edu/utsw/cda/dept353744/files/629807.html

Self-Control in Decision-Making Involves Modulation of the vmPFC Valuation System, Todd A. Hare1, Colin F. Camerer, and Antonio Rangel1,Science, 2009. DOI: 10.1126/science.1168450; http://www.sciencemag.org/content/324/5927/646

Inhaling From Just One Cigarette Can Lead To Nicotine Addiction: Kids Show Signs Of Addiction Almost Immediately, ScienceDaily. Retrieved May 14, 2011, from http://www.science-daily.com /releases/2007/07/070703171843.htm

Drugs, Brains, and Behavior – The Science of Addiction, Dr. Nora D. Volkow, 2010 National Institute of Drug Abuse

Dopaminergic Reward System: A Short Integrative Review, Oscar Arias-Carrion, Maria Stamelou, Eric Murillo-Rodríguez, Manuel Menéndez-González, Ernst Pöppel, 2010, International Archives of Medicine, 3:24;

Remember the Future: Working Memory Training Decreases Delay Discounting Among Stimulant Addicts, Dr. Warren K. Bickel, Richard Yi, Reid D. Landes, Paul F. Hill, Carole Baxter, 2011, Journal of Biological Psychiatry, 69 (3): 260 DOI: 10.1016

The End of Overeating, Dr. David Kessler, 2009, Rodale Books

The Plastic Trap: Self-Threat Drives Credit Usage and Status Consumption, N. C. Pettit, N. Sivanathan, 2010, Social Psychological and Personality Science, DOI: 10.1177/1948550610385138; http://faculty.london.edu/nsivanathan/pdf/Pettit%20&%20Sivanathan%20%282011%29.pdf

Sadness and Consumption, Nitika Garg and Jennifer S.Lerner, 2010, Harvard University; http://content.ksg.harvard.edu/lernerlab/papers/files/PSPBDraft-12-15-09.pdf

Desire to Acquire: Powerlessness and Compensatory Consumption, Journal of Consumer Research, 2008; 0 (0): 080418160208692 DOI: 10.1086/588569; http://insight.kellogg.northwestern.edu/index.php/Kellogg/article/desire_to_acquire

Genetic Anthropology, Ancestry, and Ancient Human Migration, Human Genome Project Information; http://www.ornl.gov/sci/techresources/Human_Genome/elsi/humanmigration.shtml

Gambling Severity Predicts Midbrain Response to Near-Miss Outcomes, Henry W. Chase, Luke Clark, 2010, Journal of Neuroscience; 30 (18): 6180 DOI: 10.1523/JNEUROSCI.5758-09.2010

Prolonged Rewarding Stimulation Of The Rat Medial Forebrain Bundle: Neurochemical And Behavioral Consequences, Hernandez G, Hamdani S, Rajabi H, et al. (August 2006), Behav. Neurosci. 120 (4): 888–904. doi:10.1037/0735-7044.120.4.888. PMID 16893295.

Learning

"Education comes from within. You get it by struggle and effort and thought."
– Napoleon Hill, Think and Grow Rich, 1987

If you have an Internet connection, you have the historically unprecedented ability to learn about anything and everything you wish, as superficially or as deeply as you want, from auto mechanics to engineering, from human anatomy to astrophysics. You can now learn anything with no more cost to you than your connection fees and a little investment in your time.

The worldwide Open Learning Consortium lets you to study, free of charge, under the most brilliant minds in contemporary science. In the course of bringing you this book, I studied under half a dozen Nobel-prizewinning scientists, as well as some of the most highly-regarded professors of MIT, Berkeley, Cambridge, Duke, Harvard, McGill, Stanford, and Yale – all within the comfort of my living room. You can too. If you're not studying exactly what you want to learn from some of the greatest teachers alive, you're missing the boat. Empower yourself; make a resolution to start studying at the world's greatest schools today.

The Biological Basis Of Learning

Your brain is constantly processing, updating through physical changes as it processes, evaluates and records or discards sensory input from everything you encounter. Every moment of your life, even as you dream, your brain undergoes tremendous, complex changes, and makes constant complex, usually unconscious calculations.

Your prefrontal cortex (PFC) orchestrates thoughts and actions in accordance with your goals, while your basal ganglia and limbic lobe help to coordinate motor control, cognition and emotions. All three areas are extensively connected with each other, and with the rest of your brain, to help you learn.

Learning is a neuroadaptation that physically alters your brain; dendrites sprout and migrate to nearby neurons, creating *memory traces* – synapse and receptor synthesis, and structural reinforcement, increasing sensitivity (and therefore conductivity) which makes it easier to use the same pathways in the future.

After repeated neural reinforcement, your brain becomes able to perform certain activities with significantly less energy and effort, and certain tasks can be conducted without your conscious attention. You can retain information, impressions and emotional states long-term, allowing you to modify your behavior, and adapt yourself for future improvement.

125

Learning mentally links ideas or sensory input, and generates brief neural signals which indicate whether predictions and responses are correct or incorrect. After a reward, neurons convey strong, sustained output for 4 to 6 seconds. This sustained, high-frequency stimulation can result in *long-term potentiation*, genetically-triggered formation of new synapses and receptors – the physical components of memory traces.

In 2004, Nobel winning neuroscientist Dr. Susumu Tonegawa and his MIT team discovered how neurons create these proteins: An enzyme called *mitogen-activated protein kinase* (MAPK) acts as "a direct activational signal from the synapse to the protein synthesis machinery," a molecular switch that turns on protein synthesis.

Plasticity

Your brain has a high level of *plasticity*, the ability for neurons to forge connections. These connections switch rapidly on and off, leading to a continuous adaptive rewiring as your brain constantly strengthens and prunes its circuitry. Over the course of just a few hours, connections are formed and re-formed many times. Thus, your brain's circuitry is like a social network, your neurons acting like people directly linked to only a few others. Metaphorically, your neurons are constantly "switching alliances" and linking with new circles of "friends" to better process information.

On the other hand, forgetting means you haven't used a piece of information sufficiently, so the memory is discarded to free up resources for more important information, primarily in your hippocampus.

Memory is organized in your brain in the form of *matrices*, an interconnected group of associations called *schemata*. This makes it very fast and easy to learn new information – you simply link it to pre-existing information structures in your mind. A robust pre-existing matrix of knowledge makes it easy for information to quickly be added to long-term storage.

For example, to a painter, extensive schemata exist encoding light, color, texture, perspective and other visual information. Because of this, learning photography is significantly easier than for non-artists, and the painter is more quickly able to add to her existing stock of knowledge – the synaptic connections related to that sort of information are already robust and have multiple connections.

This means that consolidating memories isn't always gradual. If new information is related to existing long-term memories (a framework of related mental schemata into which they fit) it will help new memories quickly solidify.

Similar past experiences provide a neural nexus to which new, related information can quickly be attached. Once a schema has been built in your cortex, your hippocampus can more quickly transfer related memories to the region. In a nutshell, this means the more you already know about a subject, the faster you can learn related information.

This physical wiring "shortcut" can be used to your advantage: if you can find similarities or relations between new information and things you already know, you'll much more quickly and successfully strengthen the synaptic connections that encode the new data in your brain.

Memory And Learning

Research has shown there are three broad stages to human memory:

1. ***Immediate memory*** holds sensory information a few hundred milliseconds for analysis and further processing. This immediate memory is erased by new incoming signals. With each signal, Ca2+ accumulates in presynaptic terminals; this prolongs release of neurotransmitters, allowing for synaptic potentiation.

   Immediate memory is extremely temporary, a "place-holder" where input is unconsciously sorted, either deemed unimportant and discarded, or stored until it can be processed into longer-term permanent memory. Immediate memories are believed to reside in your hippocampus. Emotional values generated by the connected amygdala can mark these memories as salient, boosting the probability they'll become permanent – information that creates strong emotions is almost certainly important for your survival.

2. ***Short-term memory*** lasts seconds to minutes, with salient information selected from immediate memory. Here too, information is erased as new items replace old data. For example, if you see a rapid sequence of slides, the last will remain in your short-term memory.

   Recent events are stored in short-term memory for seconds to minutes, possibly due to repetition – impulses recirculating in neuronal circuits for a limited time, a process called rehearsal. *Working memory* is short-term memory used while generating conscious thoughts. This is where stimuli is managed which has captured your attention and interest. Through *rehearsal*, the likelihood increases that a working memory will last; re-use of a neural pathway strengthens its synapses, enhancing future signal transmission so the information is more frequently and easily retrieved.

The average adult working memory holds about three to four pieces of information at any given instant. But by clustering multiple groups of three to four facts into larger chunks, you can process greater amounts of information. This is why telephone numbers are arranged in sequences of three and four digits – the arrangement is optimal for remembering.

Items in your working memory generally last up to 45 minutes; past this point, *cognitive fatigue* begins to set in. Your maximal attention usually lasts for only 10 minutes, which is why psychologists suggest taking regular breaks to maximize learning.

3. **Long-term memory** is potentially permanent, information received from immediate or short-term memory. Long-term memories are retained for a day or more. The likelihood of successful long-term storage increases with salience and *rehearsal* (the number of repetitions).

Long-term memory is subdivided into intermediate long-term memory, which lasts for days or weeks and can be disrupted, and longer-lasting long-term memory, which lasts for years. The longest-lasting memories are of highly overlearned information, like your own name and address. This long-term memory formation is due to protein synthesis at the synapses – an increased number of vesicles and receptors. These long term-memories are organized throughout your cortex, which maintains the synaptic modifications after several rehearsals.

Short-term memories are candidates for long-term storage if they meet two criteria:

1. The information is **personally relevant**. This appears to be the most important criterion for choosing which facts get transferred into long-term memory.

2. The information is **logical and consistent**, fitting what you already know or believe, allowing it to be integrated into existing long-term memories. A number of studies have shown memory and learning are optimized when information is logical, consistent and personally relevant. Material you deem trivial gets discarded, while information you recognize as personally important is processed for long-term storage.

Be sure not to overload your working memory; if you're new to a field of study, you'll only be able to hold three to four facts at a time in your working memory. Avoid memory fatigue by cutting your study sessions into 10- to 20-minute "chunks" with complete breaks, in which you engage in some other activity, preferably involving physical activity.

Engaging More Of Your Brain

As you've seen in book one, specific sensory processing is occurs within specific lobes of your brain and is integrated in the association areas:

Images are initially processed by your occipital lobe.

Verbal information is primarily processed in your left temporal lobe (if you're right-handed).

Reading is primarily conducted by cooperation between your occipital, left temporal and frontal lobes.

Writing mainly recruits your motor cortex in your dominant hemisphere (the left hemisphere for right-handed people) and your temporal lobe.

The more of your senses you engage when learning, the faster you'll acquire information, and the better you'll retain it. Ideally, you want to recruit all your sensory processing networks, including listening, reading, writing, watching, even gesturing. Additionally, because repetition reinforces memory traces, one of the most powerful ways to solidify memory of recently-learned material is to teach it to someone else. This will also help you articulate what you've learned for future use.

Active participation is key to deep learning, using multiple streams of reinforcement (watching, listening, reading, writing and gesturing), and deciding why it's important to you personally and how it relates to that you already know. Make sure you take your time as you study, so that you completely understand the material and the logic behind it. Writing notes in your textbooks is another excellent learning booster.

Remember What's Important To You

There are four primary factors that influence how well you remember, and you can use this to your advantage:

1. *Attention* – Make a conscious effort to focus upon what you wish to remember, repeat it, and then connect it to what you already know to strengthen the memory.

2. *Motivation* – Necessity or interest register as salience in your brain, greatly strengthening memories.

3. ***Emotional meaning*** – as you learn something, your emotional state strongly influences how well you'll remember it. Intense emotions such as excitement, tension or shock (for example at an event like the destruction of the World Trade Center) trigger stress hormone releases, increasing your arousal and recruiting your amygdala, which works with your hippocampus to forge powerful, emotionally-charged memories.

4. ***Context*** – because your brain is associative, the location, sights sounds, smells, etc. of the environment when you are memorizing a piece of information are all remembered. This means if you can't recall the information itself, remembering something linked to it, such as *I was walking on the left side of the street when I saw the building* will help you. Additionally, the more things you know related to a piece of information will more firmly affix it in your mind, with a longer-lasting, more robust neural circuit which is easier to access for recall.

Instantly Sharpen Your Focus

The single most important component of learning is focused attention. When something is salient – worth paying attention to – you'll focus upon it and relate it to yourself. Things which you believe are irrelevant to you have no salience, and are rejected as candidates for long-term memory formation.

Thus, you're more likely to remember something if you can find how it relates to you personally. Repetition will also strengthen memory traces. Finally, there is the process of *elaboration*, looking at a piece of information in a number of different ways to increase the number of synaptic connections to its memory trace. In this way, you create multiple paths from which to access that piece of information, and increase that circuit's sensitivity – lowering the threshold at which it fires.

It follows that the more senses you engage in the learning process, the stronger the synaptic connections will be, and the easier it will become to remember the information. If possible, listen to recordings or lectures, take notes, watch videos or demonstrations, discuss the material with others, and even physically act out with gestures to add additional neural "access paths".

Get the right amount of sleep: you need 7 to 8 hours if you're an adult or teen, and 9 or more if you're younger. Memory transfer and consolidation occur during sleep, so getting too little will severely impact your studies and work.

Get A Little Lazier – *Want to instantly improve your concentration? Take a break. According to the latest research, concentrating too long weakens your focus and degrades your performance. This vigilance decrement comes from a drop in attention resources, says University of Illinois psychology professor Alejandro Lleras. After a while, attention naturally wanders, and performance on a task drops.*

Something similar occurs with perception – if a stimulus like a noise remains constant, eventually you will stop noticing it – your brain becomes habituated – for example, no longer noticing the feeling of clothing on your skin or your tongue in your mouth (sorry!). Your brain has classified this sensation as unimportant, so it's erased from your awareness. Sustained attention on a mental process also eventually affects your awareness the same way.

Dr. Lleras and his team had subjects focus on a repetitive computing task for an hour. One quarter of the subjects were instructed to respond when numbers flashed onto the screen. Just as expected, the control group, which repeated their task for an hour without breaks, began to perform progressively more poorly. But the group which was distracted by the need to respond to the digits showed no performance decline. Two very brief breaks from their task (responding to the digits) enabled them to maintain the same level of focus for the entire hour.

According to Lleras, your brain is designed to detect and respond to change, and sustained attention to a single task can actually hinder your performance. Diverting and then returning your attention allows you to remain focused. This means you need to brief breaks during long tasks like studying before a major test or a presentation. These brief mental breaks, he says, will keep your mind sharp and on track.

Your attention is (usually subconsciously) focused on specific outside stimuli, selectively "tuning out" what you don't need to pay attention to, such as the constant sensation of clothing against your skin. If change or something novel occurs (a dangerous, interesting or otherwise special event), your attention will instantly lock onto it with razor-sharp focus.

Additional Focus- Improving Techniques

Usually, the inability to remember something comes from a lack of attention; your mind simply didn't believe the information was worth expending sufficient mental energy. If you really want to remember something, stop everything else and focus on just that one thing – turn off any distracting music, go someplace quiet and stop multitasking.

- Engagement – Invest a little time to really imprint an idea in your mind. Think about different aspects of it — what the sound resembles, how something might look in different circumstances, any emotions it brings up in you. The more you "tie" to this information, the better you'll remember it.

- Napping – Study or work starts to deteriorate rapidly after about 60 minutes. Afternoon naps, if at all possible, will consolidate information in your memory, however.

- Rehearsal – To maintain long-term memories, you should periodically dust them off and go over them again, reconsolidating them. This reactivates PKMzeta production (see below) so the memory remains.

- Test Yourself – Tests force you to recall and use information you've learned, making them important opportunities to solidify learning. They also give you an important opportunity to find out how well you've absorbed the material you've studied.

Neuroscience Secrets Of Success:
The Trial And Error Circuit

University of Iowa and Caltech researchers recorded the neurochemistry of the learning process in real time, in the *Iowa Gambling Task* experiment. According to *Wired* Magazine's Jonah Lehrer, the results show that developing expertise and achieving goals is simply a matter of long-term trial and error, and a willingness to embrace failure as a critical tool for self-improvement:

"Unless you experience the unpleasant symptoms of being wrong your brain will never revise its models. Before your neurons can succeed, they must repeatedly fail. There are no shortcuts for this painstaking process."

The system, says Lehrer, is based upon expectation; when you learn a cause and effect pattern – press the lever and food appears – you associate actions with the pleasurable feelings of dopamine release. In this manner, you learn to anticipate rewards when you follow certain behavior patterns.

But when such a behavior pattern unexpectedly doesn't produce a reward, error detection circuits in the anterior cingulate cortex (ACC), dense with dopamine receptors, don't receive their expected dopamine "fix". The ACC prompts the thalamus to amplify sensory signals related to the error, and your attention focuses with a jolt onto the mistaken prediction. As Lehrer expresses it, this is the neural circuitry neuroscientists commonly refer to as the "Oh, shit!" circuit.

Meanwhile, the ACC activates your hypothalamus, triggering epinephrine release, and your heartbeat increases, your pupils dilate, your blood vessels constrict and your blood and glucose stores prime your muscles for the proverbial "fight or flight".

The process is highly salient, triggering the synaptic reinforcement comprising a memory – so you don't repeat the same predictive mistake, and this is how your decision-making skills evolve and improve, through a subconscious trial-and-error process.

> *"You never learn!"* – *This exasperated accusation seems to have some neurological basis in fact – genetically predetermined reductions in ACC dopamine receptors render some people less capable of learning from negative reinforcement. People with this deficiency are also at a much greater risk of addictions – when you can't learn from your mistakes, you keep repeating them.*
>
> *The long, slender "spindle cells" of the ACC spread throughout your brain, saturating it with dopamine messages. Says Baylor University neuroscientist Read Montague, 99.9% of human behavior is driven by these dopaminergic messages. And this means your brain is constantly adjusting its neural connections in response to novel events and to the mistakes you make.*

Failing Your Way To Success

This constant comparison between expectations and results is the basis of trial and error, and exactly the process at work when the world's greatest inventor cited his personal recipe for success: embracing the power of failure.

Arguably the most famous inventor of all time after Leonardo da Vinci was Ohio's self-taught Thomas Alva Edison. He had little formal school training; his mother, discovering her son had a keen interest in chemistry and electronics, gave him books on the subject, and he pursued knowledge doggedly.

Edison personally created 1,093 patented inventions, including the microphone, telephone receiver, universal stock ticker, electric car battery, recorded music and motion pictures. He also built the first public power station, transforming civilization forever.

His most famous "invention" is the modern light bulb, which was actually an improvement of other scientists' previous designs. However, in his quest to perfect the light bulb, Edison and his colleagues tried and failed over *3000 times* (!) before they finally hit upon the correct material for the bulb's *filament*, the central wire which emits photons, glowing when electric current flows across it.

Change Your Mind

Edison's incredible perseverance shows the primary strength of character driving this remarkable man; his optimism simply didn't allow for failure. As he is quoted in the Encyclopedia Britannica,

"If I find 10,000 ways something won't work, I haven't failed. I am not discouraged, because every wrong attempt discarded is another step forward."

This powerful shift in interpretation is a life-changing skill taught by pioneering American psychotherapist Virginia Satir to her patients: *reframing* – re-evaluating a situation from a positive, growth-promoting point of view.

Edison was a master of reframing: when his factory was destroyed by fire in 1914, and a great deal of his life's work went up in flames, he amazed his son the next morning by saying, "There is great value in disaster. All our mistakes are burned up. *Thank God we can start anew.*" He was right, of course; three weeks later, he went on to create the world's first phonograph.

There is incredible power in this simple change in the way you view events. You can CHOOSE to view the glass as half-empty or half-full, and, if you choose the latter, your results will continuously improve. If you choose defeat, you may never know what was waiting around the corner. As Edison summed it up, "Many of life's failures are people who did not realize how close they were to success when they gave up."

Learning: Your Mindset Sets You Up For Success Or Failure

Success boils down to one simple process: discovering the "right way" through failure, then improving. In other words, your tolerance for failure is your capacity for success.

In fact, while it confers the initial advantage of a head start, talent is nearly irrelevant when it comes to success, according to extensive research. Successful people aren't necessarily the most talented or intelligent; they're simply thick-skinned and patient – better at learning from failure.

Michigan State University, Professor Jason Moser set out to discover the principle underlying this. What he discovered is that, while everyone fails, the critical point is what you do afterward. At the critical point of failure you're faced with a choice: do you choose to ignore your failure for the sake of massaging your ego, or do you study your failure, and learn from it?

Moser says there are two neural processes which automatically occur at the moment of failure, both of which can be measured by an EEG:

- 50 milliseconds after a mistake, an involuntary reaction called *error-related negativity* (ERN) occurs. This is thought to be the anterior cingulate cortex activating, helping monitor behavior, anticipate rewards and regulate attention;

- 100-500 milliseconds after the mistake, a second signal called *error positivity* (Pe) occurs. This is the point at which awareness of the error arises, attention focuses on the mistake, and you reflect upon the disappointing result.

Recent studies show you learn more effectively if your brain has 1) a larger ERN signal (a bigger initial response to your error); and 2) a consistent Pe signal (you're paying greater attention to your mistake, and therefore presumably learning from it).

The Power of Affirmations Revisited

Your beliefs about yourself shape these mainly involuntary error-related brain signals, both of which occur in under half a second.

Mindsets are what you believe about yourself and your intrinsic talents. When you think about your intelligence, talents and personality, you can consider them to be fixed, immutable points or subject to growth and development throughout life.

Stanford University psychologist Dr. Carol Dweck has demonstrated there are two types of people: *fixed mindset* and *growth mindset*. If you have a *fixed mindset*, you believe your traits are fixed from birth: you think you have a certain level of talent and intelligence which cannot be changed. You believe that if you're smart and talented, you're in luck, but this means you're also likely to constantly worry about how you "measure up", and constantly feel the need to prove your value, both to yourself and to others. But if you have a *growth mindset*, says Dr. Dweck, you believe hard work and perseverance will allow you to grow and develop.

Those with a fixed mindset believe (mistakenly) personal qualities like intelligence and talent are fixed traits, and that success can be achieved through talent alone, without requiring effort. Thus, they don't try to develop their talents.

People with a growth mindset, however, believe (correctly) that their personal attributes can be improved by dedicated, hard work, and that talent and ingenuity are only an advantageous starting point – a sort of head start in life. This growth mindset fosters a joy in learning and the mental toughness necessary for achieving great things.

Dr. Dweck says every great achiever has a growth mindset – and numerous studies back her up.

But can your baseline intelligence really be improved? In fact, no less than the inventor of the IQ test, Alfred Binet, said,

> *A few modern philosophers assert that an individual's intelligence is a fixed quantity, a quantity which cannot be increased... But with practice, training, and above all, method, we manage to increase our attention, our memory, our judgment and literally to become more intelligent than we were before.*

As with all other traits, your intelligence is determined by both your genetics and your environment. While you may be born with advantages or disadvantages, it's up to you to capitalize on them and even evolve. Experience, training, perseverance, a positive mindset and hard work catalyze that evolution.

How to Boost Your IQ

1. *Feed Your Head* – Oxford University studies in 2007 showed children fed Omega 3 fish oil for three months radically improved learning capacity, advancing as much as two years in reading, memory and concentration. It is believed the nutrients DHA and EHA improve synapse conductivity.

2. *Exercise Your Body* – A 2011 study at Georgia Health Sciences University demonstrated that overweight and previously inactive children aged 7 to 11 improved intelligence scores an average of 3.8 points within three months of starting a daily 40-minute exercise program. Their attention, planning, social behavior, and math and

reading skills all showed improvement, and fMRI scans showed increased prefrontal cortex activity after vigorous exercise. Researchers assume increased blood and oxygen in the brain were primarily responsible for the effects.

3. ***Train Your Brain*** – Although it's long been held that IQ is 50% to 80% predetermined by genetics, a new study suggests it's possible to improve with practice. Psychologists at the University of Michigan believe they have uncovered an effective method for boosting core intelligence with a simple mental exercise. Several dozen Detroit elementary- to middle-school children used the exercise daily for 15 minutes and showed marked gains in intelligence tests. This intelligence boost lasted three months, even after the children stopped training.

   Psychologists say intelligence is comprised of two elements: *fluid* and *crystallized intelligence*. *Fluid intelligence* is made up of dynamic, novel problem-solving and new pattern-recognition. *Crystallized intelligence*, on the other hand, is accumulated knowledge, memorized facts such as historical details, also known as *semantic memories*.

   Fluid intelligence was believed to be solely based upon genetics, but children in the study gained fluid intelligence equal to approximately five IQ points after only a month of training. This wasn't just an accumulation of facts that could easily be forgotten, but an actual sharpening of problem-solving skills.

   The exercise they used is called the *n-back task*. It begins with a visual cue – in this case, the location of a cartoon character. As the test proceeds, the cue changes—in this case, the cartoon character relocates. Volunteers press a keyboard space bar every time the character returns to a spot it has previously visited, ignoring any other locations. The locations gradually move further back in time as the test progresses, requiring sifting through an ever-greater amount of information.

   After playing the n-back game repeatedly, the children showed improved focus, requiring less short-term memory for irrelevancies – locations they didn't need to remember. In other words, according to senior author John Jonides, they became better at discriminating between what was and wasn't relevant.

   However, not every student improved dramatically from the training; those who found it overly difficult or tedious (and therefore didn't fully engage in the exercise) showed no improvement. Additionally, some psychologists question the real-world value of this improvement, asserting that all it enhances is the ability to achieve higher scores on abstract intelligence tests.

4. ***Shine a Little Light on Matters*** - 2009 government studies showed that children studying in schools with the largest classroom windows progressed 15 percent faster in math and 23 percent faster in reading than those who studied in schools with smaller windows. Their grades on standardized tests also increased 25 percent. Grade improvements to this degree could mean the difference between passing and failing.

   Bright light, particularly blue-tinged light, boosts alertness, helping with mathematics, logical reasoning and reaction times. Daylight elevates mood, boosts visibility and concentration, and regulates melatonin, the main hormone responsible for sleep cycles. Melatonin, secreted mainly during nighttime, is also responsible for a number of biochemical activities which impact immunological function, including estrogen production. Suppressing melatonin with daylight boosts general arousal, making students more alert.

   Daylight also seems to significantly affect behavior, improving sociability; children in classrooms lit by fluorescent bulbs have higher levels of cortisol production and aberrant behavior, and classrooms (and offices) without daylight appear to upset hormonal balances, with a major impact on mood, concentration and cooperativeness.

Secrets Of Expertise

Cutting-edge research shows the primary difference between experts and novices is in focus and improved pattern recognition. With experience, you improve at quickly cutting through irrelevancies to find the most useful information, and more efficiently organize data for storage and retrieval.

It's been estimated that it takes about 5,000 hours (roughly two and a half hours a day for five years) to become an expert at something, whether it's motor skills or cognitive tasks you're mastering. Largely what is occurring is the buildup of a giant memory bank of useful, relevant information and associations – sheer memorization and a massive reshuffling of data for the greatest efficiency.

Inborn talent, on the other hand, seems derived from advantageous neural connections present at birth, the result of genetics. These innate neural advantages can be capitalized upon while training, which fosters and enhances natural talent.

Learning Skills

Procedural memory is what guides you through daily mental and physical activities, usually at an unconscious level. These memories are automatically retrieved and used as needed to direct you through the steps involved in complex motor skills – from brushing your teeth to driving a car. Usually, neither conscious effort nor attention is required to access these long-term memories, created by repeating an activity until it becomes effortless.

Four resources are necessary for learning procedural skills. The greater their availability, the greater your skill can become:

1. Memory capacity and functionality

2. Knowledge

3. Problem-solving skills

4. Focus

Depending upon the skill you want to master, each of these plays a varying degree of importance – for example, memory and focus are more important when learning a sequence of dance moves, while problem-solving and knowledge are more important for a mechanic repairing a car. However, studies suggest that focus is the core component which can be manipulated to quickly improve. Psychologists believe skills are acquired in three stages:

1. Cognitive

2. Associative

3. Autonomous

1. Cognitive – In the first phase of learning, you break down a skill into discrete steps, and learn how these steps combine to perform the task correctly. At this stage, the steps are held in your short-term (*working*) memory and concentrated upon one-by-one, independently of one another. Because attention is a limited resource, at this stage, the novice can't focus upon factors which *improve* performance – being unable at this point to see the entire structure, fine-tune movements, or discern between good and bad elements.

2. Associative – The activity is practiced repeatedly until recognizable patterns emerge, and you gradually improve, as mistakes or ineffective steps are discarded, and your brain and body begin to make the process more automatic. Distinguishing relevant and irrelevant information is critical in this phase. Through repetition, procedural memory develops, and working memory is gradually less required. As the activity becomes more automatic, it frees your mind to focus on more subtle aspects of performance, fine-tuning and perfecting.

3. Autonomous – The third phase of learning is where a skill becomes polished. Recognizing missteps and irrelevancies becomes much more rapid, and progressively less conscious thought is required as the skill becomes automatic.

> **On the other hand** – *A recent. more simplistic alternative theory suggests that learning a skill doesn't require understanding steps, but is just a matter of visualizing the end result, then making attempts and analyzing failures to improve each time, until the skill has become automatic.*

The Expert Brain vs. the Novice Brain

Automaticity is when a skill has been learned and practiced to the point at which concentration on the steps is no longer required. Complex motor tasks like driving a car improve and become automatic through practice, until they can be performed without the need for conscious effort.

Called *procedural memories*, they primarily involve your basal ganglia and cerebellum. Everyday examples include speaking, walking, or riding a bicycle. After the initial learning, once the activity has been sufficiently practiced, it becomes possible to concentrate on other activities while performing it (such as talking while walking).

Recent studies have begun to shed light on how this process occurs. After practicing three to four hours a day over several years, professional *Shogi* (Japanese chess) players say the choice of the best move appears in their minds intuitively – game strategy is automatically and rapidly generated without conscious analysis or a mental searching through alternatives.

fMRI scans at Japan's RIKEN Cognitive Science Institute show this is because expert players access a different brain region than amateurs while studying patterns and planning their next moves. It appears that the more expert they become, the less conscious thought is required and the more intuitive the process becomes. The neural circuits used in automatic categorization differ from those used when a skill is first being learned. For example, categorization based on newly-learned rules initially requires heavy use of *declarative* (conscious) memory, but thousands of repetitions eventually make this mental sorting effortless.

This and similar studies show pattern analysis and planning transferring gradually from the cortex into the subcortex, mainly the striatum. The caudate in particular plays a central role, as practiced skills shift from requiring conscious thought into a state of automatic access.

This means the caudate is critical for people living in modern societies full of fast-paced information flow and constant change. By necessity, our brains learn to automatically categorize a tremendous number of objects effortlessly and instantaneously. This progressive automaticity applies to a wide variety of daily skills, including motor skills, emotional processing, logical and sensory categorization, and in switching between languages among multilingual speakers.

Choke-Proof

Choking – making a mistake at something you're skilled at when stress levels are high – can occur anytime a high-level skill is performed, when your desire to succeed or your fear of failure lead you to become overly self-conscious and start focusing once again on the step-by-step procedures.

This shift in focus from your subcortex to your cortex disrupts the natural flow of procedural memory, and therefore the performance of automatic skills. Mental control of the process has shifted back from your basal ganglia into your frontal cortex, the region used by novices when they're first analyzing and learning the steps involved.

However, numerous studies have shown that overtraining well past the point of flawless execution, is the key to making a skill "distraction-proof". Additionally, engaging your working memory with a distracting task, such as whistling a tune, can put your subcortex back in control.

Clearly visualizing success, as Jack Nicklaus described in his famous textbook, gives rise to the opposite of choking. *Clutchness*, also called "rising to the occasion", is when you perform a feat of outstanding excellence under pressure. This has been demonstrated even among the unskilled, and is highly dependent upon your mastery of visualization and positive thought.

Music Hath Charms

Musical training from an early age appears to significantly alter brain development, boosting speech, vocabulary, learning of foreign languages, reading comprehension, memory, motor skills, attention, and empathy. The effects are thought to be powerful at any point in life, but particularly before the age of seven.

2011 research has demonstrated that childhood musical ability is closely related to verbal memory and literacy, affecting auditory working memory, attention and even reading ability. Dr. Nina Kraus at Northwestern University's Auditory Neuroscience Laboratory tested children on their ability to read and to recognize words, then compared results with their auditory working memory (in remembering number sequences and then reciting them in reverse), and musical aptitude (in recognizing and producing melody and rhythm).

Brain stem activity was also measured, as the brain stem responds strongly to rhythmic sounds based on speech. Poor readers had reduced auditory brain stem responses to rhythmic sounds when compared with good readers, and this rhythmic sensitivity correlated with both reading skills and musical aptitude. Musical ability in terms of auditory working memory and rhythm went hand-in-hand with superior reading skills.

According to Dr. Kraus:

> ...music skill, together with how the nervous system responds to regularities in auditory input and auditory memory/attention, accounts for about 40% of the difference in reading ability between children. These results add weight to the argument that music and reading are related via common neural and cognitive mechanisms and suggests a mechanism for the improvements in literacy seen with musical training.

Optimized Learning

The environment in which you work or study can have a marked effect on how well you learn and perform; a stimulating, well-organized and clean environment will increase your focus and lower your stress.

It's also important to establish a routine, in which you work or study in the same place, at the same time – ideally when your attention levels peak due to your circadian rhythms. Breaking your concentration roughly every ten minutes by briefly standing, stretching, or taking a walk to another room and back will also ensure your attention stays on track.

Cortisol can impair learning and productivity. Stress from conflict, or from feeling overworked or rushed can raise cortisol levels. A safe environment, free of negative or demeaning comments and bullying will ensure cortisol levels remain low.

If you're frustrated by a particular task, you should put it aside for the time being, until you're ready to tackle it once again. This avoids imprinting negative associations with the task and keeps stress hormones in your blood at a minimum. When your energy and motivation levels return, you'll have renewed ability to master the task, and your memories of it will be more positive – and thus more beneficial to you.

When you experience a positive or negative emotion while learning, your endocrine system releases small amounts of epinephrine, increasing your attention and making more robust memories. Your amygdala has found the experience to be salient, and therefore worth your attention and of sufficient value to merit long-term storage in your memory.

Epinephrine levels can be elevated by interest in the topic at hand. Therefore, if you find something you have to do boring, try Edison's trick of reframing: think specifically about how you can benefit from it, and this will more fully engage your mind: how will this be useful to you? (If the answer is "not at all", then you shouldn't be doing it.)

Emotionally salient experiences tend to be the most strongly preserved– you can vividly remember those moments of greatest joy and deepest sadness in your life – the death of a loved one, or special events such as your wedding day tend to leave deep, abiding memories. Experiments have demonstrated humans recall vivid details about locations and activities at the time of major disasters. Animals likewise remember spots in which they receive painful shocks or the route to an escape platform in a water-filled tank.

Your adrenal glands excrete stress hormones critical to memory consolidation during events which are highly emotionally-charged. These stress hormones – glucocorticoids, epinephrine, cortisol, and their *agonists* (chemicals which make their receptors more sensitive) – enhance long-term memory consolidation after emotionally-arousing experiences.

Such emotional arousal appears to trigger the amygdala, which activates the neural circuitry responsible for stress hormone release (the hypothalamus-pituitary-adrenal gland axis). These stress hormones haven't been found to enhance non-emotional memories, however.

The hormones epinephrine and cortisol are secreted by your adrenal glands in response to stressful events, with the degree of activation dependent upon the severity and type of stress. Removing the adrenal glands, on the other hand, impairs memory consolidation of emotionally-charged events.

Directly injecting epinephrine or glucocorticoids after training enhances long-term memory retention of animal training across a variety of tasks, and appears to have the same effect on humans. Norepinephrine also influences forebrain structures which participate in learning and memory, such as the amygdala, as well as the medulla and locus coeruleus, which in turn projects back to the amygdala, hippocampus and prefrontal cortex.

Pleasant experiences including exercise trigger endorphin secretion, also resulting in enhanced learning. Positive social interaction with your co-workers, fellow students, and/or family is also known to increase endorphin levels, leading to enhanced learning and productivity.

How Not To Learn

Cramming, it turns out, is precisely the wrong way to study, particularly if it involves staying up all night. In addition to impairing the neurochemistry of memory consolidation and seriously crippling your focus and concentration, it ignores your limited window of focus.

Short-term cramming of facts into your head to take a test nearly guarantees you'll forget the information in the long run – after you've taken your test, this information will be discarded, and never transferred into your long-term memory referred to by psychologists as the *Zeigarnik Effect*.

What's more, humans and other animals learn more effectively when studies are distributed over time, instead of being performed all at once. Called the *spacing effect*, it's due to the process of long-term potentiation, as short-term memories are *consolidated* (stabilized) into long-term ones. Dr. Takehito Okamoto and colleagues at Japan's RIKEN Brain Science Institute discovered the underlying mechanism by studying eye movement responses of trained mice.

Studying mouse *horizontal optokinetic response* (eye movements which track things moving across the field of vision), the team discovered that learning is strongly dependent upon whether the training is performed all at once, or across spaced intervals. "Crammed" learning vanished within 24 hours, while knowledge acquired through spaced training lasted much longer. The spacing effect seems to be due to the transferal of memory traces from one brain region to another.

Anaesthetizing the region where these temporary memories (of eye movement sequences) were stored, Dr. Okamoto's team saw that learning had vanished in the mice which had crammed for an hour, but the mice which had studied the same amount, spaced out over a four-hour period, were unaffected by the anaesthetic – their learned memories had been transferred from the temporary region to a more permanent storage area.

Too Much or Too Little

While small amounts of epinephrine or glucocorticoids enhance emotional memory consolidation, too little – a bored and inattentive state – or too much – extreme or chronic stress – can impede memory consolidation and even lead to hippocampal damage. The effects depend upon the level of emotional arousal. Stress hormone memory effects require the amygdala, and inactivating it blocks epinephrine and cortisol memory enhancement.

Your amygdala isn't a storage site for these enhanced memory traces, but is instead involved in strengthening consolidation in other brain areas, interacting with regions such as your hippocampus, caudate, insula, cingulate cortex and prefrontal cortex in regulating memory consolidation. PET and fMRI studies have shown amygdala norepinephrine activation from emotional stimuli leads to memories that last for weeks, as the amygdala acts directly upon the hippocampus.

Categorizing

The evolutionary advantage of learning is that experience is encoded as permanent associations, allowing quick categorization and interpretation of what's being experienced in the present; this in turn allows for progressive correction, creating ever-more effective behavioral responses to ensure and maximize survival.

But recall isn't simply matching images or other sensory stimuli; often your brain needs to interpret and give meaning to unfamiliar sensory data. Because of this, your brain attempts to use *heuristics* – general, loose logic which you apply to new sensory information. Your brain doesn't just improve at tasks like spotting a familiar face in a crowd, but instead, previous experience trains your neural circuits to recognize *categories* instead of simply matching visual patterns.

University of Birmingham professor Dr. Zoe Kourtzi researched how experience assists in flexible decision-making. By using fMRI imaging, his team observed how people learn to discriminate between and classify similar visual patterns. Volunteers were taught two different rules for categorizing visual patterns, but members of one category could also be members of other categories. This meant the volunteers had to use abstract classifications for some patterns, rather than simple visual similarity.

According to Dr. Kourtzi, "Based on their findings, they believe that learned information about categories is stored in neural circuitry in the brain's posterior, where it's then fed through to the frontal lobes for use in flexible decision-making and taking appropriate actions."

Thus, your brain seems to recognize objects based not only on shape or pattern recognition, but also through recognition of a low-level set of logical rules. A related 2010 MIT study looked at how the brain applies this logic to object recognition. Take a horse for example: it may be grazing close by or far away, standing in the sunlight or in shadow. Each variation in the horse's position sends a different light pattern to your retinas, but you still recognize it as a horse.

One fundamental law of reality your brain implicitly understands is that real-world objects don't suddenly change identity, so your brain infers that when two visual patterns appear one after another in rapid succession on your retina, they're representations of the same object; these different visual patterns only mean that either you or the object have shifted in space.

There are two types of cognition involved in pattern recognition: getting a general sense of objects, or understanding the relationships between them, and your mind can only process one at a time, according to Princeton University Assistant Professor Nicholas Turk-Browne. Both types involve subconsciously calculating statistics on the fly:

In *statistical summary perception*, your brain infers general properties at a quick glance, for example, determining how many people in a group look happy, or the time of year based on the color and presence of leaves on nearby trees.

In *statistical learning*, over time your brain memorizes *relationships* – organizing the world into patterns, for example, associating a familiar face with a location, learning to predict the trajectory of a moving car, or discovering a building's layout. All three cognitive processes use statistical calculations for different purposes.

These two processes can't be performed simultaneously: as you're learning to recognize a relationship between objects, you can't learn about their general properties, and vice versa.

Learning And Memory Compete

Just as with the mental competition between two aspects of pattern recognition, learning and recall also compete.

An international collaboration between Duke and the University of Amsterdam has found this learning-memory conflict is particularly pronounced during social interactions, which require rapidly exchanging new and old information. During a typical conversation, while absorbing new information from your conversational partner, you're also retrieving memories for appropriate responses.

This 2009 study is the first clear evidence these mental processes cannot occur simultaneously, and thus compete for priority within your mind; it also suggests a single brain region resolves the conflict, efficiently and rapidly switching between memory and learning.

Using a special memory task that forces learning and remembering within a brief span of time, the researchers furnished volunteers with a set of words on a computer screen. As participants tried to quickly remember whether the words they were seeing had previously appeared or not, changing color pictures filled the background. Their brains were scanned with fMRI as they performed the exercises.

After the brain scans, they were surprised with a recall test of the background images instead of the words. The unexpected test showed that learning new images was much more difficult if the volunteers had been trying to remember words at the same time.

FMRI scans showed that as words were being remembered, cortical regions responsible for learning images became less active, demonstrating that the recall process suppressed the learning of new information. However, when the words were forgotten, learning the pictures became easier.

When volunteers were successful at both remembering and learning, a single frontal lobe region showed activity. Those who performed best showed activity in this region. This region seems to function as a mental switchboard – learning and remembering apparently cannot happen simultaneously, so the region appears to assist in rapidly switching between modes of activity.

Patients with damage to the region have difficulty in switching between tasks. They also tend to have trouble in quickly adapting to new situations, preferring to stick to old rules.

The same region also appears to lose functionality with age, but the research team believes future studies will point to methods of training and improving this mental switching circuit.

Praise Undermines Motivation And Performance

Contrary to what you'd expect, telling someone they're "smart" or "talented" may end up handicapping them. Kids in particular can grow up expecting things to come easily, and learn to easily give up when they don't.

Studies show again and again that giving someone vague praise along the lines of *"you're a natural at this"* almost immediately results in worsening their performance. Stanford University psychologist Dr. Carol Dweck says this is because suggesting something is an inborn trait removes the listener's autonomy – they have no control over a "talent". Praising specific examples of effort and improvement do boost performance, however.

In other words, a near sure-fire way to worsen someone's performance is to tell them they're naturally talented at what they're attempting. Kids in particular are very susceptible to this. "When we praise children for their intelligence," says Dr. Dweck, "we tell them that this is the name of the game: Look smart, don't risk making mistakes."

So children get silent and don't attempt difficult things to avoid the chance of being embarrassed. On the other hand, "Emphasizing effort gives a child a variable that they can control," she explains. "They come to see themselves as in control of their success. Emphasizing natural intelligence takes it out of the child's control, and it provides no good recipe for responding to a failure."

Thus, if you want them to succeed, teach your kids that intelligence can be developed through hard work, and that they need to be willing to risk falling and looking stupid if they want to excel. You can see a video of the effects here: http://www.youtube.com/watch?v=TTXrV0_3UjY

Encouraged to Fail

At the University of Bielefeld, German Psychologist Wulf-Uwe Meyer says that children as young as 12 typically believe the praise of a teacher isn't a positive sign – it actually means they lack ability, and the teacher wants to give a boost of encouragement. By the time they become teenagers, they discount praise to the degree that they think *criticism* – not praise – actually conveys a teacher's belief in a student's aptitude. This means that teachers who praise children could be inadvertently conveying the message the student has reached the limit of his abilities, while criticizing a student sends the message that he can improve.

Over 150 studies of praise and academics have shown that students who are frequently praised become *risk-averse* and feel they lack autonomy. Such students tend to engage in "shorter task persistence, more eye-checking with the teacher, and inflected speech, such that answers have the intonation of questions."

For overpraised kids, maintaining image becomes paramount, and they become more competitive and interested in shooting down others. Students praised for their intelligence tend to worry more about their class rank and reputation, rather than to use their time in preparation.

Experiments have shown that when kids are praised for their effort, nearly 90 percent choose increasingly harder tasks, but when praised for their intelligence, almost all choose simpler tasks. According to Dweck, this is because praising kids for intelligence encourages them to "look" smart, and they become concerned with avoiding the risk of making mistakes.

The effect is measurable; when retaking a test on which they scored poorly, students praised for their effort show significant improvement, raising average test scores by 30 percent, but students praised for being "smart" do worse on their tests by nearly 20 percent. Failure deflates "smart" kids so much that their performance measurably regresses. Says Harvard social psychologist Dr. Mahzarin Banaji, "Carol Dweck is a flat-out genius. I hope the work is taken seriously. It scares people when they see these results."

Praise the "process" rather than the trait: "You must have worked really hard" is much better than "You're so smart!" To be effective, researchers have found, praise needs to be specific; for example, in soccer, a team will perform well if they're complimented on something concrete such as "team communication" rather than a blanket "y'dun good!"

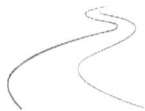

Learning Sculpts the Spontaneous Activity of the Resting Human Brain, Maurizio Corbetta, Chris Lewis, Antonello Baldassarre, et al., 2009, Proceedings of the National Academy of Sciences; DOI: 10.1073/pnas.0902455106

Evaluating the Negative or Valuing the Positive? Neural Mechanisms Supporting Feedback-Based Learning across Development, Anna C. K. van Duijvenvoorde, Kiki Zanolie, Serge A. R. B. Rombouts, Maartje E. J. Raijmakers, and Eveline A. Crone, 17 September 2008, The Journal of Neuroscience

Novel Mechanism for Long-term Learning Identified, Carnegie Mellon University (2008,

January 7), ScienceDaily. Retrieved May 11, 2011, from http://www.sciencedaily.com /releases/2008/01/080103144413.htm

Past Experience Is Invaluable For Complex Decision Making, Brain Research Shows, Dr. Zoe Kourtzi , 2009, Neuron.

When Learning and Remembering Compete: A Functional MRI Study, Huijbers et al, PLoS Biology, 2009; 7 (1): e11 DOI: 10.1371/journal.pbio.1000011

Switchboard In The Brain Helps Us Learn And Remember At The Same Time, Willem Huijbers, Cyriel Pennartz, Sander Daselaar, and Roberto Cabeza, 2009, January 16, Public Library of Science.

Schemas and Memory Consolidation, Dorothy Tse, Rosamund F. Langston, et al, 2007, Science Magazine, Vol. 316 no. 5821 pp. 76-82 DOI: 10.1126/science.1135935; http://www.sciencemag.org/content/316/5821/76.abstract

Role of Cerebellar Cortical Protein Synthesis in Transfer of Memory Trace of Cerebellum-Dependent Motor Learning, Takehito Okamoto, Shogo Endo, Tomoaki Shirao, and

 Soichi Nagao, 2011, The Journal of Neuroscience, 31(24): 8958-8966; doi: 10.1523/?JNEUROSCI.1151-11.2011; http://www.jneurosci.org/content/31/24/8958

Study Says Natural Light Boosts Learning, Kenneth J. Cooper, 11/26/99 The Washington Post

Daylighting in Schools: An Investigation into the Relationship Between Daylighting and Human Performance, August 20, 1999, HESCHONG MAHONE GROUP; http://www.coe.uga.edu/sdpl/research/daylightingstudy.pdf

Easy Ways to Gain Optimal Learning in the Classroom by Activating Different Parts of the Brain, Bruce D. Perry, M.D., Ph.D., Instructor magazine.

Unsupervised Natural Visual Experience Rapidly Reshapes Size Invariant Object Representation in Inferior Temporal Cortex, Nuo Li, James J. DiCarlo. Neuron, 2010; 67 (6): 1062-1075 DOI: 10.1016/j.neuron.2010.08.029

The User's Guide to the Brain, Dr. John J. Ratey , 2002

Executive Function and Achievement and Alters Brain Activation in Overweight Children: A Randomized, Controlled Trial, Catherine L. Davis, et al, Exercise Improves 2011, Health Psychology. 30(1):91-98. doi: 10.1037/a0021766; http://www.ncbi.nlm.nih.gov/pubmed/21299297

Working Memory Capacity Predicts Dopamine Synthesis Capacity in the Human Striatum, Roshan Cools, Sasha E. Gibbs, Asako Miyakawa, William Jagust, and Mark D'Esposito, 2008, The Journal of Neuroscience, January 30, 2008 • 28(5):1208 –1212; http://www.jneurosci.org/content/28/5/1208.full.pdf+html

The Episodic Buffer: a New Component of Working Memory? Alan Baddeley, 2000, Trends in Cognitive Sciences – Vol. 4, No. 11, November 2000, PII: S1364-6613(00)01538-2; http://www.scribd.com/doc/6164570/Baddeley-the-Episodic-Buffer-a-New-Component-of-Working-Memory

Essentials of Understanding Psychology, seventh edition, Robert S. Feldman, 2007, McGraw-Hill Primis

Integrating What and When Across the Primate Medial Temporal Lobe, Yuji Naya and Wendy A. Suzuki, 2011 Science: 773-776 DOI: 10.1126/science.1206773; http://www.sciencemag.org/content/333/6043/773

Changes in Cortical Dopamine D1 Receptor Binding Associated with Cognitive Training, Fiona McNab, Andrea Varrone, Lars Farde, Aurelija Jucaite, Paulina Bystritsky, Hans Forssberg and Torkel Klingberg, Science; http://www.sciencemag.org/content/323/5915/800.abstract

The Brain from Top to Bottom, Bruno Dubuc, 2002, McGill University; http://thebrain.mcgill.ca/flash/d/d_07/d_07_m/d_07_m_tra/d_07_m_tra.html

Local, Persistent Activation of Rho GTPases During Plasticity of Single Dendritic Spines, Hideji Murakoshi, Hong Wang, Ryohei Yasuda, 2010, Nature; DOI: 10.1038/nature09823

Learning and Memory, lecture, Frank Longo, MD, PhD, March 9, 2010 , Stanford Mini Med School, Stanford Continuing Studies, Stanford's School of Medicine; http://med.stanford.edu/minimed/winter/video_window_yt.htm?KeepThis=true&videoFile=a_HfSnQqeyY&titlecard=FrankLongo.jpg&title=Learning%20and%20Memory&TB_iframe=true&height=504&width=600

Rapid Erasure of Long-Term Memory Associations in Cortex by an Inhibitor of PKMzeta, Shema, Sacktor & Dudai, 2007, Science 317: 951-953.

Be Caught Napping: You're Doing More Than Resting Your Eyes, Maquet, P. et al. 2002, Nature Neuroscience, 5 (7); 618–619.

The Restorative Effect of Naps on Perceptual Deterioration, Sara Mednick, et al, 2002, Nature Neuroscience, 5 (7): 677–681.

Protein Essential in Long Term Memory Consolidation Identified, 2011, ScienceDaily;

Sleep Spindle Activity is Associated with the Integration of New Memories and Existing Knowledge, Jakke Tamminen, Jessica D. Payne, Robert Stickgold, Erin J. Wamsley, and M. Gareth Gaskell, 2010, Journal of Neuroscience30 (43): 14356 DOI: 10.1523/JNEUROSCI.3028-10.2010 http://www.jneurosci.org/cgi/content/full/30/43/14356

Deterioration Of Physical Performance And Cognitive Function In Rats With Short-Term High-Fat Feeding, Andrew J. Murray, Nicholas S. Knight, Lowri E. Cochlin, Sara McAleese, Robert M. J. Deacon, J. Nicholas P. Rawlins and Kieran Clarke, Journal for the Federation of American Societies for Experimental Biology doi: 10.1096/fj.09-139691;

Effects of a Saturated Fat and High Cholesterol Diet on Memory and Hippocampal Morphology in the Middle-Aged Rat, Ann-Charlotte Granholm, Heather A. Bimonte-Nelson, Alfred B. Moore, Matthew E. Nelson, Linnea R. Freeman, and Kumar Sambamurtia, National Institutes of Health, Journal of Alzheimer's Dis. 2008 June; 14(2): 133–145;

Working Memory and Academic Learning: Assessment and Intervention, Milton J. Dehn, 2008, John Wiley and Sons, Inc. ISBN-10 047014419X

Subcortical Processing Of Speech Regularities Predicts Reading And Music Aptitude In Children, Dana L Strait, Jane Hornickel and Nina Kraus, 2011; http://www.behavioralandbrainfunctions.com/

151

Effects of a 14-Day Healthy Longevity Lifestyle Program on Cognition and Brain Function, Gary W. Small, M.D., et al, 2006, American Journal of Geriatric Psychiatry 14:6; http://www.rand.org/content/dam/rand/www/external/labor/aging/rsi/rsi_papers/2007_small2.pdf

A Simple Exercise to Boost IQ, Jonah Lehrer, June 11, 2011 The Frontal Cortex, Wired Magazine; http://www.wired.com/wiredscience/2011/06/a-simple-exercise-to-boost-iq/

The 12 Pillars of Wisdom, Adrain M. Owen30 October 2010, NewScientist magazine;

Can Preference For Background Music Mediate The Irrelevant Sound Effect? Nick Perham, Joanne Vizard, 2010, Applied Cognitive Psychology; DOI: 10.1002/acp.1731

Brief and Rare Mental Breaks Keep You Focused: Deactivation and Reactivation of Task Goals Preempt Vigilance Decrements, Alejandro Lleras and Atsunori Ariga, 2011, Cognition, DOI: 10.1016/j.cognition.2010.12.007 http://www.ncbi.nlm.nih.gov/pubmed/21211793

The Surprising Connection between Two Types of Perception, Divya Menon, 2011, Association for Psychological Science; http://www.psychologicalscience.org/index.php/news/releases/the-surprising-connection-between-two-types-of-perception.html

Memory

"Good days are to be gathered like grapes, to be trodden and bottled into wine and kept for age to sip at ease beside the fire. If the traveller has vintaged well, he need trouble to wander no longer; the ruby moments glow in his glass at will."
– Freya Stark, Perseus in the Wind, 1956

It's estimated your memory holds approximately, "...58 holidays you will have taken, the 1700 friends and acquaintances you will have made in your lifetime, the 2100 books you will have read, and the 5800 films you will have seen."

Your very identity is based upon your memories of such experiences. This is largely due to the function of your hippocampus. The hippocampi – one in each brain hemisphere – never rest, but are constantly receiving information about every experience you have, recording the most important of those moments throughout your life. This ongoing recording of your environment is accomplished by making new neural connections. Throughout your brain, dendrite spines "search around", physically moving about in search of new connections. If a neuron is active, it will attract dendrites, and a new connection will form.

Your hippocampus is believed to quickly record facts and events in real-time via these connections, and when you sleep, these temporary memories are transferred to your cortex for long-term storage. If the hippocampus is damaged, however, it can impair the ability to form new memories, and thus to learn new information.

Being able to learn and form new memories is critical to daily functioning, and to preserving your identity – your persistent sense of self and ongoing understanding of the world, allowing you to adapt your behavior as necessary to meet challenges in your environment.

Your memory is believed to reach its full power when you reach the age of 25 – at which point you're capable of processing an estimated 200 separate bits of information in a single second, all while your brain is continuing to monitor and control your body. After about age 27, your memory begins to decline in capacity at a rate of about 2% per decade. Scientists believe this cellular die-off is due to reduced blood flow in the brain.

In healthy individuals, even at age 90 the majority of brainpower (over 80%) is usually retained. But half of those who live past 85 aren't so fortunate, instead falling victim to some form of *dementia* – toxic proteins build up in the brain, impairing its function and contributing to a neural die-off.

A Worm's Memory

Nobel prizewinner Eric Kandel pioneered the use of the sea slug *Aplysia californica* to study memory, because it has a relatively small number of neurons (about 20,000, compared to the estimated five million times as many in humans), some of which are visible to the naked eye. Even with this relatively simple nervous system, Aplysia is capable of learning – forming lasting memories – through the same biochemical processes as animals, including the human animal:

When touched, Aplysia reflexively withdraws its gills. As the touch stimulus is repeated, this withdrawal reflex gradually weakens to the point at which it is finally ignored. This reduction in sensitivity to a repeated stimulus is called *habituation*, a very primitive type of learning common to all animals.

Conversely, in response to an unexpected or strongly aversive stimulus, creatures become increasingly *sensitized* to repetitions over time. The first time the alarming stimulus is encountered, the mental and physical response is short-lived, for just a few minutes or less. Eventually, however, with successive repetitions, sensory responses can be heightened for days or even longer, as the sensitization becomes the basis of a long-term memory.

Making The Connection

In 1949, Canadian psychologist Donald O. Hebb first suggested memories were produced by two nerve cells strengthening their signalling across the synapse.

It was not until nearly three decades later that his theory was proven. Dr. Holger Wigström of Sweden's Göteborg University found that by electrically stimulating a presynaptic neuron at the same time as the postsynaptic neuron, he could improve synaptic signalling. A postsynaptic neuron would respond more easily to the same amount of input from the presynaptic partner. They had discovered the principle that *"nerves which fire together wire together"*, the basis of memory formation.

The NMDA receptor, a protein found on the membranes of postsynaptic neurons, was believed to be a "coincidence detector" which led to this synaptic reinforcement. This also turned out to be correct: in 2001, Princeton's Dr. Joe Tsien found that mice with few hippocampal NMDA receptors showed profound memory deficits. By boosting NMDA receptor production in the hippocampus and cortex, the team created mutant mice with the ability to learn significantly more quickly and retain memories significantly longer than normal.

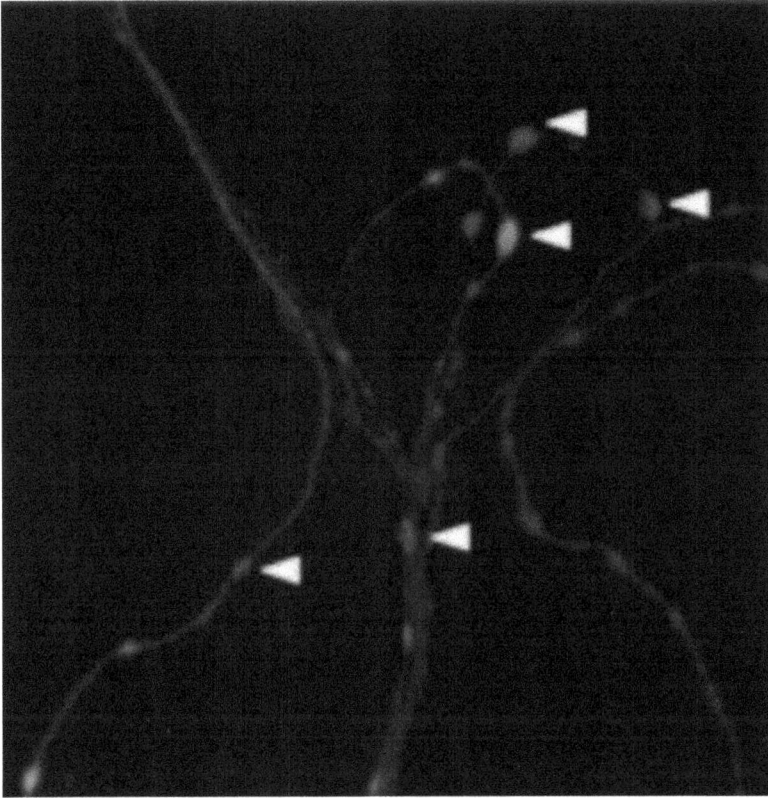

The world's first photograph of a memory trace being formed. Local translation at synapses during long-term synaptic plasticity. Dr. Wayne Sossil and Dr. Kelsey Martin, 2009. Used with permission

The Genius Gene

The transmitting (pre-synaptic) neuron which fires repeatedly creates a stronger response in the receiving (post-synaptic) neuron. This is because the (post-synaptic) neuron has been *sensitized* through new receptor and vesicle growth; the effects last from days to years, and potentially for a lifetime. Chemically, the neurotransmitter glutamate binds to an NMDA receptor, opening an ion channel in the neural membrane to allow a rush of calcium into the post-synaptic dendrite.

This activates a chain of signalling proteins that trigger *phosphorylation*, the chemical uncoiling of a length of DNA for copying. These activated genes build more receptors in the post-synaptic neuron, enhancing its ability to fire, and making signals easier to generate.

Laboratory experiments appear to show that intelligence can be significantly boosted by stimulating this receptor-encoding gene expression. In 1999, Princeton neurobiologist Dr. Joe Z. Tsien created a strain of super intelligent mice by modifying the *NR2B gene*, which encodes NMDA receptors.

Two chemical signals are necessary to trigger the NMDA receptor, the basis of your memory. For example, when you cut your finger, both visual and pain signals arrive in your brain to trigger neurotransmitter release. NMDA receptors then initiate the chemical events which result in long-term potentiation – creating the connection between neurons called a *memory trace*. Assuming you're typical, you'll find the pain to be aversive, and remember not to repeat the experience. A survival-enhancing memory has been formed.

Dr. Tsien found that limiting NR2B expression impedes learning and memory; laboratory mice without the gene were significantly less intelligent than normal. Since 2009, over 30 more proteins have been found which help enhance or impair memory and learning in this way.

Serotonin's Role in Memory

In addition the central glutamate-NMDA receptor synaptic strengthening process, scientists have only recently discovered a second, intriguing piece of the puzzle.

Dr. David Glanzman, UCLA professor of physiological science and neurobiology, has also been studying learning and memory in Aplysia for 25 years. According to Glanzman, the strengthening of synaptic connections is also bound up in serotonin, which binds to receptors on the presynaptic axon and, through a complicated process, causes the growth of new presynaptic axons.

Interestingly, the protein synthesis necessary for axon growth appears to be regulated by calcium on the post-synaptic side of the connection. According to Dr. Glanzman, serotonin binds to receptors on the postsynaptic neuron, triggering an elevation in calcium within the postsynaptic neuron, "...and somehow this elevation of postsynaptic calcium causes synthesis of presynaptic proteins. In other words, the information is going backwards. We don't know yet how that happens.... There's a complicated dance taking place between the postsynaptic cell and the presynaptic cell."

He believes this complex process might be how the brain's protects itself against mistaken learning.

Nature seems not to want your synapses to change very easily. To learn something, you have to produce fairly detailed cellular changes. It looks like you can't just change one side of the synapse if you want to have a long-term memory. You don't want long-term changes at synapses that are important for learning to occur easily. This is a way to minimize mistaken learning; it keeps synapses from changing for unimportant reasons. It's better than a lock-and-key relationship; you can put the key in, but you also have to have a code to get the key to turn to lock something in long-term memory.

In other words, synaptic change requires an interaction between both sides of the synapse; for memories lasting weeks or longer, the presynaptic and postsynaptic cell both need to talk to each other.

Wired Together

Long-term memories are formed after a pattern has been repeated frequently, or if there is sufficient reason for it to be encoded (if it's been assigned a high degree of salience by the amygdala). Every time a group of neurons fires together, the potential for those neurons to fire again increases – when a post-synaptic neuron has been triggered to fire, its surface undergoes chemical changes which make it more sensitive to stimulation from the same neighbor.

Once altered, this post-synaptic cell remains in a state of heightened sensitivity for hours or even days, even if it is not immediately stimulated again. But with each subsequent firing of the presynaptic cell, the post-synaptic cell's sensitivity to its signals increases, until the pair are so well-bound that the merest of activity in the pre-synaptic cell can trigger all the others which have been linked to it to fire, too.

This is one reason it's initially difficult to learn something new, but as signals cross and re-cross the same synaptic gaps at high frequency, the neural pathway is reinforced, and that task becomes progressively easier. After multiple repetitions, using this neural pathway (and therefore using your newfound skill) – becomes effortless, and you can do it any time you wish.

In this way, learning a new skill reorganizes your brain's neurons, reinforcing and creating new synaptic connections. Millions of new neural pathways are created each time a new task is mastered. While repeated use of a connection makes it grow stronger; lack of use can cause a connection to be lost.

Protein translation, the synthesis of new proteins (for dendrites and receptors), is the biological basis of memory storage. Repeatedly and rapidly
exciting a synapse causes a long-term increase in its sensitivity and ability
to transmit – hence the name *long-term potentiation* – an increased *potential* for activation in the future. Calcium ion concentration, an increase in
vesicles, vesicle size, and the addition of receptors can all serve to potentiate
synaptic connections, and as the potential for neurons to fire increases, less
energy is required in the future to activate the same neural circuitry.

> **Prioritizing** – *A constant wash of sensory input from your envi-
> ronment means your brain must have a way to choose what will
> be stored long-term. Professor Lars Olson, who led the discov-
> ery, said there is a neural encoding system in your brain which
> prioritizes experiences - the more important the experience, the
> more vivid and intense your memories of it will be. Prioritiz-
> ing memories determines how much the synaptic connections will
> be strengthened.*
>
> *Dr. Olson says your memories consist of two parts: "content" and
> "importance." The content is the data itself, while its importance to
> your survival determines how strong that memory will become. This
> suggests that you attach a value to everything that you learn, and
> remember or discard information based on how relevant it is to your
> success in life.*
>
> *As he explains it, the importance of a memory is encoded by the
> number and strength of neurons that process or become related to it.
> He also believes that a greater number of neurons attuned to impor-
> tant stimuli (such as the sound of your own name) helps explain why
> you focus your attention upon it in the presence of distractions (like
> at a noisy party).*

Commiting It To Memory

Long term memories last for years, some even a lifetime, comprising
physical changes to your brain, the selective creation and strengthening (or
withdrawal) of neural links. Every thought, action and memory you have is
governed by neurochemical exchanges across synapses in the staggeringly
complex neural network of your brain and body.

Any one memory is comprised of a number of physical neural connections, and some of these connections can be used for several related memories, stored within specialized brain regions throughout your cortex. Memories are links among groups of neurons, and when one fires, it can cause all neurons in the group to fire, producing a specific pattern. All higher brain functions, such as sensory perception, thoughts, ideas, and even hallucinations are composed of the same sort of physical linkage between neurons. For example, a group of adjacent neurons firing simultaneously in your auditory cortex brings about the experience of a specific note in music.

Memory includes three phases: *encoding* (biochemically "recording" important information with the formation of synapses), *storing* (transferring the memories to specialized regions, primarily in the cortex), and *recall* (reactivating the existing traces). Failure in any one of these phases results in forgetting. It's quite possible to have memories stored for years that you never access, but eventually these connections can lose strength, the dendrites withdraw, and the memories disappear.

Short-term memory, also called *working memory*, seems to reside in your prefrontal cortex. This information will be discarded unless you reuse it, link it to something you already know, or find some kind of personal relevance in it. Working memory holds the details of what your brain is currently focusing upon. It's temporary data which remains for about ten seconds, and its capacity appears limited to three to four items at a time – the reason narrative stories and learning tasks organized into groups of three are so powerful. These groups of three to four details can be linked to others and shuffled about for your immediate use. For example, working memory enables you to dial a phone number someone just told you, and is at work while you read, allowing you to keep in mind the content from the previous sentence, so there's a logical continuity with the sentence that follows.

According to Dr. Nelson Cowan of the University of Missouri-Columbia, it's possible to enhance your working memory, conferring great advantages in learning and cognition.

After a salient piece of information is saved as a trace by the hippocampus, it needs to be either discarded (if it's unimportant) or filed away in the appropriate specialized cortical region, if it's important enough for long-term storage. The chemical process of *consolidation* that stabilizes a memory trace after initial learning is LTP.

Shortly after a salient item is learned, it's consolidated through LTP for recall that lasts as long as a few days; if it's useful enough to be kept longer, it will be transferred from the hippocampus to the appropriate cortical region, where it can potentially last a lifetime. A copy of the memory remains in your hippocampus for up to a week after it's first learned, as your hippocampus "teaches" your cortex increasingly more about the memory, until it has eventually been fully transferred to your neocortex for permanent storage.

Whenever that memory is recalled, it must be reconsolidated. This means that, at the point of recall, memories are again in a *labile* (easily altered) state and can easily be wiped out, a recent discovery which has proven useful in treating patients with post-traumatic stress disorder.

The Memory Engine

Scientists have also only recently discovered that the default state of a neuron appears to be a "blank slate", in which memories are constantly wiped clean; maintaining your memory requires constant effort.

According to Reut Shema of the Weizmann Institute of Science, human memory is like a computer's RAM, needing a constant zap of protein "juice" to sustain it. If that enzyme production stops, memories are permanently lost. The protein "juice" sustaining your memories is the enzyme PKMzeta.

For memory to last, a regular "shot" of PKMzeta must be continually supplied. A single dose only lasts for a few days, after which, without another dose, a memory will fade. PKMzeta can revitalize old memories or, if it's in short supply, cause them to vanish forever. This means your synapses need a constant refreshing of this protein to stabilize long-term memories. But once the PKMzeta production cycle has been started, it continues for decades, and potentially indefinitely.

Every time you learn something new, the PKMzeta molecule appears in the synapses, boosting neural transmission across the gap. The presence of PKMzeta doubles the strength of the neural connection. Thereafter, every time that memory is recalled, the synaptic connection once again becomes "plastic", and needs to be restrengthened. But after multiple such recalls, the specific neurons preserving that memory have grown many new, strengthened synapses, and the conductivity becomes much stronger. As with a country road that's been upgraded with gravel, cognitive traffic can now navigate more easily.

Long-term potentiation (LTP) is divided into two stages: *induction*, where information is initially learned, and *maintenance*, where a memory is revitalized. PKMzeta is vital for this maintenance stage. Neutralizing it erases maze-navigating memories from mice hippocampi, and even memories of food preferences – such as dislike of an artificial sweetener – can be permanently erased from regions of the brain processing taste.

On the other hand, an injection of PKMzeta boosts even old, fading memories, in the same manner as sleeping and repetition. PKMzeta increases levels of *AMPAR*, a protein in the synapses that allows fast signals to cross. PKMzeta pushes AMPAR towards the synapse, and each arrival strengthens it further. Other proteins constantly try to pull AMPAR back in from the synapse, but PKMzeta stabilizes its presence. If PKMzeta disappears, AMPAR is pulled from out the synapse up into the presynaptic neuron ("uptake"), the synapse's signalling capacity weakens, and the memory is eventually erased.

This means, of course, that your brain is always about to be erased; PKMzeta appears to be the "memory engine" that keeps it from being turned into a blank state. In other words, your brain's default state is complete ignorance. It takes constant protein production to keep anything in there at all.

Acetylcholine Unlocks Memory Blocks

During the learning process, your brain releases acetylcholine, which functions as a *"store this now!"* command to your brain, one that's critical for new memory formation: in fact, drugs which boost acetylcholine are so far the only known effective treatment for Alzheimer's symptoms.

Acetylcholine allows the "unlocking" of NMDA receptors so synaptic strengthening can proceed. Normally, brain plasticity is held in check by chemical blocks called *SK channels*; these SK channels allow polarizing potassium ions into a neuron. This normally hyperpolarized state restricts NMDA receptor responses to glutamate - the first step in LTP.

The hippocampus appears to be responsible for consolidating short-term memories into long-term ones, but actual memory storage exists throughout your brain, particularly in your temporal lobe and association cortices. The hippocampus organizes both encoding and the retrieval, so if it's damaged, information can't be properly stored or retrieved.

If you recall, the neocortex is highly-evolved in mammals, particularly humans, but the hippocampus is a much older part of the brain, a refinement of the organ called a *pallium*, present since the first *vertebrates* (spiny animals) evolved in the sea 500 million years ago. The pallium, also called the "avian hippocampus", is the organ which birds, fish, reptiles and amphibians use to navigate. Thus, memory and learning in general are refinements of the evolutionarily ancient ability to navigate.

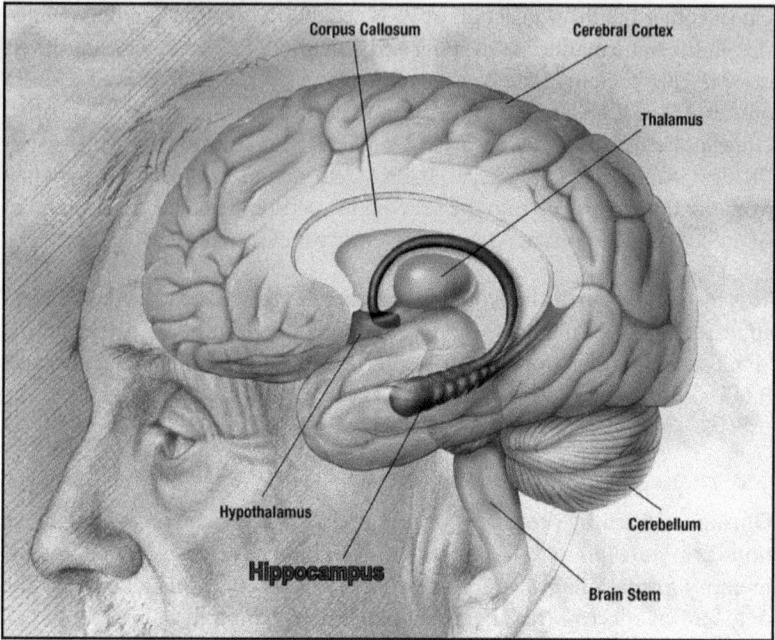

National Institutes of Health, 2009, public domain

Your hippocampus receives visual input from your occipital lobe, auditory input from your temporal lobes, tactile input from your parietal lobe, and olfactory input from your olfactory bulb via your amygdala. It's two-way communication; information comes into your hippocampus, gets processed and goes back out for long-term storage. FMRI scans show the same regions that originally encode or record a memory also reactivate when that memory is recalled, essentially replaying the information from the same cortical sensory region that originally sent the information.

Skills such as playing the piano illustrate this idea of distributed memory. There is a motor/procedural component (pressing the keys), it's tactile, visual (reading the score), and auditory. If there's memory damage, you might lose one component of the skill, but others may be intact.

During *slow wave* (deep) sleep, your hippocampus reactivates recently-formed memories and they are then organized, transferred and consolidated in the appropriate cortical regions for long-term memory storage. This transferal happens gradually (over several days), freeing up hippocampus storage capacity for new memories. Thus sleep is vital for learning and memory formation.

There are three stages of memory processing:

Encoding – (Data entering the hippocampus) When a memory is formed by having an experience or learning a piece of information. Information from among the different sensory systems is transduced, integrated and transmitted as neurochemical impulses, within the hippocampus and the cortex.

Consolidation – (Data being stored and transferred to various regions of the cortex) The information is permanently stored through the process called long term potentiation, which, through protein synthesis and reorganization, enhances the sensitivity (potential) for the synapse to fire again in the future. Potentiation means your brain requires less energy to perform a task that has been habitually repeated. Your hippocampus orchestrates this process. Memories are transferred and saved into a more durable form, stored throughout your brain, in appropriate cortical regions.

Retrieval – (Retrieving these memories from the cortex, back into the hippocampus, and back into consciousness) The process of recalling a memory, as it is retrieved at a future date. It has been suggested that your amygdala-hippocampus perform a sort of "shuffling through" stored memories to accomplish retrieval.

Neural Natural Selection

Forgetting can happen at any of these three stages. It was originally believed that over time your memories fade because of a loss in *myelination,* a wearing down of the fat-like insulation surrounding the axon of nerve cells. Because of this, the ionic charge "leaks" and impulses aren't as easily conducted by neurons. Now however, scientists have found that there's a sort of constant neural natural selection occurring in your brain. University of Michigan Health System researchers demonstrated in 2011 that memory circuits refine themselves through neural competition – a sort of neural "survival of the fittest".

Dr. Hisashi Umemori says neurons grow and extend in pathways which link brain regions, and, as your brain develops, these circuits get fine-tuned, improving their efficiency. He explained to me, however, that rather than neural *apoptosis* (programmed cell death), it's a retraction of the axons. Your brain keeps the best connections and discards bad ones – the dendrites retracting.

Using mice which had been genetically modified so neurons of interest could purposefully be shut off, Dr. Umemori's team focused on a critical link between the hippocampus and cerebral cortex. After switching off about 40 percent of that circuit's neurons, the team observed over three weeks as the mice neurons withdrew all the inactive connections, retaining only the active ones. A follow-up experiment showed that if the neurons in the entire circuit were deactivated, their connections were still preserved, however, presumably as a functional fail-safe.

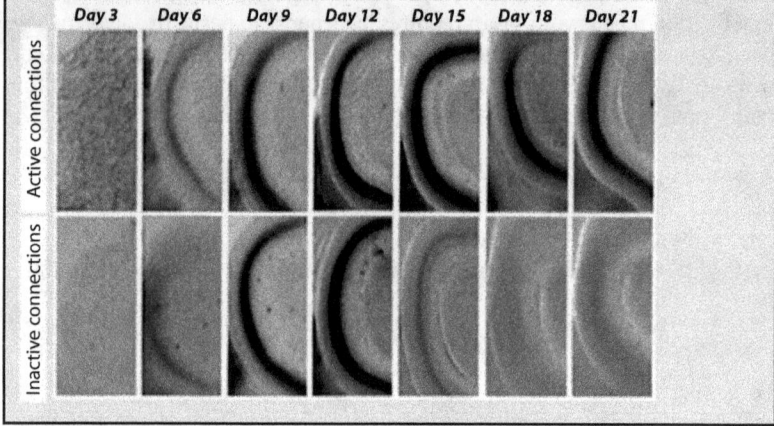

This illustration demonstrates how inactive neral connections are eliminated during development.

The top row shows the brain with all neurons kept active and the bottom row shows a brain with 40 percent of neurons that have been switched off.

As the numbers count forward in days, the dark band - derived from targeted cells that can be switched off - shows the neural connection being formed. In the lower row, the disappearance of the band demonstrates that deactivated connections have been eliminated.

	Day 3	Day 6	Day 9	Day 12	Day 15	Day 18	Day 21

University of Michigan, Dr. Hisashi Umemori. Used with permission.

Said Dr. Umemori:

> *This tells us that the brain has a way of telling among a group of neurons which connections are better than others. The neurons are in competition with each other. So when they're all equally bad, none can be eliminated.... The better the brain is at eliminating bad connections to keep the circuitry at its most efficient, the more efficient learning and memory will be as well.*

In adults, *neurogenesis* – the growth of new brain cells – only seems to occur throughout life in the olfactory bulbs and the *dentate gyrus* region of the hippocampus. All the current research indicates that you're otherwise born with all the brain cells you'll possess for life.

Dr. Umemori's team found that in the dentate gyrus, a type of "neural natural selection" was occurring, as newly-born cells competed with mature cells for survival.

Additionally, according to UCLA neurobiologists Dr. Alcino J. Silva and Sheena A. Josselyn, your brain is protected from a constant bombardment of useless information by actively memory suppression. An enzyme called *PP1* (protein phosphatase 1) naturally suppresses memories, but can be switched off when needed:

> *Like other biological processes, memory is regulated by yin-and-yang interactions between molecules with opposing functions – in this case, protein phosphatases and kinases, which respectively remove and add phosphate groups on target proteins, thereby altering their properties.*

These special molecules acts as "on/off switches" for enzymes and receptors functions. In memory, *kinases* are the "on" switch, while *phosphatases* are the "off" switch.

Types Of Memory

There are four broad categories of memory:

1. *Short-Term (Immediate) Memory*

2. *Working Memory*

3. *Declarative Memory* – Long-term declarative (conscious) memories are stored in your association areas – faces and visual features of objects in your visual association area, tunes in your auditory association area, etc.

   A. Episodic – These are memories of the events in your life – part of what makes up your unique identity.

   Long-term episodic (autobiographical) memories about time and place are stored in association areas in your frontal lobes. Spatial-navigational memories, however, remain in your hippocampus.

   B. Semantic – These are memories of dry facts, like dates or names, word definitions or historical facts. Semantic memories are distributed throughout your cortex (in multimodal association areas), but organized in categories according to the logical properties of the item in question.

4. *Nondeclarative (subconscious) memory*

   A. Procedural – These are motor program memories which allow you to do everything from waving hello to driving a car. After you have practiced to a sufficient degree, they operate without your need to focus upon them.

B. Priming – Mental preparation for later events, including the power of suggestion

C. Associative (Classical conditioning and Fear Memories) – This is when answers "jump out at you", based on associations with known data. It's also the basis of "conditioned" learning – linking of one type of information with another. This is how, for example, Pavlov trained his dogs to mentally link a ringing bell with the presence of food, so that eventually the sound of the ringing bell alone, as much as the food itself, could stimulate hunger.

D. Nonassociative – Gradual sensitization and desensitization (habituation) Please the the following illustrations.

Cliques

Six years after creating his "Einstein mice", in 2005, Dr. Joe Tsien discovered that specific aspects of experiences are encode and organized in discrete neural clusters he called *cliques*. The information ranges from the very general to the very specific, grouped into hierarchies.

Dr. Tsien and his team monitored 260 neurons in the CA1 region of a mouse's hippocampus, which encodes *episodic* (personal experiences) and *semantic* (facts) data in both mice and people. The CA1 region receives input from several brain regions and sensory systems, and then converts these sensory stimuli into memory traces. The team created simulations of distressing events such as earthquakes (shaking small containers with mice inside), owl attacks (a sudden air puff blown at their backs (simulating an owl attack from above) and free fall (using a cookie jar as a small elevator). Each mouse experienced seven episodes of each distressing event, separated by resting periods of several hours. During the events and resting periods, an EEG machine plotted the firing of each neuron from 260 separate CA1 cells.

While memories were being formed, the events would "replay" – the same firing pattern which occurred as the mouse experienced each event would repeat several times up to a few minutes after the events, gradually decreasing in amplitude (signal strength), suggesting the experiences were being recalled. This replaying of events was the mouse recalling sensory stimuli of the distressing events after they had occurred.

Each aspect of the events was recorded by a discrete clique – a separate, cluster of hippocampal neural cells, which represented one specific aspect of the experience, from the general to the specific.

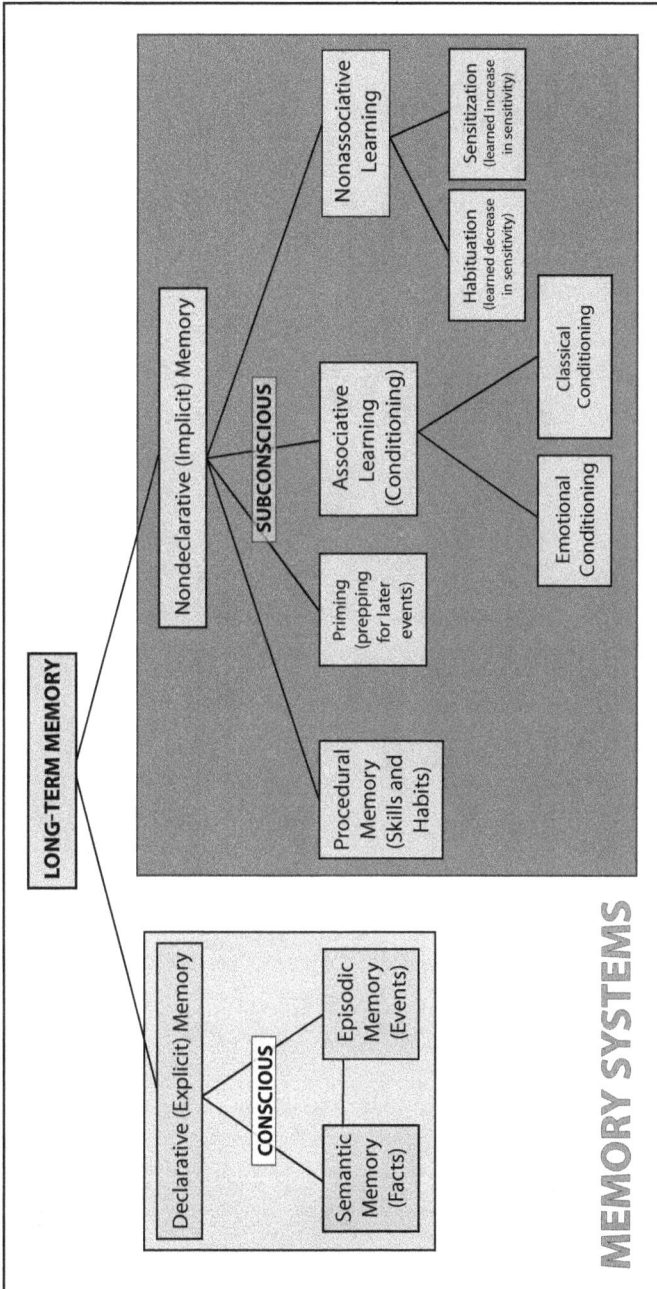

MEMORY SYSTEMS

LONG-TERM MEMORY

Declarative (Explicit) Memory
CONSCIOUS
- Semantic Memory (Facts)
- Episodic Memory (Events)

Nondeclarative (Implicit) Memory
SUBCONSCIOUS
- Procedural Memory (Skills and Habits)
- Priming (prepping for later events)
- Associative Learning (Conditioning)
  - Emotional Conditioning
  - Classical Conditioning
- Nonassociative Learning
  - Habituation (learned decrease in sensitivity)
  - Sensitization (learned increase in sensitivity)

Adapted from Learning and Memory: How it Works and When it Fails,
Dr. Frank Longo, Stanford University, 2010

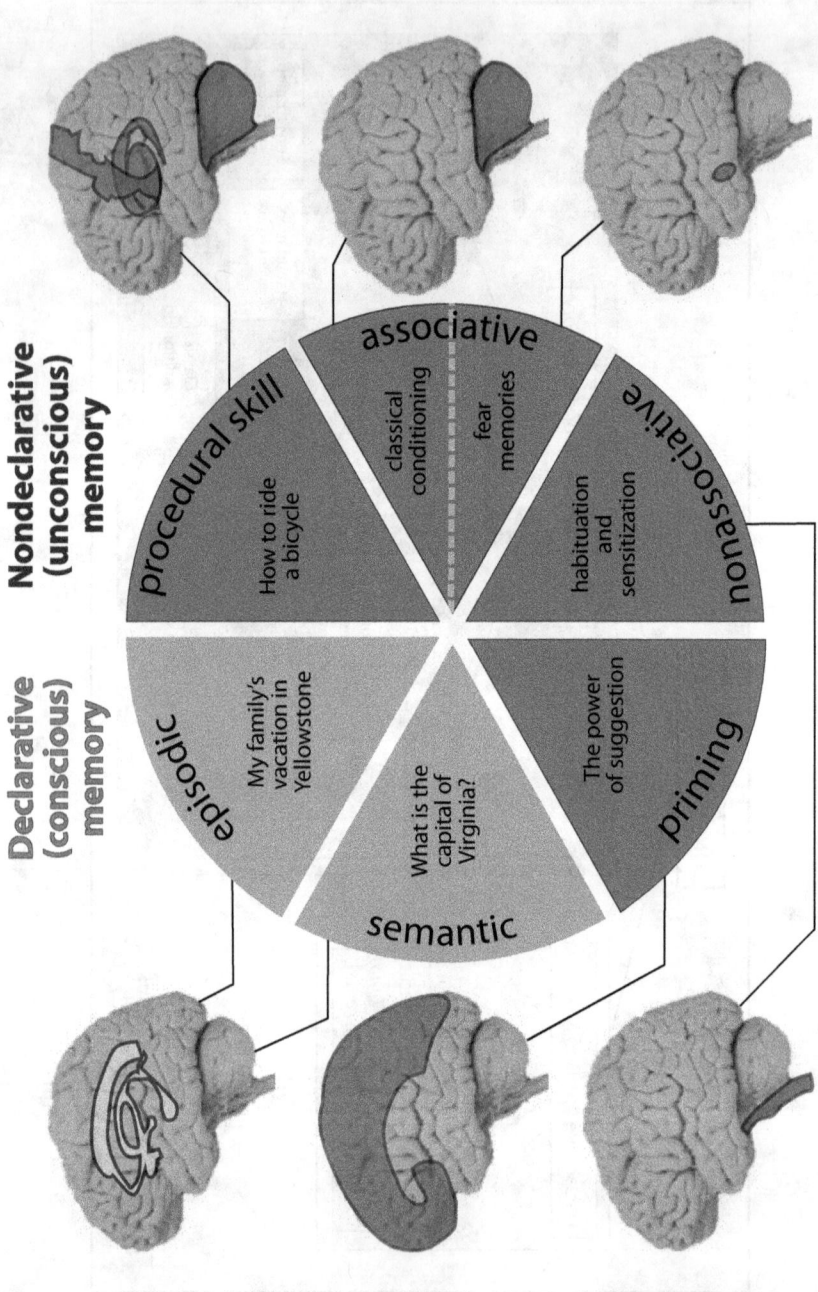

Memory storage and retrieval centers, copyright 2011, Polyglot Studios, KK

Cells in one clique share similar firing patterns, but don't participate in the activity of other cliques, each clique operating independently. Information in these cliques is organized hierarchically, with the most general at the top, and the most specific at the bottom. Each hierarchy can also be part of an even greater, more general hierarchy, representing all types of a specific category, for example "all startling events".

These functional groups operate as a unit to recreate experiences in the minds of animals like mice and humans. Each clique encodes different sensory aspects of events – some were involved in recording and replaying motion-related data, some with location, and some with the simple state of being startled. The cliques also vary in terms of content, in a hierarchy from the general and abstract to the specific and concrete. Says Dr. Tsien, the brain encodes information just like a computer's *binary code* – electrical ons and offs, which can be converted into sequences of ones and zeros, representing everything from colors to sounds to shapes, even complex movement and mathematical calculations.

This organization of encoding allows for virtually limitless flexibility, allowing for a an almost unlimited number of combinations to be generated to represent life experiences. Simple signal flow from one neuron to the next is insufficient for processing perceptions and memories. Just as computers work on the principle of "parallel processing", in the human brain, an entire network of neurons is involved in the process.

For mice, the clique – hippocampal neural group – encoding a memory of a simulated earthquake is represented by 11001. In a mouse brain, this encodes the sequence "startling event", "disturbing motion", "no air puff", "no drop", and "shake", while a sudden drop is represented by 11010: "startling event", "disturbing motion", "no air puff", "drop", and "no shake".

Says Dr. Tsein in *Scientific American:*

> *...because the memory code is categorical and hierarchical, representing new experiences might simply involve substituting the specific cliques that form the tops of the memory pyramids to indicate, for example, that the dog barking behind the hedge this time is a poodle instead of a German shepherd or that the earthquake took place in California rather than in Indonesia. The fact that each memory-encoding pyramid invariably includes cliques that process rather abstract information also reinforces the idea that the brain is not simply a device that records every detail of a particular event. Instead neural cliques in the memory system allow the brain to encode the key features of specific episodes and, at the same time, to extract from those experiences general information that can be applied to a future situation that may share some essential features but vary in physical detail. This ability to generate abstract concepts and knowledge from daily episodes is the essence of our intelligence and enables us to solve new problems in the ever-changing world.*

Consider, for instance, the concept of 'bed.' People can go into any hotel room in the world and immediately recognize the bed, even if they have never seen that particular bed before. It is the structure of our memory-encoding ensembles that enables us to retain not only an image of a specific bed but also a general knowledge of what a bed is. Indeed, my colleagues and I have seen evidence of this in mice. During the course of our experiments, we accidentally discovered a small number of hippocampal neurons that appear to respond to the abstract concept of "nest." These cells react vigorously to all types of nests, regardless of whether they are round or square or triangular or made of cotton or plastic or wood. Place a piece of glass over the nest so the animal can see it but can no longer climb in, and the nest cells cease to react. We conclude that these cells are responding not to the specific physical features of the nest—its appearance or shape or material—but to its functionality: a nest is someplace to curl up in to sleep."

This seems to be the basis of organization for all aspects of cognition and mental experience. In a fascinating aside, Dr. Itzhak Fried of UCLA even discovered an epileptic patient with one specific hippocampal clique that responds only to the actress Halle Berry.

Dr. Tsien asserts that, as technology progresses, eventually we'll likely have a means of reading enough human neurons simultaneously to reveal human thoughts – mind-reading machines. This idea will come as no surprise to Ray Kurzweil – dubbed the modern-day Edison – who has long held that you'll eventually be able to "download" your entire mind into a storage device:

Someday intelligent computers and machines equipped with sophisticated sensors and with a logical architecture similar to the categorical, hierarchical organization of memory-coding units in the hippocampus might even do more than imitate, perhaps exceeding our human ability to handle complex cognitive tasks.

In terms of duration, memory proceeds through three phases:

1. **Sensory Memory** – the brief moments a stimulus is held in your mind after its experience.

2. **Working Memory** – information held in your mind as it's used for analysis, planning, calculations, etc.,. before being either discarded or stored.

3. **Long-term Memory** – information which is salient – important enough for your brain to store – is encoded in memories by physical changes to the structure of a neuron's dendrites, receptors, and vesicles.

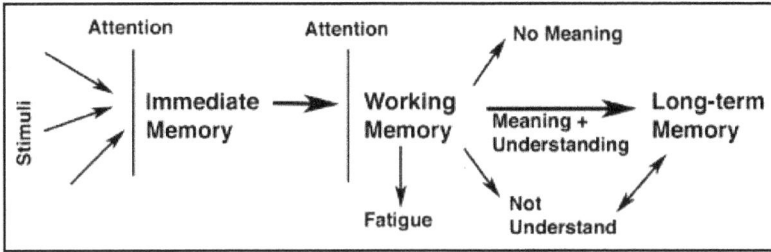

*Memory with **meaning** (salience) that's **understood***
(related to existing schema) is selected for long-term memories.

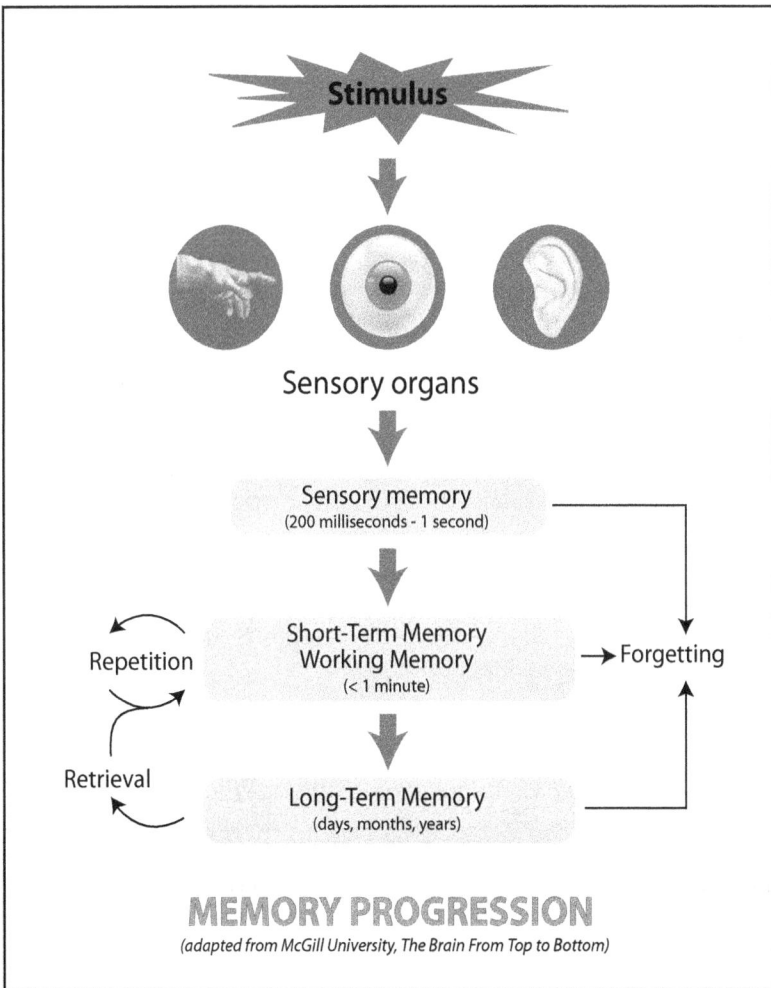

Stimulus

Sensory organs

Sensory memory
(200 milliseconds - 1 second)

Repetition

Short-Term Memory
Working Memory
(< 1 minute)

→ Forgetting

Retrieval

Long-Term Memory
(days, months, years)

MEMORY PROGRESSION
(adapted from McGill University, The Brain From Top to Bottom)

Sensory Memory

This is the brief imprint of stimulus upon your nervous system, which quickly fades. After a flash of lightning, for example, the image will still be in front of your eyes for a few seconds.

Working Memory

Working memory is a kind of mental "scratch pad", as you plan, calculate, evaluate, analyze, and compare, etc. Your prefrontal cortex seems to hold your working memory, using it for short-term calculations or tasks such as remembering a phone number just long enough to dial it.

Your limbic system connects with the part of your cortex that houses working memory, which is why, when your limbic system has you in its emotional grip, this functionality is impaired. It's difficult to concentrate or think clearly when you're under stress or excessive worry. You find it difficult to focus, learn, remember or make sound decisions: as Daniel Goleman puts it, "stress makes people stupid".

Humans can consciously process five to nine pieces of information at a time, depending upon individual capacity. While processing, these pieces of information are held in short-term "working" memory. Short-term memory capacity has a tremendous impact upon your powers of reasoning, decision-making, calculations, and even willpower – the higher your capacity, the stronger your mental abilities will be. This short-term memory capacity depends upon the relationship between two brainwave frequency ranges, according to 2012 experiments at the Polish Academy of Science's Nencki Institute of Experimental Biology. Neurotransmission occurs in brainwaves of specific patterns of frequencies, and these are classified into different frequency ranges, including the slow theta waves of reflective states and fast gamma waves of region-to-region transmission.

An electroencephalography machine (EEG) uses electrodes on a subject's scalp to record changes in neurotransmission speed (frequency) and strength (amplitude) of neurotransmission. Theta waves are very slow - 4-7 *Hertz* or cycles per second. They're strongest during moments of internal focus, including meditation, prayer, and spiritual states.

Gamma waves (above 25 Hz) are the only frequency range found throughout the brain, and allow processing between different brain regions.

Scientist have long known the two types of waves are necessary for the use of short-term memory; as people attempt memory tasks, an increase in theta and gamma activity can be observed. Short-term memory capacity depends upon how many gamma cycles can be generated in the space of one theta cycle. In other words, as few as five or as many as nine cross-regional gamma signals are sent during the same time as one slow theta signals.

An individual's neurotransmission efficiency is what determines this ratio - and the number of items he or she can hold in working memory at a time.

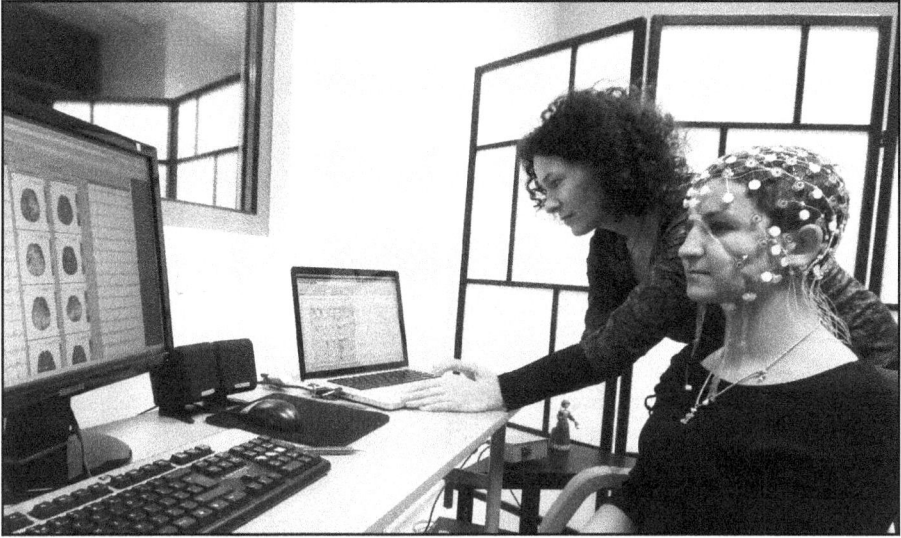

Dr. Aneta Brzezicka monitors the brainwave activity of a volunteer with an EEG machine, 2011. When an electroencephalography machine (EEG) is used, the electrodes are placed onto a subject's scalp, and they record changes in speed (frequency) and strength (amplitude) of the brain's neurotransmission. Nencki Institute of Experimental Biology, Warsaw, Poland. Used with permission.

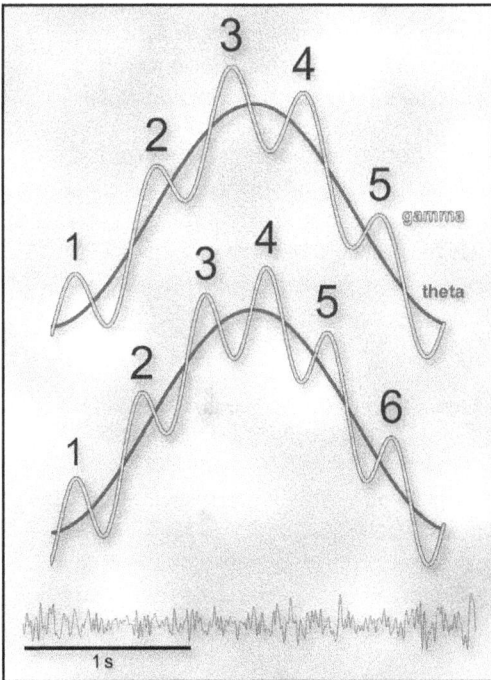

Neurotransmission occurs in brainwaves of specific patterns of frequencies, and these are classified into different frequency ranges, including the slow theta waves of reflective states and fast gamma waves of region-to-region transmission. Experiments at the Nencki Institute of Experimental Biology in Warsaw show that the more gamma cycles that fall within one theta cycle, the larger one's short-term memory capacity will be. A typical chart of brain's electric activity (EEG) is shown at the bottom. Kamiński J., Brzezicka A., Wróbel A., 2011, Short-term memory capacity (7 ± 2) predicted by theta to gamma cycle length ratio, Neurobiology of Learning and Memory) 95(1): 19-23. Used with permission.

173

"We are able to memorize as many 'bites' of information as there are gamma cycles for one theta cycle," according to lead experimenter Jan Kamiński. One such 'bite' of information can be a number, letter, idea, situation, picture or smell. The capacity of short-term memory depends upon a ratio of theta- to gamma-frequency range brainwaves.

Working memory is compartmentalized into *verbal, visual, spatial* and *nonverbal* information. The verbal component of working memory seems to use words, while another part of the memory system constantly "refreshes" it – your cingulate cortex repeatedly "zapping" the cells containing the data to keep it in memory. Nearly your entire cortex uses working memory, which can consist of information that's either just been perceived, or has been retrieved from long-term memory storage.

Working memory holds details and steps involved in actions or calculations being undertaken. It's constantly changing in content, unlike long-term memory storage, and appears to be rather limited, able to efficiently hold between three to nine specific items at a time.

This mental scratch pad appears to be used by areas distributed throughout your cortex, regions specialized for tasks such as visual analysis, verbal skills, and spatial memory working parallel. For example, when an object's *appearance* is being remembered, the temporal visual association area is activated; the object's *name* involves language-processing in regions like Broca's area; and the object's *location* activates the temporal lobe and parietal association areas.

Your prefrontal cortex appears to direct choosing and maintaining attention upon immediately useful items in working memory, but various regions contribute to this mental "scratch-pad". One area (your anterior cingulate) keeps triggering the memory "refresh" process to keep a piece of data in focus, while another (the dorsolateral prefrontal cortex) controls *attenuation* – the selective dampening down of irrelevant details.

Experiments support the theory that working memory is comprised of four components – a *central executive*, which supervises three parallel "slave systems" called the *phonological loop, visuospatial sketchpad* and *episodic buffer*:

Phonological loop – This sound-based temporary memory system allows you to remember about four to seven numbers, letters, or words in sequence. Its contents rapidly decay, so it uses *rehearsal*, the "inner voice" you hear in your head, repeating words in a loop to prevent them from fading from your memory while you need them.

The phonological loop allows for *echoic memory*, your ability to recall a few seconds of information, even if you weren't paying direct attention to it. For example, if someone's been talking to you, and you haven't been really listening, they may say to you, *"Hey! You're not listening to me!"* In your defense, you respond with, "No, I *was* listening! You said...." And are able to repeat their words back to them - even if you weren't really listening.

The phonological loop (from the Greek words for sound and words) begins in the auditory cortex when words are heard, or in the visual cortex, when words are read. Wernicke's area and the angular gyrus integrate auditory and visual information into a perceptual experience, and your memory contains a "lexicon" - a list of words (sounds) and the meanings you've attached to them.

The phonological loop varies from person-to-person in terms of capacity and strength, but it can be improved through practice. As with most brain functions, its power increases with use; those who use it frequently have it developed to a greater degree than others. You can significantly improve sound-related memory functionality by exercising your auditory recall through language study, stage acting, practicing a musical instrument, or learning musical composition. Actors and professional musicians generally have this capacity developed to a high degree; if you've ever played a major role in a stage drama, you know the amount of memory and effort involved in memorizing dialogue for an hour-and-a-half-long play.

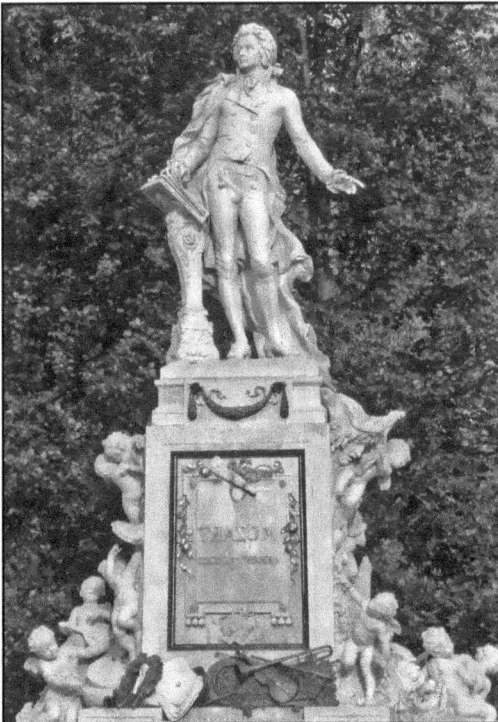

Austrian composer Wolfgang Amadeus Mozart (1756-1791) Marble sculpture, Burggarten Park, Vienna. Viktor Tilgner, 1896.

Visuospatial sketch pad (VSSP) – Complementing the phonological loop is the subsystem called the *visuospatial sketchpad*. This type of working memory holds recent information about shapes, colors, and the location or velocity of objects in space, their positions relative to one another and to the onlooker. It also appears to be involved in planning spatial navigation. In right-handers, the VSSP is mainly located in the right hemisphere of the brain in the occipital and parietal lobes.

Most people are generally able to hold in short-term memory the detailed appearance of three to four objects at a time. Like the phonological loop however, the VSSP can be dramatically improved with practice. Again, firing neural circuits repeatedly strengthens conductivity, allowing for easier access in the future, and so exercising a function strengthens it. With visualization exercises (like those in book I's meditations) or artistic training, the VSSP can be developed to produce much more vivid, detailed images.

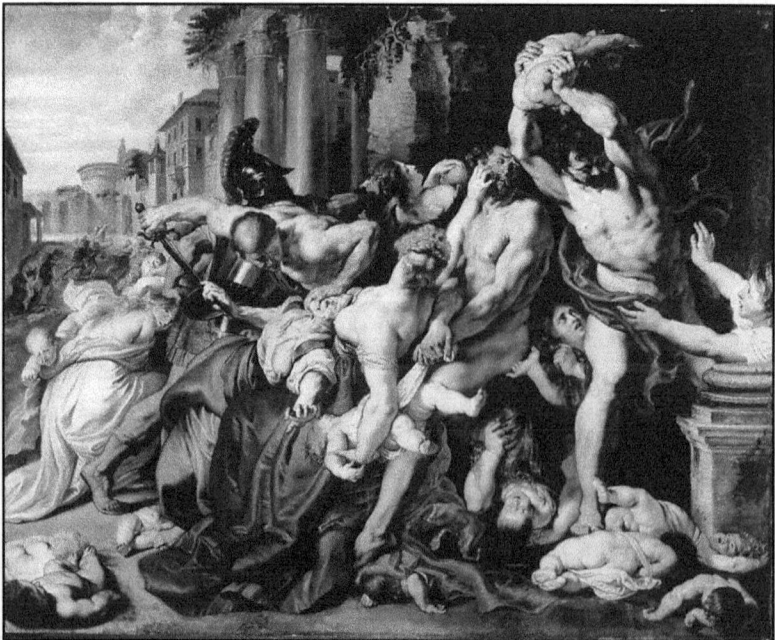

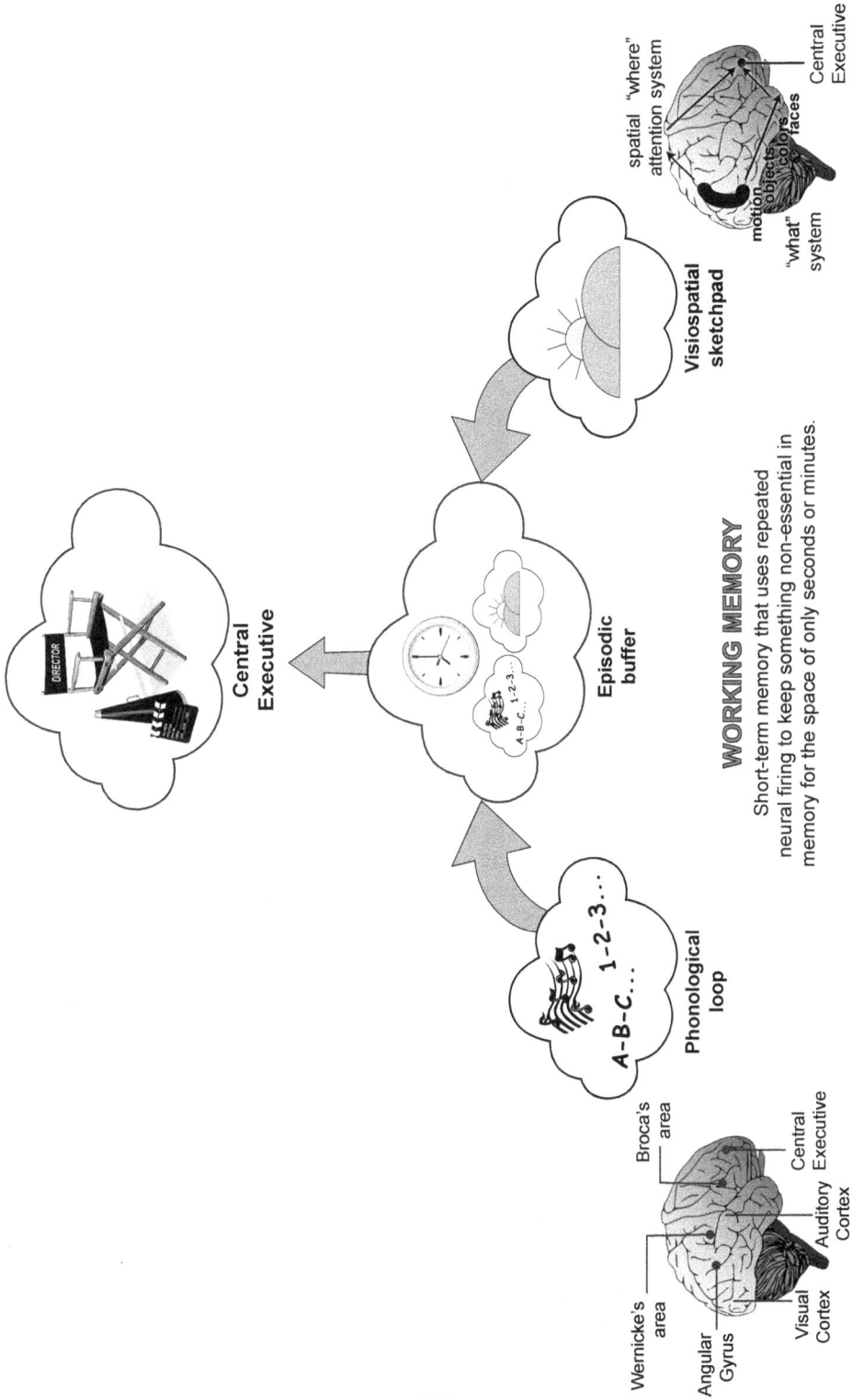

Central Executive

Visiospatial sketchpad

spatial "where" attention system

Central Executive

motion objects colors faces

"what" system

Episodic buffer

Phonological loop

A-B-C... 1-2-3...

WORKING MEMORY

Short-term memory that uses repeated neural firing to keep something non-essential in memory for the space of only seconds or minutes.

Wernicke's area

Broca's area

Central Executive

Angular Gyrus

Auditory Cortex

Visual Cortex

> **The Great Paint-Off** – *The VSSP is most highly-developed among visual artists, designers, photographers and architects; but history's greatest master of visual recall was reported to be Peter Paul Rubens, the 16th century Flemish painter, diplomat and knight, whose Massacre of the Innocents (pictured above) recently fetched £49,000,000 at a 2002 Sotheby's auction.*
>
> *Rubens was reported by his students to have an extraordinary visual memory; when criticized by a fellow artist for "lazily" wandering around observing his surroundings instead of painting, Rubens challenged his critic to a "paint off" – and rendered a more detailed version of a scene from memory alone than his critic could paint while looking directly at the same scene.*

Episodic buffer – The third parallel working memory system links visuospatial and auditory information along with logical time sequences, integrating them into "episodic" short-term memories of scenes, like story or movie scenes.

Central executive – This is the controlling function of working memory, which initiates, selects and terminates memory processing (encoding, storage, or retrieval). It's this portion of working memory which coordinates information from a variety of sources, directs focus, switches attention, organizes incoming sensory input, retrieves long-term memories and combines all the data for conscious awareness. This is the portion of memory used to perform tasks like comparison or mathematics.

Recent studies suggest the central executive may not be solely centralized in the prefrontal cortex as was formerly believed, but may be distributed, based on which type of function it's performing.

Please see the following illustration for the relationships between the subcomponents of working memory.

Subconscious (Nondeclarative) Memory

All *nondeclarative learning* is below the level of your consciousness, reorganizing your subcortical synapses. For example, conditioning of reflex reactions depends upon your cerebellum, and emotional conditioning (assigning an emotional value to something in the environment) is primarily governed by your amygdala. There are five types of nondeclarative memory:

1. *Procedural memory* – Complex motor skills like riding a bicycle or brushing your teeth, skills performed without having to consciously walk through the steps. These memories persist for life, unless there is significant brain trauma or disease. The brain regions involved in procedural memories include the cerebellum and putamen, while deeply ingrained habits are stored in the caudate.

2. *Priming* – This is a mental preparation, visual or auditory cues influencing later responses – the power of suggestion. *Positive priming* will speed up processing of related information, while *negative priming* will slow down such processing.

   This neural "prepping" occurs below the level of conscious thought, but still has a strong effect upon later responses. Priming is the principle behind subliminal advertising (which, contrary to earlier widespread debunking, has recently been demonstrated to have potentially dramatic effects).

   According to theory, the relevant neurocircuitry has been activated at a low level, so less energy is necessary to activate that circuit at a later time. Negative priming is not well understood, but it's thought that ignoring a priming trigger once means your brain assigns it low salience, so you become less sensitive to stimuli related to that trigger.

3. *Classical conditioning* – Conditioning is a mental linking of two previously unrelated cues in the environment, the basis of Pavlov's famous experiment, and one of the reasons cravings for drugs or other desires can be triggered by unrelated stimuli such as seeing a former associate, visiting a previous "hangout", or after activities such as eating or sex.

4. *Fear memory* – When delivering aversive (unpleasant) stimuli such as painful shocks, fear memories can be induced. Such overwhelming, traumatic events, or more gradual chronic exposure can build fear memories, resulting in fright in the presence of specific stimuli, such as a dog or the site of an accident you were in.

   The amygdala is central to such memories. At the extreme, there are *phobias* – excessive or unreasonable fear of objects, places or situations. *Desensitization* is an effective form of *behavior therapy* which gradually exposes phobics to fearful stimuli, while learning to calm themselves in its presence.

5. **Nonassociative memory** – *Habituation* is the gradual desensitization to an outside stimulus like a repeated sound, while *sensitization* is an increased sensitivity to a stimulus like pain.

Conscious (Declarative) Memory

Declarative or *explicit* memories are conscious memories of events from life, or of general facts. Declarative memories are retrieved on a conscious level – you recall memories about last weekend's party, for example, through conscious effort. This is the memory you call upon throughout the day to remember appointments or recall a friend from the past.

Declarative memories are either *semantic* – dry facts not necessarily tied to personal experience – or *episodic* – memories of events in your life, experiences such as taking a cruise to the Bahamas. Your brain gradually reorganizes, builds upon and improves associations between related, previous facts or experiences in your long-term memory.

The strength of these associations – actual physical neural structures – determines how easy or difficult new memories are to recall later. In practical terms, this means the more your brain reorganizes this data, the better you'll be able to remember it. Thinking about the data, writing it down, studying it and discussing it all helps to reinforce this kind of memory, and the more you repeat it (*rehearsal*), the better you'll be able to recall it.

Several neural structures are involved in declarative memory, but your hippocampus and its related support structures appear the most important for declarative memory formation and retrieval. Aside from its navigational functions, psychologists believe your hippocampus is used for three functions: overseeing episodic memory formation, finding commonalities among episodic memories, and linking these episodes based upon these commonalities. When you first experience an event, a memory link forms in your hippocampus so you can retrieve that memory in the future. Additional links are then made for details relating to the episode.

For example, when you first visit a place, a new link is created to represent it. Additional links are created for related information, such as who you were with at the time, buildings you saw in the setting, etc. The more frequently you retrieve and build upon the memory of that episode, the stronger the links become, making it easier and faster to recall the event and details related to it.

Experiences destined for long-term consolidation are first held within your hippocampus and, during sleep, replayed and transmitted to appropriate regions of your cortex; thereafter, each rehearsal strengthens a memory's permanency and mental impact. When such memories have become firmly established in your cortex, your hippocampus is no longer necessary for retrieval.

Dreams are thus thought to be a sort of replay (although unrestricted by normal logic) of the day's events, as they're relayed to your cortex by your hippocampus. The hippocampus also stores a mental "grid" of areas, and is engaged by your cortex when you decide if an event or situation is unique or similar to others.

Your PFC is involved in mental "time travel" – re-experiencing events from your past or using those memories to construct possible future events. Your amygdala is triggered for encoding and retrieving highly emotionally-tinged memories, such as the dismantling of the Berlin Wall or the explosion of the Challenger shuttle. Such memories are much more vivid than emotionally-neutral ones, and brain scans have shown amygdala activity during such recall.

The Impact of Stress

Excessive stress significantly impairs the formation of declarative memories.

Canadian neuroscientist Dr. Sonia Lupien led an experiment in three stages: In stage one, volunteers were divided into two groups that memorized the same group of words. In stage two, the experimental group gave a stressful impromptu public speech, while the control group did not. In stage 3, both groups were instructed to recall the words they had memorized.

Volunteers who had undergone the stressful task (the speech) had impaired declarative memory formation, while the control group, which had memorized the same words but not participated in public speaking, had no problem remembering the word list. This has important implications for students in particular – if you want to enhance your academic performance in areas involving semantic memory (memorization of facts such as with anatomy, history, etc.), you need to reduce your stress as much as possible.

Prolonged post-traumatic stress disorder (PTSD) in particular has been shown to lead to both a decrease in physical volume of the hippocampus, and in declarative memory performance. Cortisol, produced by stress, specifically inhibits hippocampus and PFC functionality.

Semantic Memory

This is your factual knowledge – dates, numbers, addresses, etc., filed by your brain within categories and generally involving your left temporal lobe. Because your brain is associative, semantic memories are organized by *schemata*, a web like series of related connections between facts, grouped according to categories. This is essential for understanding the underlying logic of things in everyday life.

Episodic Memory

These are the events of your life and related information such as your emotional reactions. Essentially your autobiographical memory, these are the stories you tell yourself about your past. Episodic memories can be deliberately remembered (recalled at the command of your frontal lobes), or they can be inadvertently triggered by outside stimuli, and odors in particular. This is almost certainly because of your olfactory bulb's close connections to your hippocampus and amygdala.

> *Remembering The What And When Of Events* – *New York University researchers say the medial temporal lobe (MTL) plays a central role in episodic and semantic memory. Your MTL encodes sequences – "what happened when" during an episode from your past, like the order of songs at a concert or what happened before the winning home run in the World Series. Drs. Yuji Naya and Wendy Suzuki monitored the MTL of animals as they correctly recalled sequences of visual objects, and found two main MTL areas used to integrate what and when: the hippocampus and perirhinal cortex.*
>
> *Your hippocampus supplies an incremental timing signal between events, providing information about the passage of time, while your perirhinal cortex integrates information about what and when, indicating the order of items in a sequence.*

Days of Future Past

Neural circuits used in recalling the past and imagining the future are remarkably similar. Using real-time brain scans, Washington University psychologists have found the same brain regions fire in a nearly identical pattern whether you're recalling the past or imagining the future. Scientists had previously believed imagining the future only engaged your frontal cortex – an act of pure imagination.

By measuring brain activity while college students recalled past events and then envisioned future events, they found that remembering the past and imagining the future are very closely linked, which offers hope for victims of memory loss.

According to lead researcher Dr. Kathleen McDermott, imagining yourself in the future and remembering yourself in the past activate the same neural pathways. This sort of "mental time travel", she says, heavily uses your brain's memory, whether you're reminiscing about the past or considering the future. In other words, you use your past experiences and memories to construct future scenarios.

Although your frontal cortex is also necessary for such mental activities as anticipating and planning, envisioning yourself in a future event also requires engaging your hippocampus and other memory-associated regions to recall memories.

Because exactly the same parts used for recall are also used for projecting into the future, improving your memory improves your ability to imagine, plan and project into the future as well – very important for creativity. This capability, called *mental time travel*, is key to virtually all abstract thinking: being able to link elements of your experience in novel ways is the key to creativity, language and problem-solving skills.

Sleep And Memory

In a nutshell, sleep reactivates newly-learned memory traces in your hippocampus, then redistributes and integrates them into a network of pre-existing long-term memories in your cortex. The gradual transfer of information to neocortical circuits makes those memories independent of your hippocampus, freeing it to continue encoding new information after you awaken.

Your hippocampus encodes spatial and temporal information – the "wheres" and "whens" of navigational and episodic memory, and during slow-wave sleep, navigational neurons reactivate in the same order as when you're first learning to navigate a path. In other words, your brain replays your daily experiences as you sleep. This is thought to be part of the memory transferal process from your hippocampus to your cortex for long-term storage and integration. After the short-term storage of your hippocampus has been freed by this memory transferal to more permanent cortical storage sites, when you reawaken, the now-permanent memories are shielded against interference as new information enters your hippocampus.

You cycle through light, deep and dreaming sleep states every 90 minutes, so seven and a half hours of sleep provides you with 5 complete sleep cycles. Less sleep results in fewer full cycles, resulting in a reduced opportunity to transfer and consolidate memories.

Researchers have shown there are four sleep stages which recur in these cycles: three progressively deeper stages of non-REM followed by one stage of REM (dreaming) sleep. The deepest sleep is in stage three, slow-wave sleep (SWS).

Extensive experimental evidence points to neruotransmission spikes in activity called *sleep spindles* during sleep as the transferal of memories from your hippocampus to your cortex for permanent storage: in 2010, researchers at the University of York and Harvard Medical School found mental processing during sleep cements new declarative memories in your brain much more effectively, helping you remember detailed information such as new vocabulary or numbers. This was the first time scientists had been able to monitor the specific brain activity involved when memories are reorganized during sleep.

The team taught volunteers new words in the evening, and tested them immediately afterward. Subjects then slept overnight in the laboratory while EEG machines monitored their brains. When tested the following morning, researchers consistently found the volunteers remembered more words, and at a faster pace, than immediately after they had first learned them.

NonREM sleep was the most beneficial for strengthening these new de-clarative memories, as intense bursts of activity (sleep spindles) showed neural communication – presumably memory transferral – between the cortex and hippocampus. Subjects who experienced the most sleep spin-dles performed the highest in making associations between new words they'd learned and words that were already in their memory.

According to co-author Dr. Jakke Tamminen:

> New memories are only really useful if you can connect them to information you already know. Imagine a game of chess, and being told that the rule governing the movement of a specific piece has just changed. That new information is only useful to you once you can modify your game strategy, the knowledge of how the other pieces move, and how to respond to your opponent's moves. Our study identifies the brain activity during sleep that organizes new memo-ries and makes those vital connections with existing knowledge.

Dreams during rapid-eye movement (REM), sleep appear to be free asso-ciations; an unrestricted flow and creative recombining of integrated sen-sory impressions from your association areas – the very heart of creativity.

REM sleep is triggered by a special set of nerves in the pons of your brain stem. Norepinephrine and serotonin release completely shut down, so your body goes into a state of atonia (muscular paralysis), presumably so you don't thrash around in your dreams.

Acetylcholine is at its highest levels when you're awake and in REM sleep; it's at its lowest when you're in slow-wave sleep. Thus, it's thought to may be involved in controlling memory transfer and consolidation. Since acetylcholine "releases the brakes" of SK Channels – the first step in LTP, low acetylcholine levels seem to allow hippocampus transfer, while high levels block hippocampus transfer and allow transferred memories to be reorganized and "written".

High acetylcholine in your hippocampus during dream sleep suppresses memory transfer and memory control signals to your cortex, and low levels of cortisol, norepinephrine and acetylcholine in the cortical association areas allow the unrestricted, free flow of associational activity.

Different types of memory use different memory centers: declarative, episodic, and spatial-navigational memory depend upon your hippocampus, while procedural memories and habit depend upon your striatum and cerebellum.

The structure of sleep cycles means your first 3.5 hours of sleep, dominated by SWS, offer the greatest benefit to declarative memory recall – the kind of memory you need for a test, while the latest stages, dominated by REM sleep, offer the greatest benefit to creativity and to procedural memories – the kind you need for sports, or a musical performance.

> ***Preparing for the Big Test*** *– Sleep is so critical to learning and memory formation that you're better off just reading something once and sleeping on it than you would be pulling an all-night "cram session". So if you're about to take a "killer exam", you just might want to reconsider plans to pull an all-night cram session – you'd be better off memorizing the salient points and then sleeping on it.*

Build A Super Memory

A 2008 study has found that your striatum's ability to manufacture dopamine is linked to your working memory capacity. Dopamine regulates brain activity, so it's critical to many functions. Disruptions in the supply impair working memory, making it difficult to remember details on a short-term basis.

Since dopamine is dependent upon the amino acid tyrosine, consuming foods rich in tyrosine is thus likely to improve working memory – and therefore, nearly all your mental processes.

In 2009, neuroscientists at Sweden's Karolinska Institutet University also showed that training working memory generates new dopamine receptors. Dr. Torkel Klingberg said this is direct evidence of how thought affects biochemistry. He says working memory can be improved in just a few weeks with intensive brain training, which increases cortical dopamine D1 receptors. The brain training he recommends follows a four-part system consisting of:

1. Crossword puzzles, brain teasing and exercises emphasizing verbal skills throughout the day.

2. Five regular meals rich in omega-3 fats, antioxidants and whole grains. Eating regularly (approximately every four hours) prevents spikes and dips in blood glucose, which is your brain's primary fuel.

3. Pursuing a daily physical fitness program that includes vigorous aerobic exercise.

4. Stress-reducing activities, including relaxation exercises and stretching. This reduces cortisol, found to impair memory and even erode cells in the hippocampus, the brain's primary memory center.

Method Acting

Russian theater director Constantin Stanislavski was the inventor of *method acting*, an acting system considered the industry's primary training method. His groundbreaking method encouraged actors to "live the part", striving to emotionally become the characters they were portraying.

Part of Stanislavski's technique for memorizing large amounts of material involves breaking lines down into units of action. Each unit encompasses an intention or goal of the character, with which the actor strives to empathize. His pupils were instructed to study their own emotions and use gestures and vocal inflection to convey these emotions to the audience.

This advice can also be of tremendous benefit to you. Explore your emotions deeply, and you'll learn about yourself, and how to connect more effectively with others. If you want to improve the phonological loop of your working memory, you might consider joining a local theater group. Learning dialogue and method acting can do incredible things for your mind.

The Brainy Lifestyle

Your health and lifestyle, of course, have a profound influence upon your mind. Diet in particular plays a significant role in memory and cognition. For example, researchers at the University of Cambridge demonstrated in 2009 that rats which consume a high-fat diet take 25 percent longer to solve mazes than when the same rats consume a normal diet.

University of South Carolina researchers also found that rats fed a high-fat/high-cholesterol diet perform more poorly and make more errors in maze tests when compared with rats eating a normal diet. The lesson is clear – fatty foods make you stupider.

Improper dieting can be just as bad: a 2008 study at Tufts University compared women on low-carb diets vs. those which meet American Dietetic Association recommendations, and found those on low-carb diets perform much more poorly on memory-based tasks than those who eat a standard ADA diet. Cutting carbs too much impairs your memory, robbing your brain of glucose, according to co-author Dr. Robin Kanarek. Whole grains and complex carbohydrates which digest slowly deliver a steady stream of glucose to fuel your brain.

As mentioned earlier, exercise also significantly improves mental function, increasing blood flow to your brain, supplying it with necessary oxygen and glucose, according to Dr. Sandra Aamodt, co-author of *Welcome to Your Brain*. Once-a-week strength training has additionally been shown to improve prefrontal function. Weight training provides a major boost in circulating *brain-derived neurotrophic factor* (BDNF), which Harvard psychiatrist John J. Ratey calls "Miracle-Grow for the brain."

A 2010 study published in the Journal of Neurobiology demonstrated that subjects who engaged in an intense workout were able to memorize new vocabulary 20 percent faster than those pursuing low-impact activities.

Hygiene is just as important: Flossing your teeth is critical for your gum health, and protects you from gum disease, which can allow harmful bacteria to enter your bloodstream. According to Dr. Jonathan B. Levine, author of *Smile,* bacteria from tooth decay can lead to inflammation throughout your body, including in your brain, leading to cognitive impairment.

Memory Superstars

Jill Price is a remarkable woman. Without effort, she can recall, down to the minutest detail, every moment of her life since the age of 14. The color of shoes she was wearing on the first day back in school? No problem; she can also tick off the brand name, size, location in her closet, and even the store where she bought them (and the time, date and weather) with complete ease. She can recite headlines from random dates, and tell you the weather from any time in her past. Mrs. Price is a master of episodic memory, and never forgets a moment of her life.

Jill Price's memory is mind-boggling, but it's strictly autobiographical – she has trouble memorizing poetry or other facts; her episodic memory is exceptional, but her semantic memory is typical.

She has superhuman-level episodic recall, but trouble in suppressing that recall; her prefrontal cortex – used for suppression of thought, emotion and recall – slightly under performs, and her IQ is also average, at 93.

Hyperthimesia, or super autobiographical memory (from the Greek words hyper- and thimesia – remembering), is extremely rare, but there are presently believed to be perhaps 50 with the condition in the United States.

Drs. Elizabeth Parker, Larry Cahill and James McGaugh of the University of California have discovered an unusual anatomical property of Mrs. Hill's brain which may explain her extraordinary powers. fMRI scans indicate those with this remarkable ability have greater mass in their temporal lobes – which hold the hippocampus and store facts, dates and events – and in their caudate nuclei – which hold procedural memories and allow learning and habit formation.

While it's believed hyperthimesia appears at birth, Mrs. Price specifically recalls the trauma of relocating at age eight spurred her to begin trying to "hold onto" events, writing a diary and collecting memorabilia. These aspects of her ability, along with her comparatively lower PFC functionality, resemble dysfunctions like OCD and Tourette's syndrome, where impulse control is impaired. The study of Mrs. Price makes for fascinating reading; you can find it online at: http://today.uci.edu/pdf/AJ_2006.pdf

Dr. James McGaugh, the world's leading authority on hyperthimesia, says this type of super-memory is completely new to science. However, he agrees with Stanford University Neurology Chairman Frank Longo; the implications are that human long-term memory is far, far more powerful than ever imagined. In fact, says Dr. Longo, human memory may in fact be "potentially limitless".

Build Your Own Super Memory

Much more personally useful, no doubt, is boosting your semantic memory – your ability to remember facts, names, dates and the like. The good news is that you can do this to virtually any degree you wish – memorizing entire books word-for-word, if you like. You can use it memorize faces, dates, numbers, historical facts, poetry or even random visual images if you like. Amazingly, semantic memory can be trained to superhuman levels in less than a day.

If you're not aware of it, World Memory Championships have been held every year since 1991. Perhaps the most amazing achievement to date is that of Malaysian champion Dr. Yip Swee Chooi, who memorized the entire Oxford Chinese-English dictionary – 57,000 word pairs and 1,774 pages. Call out a word, and he not only knows the definition in both languages, he can instantly tell you what page it's on. An astounding video of Dr. Chooi can be seen online:

http://www.youtube.com/watch?v=PDcVKtyryPw

You can also watch world memory champion Andy Bell learn the exact sequence of ten decks of randomly-shuffled cards. He teaches his "link method" of association step-by-step to Professor Robert Winston on BBC One's 2003 program "Get Smart". It's something you can learn to do too – in under an hour:

http://www.youtube.com/watch?v=9NROegsMqNc&feature=related

Bell associates images with locations. Because your mind is exceptionally good at remembering images and routes between locations, Bell says the method can turn an ordinary memory into an extraordinary one, and that it's "something anyone can do".

Joshua Foer, self-trained memory champion and author of the best-seller *Moonwalking with Einstein*, tells the story of how he went from being a journalist researching memory competitions, to winning America's 2006 Memory Championship. Foer started out with no special abilities, and trained his memory.

Chooi, Bell and Foer are all *mnemonists* – memory experts who use various techniques to improve their ability. Anyone without brain impairment can master the same skills, if they've got the desire. The secret lies in *mnemonic devices* – memory tricks like associating a mental image with each name, number or fact.

The Memory Master Secret Of Ancient Greece

The most powerful of all such techniques has existed since the middle ages. Called the *Method of Loci* or more commonly the *memory palace* or *mental walk*, it involves mentally constructing a house or path and placing items you wish to remember in various locations throughout it.

The discovery is said to have first been made by the Greek poet Simonides in the fifth century B.C. According to the story, a banquet hall had collapsed, and Simonides, as the sole survivor, was asked to be a witness to testify about what happened and who the victims were. To his tremendous surprise, Simonides discovered that by mentally picturing the layout of the room, he was able to recall the names and placements in exact detail.

This technique came to be known as the memory palace or method of Loci (Latin for places), a technique for learning super-memory. By constructing an imaginary building and filling it with things that you wish to recall, you can learn to use this technique within less than an hour.

In Thomas Harris' novel *Hannibal,* mad genius and serial killer Hannibal Lecter uses his memory palace to store amazingly detailed memories of years of patient records and other facts. In the real world, the Method of Loci enabled eight-time world memory champion Dominic O'Brien, for instance, to memorize 54 decks of cards in sequence (2808 cards), viewing each card only once.

The Memory Palace technique is incredibly powerful for all kinds of mental skills, like learning foreign languages, memorizing speeches you need to give, preparing for exams and more. Your Memory Palace is a mental reconstruction of any place you can easily recall, such as the inside of your house or your route to work. You can even make it a fantasy palace, if you prefer.

Build Your Memory Palace

1. *Choose the Site* – Choose where you'll store your memories. The better you're able to picture the place, the more effective this technique will be. Make not just the place, but a route, a walkthrough circuit in your house or a route you tend to walk.

2. *Note Landmarks* – Pay attention to specific details about the place you've chosen. Start with how the door looks, and what makes it "stand out". Take a mental walkthrough – what comes after you step through the door? Carefully analyze the room. What captures your mind's eye? Is it a mirror on the wall, a vase of flowers, a picture?

Each feature you add is a "memory slot" where you can store a piece of information. Continue to proceed through all the rooms of your memory palace.

3. *Imprint it on Your Mind* – The most critical point is for you to imprint the place or route 100% percent within your mind, committing it completely to memory. If you're visually-oriented this is easier. If not, some additional tips include:

   • Actually walk your route, noting out loud any distinctive features you see.

   • Write these features down on a sheet of paper and repeat them out loud as you mentally rehearse walking through them

   • Look at these features from the same viewpoint each time

   • Visualization is a skill you can develop. (See chapter 23!)

   • When you feel ready, review it one last time; overtraining is critical to the method of loci

   • When you're satisfied that your route has been deeply implanted within your mind, you can use your Memory Palace repeatedly, any time, to memorize anything you wish.

4. *Build Associations* – After constructing your memory palace, you can now put it to use. As with most mnemonic devices, the Memory Palace method uses visual associations. Use an image (a memory peg) to combine with a piece of data you need to memorize. Each memory peg comprises a distinctive feature within your Memory Palace.

The best visual associations are highly memorable – stupid, offensive, funny, crazy, or otherwise unusual. You need to construct scenes so outrageous they could never occur in the real world: just like sex, if it's boring, you're not doing it right. You can eventually use the method to commit a huge amount of information to memory, but you should start small, for example with a shopping list. Image the first item on your list is a hammer:

Visualize yourself at the start of your Memory Palace. Your first distinctive visual feature will be the front door. You need to combine the images of a hammer with your front door in an odd way. For example, how about, instead of a door knocker, there's a hammer swinging from a piece of wire? To knock, you hammer on the front door. You want to feel the solid wood of the hammer in your hands, and hear the sound of it going >tock< >tock< on the dark walnut door, the glass panes shivering at the impact.

Next you need to open your front door and continue along your path, following the exact path you first imagined. If the second item on your list is nails, perhaps this is how hats and coats are hung in the hallway. Make them visually distinctive – big and rusty, etc. In this way, proceed down your list, mentally associating items until you've included them all.

5. *Visit Your Palace* – After you've finished memorizing all the items on your list, if you're a novice, you'll need to practice, mentally reviewing your route at least once. When you start at the same place and walk along the same route, items you've committed to memory will instantly jump into your mind as you see the distinct features along the way. Walk your route from beginning to end, paying particular attention to the distinct features, and reviewing your scenes. When you've reached the end of your journey, turn around and retrace your steps in the opposite direction until you return to the start. The most important part is developing vivid imagery; additionally, you want to be as relaxed as possible, so your memorization will be easy and effective.

Alternatives

Mnemonic devices use associative techniques which are all variations of the Method of Loci; allowing the memorization of unrelated objects by mentally placing them within a mental path or building. Andy Bell, for example, mentally places objects along familiar city routes, mentally walking through them as he remembers. This deceptively simple technique allows him to, for example, memorize the position of every single playing card within six decks, so if you were to ask, "what was the 53rd card in the pile?" he can answer, "Jack of diamonds", and so forth, with 100% accuracy. This is also the same method Malaysian memory champion Dr. Yip Swee Chooi used to memorize the entire Oxford Chinese-English dictionary – 57,000 word pairs and 1,774 pages.

Other methods include substituting images for words. Seven-time German champion Gunther Karsten won a poem competition by creating a dictionary of images for two hundred of the most common words which are difficult to memorize, and he mentally navigates through his visual dictionary. Joshua Foer trained in his technique using a metronome, memorizing a card every time it clicked, and gradually setting the metronome speed higher and higher, repeating the process until he could do it flawlessly. More of his techniques and advice can be found online at Mnemotechnics.org

Final Thoughts

With experience, things you memorize via your Memory Palace can remain with you for days, weeks or more. You can also create as many memory palaces as you need, and they can be as simple or as complex as you wish. Each is your personal memory bank, available to help you recall anything, at any time.

Homework: You can take full courses from Harvard, MIT, Yale, Oxford, Cambridge, and hundreds of other top universities around the world for free. Check out the Online Open Courseware here: http://www.aussieeducator.org.au/education/specificareas/online=2.html

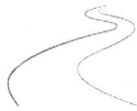

Neural Plasticity and Memory: From Genes to Brain Imaging, Boca Raton (FL): CRC Press; 2007.

Adrenal Stress Hormones and Enhanced Memory for Emotionally Arousing Experiences, Christa K. McIntyre and Benno Roozendaal; U.S. National Library of Medicine, National Institutes of Health, Bookshelf ID: NBK3907 PMID: 21204426; http://www.ncbi.nlm.nih.gov/books/NBK3907/

Synapse- and Stimulus-Specific Local Translation During Long-Term Neuronal Plasticity, Dan Ohtan Wang, Sang Mok Kim, Yali Zhao, Hongik Hwang, Satoru K. Miura, Wayne S. Sossin, and Kelsey C. Martin, 2009, Science Vol. 324 no. 5934 pp. 1536-1540 DOI: 10.1126/science.1173205; http://www.sciencemag.org/content/324/5934/1536.short

Making Smart Mice: Lab-bred "Doogie" Mice Learn Faster and Remember More Than Their Field-Born Brethren, Kristin Leutwyler, September 7, 1999, Scientific American; http://www.scientificamerican.com/article.cfm?id=making-smart-mice

The Memory Code, Dr. Joe Tsien, Scientific American, July, 2007, http://hebb.mit.edu/courses/9.03/lecture3.html

Summary: Changes in Sensory Cells in Habituation; http://www.fmrib.ox.ac.uk/~stuart/thesis/chapter_3/section3_2.html B

Cognitive Science: The Molecules of Forgetfulness, Alcino J. Silva and Sheena A. Josselyn, 2002, Nature: DOI: 10.1038/418929a

Genetic Switch Could Restore Memory, Laura Sanders, May 7, 2010 Wired Magazine; http://www.wired.com/wiredscience/2010/05/mouse-memory-switch/lab_mouse

How Does Your Memory Work? Annabell Gillings, 2008, BBC Horizon

Localization of a Stable Neural Correlate of Associative Memory, Leon G. Reijmers, Brian L. Perkins, and Naoki Matsuo, et al, August 31, 2007, Science

Memory Consolidation, Wikipedia, 2010

Exposing the Memory Engine: the Story of PKMzeta, John Timmer, Nature Neuroscience, 2011. DOI: 10.1038/nn.2751 (About DOIs).

Multiple Forms of Activity-Dependent Competition Refine Hippocampal Circuits In Vivo, Masahiro Yasuda, Erin M. Johnson-Venkatesh, Helen Zhang, Jack M. Parent, Michael A. Sutton, Hisashi Umemori, 2011, Neuron Magazine; 70 (6): 1128-1142 DOI: 10.1016/j. neuron.2011.04.027

The Effects of Stress and Stress Hormones on Human Cognition: Implications for the Field of Brain and Cognition, S. J. Lupien, F. Maheu, M. Tu, A. Fiocco, T.E. Schramek, et al, 2007, Brain and Cognition 65; http://gettingstronger.org/wp-content/uploads/2011/07/Lupien-Definition-of-Stress.pdf

What Determines The Capacity Of Short-Term Memory? press release, 15 December 2011 Nencki Institute of Experimental Biology

Hippocampus Evolution, 2011, Wikipedia

Brain Coach Answers: How can I improve my short term memory? Is there a daily exercise I can do to improve it? Caroline Latham, 2006

Superhuman: Genius, Andrew Pettie, 19 Aug 2008, ITV1

Fundamentals of Human Neuropsychology, Brian Kolb & Ian Q. Whishaw, 2003

Procedural memory, 2010, Wikipedia; http://en.wikipedia.org/wiki/Procedural_memory

Evidence for Cortical Automaticity in Rule-Based Categorization, Sebastien Helie, Jessica L. Roeder, and F. Gregory Ashby, 2010, Journal of Neuroscience; http://www.jneurosci.org/content/30/42/14225.abstract

A Neurobiological Theory of Automaticity in Perceptual Categorization, F. Gregory Ashby, John M. Ennis, and Brian J., 2007, Psychological Review DOI: 10.1037/003-295X.114.3.632; http://www.psych.ucsb.edu/~ashby/SPEED.pdf

Is Memory Consolidation A Multiple-Circuit System? Federico Bermudez-Rattoni, 2010, doi: 10.1073/pnas.1003434107 PNAS May 4, 2010 vol. 107 no. 18 8051-8052; http://www.pnas.org/content/107/18/8051.full

Slow-Wave Sleep, Acetylcholine, and Memory Consolidation, Ann E. Power, February 9, 2004, doi: 10.1073/pnas.0400237101 PNAS February 17, 2004 vol. 101 no. 7 1795-1796 ; http://www.pnas.org/content/101/7/1795.full

A Cortical Neural Prosthesis for Restoring and Enhancing Memory, Berger et al, 2011, J. Neural Eng. 8 046017

194

Reactivation and Consolidation of Memory During Sleep, Björn Rasch and Jan Born doi: 10.1111/j.1467-8721.2008.00572.x Current Directions in Psychological Science June 2008 vol. 17 no. 3 188-192; http://cdp.sagepub.com/content/17/3/188.abstract

Brisk Stroll Every Day Helps Improve Memory In Old Age And Wards Off Dementia, A Study Finds, Richard Alleyne, 2011, http://news.bbc.co.uk/2/hi/health/3152502.stm

Fitness: A Walk to Remember? Study Says Yes, Paula Span, February 7, 2011, New York Times

Synapse- And Stimulus-Specific Local Translation During Long-Term Neuronal Plasticity, Dan Ohtan Wang, Sang Mok Kim, Yali Zhao, Hongik Hwang, Satoru K. Miura, Wayne S. Sossin, and Kelsey C. Martin; 2009, Science 19 June: 1536-1540 http://www.sciencemag.org/content/324/5934/1536.abstract

The Memory Virus: Gene Boosts Memories Made Weeks Earlier, John Timmer March 4, 2011, Ars Technica; http://arstechnica.com/science/news/2011/03/the-memory-virus-gene-boosts-memories-made-weeks-earlier.ars

Enhancement of Consolidated Long-Term Memory by Overexpression of Protein Kinase M? in the Neocortex, Reut Shema, Sharon Haramati, Shiri Ron, Shoshi Hazvi, Alon Chen, Todd Charlton Sacktor and Yadin Dudai. Science, Vol. 331, March 3, 2011. DOI: 10.1126/science.1200215

Labile Or Stable: Opposing Consequences For Memory When Reactivated During Waking And Sleep, 2011, Diekelmann, S., Büchel, C., Born, J., & Rasch, B., Nature Neuroscience DOI: 10.1038/nn.2744

A Critical Role for IGF-II in Memory Consolidation and Enhancement, Chen, D., Stern, S., Garcia-Osta, A., Saunier-Rebori, B., Pollonini, G., Bambah-Mukku, D., Blitzer, R., & Alberini, C. (2011). Nature, 469 (7331), 491-497 DOI: 10.1038/nature09667

A Case of Unusual Autobiographical Remembering, Elizabeth Parker, Larry Cahill and James L. MacGaugh, 2006, Neuroscience 12, 35-49; DOI: 10.1080/13554790500473680

Get Smart, Dr. Robert Winston, 2007, BBC One

Endless Memory, Shari Finklstein, December 19, 2010, 60 Minutes, CBS News

Mnemotechnics.org, Josh Cohen, March 15, 2011, http://mnemotechnics.org/

Method of Loci, Wikipedia, 2010

Endless Memory, Shari Finklstein, December 19, 2010, 60 Minutes, CBS News

Secrets of a Mind-Gamer: How I Trained My Brain and Became a World-Class Memory Athlete, Joshua Foer, Feb 15, 2011, New York Times; http://www.nytimes.com/interactive/2011/02/20/magazine/mind-secrets.html

Develop Perfect Memory with the Memory Palace Technique, Luciano Passuello, 2008, http://www.litemind.com/memory-palace/

195

Plastic

"I saw an angel in the block of marble and I just chiseled until I set him free."
– Michelangelo, on the creation of his masterpiece "David", 1501 AD

Scientists used to believe that, with the exception of memory formation, brain structure was fixed after puberty, and new neural growth did not occur in adults to any great degree, but modern science has disproven this in spectacular fashion, showing conclusively that the brain changes "physically, chemically and functionally", throughout life, even through the power of thought.

Said to be "the most important breakthrough in our understanding of the brain in 400 years", this is the new frontier science of *neuroplasticity*. A landmark 1998 study published in Nature Medicine by Dr. Peter S. Eriksson of the Swedish Institute of Neurology first announced the discovery that the human brain had the ability to generate new brain cells. Previously, scientists had believed that the human brain was fixed, with no capacity to generate new cells; that humans were born with all of their brain cells, lost them on a daily basis, and could not generate or replace lost cells with new ones.

Rewiring Your Brain

In *How Brain Research Relates to Rigor, Relevance and Relationships: Emerging Evidence of the Ability to Manage 'Brain Health'*, Drs. Willard Daggett and Paul Nussbaum say, "The brain has plasticity. As such, there is no finite capacity or limitation. In this way, every 'normal' brain is distinct and actually much superior to the fanciest of all computers, because computers will always have built-in limitations and finite capacity."

Dr. Norman Doidge, author of *The Brain That Changes Itself: Stories of Personal Triumph from the Frontiers of Brain Science* asserts that you have some control over the process as well: "our thoughts can change the structure and function of our brains, even into old age". According to Doidge, investigation into this kind of neurogenesis was first prompted by psychiatrist Eric Kandel, who won the Nobel Prize for demonstrating how neurons form new connections in response to learning. There are three circumstances in which neuroplasticity is known to occur:

1. When an infant's brain undergoes initial organization

2. When there is severe trauma and other portions of the brain are reorganized to provide lost functionality

3. When new information is learned and memorized

So how can you put this information to practical use?

Mental Rehearsal

In 1996, Harvard Neurology professor Dr. Alvaro Pascual-Leone published the results of a sensational new study: A group of non-musicians were taught a five-finger piano training exercise, which they practiced repeatedly at a keyboard for two hours over five days. Because they were learning something new, scans showed substantial changes in their motor cortices, the area of the brain which handles finger movement, as new neural connections were forming.

A second group of volunteers learned the same exercise, but didn't actually move their fingers, simply practicing mentally for the same amount of time. Amazingly, the motor cortex changed significantly among both groups during the five days. The scans, which you can see online at the link in this chapter's references, are startling. In other words, the volunteer's brains essentially didn't distinguish between physical practice and mental visualization. These findings mean, as Dr. Pascual-Leone explains, "Just thinking will change your brain. And what that ultimately means is that one needs to be careful with what one thinks."

How Does It Work?

There are two types of changes in the neural network of your brain. The first is a functional reorganization, which reassigns tasks among neural circuits. As you've learned, specialized areas of your brain have developed to handle specific tasks, both conscious and unconscious. And when a patient suffers serious brain injury, areas previously dedicated to handling other tasks can take over work for the damaged areas. One example of this is how the visual cortex of blind patients develops to recognize patterns of raised dots when reading braille.

The second type of plasticity is synaptic plasticity, which includes

1. neural migration, neurons extending connections to distant brain areas

2. pruning, the normal removal of inefficient or unused neurons

3. neurogenesis, the creation of new neurons

4. Long-Term Potentiation, strengthening of neural connections through repeated use

Brain Training

As you repeat a certain activity, long-term potentiation strengthens the brain region under constant use, like muscle growth in response to exercise. As your expertise grows, so does the neural development in that region of your brain. This was demonstrated in the year 2000, when a group of London researchers compared brain scans between taxicab drivers and non-drivers:

> Taxi drivers in London must undergo extensive training, learning how to navigate between thousands of places in the city. This training is colloquially known as 'being on The Knowledge' and takes about 2 years to acquire on average.

The researchers concluded that

> ...there is a capacity for local plastic change in the structure of the healthy adult human brain in response to environmental demands. Significantly increased gray matter volume was found in the brains of taxi drivers compared with those of controls in only two brain regions, namely the right and the left hippocampi. No differences were observed elsewhere in the brain.

The hippocampus is used by humans and other animals for navigation and creating mental maps of an area. When it's not functioning properly, as with amnesia or Alzheimer's disease, people lose track of where they are and may not even remember where they were going.

In February of 2011, researchers found learning motor skills created as much as an additional 22% dendrite growth in the motor cortices of laboratory rats. By studying as the animals learned to reach for and grab food pellets – the human equivalent of learning to drive or to play the guitar – the researchers found that everyday learning apparently results in significant neural plasticity.

Said University of California neuroscience professor Mark H. Tuszynski, MD, PhD, (director of UC San Diego's Center for Neural Repair:

> Our findings show... a dramatic increase in the size and complexity of the affected neurons – and yet highly restricted to a small subset of cells. And all of this structural plasticity is occurring in the context of normal learning, which highlights just how changeable the adult brain is as a part of its normal biology.

But it's not just the learning of practical skills that stimulates neuroplasticity: "We can think of emotions, moods and states such as compassion as trainable mental skills," says University of Wisconsin Neuroscientist Dr. Richard Davidson, who leads an ongoing study of meditation's effects on the brain, in cooperation with the Dalai Lama. Brain scans during his research show that meditating on compassion changes brain regions associated with focus, anxiety, sadness, fear, anger, and even the body's healing functionality. Among Buddhist monks with years of training, the changes were much more marked and lasting.

Armed with new knowledge about the constantly-changing human brain and its mechanisms means every waking moment of your life you can choose to either reinforce old thought and behavior patterns or create new ones – the choice is yours. The process of creating new neural connections is a double-edged sword: the more frequently you strengthen the neural connections of fear, anger, laziness, addiction and obsession, the stronger those connections become, and the greater the grip those thought processes will have on your life. However, because every waking moment you have the choice of freewill, you can begin the process of inner change at any moment. How about right now, for instance?

The Healing Brain

Neuroscientists can pinpoint general brain function using brain maps – depicting regions which specialize in specific functionality. And recent studies show that in cases of severe injury to one part of the brain, other regions can take over the damaged region's functions, "remapping" or "rewiring" the neural connections.

Eye surgeon and classical pianist Michael Bernstein is a dramatic real-world example of this mechanism in action. At the age of 54, Bernstein suffered a massive stroke, resulting in a loss of speech and paralysis of his left arm, hand and leg. Dr. Edward Taub of the University of Alabama took Dr. Bernstein as a patient, and began using his newly-developed rehabilitation technique called *constraint-induced therapy* to see if he it would have a helpful effect. The technique involves restricting the movement of a patient's fully functional limb so that he's forced to use the impaired limb in its place.

Bernstein, whose personal doctors had given him very little chance of even partial recovery over the course of years, recovered nearly full mobility and speech within a matter of days, to the point at which he can now give concert recitals and resume work as before. Significant, physically measurable neural changes had occurred, as his brain remapped functionality to other regions.

The most remarkable story of brain remapping however, is of Michelle Mack, *born with the entire left hemisphere of her brain missing*. By all accounts, Michelle shouldn't even be alive, but her brain remapped all its critical functions to the point at which she can speak like any other adult, and has exhibited the remarkable ability to recite the exact date when random events occurred, even years in the past. Amazing video interviews of her can be found online at the links following this chapter.

Addicted To Your Emotional Neurochemistry

Just as your brain can heal itself to a remarkable degree, it's also integral to healing your body. As Joe Dispenza, author of *Evolve Your Brain – The Science of Changing Your Mind* points out, the connection between your brain and body's physical state means that your thoughts and feelings (which are encoded by brain and body chemistry) can send you into a lifestyle feedback loop, for better or for worse. Essentially, you can become addicted to your own emotional (chemical) states. And, in turn, you then "...see reality based on how you're chemically feeling".

He cites two experiments to illustrate his point. In the first, a group of subjects were shown a series of slides, half of which were scenes of funerals, and half of which were scenes of weddings. Although there was an equal number of each kind of slide, when asked to report what they saw, depressed subjects would always report seeing many more funeral scenes, while optimists reported a greater number of wedding scenes.

In the second experiment, a group of subjects were given special tinted glasses to wear constantly for two weeks. One lens was tinted yellow, the other blue. At the end of two weeks, while still wearing the colored glasses, the subjects were asked to look at a white sheet of paper, looking first to the left, and then to the right. When asked what color they saw, all the subjects responded that they didn't see any color – the paper was white. In other words, their brains had come to accept this altered perception of reality as "normal" and adjusted themselves accordingly.

This is the manner in which your emotions "color" reality, but you're unable to recognize it. Your brain sends neurochemical signals to your body on a constant basis, and reads your body's states as you react to the world, profoundly changing your interpretation of it. Dispenza describes how this relates to the process of creating your own permanent inner, subjective reality:

Every time you make a thought, you make a chemical; if you have happy thoughts, you make chemicals that make your body feel happy. If you have negative or self-deprecating thoughts, in a matter of seconds, you begin to feel unhappy. The brain reads our body's feelings, and we think the way we feel; so we create a loop. Eventually, this chemical loop becomes a permanent personality trait by which we define ourselves. This is how we condition ourselves. Our body becomes used to that chemical state.

The body you've trained and conditioned to expect this constant chemical feeding (feeling) for twenty years or more wants to maintain the chemical state it's used to. We're allowing our bodies to control us rather than our conscious thought and will.

So once you've become comfortable with a chemical state (such as depression or anxiety), it requires a conscious act of will to change into a more positive chronic chemical state (such as happiness or enthusiasm), a process he calls reinventing yourself.

Dispenza spent decades studying patients who had *spontaneous remissions* from diseases – those with conditions like diabetes and cancer, whose survival or recovery defied medical science. He says he discovered four attitudes and activities they all shared that were at the heart of their recovery. All the patients (both agnostic and religious) had four things in common:

1. They believed there was a greater, conscious force at work giving them life and by "surrendering" the healing process to this greater Being (be it God, Buddha, the Universal force, or even just the spiritual side of themselves), they would begin to heal;

2. They accepted that their own thoughts and attitudes were responsible for their illness; the chemistry in their bodies caused by their negative thoughts, emotions and unhealthy lifestyle choices led to a breakdown in their health: "My 20 years of hatred, and my 10 years of suffering, and my five years of anger – I was really an unhappy person, and that was what gave me my disease."

3. They decided they could no longer "be themselves", that, to survive, they had to reinvent themselves. He says the questions they would typically ask were, for example, "What would it be like to be happy?", "Who do I know in my life that's a happy person?", "What would I have to change about myself to experience joy?", "Who in history do I admire?", and "Who in history do I want to be like?"

4. They began to deliberately mentally rehearse their new thought patterns with absolute commitment on a daily basis, putting aside daily trivial tasks and socializing when necessary. At the peak moments, upon awakening and just before going to bed, they would practice. As a result of the daily, constant repetition, neuroplasticity would take place in their minds, with neurons strengthening connections and creating new ones for those thought patterns, and, in a manner similar to muscle exercise, through thought alone, their mind and body would adapt and their new identity choices would take deep root. He echoes what many other psychologists, counselors and biologists suggest: gratitude to whatever moves the universe (thankfulness for being alive, and a conscious "counting of one's blessings") is one of the most effective thought processes for this daily repetition.

By focused concentration, you can make your inner reality stronger than your external one – signals from the environment or worries about external events. This is a core benefit of mindfulness meditation, where you focus, for example, on your breathing, and learn to tune out distracting thoughts. This training, among other things, allows you to master your emotions – amygdala activity has been shown to decrease significantly, accompanied by significant drops in stress hormones, heartbeat, blood pressure, and a number of other beneficial effects. Despanza has a wealth of other advice, including:

1. Deliberately decide who it is you want to become and construct a very vivid picture of that "ideal you" to keep firmly in your mind

2. Reflect inwardly to discover what attitudes and negative emotional and cognitive habits your brain has become addicted to and "interrupt the flow" of these thoughts when you find yourself engaging in them (one psychologist suggests mentally shouting "Stop!" and deliberately switching to a more positive train of thought)

3. Decide to stop dwelling upon past events that leave you feeling like a "victim" instead of an active participant in your own destiny, and stop blaming others for your circumstances and behaviours.

4. Substitute positive thoughts – such as interest and gratitude – in place of negative ones

5. Cultivate new experiences, such as travel, and try things you've never done before

6. Use all your spare moments to focus on becoming the "new you"

7. Engage fully in the present, pushing out regrets or worries; focus deeply upon what you're doing at any given time, pushing out distractions

8. Find a mentor to help guide you

9. Make healing and changing the most important thing in your life.

Dispenza admits to being heavily influenced by the work of Dr. Leo Galland, one of the pioneers of integrated medicine, whose groundbreaking book *The Four Pillars of Health* teaches how the mind influences recovery. Director of medical research at the Gesell Institute for Human Development in New York, Dr. Galland talks about the treatment he developed over years of working with patients whose illnesses were particularly difficult to treat. He explains that there are *mediators, triggers,* and *antecedents* to illness.

Mediators, including stress hormones and your thoughts and feelings, produce symptoms and can cause physical damage to your body, or change your behavior.

Triggers may be *physical* (such as an infection, a drug or a toxin) or *situational* (worry or social problems)

Antecedents are risk factors like genetics and age, which make you more likely to contract a specific illness

His "Four Pillars" teach how to identify your mediators, triggers, and antecedents, then how to use four healing principles for recovery and optimal health:

1. creating strong, healthy relationships (the most important of the four)

2. designing a custom program of exercise, nutrition and rest

3. cleaning and purifying your external environment

4. cleaning and purifying your internal environment

Perils Of Plasticity

The incredible adaptability of your mind can also work against you. McGill University psychologists Alain Brunet and Karim Nader, along with Harvard psychiatrist Roger Pitman are developing a new method of treating sufferers of Post-Traumatic Stress Disorder, where neuroplasticity has altered the nervous system in response to a tragic, life-altering event.

"Traumatic events can be human-made or natural accidents," explains research partner Alain Brulet. "Events that are human-made really shatter people's expectations of others. The world becomes a very dangerous place."

Brulet estimates that there are about one million Canadians with PTSD. Rape and other trauma resulting from the actions of others are the most common causes in 50% of the cases.

PTSD is triggered by the mind perceiving a brush with death. The traumatic event is so overwhelming that your brain is unable to process it normally into memory, so you keep re-experiencing the event as if it were occurring in the present. The more often you relive the event, the stronger the neural connections become, until the condition begins to seriously disrupt your life.

Curing PTSD

Dr. Karim Nader was inspiration for the 2004 hit movie *Eternal Sunshine of the Spotless Mind*. He explains that memories are *labile* (highly plastic, unstable and easily changed) at the moments of formation and recall, before they're fixed into long-term memory in the process called *consolidation*. Even long-established memories can be easily reshaped or completely wiped out during this unstable phase.

Through laboratory experiments, Nader discovered that recalling and re-consolidating emotional-based memories in the hippocampus requires the amygdala to synthesize specific neurochemicals. By blocking this chemical formation with a blood-pressure medication called *propranolol*, the strong emotions and release of stress hormones were dampened. In effect, his patients could be calmed during the labile phase of memory recall, when the link between fear and past events was weak. Thus, the memory's power could be remolded and reconsolidated in less traumatic forms, freeing the patients from having to relive the trauma endlessly.

Dr. Brunet began to use propranolol in therapy with his PTSD patients, directing them to write down the traumatic memories that led to their conditions in vivid detail, and then, while under the calming effect of propranolol, they would reread the events every week. This allowed them to properly analyze the events without the sympathetic nervous system arousal and neurohormonal changes of anxiety. In this state of calm, they were then able to store their memories properly, so they were no longer being re-experienced as if in the present.

The results appear to be excellent; patients report the ability to recall the traumatic events with a sense of emotional detachment for the first time, fully recognizing that these events are in the past. Nader says it's important, however, not to completely erase the memories, as they're a fundamental part of the patient's identity.

One of the "takeaway" lessons from this is that life experiences are interpreted within your mind, just as thoughts are generated within your mind, and both have the power to change your brain and body chemistry. In this sense, reality is subjective, and you can choose to make it what you wish within your own mind.

Unable To Stop

Another example of the destructive side of neuroplasticity is OCD, or obsessive compulsive disorder. This is an extreme form of worry, in which sufferers try to calm themselves through a set of repeated behaviours called *rituals*. For example, an OCD patient might have such an excessive fear of disease and contamination that he washes his hands hundreds of times a day, even scrubbing them with bleach and steel wool. After hundreds of repetitions, the neurological connections are so strongly reinforced that he can no longer escape the thoughts, even by performing the cleansing ritual.

Psychologists have recently unravelled the underlying principles of this disorder:

1. The orbitofrontal cortex (located just behind your forehead) notices a mistake has been made

2. It signals the error-processing anterior cingulate cortex, which directs the hypothalamus to release stress hormones, raising anxiety and increasing focus on the mistake until it's corrected

3. After the mistake has been corrected, the caudate shifts attention onto other things

The problem arises in the third phase of the correction sequence; a malfunctioning caudate is unable to shift attention away from the perceived error, so the sufferer cannot stop thinking about it (obsessing), and repeating the ritualistic behavior against his will (compulsion).

The Observing Ego

UCLA's Dr. Jeffrey Schwartz has been teaching OCD patients to use mindfulness meditation to gain control over the endless neurological loop of OCD, and found the results just as effective as conventional drugs. He trains sufferers to use their minds as impartial spectators, observing the mental processes of OCD as if they were happening to someone else, and then redirecting their thought processes in more positive ways.

When an obsessive thought begins to take over a patient's mind, Dr. Schwartz directs them to observe, "My brain is generating another obsessive thought. I know it's just some garbage thrown up by a faulty circuit."

He advises patients to follow a four-step process when obsessive thoughts arise:

1. Stop and observe the thought process, recognizing it as a symptom of OCD

2. Recognize the illogical nature of the thought process – that it's a form of "brain lock"

3. Direct your attention and focus onto something else

4. Observe over time as the power of the compulsions fades

In experiments, 65% of Dr. Schwartz's patients showed significant improvement after ten weeks of training in mindfulness meditation, and scans of their brains showed orbital frontal cortex activity had quieted dramatically.

Similar results were found in 2006 at the University of Toronto, where Dr. Zindel Segal and colleagues found mindfulness meditation "just as effective as antidepressants" in preventing relapses among patients with depression. Dr. Segal's training focuses on teaching patients to view key life experiences in different ways, for example perceiving a failed date as a minor unsuccessful event instead of devastating proof that they can never find love. Mindfulness meditation training quieted frontal cortex hyperactivity, showing the endless cycle of worry over the event had ended.

Suckling At The Glass Teat

Modern technology is reshaping your brain.

Neurobiologist Susan Greenfield, Director of the Oxford Centre for the Science of the Mind, says that the constant bombardment of "instant sensory and information gratification" from television, movies and computers is fundamentally reshaping human brains, and not entirely for the better. While computers, movies and television train you for incredibly fast information-processing, she contends that they stunt your emotional, empathic, communication and deep-thinking capacities.

Children are particularly susceptible, and the effects include shortened attention spans, a preference for instant gratification, and the development of self-centered thinking. It's also, she says, impairing the ability of young people to communicate and concentrate in the real world. Adbusters Magazine, aware of the problem, sponsors an annual TV Turn-off Week to heighten awareness of the profound negative effects of television in particular.

Building Your Brain Reserve

The effects of modern technology, stress, aging, and negativity can all increasingly impair your brain. But extensive research shows you can improve brain function substantially through daily memory exercises – a mental "fitness program".

In *How Brain Research Relates to Rigor, Relevance and Relationships*, Drs. Willard Daggett and Paul Nussbaum give an overview of what specifically promotes "brain health" and how this knowledge can help you reach your full potential.

The key to lifelong brain health, they say, lies in creating sufficient *brain reserve* through *neurogenesis* and synaptic density. They say a healthy brain reserve is like a dense jungle, rich in synaptic connections. Insufficient brain reserve is like a single palm tree in a desert, with few synaptic connections.

Dense connections add cognitive flexibility, protecting brain function when injury or diseases like Alzheimer's destroy large numbers of neurons. If there are few "reserve" synaptic connections, brain damage cannot be mitigated, and life quality and health rapidly diminish.

University of New South Wales Psychiatry Senior Research Fellow Dr. Michael Valenzuela, who won a 2006 Eureka Prize for research into how maintaining an active mind wards off dementia, adds:

...people with high brain reserve have almost half as much risk of developing dementia as those with low brain reserve. In one sense the brain appears to be no different from the muscles of the body. It's a case of use it or lose it.

Your Personal (Brain) Trainer

By providing the brain with an "enriched environment", you can trigger physiological changes, and increase your synaptic connections. So what constitutes an "enriched environment"? Drs. Daggett and Nussbaum say there are three criteria to creating the necessary environment:

1. Socialization – others to relate to

2. Physical Exercise – inactivity in one's 40s increases the risk of Alzheimer's in later life

3. Mental Stimulation

Incorporating mental exercise into a daily health regimen can help people of all ages grow "cognitively, creatively, physically, emotionally, and academically to their fullest potential", but it's especially critical at a young age.

Stimulating the brain with daily novel and complex, new or unfamiliar activity triggers positive changes in your brain, while environments that only allow rote, passive memorization aren't nearly as effective in stimulating neural change.

Dr. Daggett has developed a measure of mental benefits based upon a "Rigor/Relevance" scale. Activities requiring the most complex thinking, coupled with real-world applicability, maximize mental stimulation. Additionally, skills and knowledge are most easily acquired when people feel connected with what they're learning, when the concepts are well understood, and when the relevance is recognized. Socializing within strong relationships is also critical to sharing and exchanging ideas, fostering creativity, mental growth, and language development.

Because of this, for example, Daggett suggests reconceiving schools as *Brain Health Centers*, where, instead of lecturing and other traditional instruction, teachers

> ...engage students, treating them as active learners rather than empty receptacles into which knowledge can be delivered, and make school a place where students work and teachers observe, not the other way around. Rather than being sedentary, passive, and aligned in neat rows of desks, learners are allowed to be tactile, experiential, interactive, and social and to move purposefully around the classroom as part of the learning process. Active learning provides multi-sensory stimuli to the brain.

Design Your Own Brain

Consultant and futurist Don Tapscott, author of the best-selling *Wikinomics* and *Growing Up Digital*, says that neuroplasticity means you can progress beyond merely learning new facts or skills, to deliberately "planning" and "designing" how you think, remember and communicate:

> *You might aspire to have a strong capacity to perceive and absorb information effectively, concentrate, remember, infer meaning, be creative, write, speak and communicate well, and to enjoy important collaborations and human relationships. How could you design your use (or abstinence) of media to achieve these goals?*

Among his suggestions:

1. Take a speed-reading course to increase how much information you can absorb without losing comprehension.

2. Selectively memorizing only information you can't look up.

3. Schedule periods of "unplugging", much like *Adbusters Magazine*'s famous "TV Turnoff Week".

Scientific American also lists the six most effective ways proven to improve the brain:

1. ***Exercise*** – Mice allowed to exercise on wheels improve learning and memory, and increase hippocampus mass. Humans also display improved mood and executive brain functions such as planning, organizing and multitasking through exercise.

   Exercise promotes neural growth, communication and survival by increasing blood flow, oxygen, and nutrients, including brain-derived neurotrophic factor (BDNF). As little as 20 minutes of daily walking is enough to improve brain health.

2. ***Diet*** – Avoid eating saturated fat (animal fats), which degrades learning and memory, and puts you at risk for dementia. Better choices for fatty brain tissue health are omega-3 fats, found in fish, nuts and seeds. Low levels of Omega-3s have been linked to Alzheimer's disease, depression, schizophrenia, and other disorders.

   Antioxidants from fruits and vegetables bind to *free radical molecules* (ions of oxygen molecules thought to break down cells and disrupt DNA, implicated in aging and cancer) allowing them to pass harmlessly out of your body. These nutrients also help maintain learning and memory in aging brains and can even mitigate brain damage from strokes.

Additionally, restricting caloric intake by 25 to 50 percent has also been found to promote longevity and improve brain functionality, specifically in terms of memory and coordination.

3. **Stimulants** – Focus and alertness can be boosted by chemicals that boost blood pressure, energy, heart and respiratory rate, etc. Caffeine – the world's most popular drug – can also boost attention, short-term memory and reaction speed, although too much can lead to overstimulation, anxiety and insomnia. In addition, caffeine may protect aging women from memory decline.

4. **Video Games** – Video games improve attention span, visual perception, information processing, hand-eye coordination, depth perception, pattern recognition and rapid decision-making and deduction. Studies have also shown that surgeons who play video games a few hours a week make 30% fewer operating room errors and videogame-playing white-collar professionals have more confidence and sociability.

On the negative side, it's been demonstrated that young male gamers who frequently play violent video games exhibit lower responses to violent images, suggesting they have become desensitized, and they show aggressive brain patterns while playing first-person shooter games; however, it has not yet been conclusively demonstrated that violent entertainment leads to an increase in real-life violence.

5. **Music** – Listening to music activates the auditory cortex, which processes complex sound patterns – speed, pitch, volume, melody, rhythm and timbre. This releases dopamine, serotonin and endorphins, and quiets the amygdala, resulting in a reduction of fear and other negative emotions.

Although it's commonly believed that listening to Mozart boosts learning, the study responsible for the belief has since been debunked – any boost from listening to music is minimal and fleeting. However, music *has* been shown to lower blood pressure, soothe patients with dementia, promote weight gain and early hospital discharge for premature babies, and has been used for treating anxiety and insomnia.

Music study also develops your cerebellum, corpus callosum and motor cortex, which are all more developed in musicians than in non-musicians. Studies have also demonstrated that it improves spatial navigation in children, and the very latest research seems to indicate that learning a musical instrument helps with language acquisition substantially.

6. Meditation – Researchers have discovered amazing powers in meditation; for example, neurons typically fire at different times, but during meditation, they fire in synchronization. Expert meditators also show superior immune system function. It's been shown to improve focus, attention and higher thinking capacities, to reduce pain and to help alleviate a wide range of ailments, including anxiety, asthma, insomnia, diabetes, depression, high blood pressure, and even skin diseases. Practiced meditators also report being calmer and more creative than non-meditators. Anatomically, meditation has been shown to promote prefrontal cortex growth.

The extent to which meditation has come to be recognized as a powerful tool for health and well-being can be seen in its recent acceptance by the scientific community: in 2005, the Dalai Lama was a distinguished speaker during the world's largest brain research conference for the Society for Neuroscience. Even the Pentagon has begun a multimillion-dollar, decade-long training program in mindfulness meditation for marines about to be deployed into battle.

Neurogenesis

Adult neurogenesis is a term which means new neurons have formed. In humans, adult neurogenesis has thus far only been found to occur in the olfactory bulb and hippocampus. Hippocampal neurogenesis occurs in the dentate gyrus (DG), the input portion of the hippocampus. These two areas – the dentate gyrus and olfactory bulb – continue generating new neurons throughout life.

Nobel Prize-winning neurobiology pioneer Dr. Eric Kandel explains neurogenesis thusly:

The most interesting theme that has emerged and one that exists without question in neurogenesis in the hippocampus is that it has some role in depression. It's been known for a very long period of time that people are depressed have a somewhat smaller hippocampus than people who are not depressed. Now, what one does not yet know, is whether people with depression have a smaller hippocampus because they were born with a smaller hippocampus and therefore are prone to depression, or whether the hippocampus shrank as a result of the depression.

We have... a lot of evidence that antidepressant medicines – selective serotonin uptake inhibitors – like Prozac – stimulate neurogenesis. New cells form and get incorporated into these neural circuits.

Exercise appears to be the most powerful stimulus for neurogenesis, however. And exercise is a tremendous enhancer of cognitive function. In fact, the single best advice for people as they age is to continue to be active, not only intellectually, but physically – to be in good condition.

Inflammation is a cellular swelling, an immune response to tissue damage or to foreign invaders. In the brain, it's believed to arise from overactivation of microglia, support cells which are typically dormant, but migrate to brain injuries. In trying to preserve and repair brain tissue, microglial cells create and transmit chemical distress signals to other cells. These signals trigger a cascade of reactions, including activating genes which express proteins, and other stress-related neurochemicals to assist in cleaning up cellular debris.

Amyloid beta activation of microglial cells is believed to be central to the progression of Alzheimer's. The natural defense system becomes toxic, stuck in a constant looping response to plaque buildup. Research suggests, however, that blueberry extract may prevent inflammatory signals from overactivating microglia cells. In recent experiments, the highest blueberry extract concentrations reduced inflammatory enzymes to almost nonexistent levels, just as in healthy cells.

Radical Dangers *- Prevailing theories say that as brains age, neurons become gradually more vulnerable to both oxidative stress and inflammation. Oxidative stress is cellular damage from free radicals, potentially highly-damaging ionized oxygen molecules you encounter every day. Free radicals lack an electron and seek to stabilize by tearing one away from neighboring molecules. This can lead to a destructive chain reaction of atomic damage in DNA, RNA, proteins and cell membranes. The brain is believed to be particularly vulnerable to this sort of oxidative stress. Although the brain is just 3 pounds – only 2 percent of the body's mass – it uses as much as 50% of the total oxygen consumed by the body, according to Dr. Joseph. Phytochemicals and other vital antioxidants can bind to free radicals, preserving and possibly even boosting neural function and neutralizing these potentially harmful molecules.*

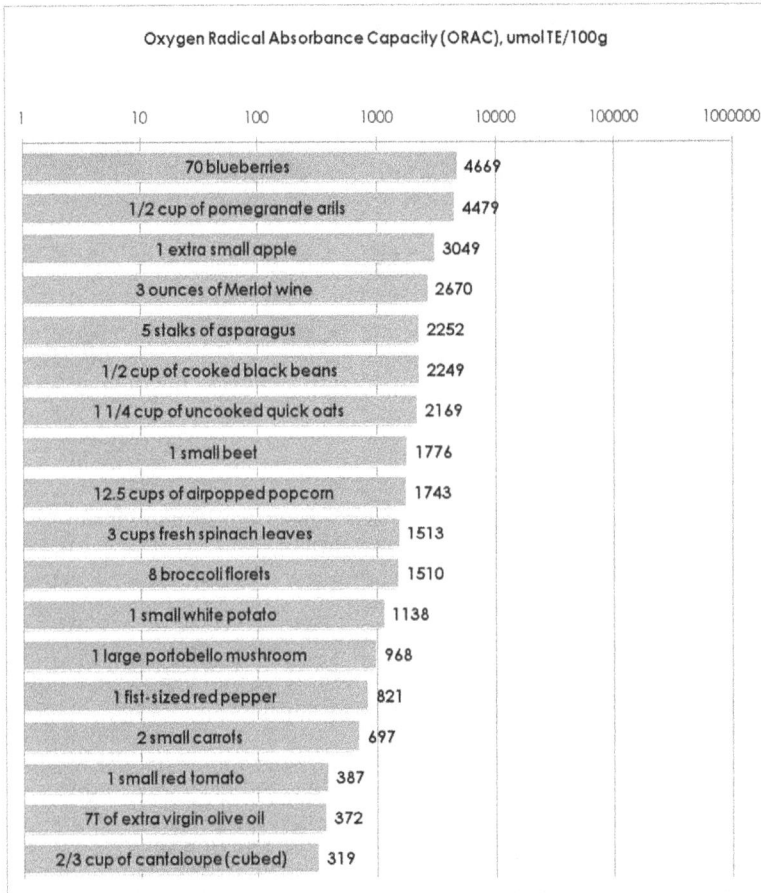

Oxygen Radical Absorbance Capacity (ORAC), umol TE/100g

70 blueberries	4669
1/2 cup of pomegranate arils	4479
1 extra small apple	3049
3 ounces of Merlot wine	2670
5 stalks of asparagus	2252
1/2 cup of cooked black beans	2249
1 1/4 cup of uncooked quick oats	2169
1 small beet	1776
12.5 cups of airpopped popcorn	1743
3 cups fresh spinach leaves	1513
8 broccoli florets	1510
1 small white potato	1138
1 large portobello mushroom	968
1 fist-sized red pepper	821
2 small carrots	697
1 small red tomato	387
7T of extra virgin olive oil	372
2/3 cup of cantaloupe (cubed)	319

Among fruits and vegetables, blueberries score highest on the Oxygen Radical Absorbance Capacity (ORAC) scale. Measurements are reported in micromoles Trolox equivalents (TE) per 100 gram sample (umol TE/g). A micromole is a chemical unit describing a comparative amount of a substance. Sheila Viswanathan, 2012, "Does Your Food Have ORAC?" GoodGuide. Used with permission.

The USDA's Radical Study

Specific nutrients and chemical compounds have long been understood as essential for the human brain, and deficiencies in some, like iron or vitamin B12, can result in impaired neural function.

The US Department of Agriculture has been researching dietary effects on the brain throughout the human lifespan. Brain cells are naturally lost throughout life, but the process, say USDA researchers, does not necessarily have to accelerate with aging; the effects will vary from person to person.

According to Dr. James Joseph, age-related mental decline can be due more to poor cellular communication than to a loss of neurons. Dr. Joseph is head of the Neuroscience Laboratory at the USDA's Jean Mayer Human Nutrition Research Center on Aging (HNRCA) in Boston, where his team studies the effects of dietary plant compounds on brain function. He was one of the first to study the protective benefits of dietary antioxidants.

Vegetables, seeds, grains, nuts and fruits provide vitamins, minerals, and protective antioxidants, but they contain thousands of additional compounds which contribute significantly to your body's ability to absorb antioxidants. To measure overall impact, the USDA designed the ORAC (Oxygen Radical Absorbance Capacity) system, which is just starting to be used on food and beverage labels.

Dr. Joseph and his colleagues have long studied connections between diet and cognitive loss in the aging brain, and made some groundbreaking discoveries which challenge long-accepted dogma. For example, it has long been held that the CNS is not capable of regeneration. But Dr. Joseph's team, along with separate teams at the Salk Institute, demonstrated the brain does produce new neurons (neurogenesis) throughout life, but it slows with age. His follow-up studies have also demonstrated how such age-related cognitive decline can actually be reversed through diet:

Laboratory rats fed from adulthood a diet of vitamin E, strawberry, blueberry or spinach extract (all of which have similar ORAC scores) avoided the normal age-related cognitive decline seen in rats fed a standard diet. Three groups of elderly rats, equivalent to 63-year-old humans, were fed different high-antioxidant extracts, while a control group ate a standard diet. After just two months (the equivalent of 10 human years) the rats were tested for balance, coordination and navigation on a rotating rod.

The rats which ate spinach, strawberry, or blueberry extracts *reversed* their age-related neuronal and cognitive deficits, with the blueberry-fed group far outperforming all others. Although they had physically become rodent senior citizens, these super-rats had "remarkable stamina and neuromotor function" according to co-author Barbara Shukitt-Hale. The brain tissue of the blueberry-fed rats contained much greater concentrations of dopamine than those of the other groups, which is thought to have contributed to their superior coordination, balance and stamina.

Sweet Blueberries

The single dietary change which radically transformed laboratory animals with inherited Alzheimer's disease, enabling them to perform as well or better than their healthy peers at navigating mazes, was feeding them blueberry extract from early adulthood.

Dr. James Joseph's USDA Neuroscience Laboratory has bred rats with a genetic mutation that promotes increased *amyloid beta proteins* in the brain. The exact causes of Alzheimer's are still not fully understood, but an insufficient breakdown and recycling of amyloid protein is believed to be the central cause. Normally harmless amyloid proteins fragment into *amyloid beta particles*, hardening and accumulating into a neural plaque instead of being recycled by the brain. This plaque eventually leads to impaired neural communication and cell death.

Beginning with rats which were four months old (equivalent to early human adulthood), half the test group bred with brain plaques were fed a diet which included blueberry extract for the rest of the year, while the other half ate standard rat food, along with a control group without the plaque-producing mutation.

When the rats reached a year of age (equivalent to early human middleage), all groups were tested for maze navigation. The rats with brain plaque which had eaten blueberry extract performed just as well as the normal control mice, and significantly outperformed their brain-plaque-impaired rat peers who had eaten a standard diet.

Interestingly, autopsies showed the same amount of amyloid beta plaques, but the mice fed blueberry extract had increased kinases, which are very important for brain functions like the conversion of short-term memories into long-term ones – if you recall, kinases are used as "on switches" by your neurons, allowing long-term potentiation to proceed.

Dr. Joseph believes the combined antioxidants within blueberry extract also reduce inflammatory compounds in the animals' brains; such inflammation is a major contributor to age-related neuronal and behavioral decline. Blueberry compounds are able to cross the blood-brain barrier to affect neural tissue; polyphenols in the extract protect the CNS from oxidative and inflammatory stress.

Genesis

A similar study by the team focused upon links between nutrition and the hippocampus in aging rats. After birth, nearly all neurons have been formed, but synaptic changes regularly occur. From that point, it largely becomes a matter of "use it or lose it" – synapses which are seldom used are eliminated in a "synaptic pruning", while those used most frequently form stronger connections, and become easier to trigger with each use.

Although the hippocampus' ability to generate new neurons has long been believed to decline significantly with age, this experiment found aged rats which ate blueberry extract for just a short time significantly increased neurogenesis in the dentate gyri of their hippocampi. And there was a direct link between this growth of neurons and better real-world memory performance: in maze navigation tests, those rats which ate blueberry extract showed improved cognition relative to their peers who ate a normal diet.

To measure rat cognition, scientists typically use a pool with a submerged platform to track rodent learning. Rats fed standard food take longer to locate this platform and show little to no progress in remembering, when compared with those fed blueberry extract. Although it's not yet clear if the cognitive improvement from blueberry extract also occurs in humans, it seems highly probable.

Antidepressants Spur Neurogenesis

Proof that antidepressants boost brain cell formation has also recently emerged. There are only two brain regions known to form new neurons throughout life, of which the hippocampus is one. For people suffering from depression, this process is disrupted, though whether this is a symptom or cause is not yet clear.

Dr. Christoph Anacker at King's College London has demonstrated, however, that antidepressants clearly boost hippocampus neurogenesis. He says the antidepressant *sertraline hydrochloride* (brand names *Zoloft* and *Lustral*) – a selective serotonin reuptake inhibitor – has been shown to increase human hippocampal neurons by as much as a 25 percent or more within 10 days.

Homework: Visit McGill University's free Interactive tour of the brain online here: http://thebrain.mcgill.ca/flash/index_d.html

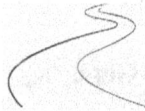

The Brain: How The Brain Rewires Itself" Friday, Jan. 19, 2007, Time Magazine;

How the 'Plastic' Brain Rewires Itself, Nikhil Swaminathan, February 28, 2007, Scientific American;

The Brain That Changes Itself, The Nature of Things, David Suzuki, Dr. Norman Doitsch, 2009, Canadian Broadcasting Corporation (online here: http://www.cbc.ca/video/#/Shows/The_Nature_of_Things/ID=1233752028);

The Plastic Human Brain Cortex, Dr. Alvaro Pascual-Leone, Amir Amedi, Felipe Fregni, and Lotfi B. Merabet, 2005, Annual Review of Neuroscience http://brain.huji.ac.il/publications/Pascual-Leone_Amedi_et%20al%20Ann%20Rev%20Neurosci%2005.pdf;

Evolve Your Brain The Science of Changing Your Mind, Joe Dispenza, 2007;

Changing Your Mind, The Nature of Things, David Suzuki, Dr. Norman Doitsch, 2010, Canadian Broadcasting Corporation (online here: http://www.cbc.ca/documentaries/natureofthings/2010/changingyourmind

The Brain That Changes Itself (book), Dr. Norman Doidge, MD, 2007;

Structural Plasticity within Highly Specific Neuronal Populations Identifies a Unique Parcellation of Motor Learning in the Adult Brain, Ling Wanga, James M. Connera, Jessica Rickerta, and Mark H. Tuszynski; Proceedings of the National Academy of Sciences, 2011; DOI: 10.1073/pnas.1014335108 http://www.pnas.org/content/early/2011/01/20/1014335108;

Navigation-Related Structural Change in the Hippocampi of Taxi Drivers, Eleanor A. Maguire, David G. Gadian, Ingrid S. Johnsrude, Catriona D. Good, John Ashburner, Richard S. J. Frackowiak, and Christopher D. Frith, 1999, Proceedings of the National Academy of Sciences; http://www.pnas.org/content/97/8/4398.full;

The Four Pillars of Healing, Dr. Leo Galland, M.D., 1997;

When Memory Lane Takes a Wrong Turn: Alleviating PTSD, Beverly Akerman, 2006, McGill Reporter, March 2 – Volume 38 Number 12;

Mindfulness CBT as Effective as Antidepressants in Preventing Depression Relapse, Dr. Zindel V. Segal, PhD, et al, 2010, Archives of General Psychiatry 67:1256-1264 http://www.medscape.com/viewarticle/733931;

Tomorrow's People: How 21st Century Technology is Changing the Way we Think and Feel, Susan Greenfield, 2003;

How Brain Research Relates to Rigor, Relevance and Relationships, Dr. Willard R. Daggett, Ed.D., Dr. Paul David Nussbaum, Ph.D., 2008, International Center for Leadership in Education; http://www.leadered.com/pdf/Brain%20Research%20White%20Paper.pdf;

Designing Your Mind, Don Tapscott, 2011, Huffington Post, http://www.huffingtonpost.com/don-tapscott/designing-your-mind_b_811989.html

Six Ways to Boost Brainpower, Emily Anthes, February/March 2009, Scientific American Mind; http://www.sciamdigital.com/index.cfm?fa=Products.ViewIssuePreview&ARTICLEID_CHAR=2311D3BC-3048-8A5E-10D8547B7E4FB645)

The Nervous System in Action, Michael D. Mann, Ph.D. 2011, textbook, University of Nebraska Medical Center; http://www.unmc.edu/physiology/Mann/index.html

The Posterior Parietal Cortex Remaps Touch into External Space, Elena Azañón, Matthew R. Longo, Salvador Soto-Faraco, Patrick Haggard, Current Biology, 15 July 2010 DOI: 10.1016/j.cub.2010.05.063

217

3-D Movie Shows What Happens in the Brain as it Loses Consciousness, press release, Emma Mason, 11 Jun 2011 University of Manchester

Adult Neurogenesis, Dr. James B. Aimone, The Salk Institute of Biological Studies, San Diego, California, 2007, Scholarpedia, 2(2):2100 doi:10.4249/scholarpedia.2100 revision #80231; http://www.scholarpedia.org/article/Adult_neurogenesis

Severe Trauma May Damage the Brain as Well as the Psyche, Daniel Goleman, 1995, NY Times

Target-Specific Encoding of Response Inhibition: Increased Contribution of AMPA to NMDA Receptors at Excitatory Synapses in the Prefrontal Cortex, Scott J. Hayton, Matthew Lovett-Barron, Eric C. Dumont, an Mary C. Olmstead, 2010, Journal of Neuroscience; 30 (34): 11493 DOI: 10.1523/JNEUROSCI.1550-10.2010; http://www.jneurosci.org/content/30/34/11493.full

Differences in "Bottom-Up" and "Top-Down" Neural Activity in Current and Former Cigarette Smokers: Evidence for Neural Substrates Which May Promote Nicotine Abstinence Through Increased Cognitive Control, Liam Nestor, Ella McCabe, Jennifer Jones, Luke Clancy, Hugh Garavan. NeuroImage, 2011; DOI: 10.1016/j.neuroimage.2011.03.054

The Skinny on Memory Loss, University of Texas press release, 2011, author unattributed http://www.utexas.edu/features/2011/05/02/dementia_obesity/

Food for the Aging Mind, Rosalie Marion Bliss, 2007, US Department of Agriculture; http://www.ars.usda.gov/is/AR/archive/aug07/aging0807.htm

Blueberry Extracts Boost Brain Function, Rosalie Marion Bliss, 2007, US Department of Agriculture

How Antidepressants Boost Growth of New Brain Cells, Jessica Hamzelou, 17 April 2011, New Scientist Magazine.

PART III: BODY

Superhuman

"When your desires are strong enough, you will appear to possess superhuman powers to achieve." – Napoleon Hill, Think and Grow Rich

The Superhuman In You

Let's talk about potential for a moment. There are some things you may not realize about yourself that are... surprising and tremendously inspiring.

Start with strength. Man or woman, whether you realize it or not, your body is an incredibly powerful and efficient biological machine. Your bones, for example, are an astounding evolutionary development, light, flexible and porous, made up of 22% water, but stronger than the best steel-reinforced concrete. Your thighbone, for example, can withstand about 2000 pounds of compression before snapping.

Your heart is a biological marvel – pumping your blood through 50 thousand miles of blood vessels, at a rate of 1.3 gallons per minute, or 700,000 gallons per year, for decades. In an extreme emergency, your heart has a *cardiac reserve* – the ability of to deliver as much as five to eight times the normal volume.

Your heart is comprised of four chambers and made up of individual cells which can, incredibly, continue to beat rhythmically through the mechanisms of a special contractile protein, even if removed from the heart and placed in an oxygen-rich environment.

No less incredible is your liver, which breaks down toxic substances and works in tandem with your pancreas to regulate your blood sugar, and to help deliver it via your bloodstream to virtually every cell in your body.

Your kidneys, meanwhile, are a multifunctional marvel, regulating water retention, re-absorption of substances into your blood, maintaining blood salt, acidity and ion levels, and excreting urea and other wastes.

Superstrength

All those stories you've heard about superhuman strength? Anecdotal grannies flinging Mack trucks out of the path of their progeny may be slight exaggerations, but a genuine phenomenon exists called *hysterical strength* – a massive, unnatural burst of power which can surface during the most extreme stress.

It appears it really is possible for you to move as much as four times your own bodyweight or more, given the right circumstances. Fortunately, those circumstances don't occur very often – fear-induced adrenaline allows you to lift huge amounts, but at the cost of ripping the muscles from your bones.

Under normal circumstances, you engage less than half your muscles at a time, even under extreme exertion. In a life-or-death emergency, however, your body can trigger all its muscle fibers in one massive synchronized contraction, giving you a single, tremendous burst of power, and overriding your body's built-in protective system. Here's how it works:

Danger prompts your *HPA axis* (hypothalamus-pituitary-adrenal system) to trigger a release of cortisol, epinephrine and norepinephrine, hormones which activate your body's emergency-responses. This state helps you confront danger: heartbeat and breathing speed up, pupils dilate, digestion slows and glucose stores are freed up for quick muscle energy. The surge of oxygen and glucose provides a burst of super-fuel.

The reason you can't toss cars about with whimsical abandon, however, is that the muscles in your body are protected by a process called *autogenic inhibition* – the amount of tension (muscular force) your muscles are allowed to generate is limited, to prevent exertions beyond what your bones and connective tissues are able to withstand.

As discussed in book I, within your muscles, joints and tendons are a number of proprioceptors - nerves that signal the position of your body parts to your cerebellum and cortex.

Your cerebellum helps orchestrate coordinated movement between all your muscles, providing a sort of synchronizing timer, and acting as a comparator between your intended movement - the sequence of muscle contractions known as a motor program, generated by your motor cortex and selected, initiated and stopped by your basal ganglia - and your actual movement, based on the locations of these position-sensing nerves.

Your muscles fuse onto your bones via tough tendon fibers, and it's here where muscles and tendons meet that your body has special overload protection devices. If the tension of a muscle fiber is too high, the golgi tendon organ triggers nerves which inhibit further muscle contraction.

Stretching the muscle fiber compresses nerve terminals. This compression opens channels in the terminal membrane, and ions can flow through, changing the neuron's polarity, and the nerve fires a signal to the spine.

To protect the muscles and tendon from tearing away from the skeleton, your spine generates a reflexive response - one that happens at the site of the spine, without requiring brain input - sending an inhibitory signal back to the muscle that prevents further tension, an automatic response called autogenic inhibition.

However, in a life-or-death emergency, your limbic system can trigger an "override" signal that shuts off the golgi tendon organ response, and you're able to place dangerously high tension upon your nerves, tendons and bones, and recruit all the available motor units simultaneously in a massive, synchronized burst – the superhuman state called hysterical strength. This power is within you at all times, and can be accessed in the direst of emergencies, but at the cost of crippling injuries.

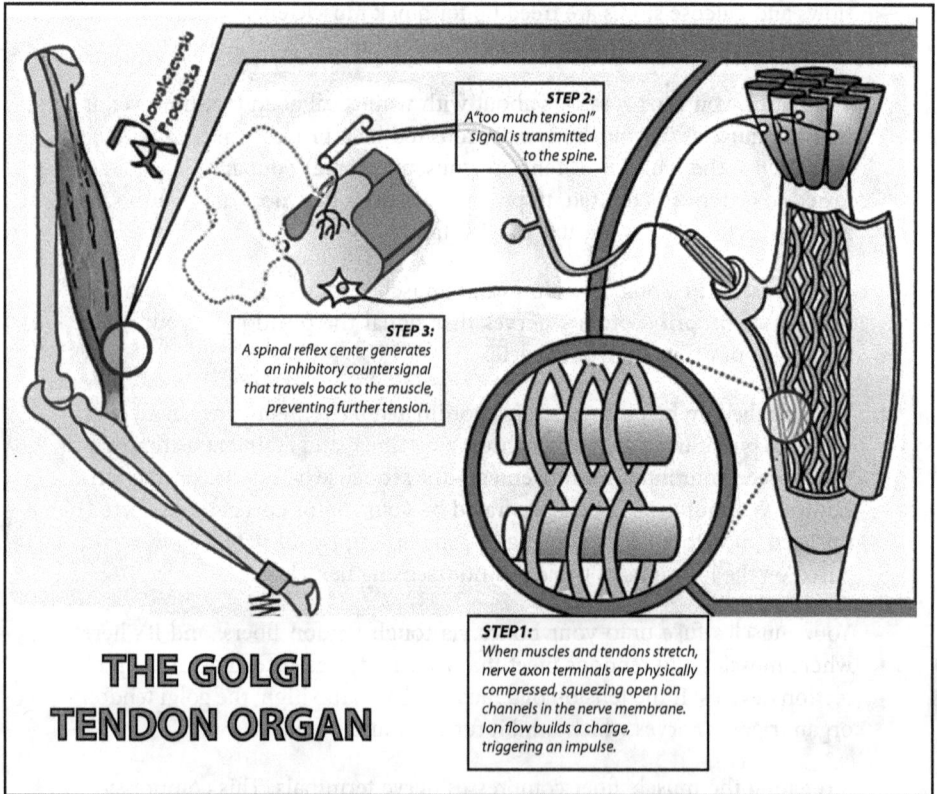

STEP 2:
A "too much tension!" signal is transmitted to the spine.

STEP 3:
A spinal reflex center generates an inhibitory countersignal that travels back to the muscle, preventing further tension.

STEP 1:
When muscles and tendons stretch, nerve axon terminals are physically compressed, squeezing open ion channels in the nerve membrane. Ion flow builds a charge, triggering an impulse.

THE GOLGI
TENDON ORGAN

Adapted from Wikipedia, 2012. Public domain image.

A second inhibitory mechanism at work in your body is your opposing musculature For every *agonist* (pushing) muscle, there is an opposing *antagonist* (pulling) muscle. One example would be the biceps-triceps musculature of your arms. While you lift with your biceps, your triceps relax, holding your bones in place and limiting the range of movement.

These twin protective mechanisms insure you don't injure yourself by tearing your tendons from your skeleton. But through progressive strength training, the inhibitory mechanisms of the Golgi tendon organ can gradually be overridden, and you can engage in greater synchronized muscle recruitment.

Power-lifters have physically adapted themselves to lift the maximum amount of weight their bodies can sustain, first by increasing muscle mass and strength, and secondly by training themselves to override natural inhibitory responses. But even a simple shout has been shown to instantly increase physical power by as much as 31%, according to a 1961 study in the Journal of Applied Physiology.

Superspeed

Your body is also equipped for short bursts of explosive superspeed. In the direst of emergencies, you can activate a very special type of muscle tissue called *Fast-Twitch Phosphagenic* (FTP) Fibers. Normally you can't voluntarily activate these fibers, but in the height of intense emotion, enzymes activated by epinephrine can enable you to recruit the muscle tissue for about a ten-second burst of super speed – allowing you to run at a pace which, for a very short time, can match that of a professional racehorse.

Your fight or flight response grants you the capacity to fight for your life – and win – against seemingly impossible odds. Take, for example, 20-year-old Megan Halavais, who fought off a 14-foot Great White shark that had sunk its teeth into her leg and dragged her into the waters of Bodega Bay on the morning of October 19, 2005. And then there's 68-year-old Alan Garratt, who successfully fought off two masked robbers attacking him with samurai swords. Anger, as you've seen, can boost courage and strength and even shut down pain until you've dealt with the danger.

In theory – you could also, if you needed to – survive on nothing but water for many weeks (please don't though, as it has a high potential of permanently injuring or even killing you): ten and a half weeks is the longest documented period anyone's survived without food – in the case of 1981 IRA hunger-striker Thomas McElwee (who died on the 73rd day).

When your body first goes into starvation mode, it triggers a release of *orexins*, hormones that heighten attention, critical thinking, memory and planning skills to help you find food. After this period however, your body will slow down metabolism to conserve energy, putting you into a state of enforced efficiency. After three weeks without food, your brain orders your body to begin *autophagia* – eating its own proteins. You can survive a loss of about half of your musculature in this gruesome manner before dying.

All of these superhuman feats lie dormant within you right now, but here are just a few more of the myriad miraculous natural feats your body is capable of:

- *Regeneration* – Your skin cells, for example, divide every 20 hours.

- *Super-vision* – It's estimated your eyes can distinguish up to 10 million different colors.

- *Super-digestion* – The substance that breaks down food in your body – hydrochloric acid – is strong enough to eat through metal.

- *Pain Immunity* – It's possible to shut down your pain responses through meditation, just as effectively as with a shot of morphine. Natural pain tolerance varies from person-to-person, but can be trained, as shown by 2010 studies at Oxford University.

- *Super endurance* – The average untrained person can, if needed, engage in mild to strenuous exercise for about two to three hours, using food that's been recently consumed. Past that point, you'll hit what endurance athletes call the wall, a point of fatigue and a drop in serotonin that leads to a deep crash in mood and willpower. At this point, your body starts to require extra oxygen and begin draining fat stores for fuel.

  The ability to continue exercising past this two- to three-hour point becomes a conscious act of willpower. Trained athletes learn to anticipate and minimize the effects of pushing through this wall, allowing them to, for example, complete marathons.

- *Super-durability* – Your knee cartilage, which functions like a shock absorber, or a water-filled cushion, can bear seven tons of compressive load before giving way; this enables your knees to bear hundreds of millions of shocks over the course of your lifetime.

> *Shrinkage* – *Then there's British lawyer, environmentalist and motivational speaker Lewis Gordon Pugh, who swam a kilometer in 18 minutes across the geographic North Pole (now iceless due to global warming) through -1.7 degree ocean waters, wearing only a speedo. Through mental imagery and gradual endurance training, Pugh has learned, like Hof, to regulate his heart rate and body temperature, and can demonstrably send his pulse from 70 to 160 bpm, and his temperature from 37°C to 38.4°C, while motionless. Laboratory tests show that Pugh, like Hof, can mentally control his metabolism, apparently tapping into hormonal releases to keep his core temperatures high.*

- *Super-cognition* – Your brain is far, far faster than any computer, by several orders of magnitude. In fact, in a single second, your brain executes many as 100 trillion instructions, equivalent to every computing device on the planet – from IC chips to pocket calculators to giant supercomputers – combined – an estimated 6.4 × 1018 instructions per second.

- *Superstrength* – Martial artists such as the shaolin monks train by repeatedly striking wood, stone and iron objects. Not only does this desensitize them to pain, it causes micro fractures in the bones of their hands and feet. These tiny cracks fill with calcium deposits, healing and hardening into deadly weapons.

Raising The Bar –
From The Jaw-Dropping…

Those are just a few of your *natural* capacities. As for limits, with genetic luck, iron mental will and two to three years of intense training, you can conceivably:

- Run 350 miles without stopping

- Swim across the Atlantic Ocean in 3.5 weeks

- Run a marathon every day for an entire year with no days off

- Bench press 1075 pounds

- Run a mile in under four minutes

- Jump 8.95 meters (29.4 feet) in length, or 2.45 meters. (8.03 feet) in height

…To The Miraculous

On September 19, 2008, free diving world champion Tom Sietas held his breath underwater on live television for *17 minutes and 19 seconds* on ABC's Regis and Kelly Live. It was an astounding feat, and, according to all accounts, absolutely real. Since then, the Guinness Book of World Records lists the current world record in *static apnea* (underwater breath-holding after preparation with pure oxygen) at 20 minutes, 21 seconds.

But 11-year-old Alvaro Garza Junior has these records beat by nearly half an hour: On December 4, 1987, in Fargo, North Dakota, Alvaro plunged through 2 inches of ice and was trapped underwater with no oxygen for 45 minutes. The live rescue footage and testimony of Dr. William Norberg, who resuscitated Alvaro at St. Luke's Hospital, is available online. Now a healthy father of four, Alvaro is fine, if a tad more cautious. (Please, please don't try either of these stunts!)

Humans still possess primitive protoreptilian and protomammalian brains. These neural centers grant animals like seagulls and seals a *diving reflex*, allowing them to plunge to great depths and stay underwater for extended periods of time. When they hold their breath and dive into cold water, their brains shut off all but the most critical functions throughout the body. The diving reflex seems to only occur in cold-water conditions, presumably because of metabolic slowdown.

According to Montana State University professor Anthony Goodman, humans possess a similar diving reflex. It's not quite as efficient, but still exists in vestigial form. Its existence was discovered by accident when Alvaro Garza was trapped under the ice in 1987, generating shock in the medical community. Garza was resuscitated with virtually no brain damage; normally, brain death begins after four to six minutes.

The Icemen Cometh

For centuries, religious and cultural rituals have included dives into icy waters in Russia, China and a number of northern European countries; and Japanese and Korean pearl divers can swim without wetsuits in near-freezing waters for up to half an hour at a time.

But Dutch Iceman Wim Hof, 52, is a rather more surprising example of such endurance. At the time of this writing, he holds eighteen world records for extreme cold endurance, reportedly using *Tantric Tummo meditation* to control his body temperature – "using his brain to turn up his body's thermostat", as he puts it.

In 2009, National Geographic taped him live, as Hof ran his first marathon (26.2 miles or 42.2 kilometers) 120 miles north of the Arctic Circle through -20 °C (-4 °F) snow, dressed only in shorts and sandals.

Exposure to such extreme cold normally kills quickly, triggering a massive shock response. When your skin surface senses a sudden intense temperature drop, it triggers involuntary hyperventilation, and your blood vessels constrict to restrict blood flow and protect your body's vital organs. This sudden massive increase in blood pressure can easily trigger a heart attack. But Hof completed his incredible endurance race in 5 hours and 25 minutes, a stunning feat that was captured live in 2009's *Daredevils: The Ice Man* for the BBC and National Geographic. Hof says, and appears to have demonstrated, that the human mind can be developed to such an extraordinary degree it can allow you to physically resist sub-zero temperatures.

Wim Hof is the first non-member to have trained with Tibetan monks in *Tummo* (Tibetan for inner fire), a branch of Tantric meditation that deals with energy control in the body. Coupled with breathing techniques and endurance training that consists of standing in freezers to adapt his body to severe temperatures, Hof is, doctors say, able to mentally control his blood pressure and core body temperature.

Dr. Juha Oksa of the Finnish Institute of Occupational Health has published a number of studies in his area of specialty, cold physiology. Initially skeptical, he also personally examined Vim Hoff, apparently further establishing his legitimacy: http://www.biomedexperts.com/Profile.bme/1049754/Juha_Oksa

Hof gave a live presentation of his ability at a 2010 TED conference in Amsterdam, standing immersed in ice for an hour and twenty minutes as Dr. Maria Hopman of Radboud University monitored his vital signs for the audience. She shows how, although his skin surface temperature drops to freezing levels, his core temperature remains stable. He is also apparently able to maintain his heart rate, while doubling his metabolism.

Although the precise mechanisms aren't known, Hof appears to have trained his hypothalamus and pituitary to control his autonomic nervous system, mentally regulating his heartbeat, blood pressure, vessel dilation, metabolic rate and even immune function. In the spring of 2011, a team of doctors led by Peter Pickkers of Radboud University injected Hof with *endotoxin*, a harmless bacterial component that triggers an immune response.

Normally, endotoxin triggers flu-like symptoms: fever, headache, and muscle pain lasting several hours, but with no long-term effects. Hof, who reported only a mild headache, had his blood immune response measured, and the results showed he produced only half the immune-system proteins of over 200 other healthy men. Professor Pickkers said this was due to a sharp rise in cortisol, which suppresses the immune system. A video of Pikkers' tests on Hof, broadcast on Dutch National Television, can be seen online here: http://www.youtube.com/watch?v=nRsNh0eB-Io

The Medical Center is assembling 10 more subjects, all to be trained in Hof's techniques, to see if the results can be duplicated. In the meantime, Hof has begun training students in Tummo meditation. Among his students is 31-year-old world judo champion Edith Bosch, who won the silver medal at the 2004 Summer Olympics, and is hoping Hoff can give her the mental "edge" she needs to win the gold.

The Supersenior

Bob Keller competes in world championship triathlons and duathlons. He's already participated in nearly 850 racing events, and his goal is 1000. What's most surprising about him, however, is his age – born in 1934, Keller is fast approaching his *80th birthday*. Although he played team sports in school and the Navy, he only got serious about fitness at age 50. He now trains at least four days a week, on weekends biking as much as 35 miles, running another nine, then swimming 1,400 yards.

The Olympic Triathlon, in which he competes, is particularly daunting – an endurance event which includes a 1.5 km swim, 40 km ride and 10 km run (one mile swim, 24.8 mile ride and 6.2 mile run, respectively) one after another with no rest. Keller's a veteran of the event, and he's not alone: in 2011, he was one of *over 15,000 triathletes aged 50 to 85* who registered to compete in the National Senior Games.

If age needn't be a barrier to realizing your potential, what's your excuse? Given your extraordinary potential, conferred upon you just by virtue of being human, isn't it just possible that you're settling for significantly less than you're capable of? If your answer is "yes", I invite you to join me as we continue down the path to success in life.

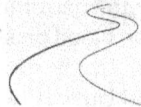

Chapter 11, *The Nervous System In Action*, Michael D. Mann, Ph.D. 1997-2012; http://www.unmc.edu/physiology/Mann/mann11.html

Superhuman: The Secrets of the Ice Man, Duncan Graham-Rowe, 2009, *New Scientist*

The Great Courses: Understanding the Human Body: An Introduction to Anatomy and Physiology, Professor Anthony Goodman, 2003, the Teaching Company Limited; http://www.thegreatcourses.com/greatcourses.aspx

Neural Adaptations to Exercise: A Practical Approach, Jacob Wilson, 2007, Journal of Hyperplasia Research 7(1); http://www.abcbodybuilding.com/neuraladaptations.pdf

Coaching Pitchers, Dr. Michael G. Marshall, 2003; http://www.drmikemarshall.com/ChapterThirty-One.html

The Human Body – Pushing the Limits: Episode 2, 2009, Discovery Communications http://www.yourdiscovery.com/video/human-body-us-vo-strength-bones/

Features of a Successful Therapeutic Fast of 382 Days' Duration, W. K. Stewart and Laura W. Fleming, Postgraduate Medical Journal 1973;49:203-209 doi:10.1136/pgmj.49.569.203; http://pmj.bmj.com/content/49/569/203.abstract

http://www.irishhungerstrike.com/

http://www.youtube.com/watch?v=x3xVQmiwGtY

http://www.youtube.com/watch?v=CCt8p_v-FU0

Cell Longevity, US Department of Energy, 2004; http://www.newton.dep.anl.gov/askasci/mole00/mole00482.htm

Color in Business, Science and Industry, Judd, Deane B.; Wyszecki, Günter 1975, p. 388. ISBN 0471452122

Digestive System, UC-Clermont College Biology, 2010; http://biology.clc.uc.edu/courses/bio105/digestiv.htm

US Army Survival Manual; http://www.equipped.com/21-76/ch2.pdf

Edward Payson Weston, Wikipedia, 2011; http://en.wikipedia.org/wiki/Edward_Payson_Weston

How Far Can You Run? Jane Hoskyn, 8 September 2006, Runner's World; http://www.runnersworld.co.uk/general/how-far-can-you-run/2387.html

Incredible Feats of Endurance, I Swim, Bike, Run, 2009; http://iswimbikerun.wordpress.com/2009/02/11/incredible-feats-of-endurance/

Orexin/Hypocretin: Wired for Wakefulness, Takatoshi Mochizuki and Thomas E. Scammell, 2003, Current Biology; doi: 10.1016/S0960-9822(03)00474-3; http://www.cell.com/current-biology/retrieve/pii/S0960982203004743

Surfer Fights off Shark, Escapes with Bitten Leg, Michael Cabanatuan and Simone Sebastian, October 19, 2005, San Francisco Chronicle; http://articles.sfgate.com/2005-10-19/news/17396469_1_salmon-creek-beach-shark-deputies

CCTV: Bypass Grandfather Fights Off Samurai Sword Post Office Raiders, UK Telegraph, December 3rd, 2008; http://www.telegraph.co.uk/news/uknews/3545532/CCTV-Bypass-grandfather-fights-off-Samurai-sword-post-office-raiders.html

Hicham El Guerrouj sets a world record in the mile (YouTube video): http://www.youtube.com/watch?v=XvCsj7eJKKA

Mike Powell vs. Carl Lewis – Long Jump – World Record (YouTube video): http://www.youtube.com/watch?v=ybEs3j_MmrA&feature=related

Strongest Man-world record set by John Wooten, World Records Academy, 2011, http://www.worldrecordsacademy.org/strength/strongest_man_world_record_set_by_John_Wooten_70849.htm

Long Distance Running World Record, 24hr 243,656 m, Sigrid Lomsky GER, IAU European Championships SUI 05/01/93; http://www.athleticsweekly.com/stats/records/world-records-and-best-performances-womens-road-running/

'Marathon Man' Completes Remarkable Feat, Ryan Hepworth, February 10, 2011, Washington Square News; http://nyunews.com/sports/2011/02/11/11marathon/

Mystery of the Iceman, TED Amsterdam, 2007 Nov. 30, 2010; http://www.tedxamsterdam.com/2010/the-mystery-of-the-iceman-remains/

Mental Fatigue Impairs Physical Performance In Humans, Samuele M. Marcora, Walter Staiano, and Victoria Manning, 2009, Journal of Applied Physiology; http://jap.physiology.org/content/106/3/857.full.pdf+html

The Limits of Endurance Exercise, T. D. Noakes, 2006, Basic Research in Cardiology, Volume 101, Number 5, 408-417, DOI: 10.1007/s00395-006-0607-2; http://www.springerlink.com/content/t77763720815w656/

Daredevils: The Ice Man, Channel 4, 21/09/2009; http://www.firecrackerfilms.com/broadcast/daredevils-the-ice-man/

Remarkable Results in Research on "Iceman" Wim Hof, Press release, Radboud University, 2011, http://www.alphagalileo.org/ViewItem.aspx?ItemId=101486&CultureCode=en

Wim Hof, Dutch 'Iceman,' Controls Body Through Meditation, Toby Sterling and Aleksandar Furtula, Associated Press, /22/11; file:///C:/Users/Elric/Desktop/wim-hof-dutch-iceman-cont_n_865203.html

Utter Endurance: 'Iceman' and 'Ultramarathon Man', Joseph Diaz and Ruth Chenetz, May 27, 2010, ABC News 20/20; http://abcnews.go.com/2020/iceman-marathon-man-feats-human-endurance/story?id=10731229&page=2

Body Temperatures During Three Long-Distance Polar Swims in Water of 0–3 °C, T.D. Noakesa, et al, Journal of Thermal Biology, Volume 34, Issue 1, January 2009, Pages 23-31; doi:10.1016/j.jtherbio.2008.09.005; http://www.sciencedirect.com/science/article/pii/S0306456508001010

Extreme Breath-Holding: How It's Possible, Emily Sohn, Feb 17, 2010, Discovery News; http://news.discovery.com/human/breath-holding-human.html

The Great Courses, Lecture 7 – Anatomy of the Brain, Dr. Anthony Goodman, 2003, The Teaching Company

World Record High Jump, Javier Sotomayor, 1993; http://www.youtube.com/watch?v=vWde8s Mxe1w&feature=related

Some Factors Modifying the Expression of Human Strength, Michio Ikai and Arthur H Steinhaus, 1961, Journal of Applied Physiology vol. 16 no. 1 157-163; http://jap.physiology. org/content/16/1/157.short

Tuning The 'Fight-Or-Flight' Response: Molecular Memory Of Stress Prompts Adrenaline Surges, Cornell Study Shows. Science Daily. April 22, 1998, author unattributed; http://www. sciencedaily.com/releases/1998/04/980422065736.htm

National Space Biomedical Research Institute; http://www.nsbri.org/HumanPhysSpace/ focus6/ep_development.html

Hold Your Breath for a Really Long Time, Wired Magazine, 2007; http://howto.wired.com/wiki/Hold_Your_Breath_for_a_Really_Long_Time

Discovery Channel The Human Body – Pushing the Limits: Episode 1 – Strength, 2009; http:// www.yourdiscovery.com/video/human-body-strength-superhuman/

This Septuagenarian Will Run, Swim and Bike Laps Around You, Jim Henry, February 23, 2011, AOL News; http://www.aolnews.com/2011/02/23/this-septuagenarian-will-run-swim-and-bike-laps-around-you/

History of NSGA; http://www.nsga.com/about-nsga/history-nsga

North Florida Olympic Triathlon race results; http://www.coolrunning.com/results/09/fl/ May30_NorthF_set2.shtml

Exercise

Looking back at Maslow's Hierarchy of Needs, you'll see that self-development begins with building upon your health. In this section, you're going to see the latest cutting-edge scientific findings on the best exercise, nutrition and supplementation. Let's start with exercise:

Why Bother?

In *The 4-Hour Body*, Timothy Ferriss tells the story of his meeting with Richard Branson. Branson, of course, is the founder of the global Virgin empire, now worth an estimated 20 billion dollars. At an exclusive training camp, the number one productivity secret Branson imparted to Ferriss and other attendees can be boiled down to two words: "work out".

Branson says the energy he gets from exercise gives him an estimated four extra hours a day of productivity. But here are a few more very compelling reasons to exercise regularly:

- A recent Harvard University study found that strenuous aerobic exercise reduces heart disease risk by 20%. Aerobic exercise dilates blood vessels, reduces hardened fatty arterial buildups and enhances blood circulation.

- A 2008 study of 64,777 women also found that when women aged 12 to 35 exercised regularly, their risk of breast cancer lowered up to 33%.

- Lifelong exercise also builds and maintains healthy bones, preventing osteoporosis, a common bone degeneration disease.

The most highly recommended exercises include brisk walking, jogging, hiking, yard work, volleyball, soccer, baseball, basketball, dancing, step aerobics, swimming, stair climbing, tennis and other racquet sports, skiing, skating, karate and bowling.

A Significant Brain Boost

A 2011 study at Georgia Health Sciences University has shown that daily exercise improves cognitive ability in inactive, overweight children, significantly improving behavior, focus, planning and analytical and mathematical skills.

171 overweight 7- to 11-year-old subjects had all been sedentary prior to the study. Dr. Catherine Davis and her team had the children take tests before and after the program started, combined with fMRI scans.

The program consisted of vigorous workouts: running, jumping rope, and hula hoops, raising the children's heart rates to 79 percent maximum – research within the last decade has found that such aerobic exercise increases growth factors such as BDNF in the brain. The effects seem to benefit people of any age.

The study showed that the more children exercised, the more they improved, and intelligence scores increased 3.8 points on average among those who exercised 40 minutes daily for three months. fMRI scans showed increased activity in the prefrontal cortex – the region responsible for analytical thinking, decision-making, moral judgment, and suppressing inappropriate behavior. Unsurprisingly, the program significantly improved their focus and behavior.

The *Pediatric Anger Expression Scale,* which measures behaviours like hitting and door slamming, was administered prior to and after the program. Earlier studies by Dr. Davis and her colleagues had shown exercise minimizes angry behavior in overweight children, raises their self-esteem and reduces the effects of depression. There is also evidence that exercise reduces anxiety.

Stronger Immunity

Exercising regularly gives you fewer and milder colds, according to the British Journal of Sports Medicine, which tracked 1,000 adults up to age 85 for 12 weeks during the 2008 autumn/winter season. Older married men seemed to have the fewest colds, but the most important factors were overall exercise amount and perceived fitness.

Those who reported feeling fit and exercising five or more days a week had 43% to 46% fewer cold symptoms than those who exercised only once a week or less, and the severity of their symptoms fell by 41%. The average adult catches a cold two to four times every year, while children catch six to ten a year, on average. (I've been exercising regularly since childhood, and suffer a cold perhaps twice a decade, if that.)

The authors of the study say exercise triggers an increase in immune system cells. These levels return to normal a few hours after exercise, but each short-term growth increases the likelihood of enhanced microbe surveillance, thereby reducing the occurrence and severity of infections.

Protecting Your Heart

Exercise protects your heart from cardiac arrest risk, and from injury if such heart attacks do occur, boosting levels of an enzyme which produces nitric oxide. In Spring, 2011, Emory University School of Medicine researchers identified this capacity to produce and store nitric oxide as the key to the heart's self-protection. Nitric oxide is a gas naturally produced by your body. When you lack oxygen, nitric oxide triggers chemical reactions that dilate blood vessels, increasing blood flow.

Your body appears to maintain emergency nitric oxide reserves, nitric oxide gas bound to proteins. Nitric oxide is generated during exercise, then stored in your bloodstream and heart in the form of nitrite and nitrosothiols. The protective benefits emerge after about a month of regular exercise, and fade after about a week, so it's important to maintain a regular schedule. Doctors recommend at least 30 minutes a day, three to five days a week.

A Completely Different Person

Aerobic exercise improves bone and muscle strength, blood circulation and oxygen uptake, boosts coordination and balance, lowers cholesterol, fights arteriosclerosis, enhances organ function, promotes sleep, strengthens the heart, reduces blood pressure, regulates hormone and blood sugar levels, improves mood, learning and concentration, strengthens immunity from disease, and may help prevent Alzheimer's. It also significantly reduces the risk of heart attacks, high blood pressure, stroke, diabetes, obesity, anxiety, depression, and breast and colon cancers. Finally, it keeps you slim, clear-skinned and energetic.

Anaerobic exercise includes weight-lifting or sports machine training, and is very effective for creating and maintaining weight loss in both men and women. Although women worry about becoming "muscle-bound" and "bulky" if they lift weights, such muscle growth is biologically impossible, unless a woman receives illegal steroid injections. Here's why:

Sex hormones determine gender differences and stimulate growth in human beings. Women and men produce both testosterone and estrogen, but the ratios vary widely. Women produce 10 times as much estrogen and one-tenth the testosterone. Estrogen causes the pelvis to widen, breasts to form, and the body to store fat. Its production tends to taper off after adolescence, so women grow rapidly for a short time after puberty, and then body growth largely stops.

In contrast, men have a longer growth period and 10 times higher testosterone levels, resulting in greater height, muscle and bone mass, broader shoulders, narrower hips and a larger chest circumference. It's this much higher concentration of testosterone that allows massive muscle growth in professional bodybuilders, but the much lower testosterone levels in women make it impossible to grow as muscle-bound as men without illegal steroid injections.

The average female body is 24% muscle mass, compared to 40% or more in men. Because of their testosterone levels, men have much higher upper body strength; however, both sexes have similar lower body strength, and women tend to have greater endurance in sports such as marathon running.

Women also tend to live, on average, as much as ten years longer than men. According to the United Nations, the current average life expectancy for women in Japan is 87 years, the highest in the world. But because we have moved away from physically strenuous lifestyles toward more sedentary ones, you need to maintain regular levels of exercise if you want to live such a long and healthy life.

Melting Away Fat Like Butter:
High Intensity Interval Training

Research over the last 15 years has shown a method of weight loss that burns 300% the fat in half or less time than typical long-distance or endurance sports. Based upon Swedish *Fartlek* training (cross-country running with short bursts of speed), it involves cardiovascular training at a moderate pace, mixed with regular intervals of high intensity. The catch? It ain't easy. But it works, and amazingly well, as you'll see after only about four sessions.

Your body is a miraculous machine, which quickly adapts to all kinds of conditions to help you survive. This adaptation is *homeostasis* – a balance of your body's various biochemical and metabolic processes. But this survival mechanism works against you when you're trying to lose fat. For example, if you "crash diet" and eat nothing, your body will adapt by bringing you into starvation mode, slowing your metabolism so you burn fewer calories. One way to combat this is by eating small, palm-sized amounts of healthy food regularly all day long, to keep your calorie-burning rate maximized. Professional athletes call this *grazing*.

When you train at the same level of intensity for a long time (e.g., running at the same speed for 30 minutes or more), your body adapts to that intensity and conserves its energy stores, burning fewer calories than before. To absolutely maximize your ability to burn fat, researchers have discovered the best means is by varying intensity constantly as you exercise.

High Intensity Interval Training can be performed with any kind of cardiovascular exercise, including swimming, jogging, skiing, cross-training machines or cycling. A 15- to 20-minute HIIT workout has been shown to burn up to three times as much fat as working out at a steady pace, and boosts your metabolism for 24 hours, burning fat while you're at rest.

The high intensity phase should be at your near-maximum intensity, and the medium-intensity exercise at about 50% of your maximum intensity. Modern treadmills usually have heart monitoring systems, or you can buy a cheap pacemaker, if you prefer.

To determine the intensity of your workouts, you can calculate your MHR (maximum heart rate) as follows:

MHR = 206.9 – (0.67 x age)

If you're a conditioned athlete, the threshold is higher:

Athletes (male) – MHR = 202 – (0.55 x age)
Athletes (female) – MHR = 216 – (1.09 x age)

If you prefer, a number of online automatic calculators are also available. Once you make the calculation, you can constantly reuse it, so it's worth the effort.

One HIIT session consists of a warm-up, six to twelve cycles of high-intensity exercise separated by medium-intensity exercise, and a final cool-down. The entire session lasts only 12 to 30 minutes.

Here are the three most powerful HIIT programs, according to recent research:

1. Standard Variation

- *Warm-up* (three to five minutes): low intensity jogging, cycling, etc., gradually increasing speed.

- *Intervals* (six to eight repetitions) one minute high intensity followed by one minute low intensity

- *Cool down* (three to five minutes): low intensity jogging, cycling, etc., gradually decreasing speed.

2. The Little Method – The newest regimen, based on a 2009 study

- Warm-up (three to five minutes): low intensity jogging, cycling, etc., gradually increasing speed.

- Intervals (eight to twelve reps): one minute high intensity followed by 75 seconds low intensity.

- Cool down (three to five minutes): low intensity jogging, cycling, etc., gradually decreasing speed.

3. The Tabata Method – This is a very advanced program, and you'll require the assistance of a trainer or doctor to measure your VO_2 max (maximal oxygen absorption). The plus side is that it is very short and provides the best results of all. The Tabata Protocol consists of 20 seconds of ultra-intensity activity (170% of VO_2 max) followed by 10 seconds of rest, repeated over eight cycles – four minutes total.

Toughen Up – Weightlifting For Men And Women

The latest studies have proven that weightlifting is a superior means of burning fat, sculpting your physique, and speeding up your metabolism, and for the reasons outlined above, women needn't worry about becoming big and bulky without steroid use. Weightlifting two to three times a week, coupled with High Intensity Interval Training on "off days" two to three times a week, is a fat-burning furnace, which provides the best body-conditioning combination discovered to date.

For your safety and maximum benefit, it's critical to learn proper form for each exercise from a trained, certified instructor, and to concentrate 100% on maintaining that form during each repetition. Please be sure to schedule an appointment with a trainer the first time you visit a gym.

Although this aerobic-anaerobic routine can get and keep you in excellent shape for the rest of your life, to help your body reach its maximum potential – advanced levels of fitness – you should vary your program, and keep a log book, in which you track your exercises, weight, repetitions and sets. Because your body will adapt to the levels of work you subject it to, to keep improving, you also need to change your routine every six months or so.

To avoid overtraining, where you risk fatigue, injury, immunity suppression and the inability to function well, you should also take one week off completely every two months.

As an additional energy burner, you can use a circuit training schedule, where you move immediately from one exercise to the next until you've completed an entire circuit. Three to four complete circuits is your total workout. Generally half an hour to one hour will give the greatest benefits; only professional elite bodybuilders or competitive athletes need to spend more than an hour a day exercising.

Fitness experts recommend a program that starts with *compound exercises* – resistance movements that engage a combination of the largest muscle groups simultaneously – such as the bench press, which uses your chest, arms and shoulders – before moving to *isolated exercises* which target only one muscle group, such as curls, which only use your biceps. You want to start with compound exercises, because using more muscles simultaneously requires greater effort, tires you sooner, and uses the most energy to produce the fastest results.

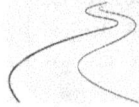

Exercise Helps Overweight Children Reduce Anger Expression, Medical College of Georgia, 2008; http://www.sciencedaily.com /releases/2008/11/081124130951.htm

Exercise Improves Executive Function and Achievement and Alters Brain Activation in Overweight Children: A Randomized, Controlled Trial, Dr. Catherine Davis, Dr. Jennifer E. McDowell, and Dr. Phillip Dr. Tomporowski, et al, 2011, Health Psychology, Vol 30(1), 91-98; http://www.ncbi.nlm.nih.gov/pubmed/21299297

Regular Exercise Reduces Depressive Symptoms, Improves Self-Esteem In Overweight Children, Mar. 18, 2009, ScienceDaily; http://www.sciencedaily.com/releases/2009/03/090318104330.htm

Upper Respiratory Tract Infection is Reduced in Physically Fit and Active Adults, David C Nieman, Dru A Henson, Melanie D Austin, Wei Sha, British Journal of Sports Medicine, 2010; DOI: 10.1136/bjsm.2010.077875; http://bjsm.bmj.com/content/early/2010/09/30/bjsm.2010.077875.abstract

Exercise Protects Against Myocardial Ischemia–Reperfusion Injury via Stimulation of β3-Adrenergic Receptors and Increased Nitric Oxide Signalling: Role of Nitrite and Nitrosothiols, John W. Calvert, Marah Elston, Juan Pablo Aragón, Chad K. Nicholson, Bridgette F. Moody, Rebecca L. Hood, Amy Sindler, Susheel Gundewar, Douglas R. Seals, Lili A. Barouch David J. Lefer, 2011, doi: 10.1161/CIRCRESAHA.111.241117; http://circres.ahajournals.org/cgi/reprint/CIRCRESAHA.111.241117v1

Women's Body Bible: Training, Diet & Supplementation, Katie Lobliner and Derek Charlebois B.S. CPT, 2008

Social Indicators, United Nations Statistics Division, 2010

A Practical Model Of Low-Volume High-Intensity Interval Training Induces Mitochondrial Biogenesis In Human Skeletal Muscle: Potential Mechanisms, Jonathan P Little, Adeel S. Safdar,

Geoffrey P. Wilkin, Mark A. Tarnopolsky, and Martin J., 2009, Gibala Journal of Physiology

Effects Of Moderate-Intensity Endurance And High-Intensity Intermittent Training On Anaerobic Capacity And VO₂max, Tabata I, Nishimura K, Kouzaki M, Hirai Y, Ogita F, Miyachi M, Yamamoto K., Medical Science Sports Exercise vol. 28 , 1996

Harvard Men's Health Watch, August 2009

Plan Your Cardio Workout, David Zinczenko, June, 2004, Men's Health Magazine

A Prospective Study Of Age-Specific Physical Activity And Premenopausal Breast Cancer, Maruti SS, Willett WC, Feskanich D, Rosner B, Colditz GA, 2008, Journal of the National Cancer Institute

Workout

"Those who think they have not time for bodily exercise will sooner or later have to find time for illness." – Earl Edward Stanley, Liverpool College address, 1873

Please see the illustrations in the following pages for a complete workout that targets all the major parts of your body and provides the greatest benefits in return for your efforts. If you're a beginner, you'll want to spend the first session learning careful technique and your maximum weight for each exercise. You'll use this to calculate how much weight to use in the future. This is initially time-consuming, but only needs to be done once. You can expect your total training session to take less than one hour, and the results will come extremely quickly if you combine the work with HIIT. Expect significant changes within about three weeks.

The Most Effective Exercises

You can use machines, dumbbells or barbells. Machines are much safer for your joints, and lower the risk of injury significantly, but you lose balance development and limit the amount you can eventually lift. Additionally, exercises that use your own body weight, such as pushups, chin-ups and dips are arguably better for you than machines or free weights, so if you are interested in such a workout, I recommend you seek out a Pilates program.

There are two types of exercise movements, *agonistic* (pulling) and *antagonistic* (pushing). Switch between the two types per body part for maximum energy throughout your workout.

For example, perform a bench press followed by a seated row (see the following illustrations). This circuit program has been designed to target all the muscle groups, and is to be performed in order, using the largest muscle groups first (compound exercises) and working down to the smaller muscle groups (isolated exercises).

Because abdominal fitness is one of the best ways to enhance your appearance and add to your overall physical strength and health, I've devoted a section specifically to abs exercises. The top three have been included for a basic circuit workout, but the section that follows, on posture and core training, will be of even greater benefit to you if you're willing to invest the time and effort (and you should!).

To date, the most thorough research has been conducted at the Biomechanics Lab of San Diego State University (published by the American Council on Exercise), where researchers examined the most common abs exercises and

240

machines (wheels, rockers, pushers, etc. using EMG machines to measure and compare actual muscle use and stimulation. When done correctly, the best exercises use the abdominal and oblique muscles, without "cheating" – getting assistance from the hips and thighs.

Surprisingly, though most people believe basic crunches are the best exercise, they're actually one of the least effective. Add a stability ball, however, and they rank #3 for effectiveness. Bicycle crunches, which topped the list in terms of effective muscle use and stimulation, are 2.5 times as effective as the basic crunch, followed by hanging leg raises (also called the "Captain's Chair"), stability ball crunches and reverse crunches. Because many neglect to exercise the lower back, I recommend including hyperextensions with your abs exercise program.

For the full study data, the American Council on Exercise published a free online article showing the detailed results at http://www.acefitness.org/getfit/studies/bestworstabexercises.pdf

Your Body Remembers

Physiologists have long believed that after extended periods of disuse, muscles would lose all the benefits of exercise, a withering called *atrophy*. But *muscle memory* describes how motor tasks are easier to perform after previous practice, even after a lapse of years, almost as if the muscles themselves could somehow "remember".

It's been demonstrated that because of this, everything from proficiency with a musical instrument to strength acquired from years of weightlifting can be rapidly regained, even after long periods of inactivity. It was thought until 2010 that these effects were entirely due to procedural memory, and that the seat of such "muscle memory" was in the CNS, but a team of researchers in Oslo Norway demonstrated that long-term effects are due to changes within muscle fibers themselves.

Muscle cells are the largest in the human body, several thousands of times larger than most others. Because of their large volume, they are special, in that they contain multiple cell nuclei, a property called *syncytia*.

During strength training, as ever-increasing loads are placed upon your muscles, muscle fibers swell, rather than increasing in number, a process known as *hypertrophy*. This generates new cell nuclei which endure "...for a considerable period of the animal's lifespan." Contrary to conventional wisdom, these myonuclei persist even when muscle cells shrink and lose power from prolonged disuse. Because of this, upon retraining, the extra myonuclei are able to more rapidly resume the protein synthesis needed for rebuilding muscle mass and strength.

This ability to generate myonuclei declines with age, however, so strength training is best begun at an early age. The finding has important implications for professional sports, because it means that, even after long periods of abstinence, the use of "doping" substances such as anabolic steroids can stimulate essentially permanent advantages in myonuclei increases, even long after doping substances are untraceable.

Your Ultimate Fitness Program

On the following pages, you'll find a complete workout that targets all your major muscle groups, and can get you started on a lifetime of supreme fitness.

Instructions:

You should weightlift twice a week and do aerobic exercise (aerobics, dance, running, martial arts, swimming, cycling, etc.) for half an hour or more on the days in between. Abdominal exercises, however, are best performed every exercise day. This is a weekday-only program, so you're free to enjoy your weekends however you like.

On your lower body days, because your legs are stronger and you will be performing fewer exercises, it's recommended that you increase your sets to four or even five.

- Spend one session practicing smooth form with a trainer

- Find your maximum single lift for each exercise

- Print out the training log (at the end of this section) to keep track of your progress.

- Warm up with a single set of minimal weight – ¼ of your maximum. This is to begin blood flow.

- Next, perform three sets of 5-10 reps (75% your single maximum lift) of each exercise.

- The movement should be rapid on exertion, and then slow and controlled on release (1/2 speed).

- Breathe OUT HARD while EXERTING, and IN SLOWLY while RELAXING.

- Rest about 30 seconds between each exercise, less to maximize calorie burn.

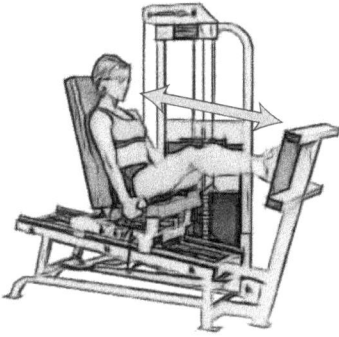

1. Leg Press

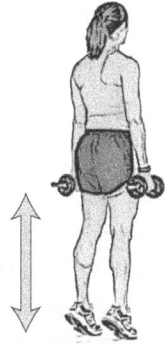

2. Calf Raises

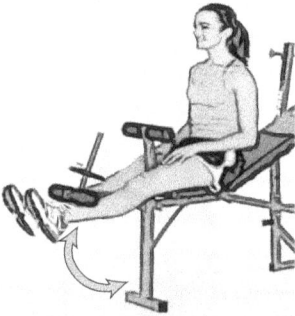

3. Leg Extensions

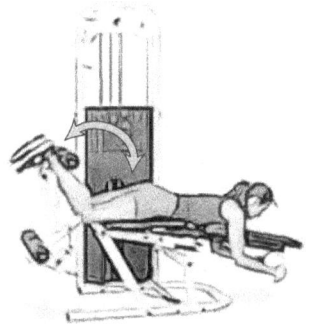

4. Leg Curls

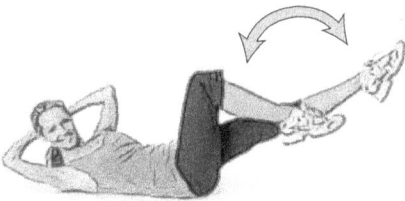

Abs 1. Bicycles

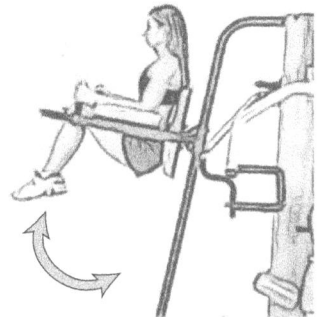

Abs 2. Hanging Leg Raises

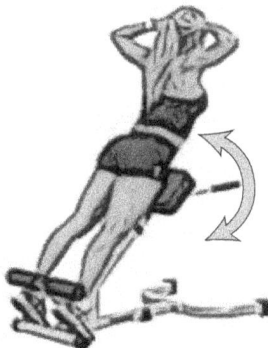

Abs 3 Hyperextensions

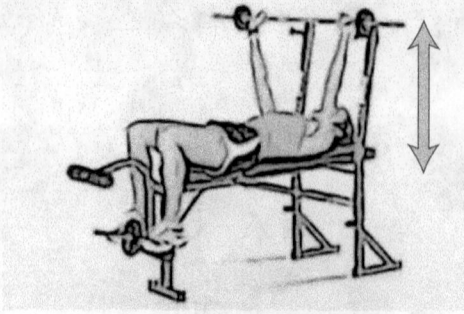
1. Bench Press

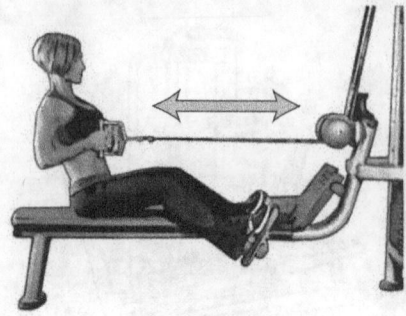
2. Seated Cable Rows

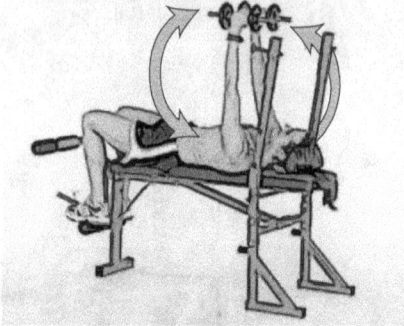
3. Dumbbell Chest Flyes

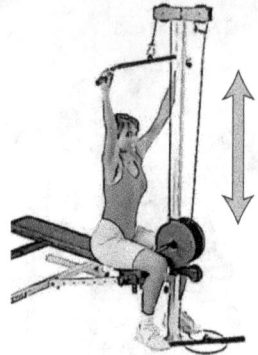
4. Lat Pulldowns

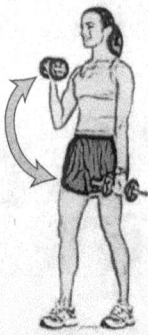
5. Dumbbell Curls

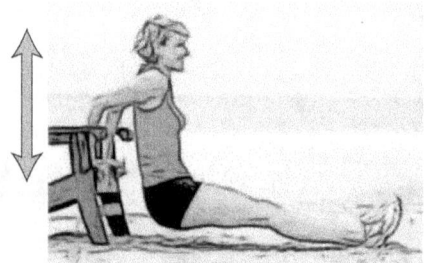
6. Dips

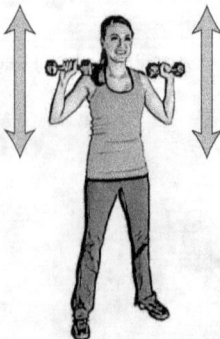
7. Dumbbell Shoulder Press

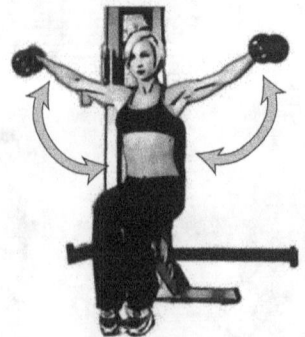
8. Lateral Raises

PERSONAL TRAINING LOG

DATE:	DAY:									
EXERCISE	**SET 1**		**SET 2**		**SET 3**		**SET 4**		**SET 5**	
Upper Body	WEIGHT	REPS	WEIGHT	REPS	WEIGHT	REPS	WEIGHT	REPS	WEIGHT	REPS
1. Bench Press										
2. Seated Cable Rows										
3. Dumbbell Flyes										
4. Lat Pulldowns										
5. Dumbbell Curls										
6. Dips										
7. Shoulder Press										
8. Lateral Raises										
9.										
10.										

PERSONAL TRAINING LOG

DATE:	DAY:									
EXERCISE	**SET 1**		**SET 2**		**SET 3**		**SET 4**		**SET 5**	
Lower Body	WEIGHT	REPS	WEIGHT	REPS	WEIGHT	REPS	WEIGHT	REPS	WEIGHT	REPS
1. Leg Press										
2. Calf Raises										
3. Leg Extensions										
4. Leg Curls										
5. Bicycles										
6. Hanging Leg Raises										
7. Hyperextensions										
8.										
9.										
10.										

PERSONAL TRAINING LOG

DATE:	DAY:									
EXERCISE	**SET 1**		**SET 2**		**SET 3**		**SET 4**		**SET 5**	
Core	WEIGHT	REPS	WEIGHT	REPS	WEIGHT	REPS	WEIGHT	REPS	WEIGHT	REPS
1. Bicycles										
2. Ball Extensions										
3. Trunk Rotations										
4. Planks										
5. Supermans										

When can perform more than eight repetitions, add weight the next session.

Upper Body Workout (Mondays)

>   *Chest:* Bench press, dumbbell flyes
>
>   *Back:* lat pull-downs, seated cable rows
>
>   *Arms (front):* Bicep curls, chin-ups
>
>   *Arms (back):* Dips, triceps pushdowns
>
>   *Shoulders:* Lateral raises, shoulder press

Lower Body Workout (Thursdays)

>   *Legs (quadriceps):* leg press machine, squats and lunges
>
>   *Legs (calves):* Calf raises
>
>   *Legs (hamstrings):* leg curl machine
>
>   *Legs (thighs):* leg extensions machine
>
>   *Abdomen:* bicycles, hanging leg raises, hyperextensions. I recommend doing these every weekday, or substituting the special 12-minute core training session (see Posture and Core training)

Training at home – *Joining a gym is really the best idea, as they have superior equipment and professionally-trained instructors to teach you, but as a last resort, a step, a set of dumbbells and resistance bands can be used at home (I've also heard great things about the "Wii Fit" machine!).*

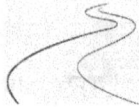

New Study Puts Crunch on Ineffective Ab Exercises, M. Anders, American Council on Exercise, 2001

Arnold's Bodybuilding for Men, Arnold Schwarzenneger, 1984

Myonuclei Acquired By Overload Exercise Precede Hypertrophy And Are Not Lost On Detraining, J. C. Bruusgaard, I. B. Johansen, I. M. Egner, Z. A. Rana, and K. Gundersen, Department of Molecular Biosciences, University of Oslo, 2010

Breathe

The air is precious to the red man, for all things share the same breath - the beast, the tree, the man, they all share the same breath. The white man does not seem to notice the air he breathes. – Ted Perry, Home, 1972 (misattributed to Chief Seattle)

How Not To Exercise

One of the keys to maximizing exercise and health in general – a kind of "open secret" that most people aren't even aware of – is the incredible power of your breath.

For thousands of years, mystics and scholars have pointed to the deep belly, diaphragm area as the Seat of Power, the source of *chi energy*. Alternative medicine and spiritualism worldwide nearly unanimously share the principle of *vitalism*, a belief that there's an unseen energy in the world. Hindi religion calls it *prana*, the Chinese call it *chi*, and the Japanese call it *ki*, although it's referred to throughout history and in nearly 100 diverse cultures around the world. This life essence has been associated with the soul, spirit, and mind. It's been associated with breath since ancient times, the Hebrews calling it *ruach*, the Greeks *psyche* or *pneuma* (breath of the gods), and the Romans *spiritus*.

This unseen energy is central to Chinese martial arts and alternative medicine. Chi is the life force believed to flow through your body's *meridians* in a rhythmic fashion. Acupuncturists believe chi flow can be enhanced by stimulating special points within these meridians. This force is said to flow not just through the body, but throughout the environment. This is the basis of *feng shui*, where the placement of your house and belongings is believed to either enhance or impede energy flow. Whether or not there is any scientific basis to this is dubious to say the least, but again we see a ubiquitous belief that a force exists in all things, and that you can be trained to harness its power.

Martial artists learn to use chi to add incredible power to their strikes. If you doubt the effectiveness of channelling chi, please watch this seven-minute documentary of Bruce Lee's "One-Inch Punch". With concentration and training, it's possible to send a full-grown man literally flying backward with a single strike from a distance of only an inch: http://www.youtube.com/watch?v=Kx9iPFMriz0

The value of harnessing your breath cannot be overemphasized. If you walk into a typical gym, you'll always run across some poor red-faced fellow, with his cheeks puffed out like a puffer fish, straining at a (kind of puny) weight.

If that poor fellow would only open his mouth and let in some oxygen, he would be able to perform the same exercise easily. The difference is stunningly powerful if you've never used correct breathing techniques during exercise:

1. Breathe in deeply and fully expand your lungs

2. Push or pull the weight quickly and smoothly (never lock your joints at the end!) while forcing your air out explosively

3. Slowly return to the exercise starting position while breathing in fully

4. Repeat for 5 to 10 repetitions

You've seen repeatedly throughout this book the power of using visualization. Here's an example to take you to the next level in your strength training:

Before you begin a tough exercise, close your eyes and imagine a bolt of golden sunlight shooting down from the sky to bathe you in light. Feel it coursing through your body, and visualize power, like crackling electricity, suffusing the body part you're about to exercise. Coupled with proper breathing, the results of this will amaze everyone around you. Try it once as an experiment – you'll soon be easily able move two to three times as much weight as anyone around you.

Jogging Beside City Traffic

Your red blood cells are composed primarily of *hemoglobin*, a molecule of folded amino acids which transports oxygen to every cell of your body (with the exception of the lenses and corneas of your eyes, where blood would obscure your vision).

Your cells use this oxygen to break down nutrients, producing energy to fuel cellular functions. These chemical reactions produce waste, including carbon dioxide, which is then removed by your hemoglobin and pumped by your heart to your lungs, where you exhale it.

Hemoglobin naturally binds with oxygen or carbon dioxide, depending on pH. pH levels in cells which need oxygen trigger hemoglobin oxygen *release*, then carbon dioxide to hemoglobin. When blood returns to the *lungs*, pH levels trigger the opposite – carbon dioxide release and oxygen binding.

Carbon monoxide is released when organic matter – for example wood or fossil fuels – burns with insufficient oxygen to fully consume it. The reason CO is so deadly to humans and other animals is that it binds with hemoglobin in your red blood cells 230 times more efficiently than oxygen. This "bound up" hemoglobin continues to circulate, but can no longer absorb oxygen; the cells in your body become starved for oxygen and die.

The carburetor in your car is a device which mixes gasoline and oxygen for your engine to burn. If it's badly tuned, it releases carbon monoxide into the air. Normally a catalytic converter attached to your engine's exhaust will convert emissions into less toxic forms, but in cold weather, or when a car is old or in need of a tune-up, carbon monoxide output climbs, along with other toxic hydrocarbon emissions.

Charcoal and wood burning stoves that are poorly ventilated also produce high levels of carbon monoxide and other toxic hydrocarbons. Car exhaust in cities is, of course, full of toxins, which is why it's a very bad idea to be jogging alongside busy city streets. Car exhaust has a number of deadly toxins, among them:

- Carbon Monoxide

- Nitrogen dioxide

- Sulphur dioxide

- Benzene

- Formaldehyde

- Polycyclic hydrocarbons

On November 18, 1994, the National Association of Physicians for the Environment hosted the first conference on *Air Pollution: Impacts on Body Organs and Systems* in Washington, D.C. They noted that blood, which flows through all the internal organs, carries toxins just as efficiently as oxygen, nutrients, hormones and other beneficial substances. Air pollution from vehicles burning gasoline and diesel deliver these deadly toxins into your bloodstream via your nose, mouth, skin, and digestive system. All the above pollutants have been proven to harm the blood, bone marrow, spleen, and lymph nodes.

Airborne pollutants enter your lungs as *volatile gas* (benzene), liquid droplets (sulfuric acid and nitrogen dioxide), or as *particulates* (diesel exhaust). These pollutants have been demonstrated to interact with the immune system, and may cause immunosuppression or overactive immune responses.

Disorders which can occur as a result of these respiratory system pollutants include immunosuppression and hypersensitivity – reactions such as asthma following exposure. Genetic susceptibility to pollutant-induced immune disorders has also been demonstrated, though studies are as yet premature.

As noted above, carbon monoxide binds with hemoglobin two hundred and thirty times more easily than oxygen, causing a form of slow suffocation. It can also worsen cardiovascular disease: additional airborne pollutants can overstimulate your immune system, producing tissue damage in the cells lining blood vessels. The combined effects are very unhealthy for your heart.

Lead sabotages blood cell formation, inhibiting enzymes and rupturing blood cell membranes. It also interferes with cellular *metabolism*, shortening each cell's survival. All of these effects can lead to *anemia*, a dangerous shortage of red blood cells. Lead and other heavy metals also impair the central nervous system, causing proven changes in behavior and cognitive function in children at much lower levels than previously realized. Nor are adults immune; they also display similar declines in learning and memory.

It's also becoming apparent that heavy metals and other air pollutants may be at the heart of rising cancer rates, as well as significant alterations of mood, cognition and behavior. A number of studies have shown that increased air pollution is accompanied by increased admissions to hospitals and psychiatric units, by behavioral changes, and by decreases in well-being. Irritating odors and airborne pollutants like tobacco smoke have been demonstrated to increase aggression, decrease altruism and degrade social interactions.

Benzine has been listed as a carcinogen by the U.S. Department of Health and Human Services. Workers exposed to benzene for periods of four years or more have died from leukemia, and it's believed that long-term exposure can lead to anemia and internal bleeding. Studies have also shown that benzene harms the immune system, increasing risks of infections and possibly lowering resistance to tumors. Benzene exposure has been linked to genetic mutations, including low birth weight, delayed bone formation, and bone marrow damage, even in concentrations as low as 10 parts per million.

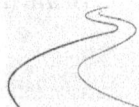

Understanding the Human Body – The Great Lectures, Dr. Anthony Goodman, 2003, The Teaching Company

Air and Breathing, Stephen Gislason MD, Alpha Online, Environmed Research, 2011; http://www.nutramed.com/environment/carschemicals.htm

Stand

There is so much to gain from improving your posture. Everybody's interested in the way they look, and then they're astounded to find the other benefits.
– Janice Novak, Posture, Get It Straight! 2006

Over time, your poor posture takes a tremendous toll on your spine, shoulders, hips and knees. – Bill Hartman, Men's Health, 2006

Stand Up For Yourself

The advice "keep your chin up" appears to have measurable effects upon your endocrine system, helping you cope with not just physical, but also emotional, pain. Your body language can enhance your performance and success, by actually altering your hormonal chemistry. Adapting open, confident body language boosts your body's testosterone release and lowers cortisol release. Insecure or defensive postures have the exact opposite effect – raising cortisol and lowering testosterone. In addition, by speaking and carrying yourself in a confident manner, you naturally increase your feelings of power, risk and pain tolerance.

A joint 2011 study at Columbia and Harvard Business School found:

> *The results of this study confirmed our prediction that posing in high-power nonverbal displays (as opposed to low-power nonverbal displays) would cause neuroendocrine and behavioral changes for both male and female participants... these findings suggest that embodiment extends beyond mere thinking and feeling, to physiology and subsequent behavioral choices. That a person can, by assuming two simple 1-minute poses, embody power and instantly become more powerful has real-world, actionable implications.*

On the other hand, poor posture doesn't just make a poor impression; it weakens you, according to Drs. Scott Wiltermuth at the University of Southern California, and Vanessa K. Bohns of the University of Toronto. What's more, having a submissive posture increases your pain sensitivity. Simply adopting a more dominant pose subconsciously boosts your sense of control, power and your capability to withstand distress: those with the most dominant posture were found to comfortably handle greater amounts of pain than those made to stand in a more neutral or submissive stance.

This builds upon earlier research which shows that the posture of someone with whom you interact also affects your own pose and internal environment. Adopting a submissive pose in response to a dominant pose from a partner increases your pain sensitivity.

A typical pain response might be to curl up into a fetal position, but research suggests that the opposite is more effective. Curling up can actually heighten pain, giving you feelings of a lack of control, intensifying pain anticipation. Sitting or standing up straight, pushing out your chest, and expanding your body is more effective, creating a sense of power and control which can lead to making pain more tolerable. A powerful, expansive posture instead of a passive, constrictive one increases testosterone, resulting in greater pain tolerance, and decreases cortisol, possibly reducing stress.

And just as physical pain relievers are used to reduce emotional pain, Drs. Wiltermuth and Bohns believe a dominant posture also reduces emotional pain from events like a breakup. They also suggest that, all too often, parents and other caregivers often coddle those under their care, trying to make things easier and reduce stress, but this forces those under their care to adopt more submissive roles, heightening susceptibility to pain. This research suggests caregivers should take a more passive role, surrendering control to those about to experience pain, to lessen its intensity.

Walking Tall

Having correct posture is arguably the single most valuable way to improve your physical appearance. Walking with a talk, erect spine can mean the difference between being noticed and being overlooked in every situation. Additionally, it enhances oxygen and blood flow throughout your body, increasing energy and promoting spinal health.

Here is a side view of correct posture. Imagine a cable holding you erect, so that your head is balanced over your shoulders.

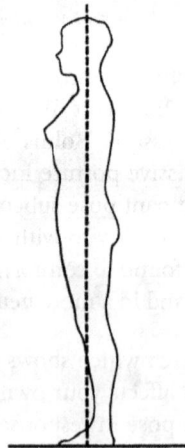

Posture & Foundation Garments, Wikisource, public domain

From the front, your shoulders and hips should be level, your head, knees, and ankles straight. When seen from the front, the vertical line passing through your body's center should cut your body into two halves, with your weight equally on both feet, and your knees facing forward. Ask a friend to check your posture for you.

The most common posture mistakes are:

- Head jutting forward

- Shoulders rounded forward

- Lower back arched

- Pelvis tilting backward (protruding backside)

- Pelvis tilting forward (protruding abdomen or pelvis)

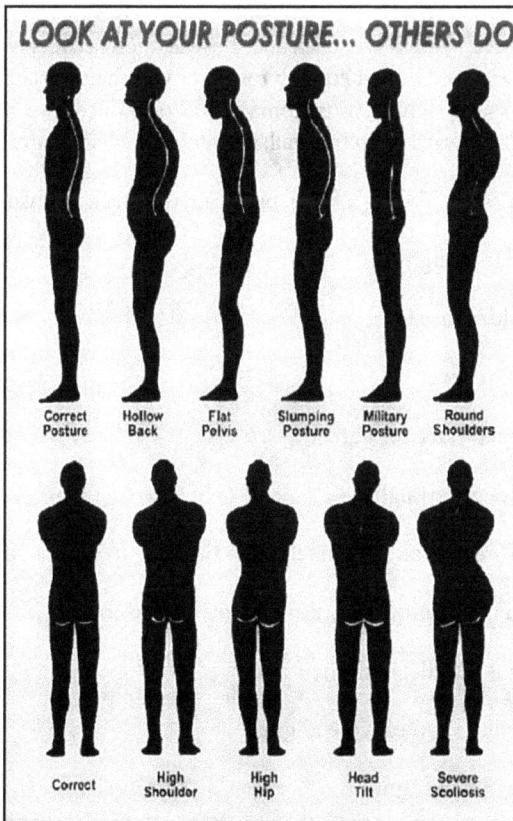

Poor posture, public domain, 1927

Conversely, good posture means:

- Chest high.

- Shoulders back and relaxed

- Abdomen and buttocks tucked in

- Feet parallel.

- Head level and straight

- Knees relaxed and not locked.

Check Yourself

Wall Test – Stand with your back against a wall. Your head, shoulder blades, and buttocks should touch the wall, with your heels 5 to 10 cm away. Slide your hand between your lower back and the wall, then between your neck and the wall. There should be just enough room for your hand to slide through. If there is more space, tighten your stomach and/or reduce your neck tilt, then stand and walk forward from the wall, maintaining this posture.

Mirror Test, Front – Facing a full-length mirror, check to ensure your:

- Head is straight

- Shoulders are level

- Hips are level

- Kneecaps face forward

- Ankles are straight

Mirror Test, side – Look at yourself from the side, to ensure your:

- Head is straight – not tilting in any direction

- Chin is parallel with the floor

- Shoulders and ears are aligned

- Knees are straight

- Lower back curves slightly forward

Improving Through Exercise

Among the exercises I'd like to recommend to you, those which train your "core muscles" are the most critical to your overall posture. These should follow your cardio and weightlifting training. You'll see noticeable improvement within a few short weeks, and if you consistently practice, you will definitely sit and walk taller – and people will take notice.

The major muscles of your "core" include:

Rectus Abdominis – A long muscle extending along the front of your abdomen. This creates six-pack abs once you reduce enough body fat.

Erector Spinae – A collection of three muscles extending from your neck to your lower back, used keep your spine straight.

Transverse Abdominis (TVA) – This muscle wraps around your spine, giving it protection and stability.

External Obliques – The muscles around your waist, on the front and side of your abdomen.

Internal Obliques – The muscles under your external obliques, facing the opposite direction.

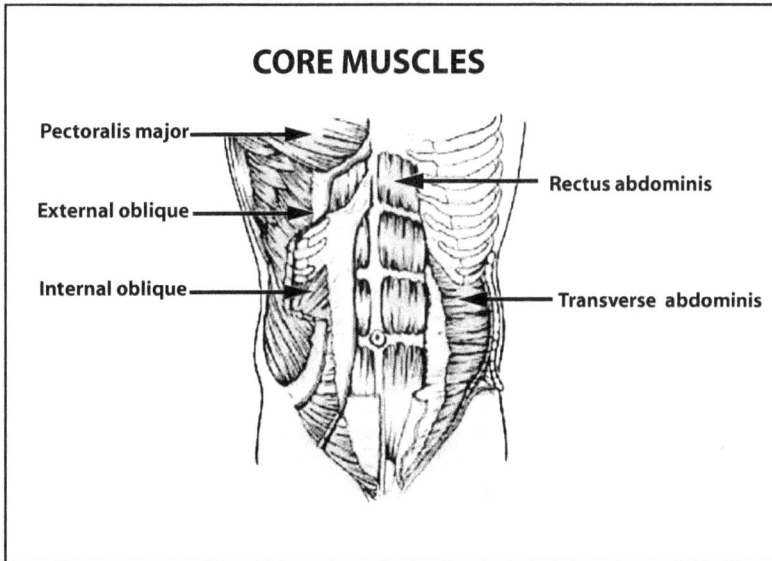

National Institutes of Health, public domain

Your *rectus abdominus* muscles – your "abs" – are just a small part of the total picture. Most people believe strengthening the abdominal muscles is sufficient for core training, but the abdominal muscles play only a very limited role in your body's core musculature, including the *erector spinae*, which run the entire length of your back. Because your core muscles run the length of your spine and stabilize it, weak core muscles will result in deformed posture and cause lower back pain.

Your "core" enables you to stand erect and walk on two legs. Its muscles help you control movement, shift your body weight, and transfer energy to your limbs, which is why a strong core is of tremendous benefit if you play team sports. Core stability creates a solid foundation and allows excellent energy transfer from your trunk out to your limbs, so this conditioning is of great value to professional athletes and dancers.

Please the illustrations on the following page. Professional trainers recommend the following exercises, which can all be performed at home. The workout focuses on strengthening all of the core muscles in your abs and back. These moves will also improve your balance, stability and coordination, making it an excellent overall workout. I highly recommend visiting the YouTube channel called "Livestrong.com" for some excellent free videos on correctly performing these exercises.

Core Exercises

Work up to performing three sets of each exercise, making sure your form is correct. Immediately stop any activity that causes pain or discomfort. Hanging leg raises (also called the "Captain's Chair") are by far the best abs exercises, but the following can be performed at home with no special equipment other than an optional stability ball and floor mat.

Bicycle Crunches – As the diagram shows, lying on your back, touch your elbow to your opposite knee and then switch, extending your leg out fully, for a total of 20 to each side (or more if you're able). This is the number one exercise for the rectus abdominus (frontal abs), proven by researchers at San Diego State University to be 250% more effective than traditional crunches.

Stability Ball Crunches – Lie back with your shoulders on the exercise ball, clasping your hands behind your head. Your feet should be planted flat on the floor and your neck and back in a straight line. Roll your trunk upward without bending your neck or lifting your feet from the floor. Look upward toward the ceiling and keep your neck and back aligned throughout this exercise. Pause in a half-sitting position (not sitting straight up) for five beats, then SLOWLY lower your trunk back to the starting position, resisting the pull of gravity. Repeat at least 20 times, increasing the number of repetitions as you improve.

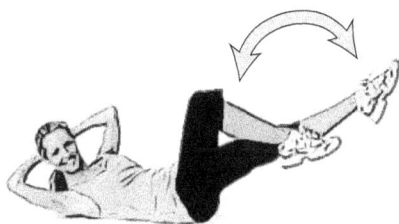

Core 1. Bicycles

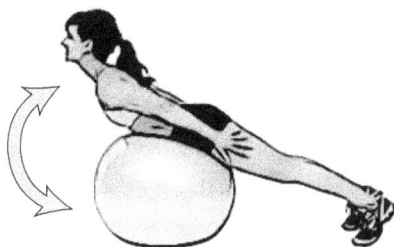

Core 2. Ball Extensions

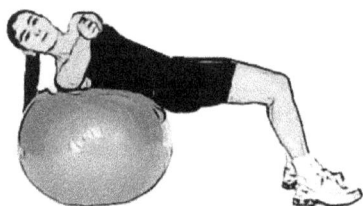

Core 3. Trunk Rotations

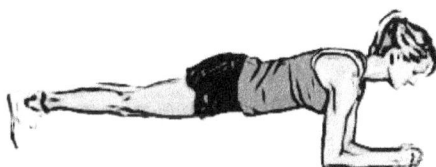

Core 4. Planks

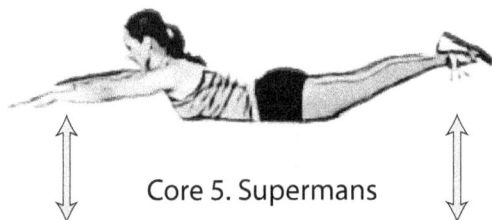

Core 5. Supermans

2011, Polyglot Studios, KK

Trunk Rotations – You can optionally use a dumbbell or medicine ball to increase the intensity of this exercise. Begin with your upper back and shoulders resting on the Stability Ball. Your legs should be bent at a 90-degree angle, with your knees over your ankles. With your arms together and straight out toward the ceiling, slowly swivel your upper body first to one side, then back. Repeat in the opposite direction. One set consists of 12 repetitions, though you can, of course, do more.

Planks – Lying face-down on the mat, rest your weight on your forearms, with your palms flat on the floor. Raise your body in a straight line onto your toes and elbows. Make sure your bottom doesn't stick up in the air or droop down. Breathing normally, hold this position for 30 to 60 seconds, and then lower yourself back to the starting position. Repeat for three or more sets.

Supermans – Start this exercise by lying face-down on the mat with your arms and legs extended straight out together. Lift both your straightened arms and legs simultaneously up toward the ceiling, creating a gentle curve with your body. Breathing steadily and evenly, hold this position for 30 seconds (or more as you get stronger). Finish the move by lowering to the floor again. Repeat for three or more sets.

Additional excellent posture exercises can be found in yoga and Pilates training. The *Alexander Technique* is also a medically-recognized course aimed at teaching excellent posture. Although the courses are not free, the website has links to a huge number of free training resources: http://www.alexandertechnique.com/onyourown.htm

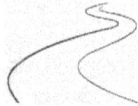

Prevent Back Pain with Good Posture, Mayo Clinic, 2009

Strengthen Your Core – Posture, Paige Waehner, About.com, 2010.

Power Posing – Brief Nonverbal Displays Affect Neuroendocrine Levels and Risk Tolerance, Dana R. Carney, Amy J.C. Cuddy and Andy J. Yap; http://pss.sagepub.com/content/early/2010/09/27/0956797610383437.abstract?rss=1

It Hurts When I Do This (or You Do That): Posture and Pain Tolerance, Vanessa K. Bohns, Scott S. Wiltermuth, 2011, Journal of Experimental Social Psychology, 2011; DOI: 10.1016/j.jesp.2011.05.022; http://www.sciencedirect.com/science/article/pii/S0022103111001612

Contraction Of The Abdominal Muscles Associated With Movement Of The Lower Limb, Dr. Richardson Hodges, Physical Therapy, February 1997;

Relationship Between Limb Movement Speed And Associated Contraction Of The Trunk Muscles, Ergonomics. November, 1997.

New Study Puts the Crunch on Ineffective Abs Exercises, Mark Anders, 2001 http://www.acefitness.org/getfit/abstudy_results.aspx).

Eat

"Tell me what you eat, and I will tell you what you are."
– Jean Anthelme Brillat-Savarin, *The Physiology of Taste, 1825*

Nutrition terms are constantly tossed around by the media without adequate explanation. The following is a complete rundown of what these terms mean, and will teach you precisely how your body uses food.

There are two categories of nutrients: *macronutrients* and *micronutrients*. Macronutrients are substances you consume in large quantities: carbohydrates, proteins and fats; micronutrients are all the other dietary substances, vitamins, minerals, fiber and phytochemicals.

Metabolism

Metabolism is a term for the chemical processes which sustain life. Living organisms use food by breaking molecular bonds to extract energy, which they then use to drive life processes. This energy, along with amino acids and various micronutrients, is used to build proteins for growth, regulation, maintenance and repair.

Special proteins called *enzymes* control metabolism, transforming chemicals, and releasing energy and waste in the process. In your body, every waking and sleeping moment, trillions of these metabolic reactions occur simultaneously, keeping all your cells functioning.

For you (and almost all life on Earth), these life processes are ultimately driven by trapped sunlight: plants use the molecule *chlorophyll* to extract and store sunlight energy within the chemical bonds of *sugars* (carbohydrates) in a process called *photosynthesis*, Latin for light and manufacturing. When you eat plants, or the meat of animals which have eaten plants, you extract this trapped sunlight energy in the form of sugars. Your body then breaks these sugar molecules down, releasing energy for distribution via your bloodstream to all the cells in your body.

There are two types of metabolism:

Catabolism – *destructive* metabolism – produces energy for all cellular activities, breaking down complex molecules – proteins, carbohydrates and fats – to extract energy and chemical components. This energy provides fuel for body heat, for muscle contraction, and for protein production, called *anabolism*. The energy is ultimately converted into the molecule *adenosine triphosphate* (ATP), which drives anabolic processes.

Breaking down nutrients to free chemical energy also creates molecular waste products – carbon dioxide, ammonia, urea, lactic acid, and acetic acid – which are expelled via your kidneys, skin, bladder, lungs, and intestines.

Anabolism – constructive metabolism – is the creation of complex molecules such as proteins and ribonucleic acids, used for growing tissues and organs. Anabolism includes new cell and tissue growth, tissue maintenance, and energy storage in *adipose* (fat) cells for future use. This process is the reverse of catabolism; in anabolism, simple molecules are combined into complex carbohydrate, protein, and fat molecules.

You may have heard of *anabolic steroids* – illegal growth-triggering hormones like *testosterone*, which can be injected to promote anabolism, but at a terrible price – side effects can include sterility, cholesterol buildup, liver damage, baldness, *hirsutism* (body hair growth), liver and heart damage, addiction, aggression, mania, and even psychosis and suicide. Professional athletes sometimes use *PEDs* – dangerous Performance-Enhancing Drugs like anabolic steroids, which can rapidly promote muscle growth, but at the risk of their health and careers.

Your metabolic rate influences how much food you require. *Basal metabolic rate* (BMR) is the "base" speed at which your body uses food energy in *kilocalories*, while resting.

Your BMR can affect both your energy levels and your weight. Someone with a low BMR (who burns fewer calories while resting and sleeping) tends to gain body fat more quickly than someone with a higher BMR eating the same amount of food and getting the same amount of exercise. BMR is largely hereditary, and can be affected by health problems, but it's possible to raise your BMR by exercising and increasing your overall fitness. A greater muscle-to-fat ratio will burn more calories while you're at rest, for example.

Hormones, the chemical messengers in your bloodstream, regulate processes such as your BMR, determining how quickly and in what ways your food energy is used or stored, and thus, how much food you require. Your thyroid (Greek for shield, based on the shape of the cartilage protecting it) is a gland found just under your Adam's apple, which helps control your BMR and physical development via the hormone thyroxine. Your thyroid also synthesizes proteins, and controls sensitivity to other hormones, in this way significantly affecting the function and growth rate of many body systems.

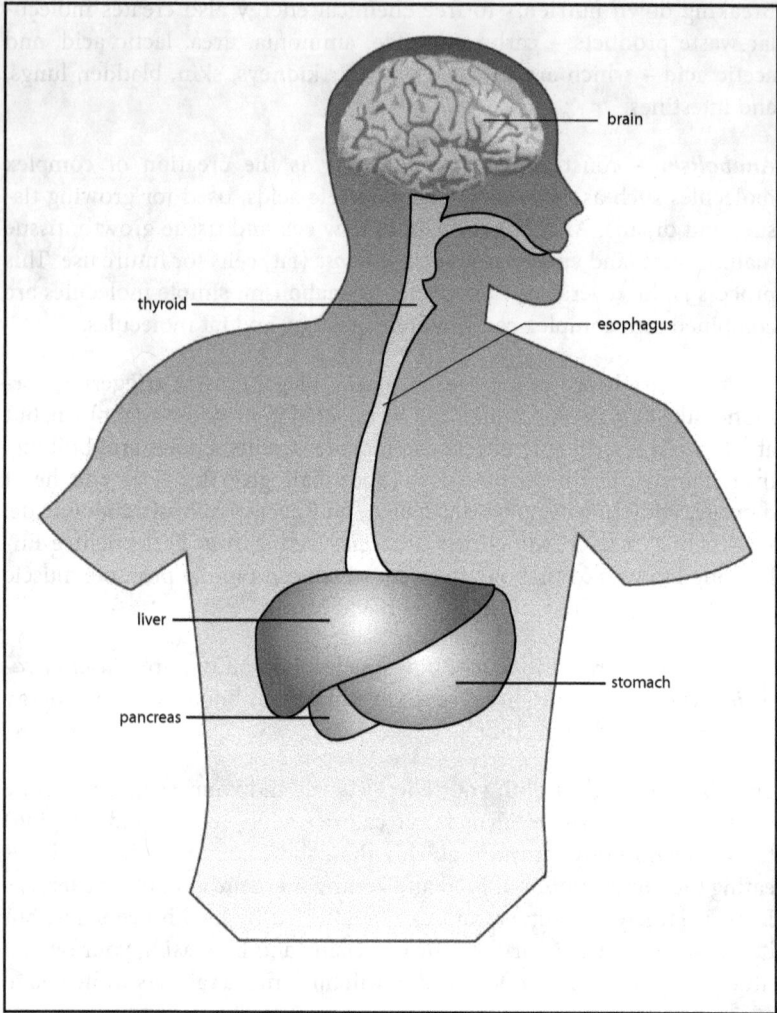

Metabolic control systems, Polyglot Studios, 2011

Twin Sugar Regulators

Insulin and *glucagon* are two hormones produced by your *pancreas*. They work in opposition to one another, helping determine whether you engage in anabolism or catabolism at any given moment. Pancreas *beta cells* constantly monitor your blood glucose levels. After you eat, digested food moves through your intestines, which release glucose into your bloodstream. In response to a rise in your blood glucose, your pancreas releases *insulin*. This triggers energy uptake and storage for daily activities like protein production and muscle contraction.

The released insulin flows through your bloodstream, then binds to receptors on liver, muscle, fat and other cells, triggering absorption of excess blood glucose. In your liver and muscles, simple-sugar (small structure) glucose molecules are chain-linked into the *polymer* (long chain) molecule *glycogen*, human starch, for energy stores. After your muscles and liver are saturated with maximal glycogen, your liver converts any remaining blood glucose into fat.

Insulin acts like a key, opening cellular "doors" to allow glucose to enter cells from the bloodstream, for metabolic energy. When insulin binds to cell receptors, *transporter proteins* floating dormant in the cell cytoplasm (inner cellular fluid) are attracted to the cell membranes, where they can then pump free-floating glucose from your bloodstream into your cells. Insulin also simultaneously inhibits the release of its hormonal opposite, *glucagon*, which could reverse insulin-triggered glycogen absorption and storage triggering glycogen breakdown into glucose to distribute in the blood.

The Effect of Insulin

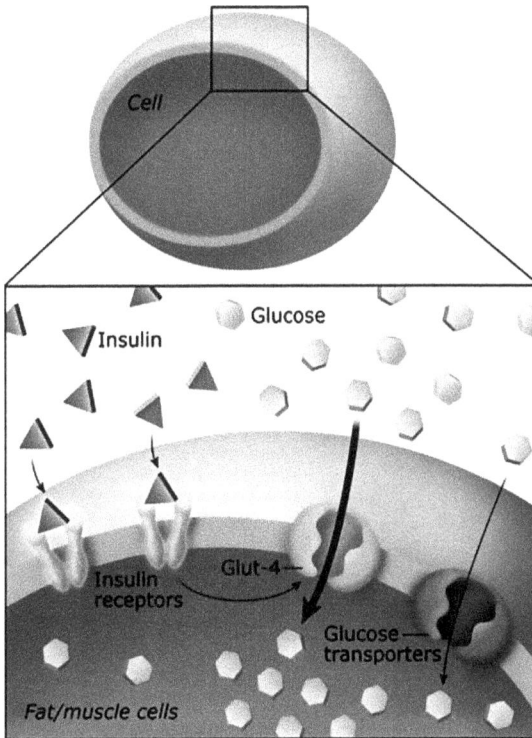

Insulin's Effects – Insulin binds to receptors on the outside of cell membranes. These receptors penetrate through the cell membrane into the cell's inner fluid (cytoplasm).

When insulin binds to these receptors, it triggers a chemical reaction down through the membrane into the cell. This chemical reaction makes glucose transporter proteins floating in the cytoplasm move up to and fuse with the cell membrane, creating openings into the cell. Glucose floating freely in the bloodstream outside the cell can now move through these opened channels into the cell. Insulin Effects, Diabetes Teaching Center, University of California, 2011, Used with permission.

As glucose is absorbed, blood glucose levels drop again, and insulin stops binding to cell receptors. The glucose transporters detach from the inner surface of the membrane and move back down into the cellular cytoplasm.

Depending upon the target cell, absorbed glucose can be used for either :

1. *Glycogen synthesis* - long-term fuel storage or

2. *Cellular respiration* - breakdown into ATP energy units.

1. During *glycogen synthesis,* insulin stimulates the liver and muscles to chain-link the simple sugar glucose into a storable complex sugar, the polymer glycogen. This glycogen constitutes an energy reserve which can be quickly mobilized to meet sudden glucose energy needs, broken down and reconverted into glucose. Over 8–12 hours, glycogen stores in the liver and muscles are slowly broken down and provide the main source of blood glucose used by the rest of the body for fuel.

2. During *cellular respiration,* energy factories in the cell called *mitochondria* break down glucose to create *ATP,* the universal energy molecule that drives biochemical processes.

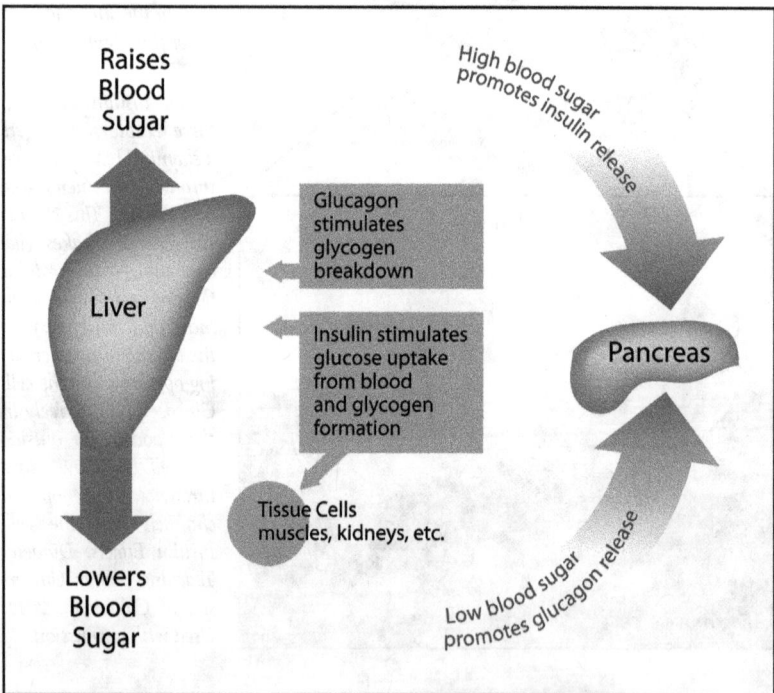

Glucose regulation, Polyglot Studios, 2011

The pancreas secretes insulin to lower blood glucose levels, and glucagon to raise them. Thus, when blood glucose levels are low, the pancreas secretes glucagon, which makes the liver break down stored glycogen into glucose, to be released into the bloodstream. So glucagon increases blood glucose, while insulin decreases it.

From the perspective of your entire body, insulin has a fat-sparing effect, causing most cells to use carbohydrates instead of fatty acids for energy, and indirectly stimulating fat accumulation – insulin inhibits the enzyme *lipase*, which breaks down fat.

Unless you suffer from diabetes or metabolic syndrome, insulin is constantly produced to remove excess blood glucose, which could otherwise kill you. *Hyperglycemia* – too much blood sugar – can be toxic. Your body tries to excrete excess glucose, drawing water from your blood and organs so you can urinate the glucose out. This severely dehydrates the body.

Meanwhile, the cells cannot normally receive glucose for energy, and unused blood glucose accumulates and clumps up, damaging veins and arteries, potentially resulting in blocked blood circulation, blindness, heart attacks, strokes, and kidney failure. That's why diabetics – who either cannot produce enough insulin or have lost sensitivity to insulin signals – have to regularly inject insulin and carefully monitor their blood sugar levels.

Insulin influences other functions as well, including cognition. In your brain, insulin enhances learning and memory, particularly verbal memory. Insulin in the brain also appears to aid in thermoregulation, thus playing a central role in maintaining your entire body's homeostasis.

A Constant Cycle

Glucagon is also secreted by your pancreas, with the opposite effect of insulin, raising your blood glucose levels by triggering glycogen breakdown when blood sugar is too low. Glucagon binds to receptors, signalling your liver to break down glycogen stores back into simple glucose, to be distributed through your blood for energy use. When both free glucose and glycogen stores have run out, your body turns to its fat stores for energy, transferring lipids (fats) to your liver for breakdown for energy use.

When blood glucose levels again become high after eating, insulin release is once more stimulated, and thus the two opposing hormones act cooperatively to stabilize your blood sugar.

Fat And Sugar Metabolism

Depending upon food availability and your BMR, fat and sugar are converted to and from one another through a series of enzyme reactions. It's this conversion that turns unused carbs and sugars into fats – and this is the basis of most weight gain.

Conversion of Sugar to Fat – Glucose is immediately available for energy needs during and after eating, but any unused glucose is converted by your liver into glycogen for reserve energy. When the "tank is full" so to speak, remaining glucose is converted into triglycerides (fat) and stored throughout your body.

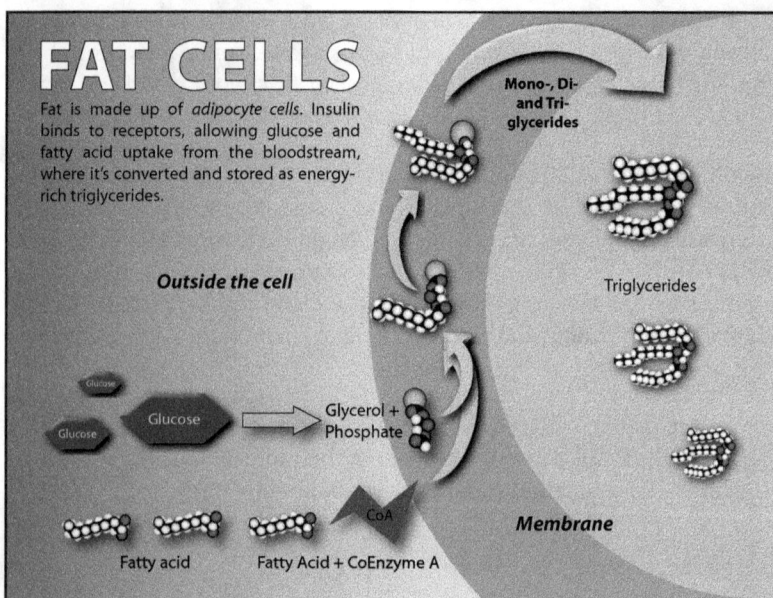

FAT CELLS

Fat is made up of *adipocyte cells*. Insulin binds to receptors, allowing glucose and fatty acid uptake from the bloodstream, where it's converted and stored as energy-rich triglycerides.

Outside the cell

Mono-, Di- and Tri- glycerides

Triglycerides

Glucose

Glucose

Glucose

Glycerol + Phosphate

CoA

Membrane

Fatty acid

Fatty Acid + CoEnzyme A

Lipogenesis (fat storage) 2011, Polyglot Studios

Conversion of Fat to Sugar – As you go about your daily affairs, glycogen stores are broken down to provide you with energy, until you "refuel" at mealtimes. But if your metabolic needs require it, fat stores can also be broken down into fatty acids and glycerol, and then broken down further into glucose, for immediate energy.

Food Energy

Your body uses three primary energy sources – glucose, glycogen and fat, converted from one form to another as needed. Fat's the most energy-dense, with about 2.5 times the stored energy of glucose, making it an excellent fuel source.

266

> **Calories** – *Food specifically provides the energy your body needs to conduct the chemical processes of life. This energy is measured in calories, the energy required to heat one cubic centimeter of water one degree Celsius. You will also hear the term kilocalories, 1,000 times the energy of one calorie – a larger-scale unit which is much more convenient for general measurement. Thus, calories on food labels describe the amount of energy released when your body digests a particular food.*

Relative Energy of Nutrients:

- *Typical carbohydrates:* 3.75 calories per gram

- *Typical proteins:* 4 calories per gram

- *Typical fats:* 9 calories per gram.

Macronutrients – Carbohydrates, Fats, Proteins

I. CARBOHYDRATES

Carbohydrates are the most abundant organic molecules in nature. The name reflects the molecular structure – generally a ratio of one carbon and one oxygen atom for every two hydrogen atoms. In other words, carbon bonded to hydrates, water molecules, with carbon, hydrogen and oxygen in a ratio of 1:2:1.

In biochemistry, they're referred to as *saccharides*, which means sugars. Sugars are multiples of the CH_2O carbohydrate ratio, such as $C_6H_{12}O_6$, the chemical basis of *monosaccharides*. These are single-molecule sugars like *fructose* and *glucose*, the most common energy source for living cells.

Carbohydrates are very versatile molecules: the chemical structure can be easily converted for energy storage and release, which is why these molecules are so plentiful in living matter. Energy from the sun, absorbed by plants, algae, and some bacteria during photosynthesis, is trapped within carbohydrate bonds.

Carbohydrates provide both metabolic fuel and structural components for nearly all organic molecules. Breaking down carbohydrate yields life-sustaining energy, but carbohydrates can also bond with a variety of other molecules: *glycoproteins* are proteins linked to carbohydrates, and *glycolipids* are carbohydrates linked to lipid molecules, common components in cell membranes. These two molecules are important structural components in plants, animals, and bacteria.

In addition to structural roles, carbohydrate molecules also assist in cell "recognition" by other molecules, a function central to growth, fertilization, cell transformation, and other processes. These functions rely upon three special molecular features of carbohydrates:

- the ability to form multiple hydrogen bonds with water or other environmental molecules;

- the ability to exist in either linear or ring form; and

- the ability to bond with fats and proteins in *polymeric* (long chain) structures.

High-carbohydrate foods include fruits, candies, soft drinks, white breads, pastas, potatoes, and grains. In humans and other animals, carbohydrates are used to provide quick energy in the form of glucose – blood sugar.

Usually when people talk about "carbs", they're referring to foods high in starch, like grains, bread, or pasta, or the monosaccharides found in sugary desserts and candies. But carbohydrates constitute a wide range of substances, and there are three broad categories found in food:

Complex carbohydrates (polysaccharides or plant starch) – found in grains like oats, rice, and wheat, vegetables like corn, peas and potatoes, and legumes like beans and lentils. These are chains of linked, simple sugar molecules. Examples include *plant cellulose* and *starch*. These complex carbohydrates occur naturally in fruits, vegetables, and whole grains; in contrast, there are *refined carbohydrates* – synthetic, sugary foods such as white rice, white bread and soda pop. The government usually recommends you obtain a large portion of your daily calories from *complex* carbohydrates, from sources such as legumes, brown rice, whole grains, broccoli and spinach.

Simple carbohydrates (monosaccharides or sugars) – found in candy, fruit, honey, milk products and vegetables. Monosaccharides consist of single sugar molecules, usually ending with the suffix *–ose*, as with glucose, *sucrose* (table sugar), *fructose* (berry sugar) and *lactose* (milk sugar).

Dietary fiber – found in whole grains: cereals, vegetables, fruits and legumes. Many living creatures can break down starch into glucose, but generally cannot metabolize structural polysaccharides like plant cellulose or shellfish chitin. But even though these complex carbohydrates cannot be fully digested by the human digestive system, plant cellulose still provides dietary fiber, to sweep intestinal walls clean, among other functions.

Carbohydrates are chemically classified into four categories, depending upon their complexity: monosaccharides linking to form progressively more complex polymers: mono- (single), di- (two), oligo- (Greek for few, so up to ten), and poly- (many) saccharides. Glucose is a nearly universal, easily accessible source of calories; many organisms can also metabolize other monosaccharides and disaccharides, though glucose is preferred.

Description	Chemical Description	Formula
Cane Sugar	Saccharose	$C_{12}H_{22}O_{11}$ (= 2 x $C_6H_{12}O_6$ – H_2O)
Dextrose (Grapes)	Glucose	$C_6H_{12}O_6$
Fruit Sugar	Fructose	$C_6H_{12}O_6$
Milk Sugar	Lactose	$C_{12}H_{22}O_{11}$
Barley Sugar	Maltose	$C_{12}H_{22}O_{11}$

Common simple sugars: Mono- and di-saccharides

In addition to the sugars listed in the chart, there are many others, with similar structures. Their common underlying structure is the basic formula $C_6H_{12}O_6$. Thus, a simple sugar molecule consists of six carbon, 12 hydrogen, and six oxygen atoms.

Monosaccharides – these are single, simple sugars such as glucose and *galactose* (part of milk sugar). Though the basic underlying formula of monosaccharides is CxH_2O, their structures can vary widely. Glucose, for example, can exist in both straight-chain and ring forms.

Monosaccharides typically contain three to seven carbon atoms. They're the primary source of fuel for metabolism, used for locomotion and biosynthesis. When monosaccharides are not immediately needed, they're usually converted into more efficiently compact and stable forms, as chain molecule polysaccharides. In many animals, including humans, the chief polysaccharide storage form is *glycogen*, stored in liver and muscle cells. In plants, *starch* is used for the same purpose. *Ribose* is another vital monosaccharide, which bonds with phosphates to form the backbone nucleic acids join to form RNA and DNA.

Disaccharides – These are twin-structured saccharides, formed from two joined monosaccharides. Among them are *sucrose,* commonly known as table sugar, and *lactose*, which is mammalian milk sugar.

Oligosaccharides – chains of three to ten monosaccharide units.

Polysaccharides – Natural complex saccharides are formed from chains of monosaccharides. These polymers of over ten monosaccharides can be either linear or branched in structure. They're very stable molecules, good for solid extracellular structures and energy storage. Polysaccharides can contain hundreds or thousands of monosaccharide units, linked by enzyme activity through *dehydration synthesis* – water removal.

Polysaccharides can again be broken down into monosaccharides by a different enzyme using *hydrolysis*, the addition of water. The most common polysaccharides include starch, *cellulose* and *chitin*.

While starch is used for energy storage by plants, in animals, the functionally analogous glucose polymer is glycogen, sometimes called "animal starch". Unlike starch, glycogen can be quickly metabolized, which suits the active lives of moving creatures as opposed to immobile plant life. Smaller monosaccharides and disaccharides can serve as more immediate energy sources.

Cellulose, used in the cell walls of plants, is said to be the most abundant organic molecule on Earth. Industrially it's used to create paper and fabrics. Chitin has a similar structure, but with nitrogen-containing side branches, which increase its strength. It's found in *arthropod* (insects and shellfish) exoskeletons and in some fungi cell walls. Saccharide components are also used in a number of critical biological functions, within the immune system, reproduction, and blood clotting.

Currently, the Food and Agriculture Organization and World Health Organization jointly recommend adults obtain 55 to 75% of dietary calories from carbohydrates, but only 10% directly from simple sugars (mono- and disaccharides). The complex carbohydrates they recommend are supplied by fruits, vegetables and whole grains, along with fiber, vitamins and minerals. Processed carbohydrates tend to provide fast saccharide energy in the form of calories, but without the presence of fiber or other nutrients such as vitamins or minerals. An excess of processed carbohydrates like potato chips, candy, soft drinks and pastries are obviously unhealthy; fiber-rich vegetables and whole grains are much healthier, and whole vegetables and fruits much healthier than fructose-high, fiber-deficient fruit juices.

The *glycemic index (GI)* and *glycemic load* describe how food behaves during digestion, ranking carbohydrate-rich foods upon the speed and strength of their effects on blood glucose: the glycemic *index* is the *speed* at which glucose can be absorbed from various foods; glycemic *load* is the *amount* of glucose present in food. The *insulin index* is similar though more recent, ranking foods based upon their blood insulin effects, caused by glucose, starch or some amino acids.

Food Values: Glycemic Index/Glycemic Load

	Low GI	Med GI	High GI
Low GL	All-bran cereal (8,42) Apples (6,38) Carrots (3,47) Peanuts (1,14) Strawberries (1,40) Sweet Corn (9,54)	Beets (5,64) Cantaloupe (4,65) Pineapple (7,59) Sucrose, i.e. table sugar (7,68)	Popcorn (8,72) Watermelon (4,72) Whole wheat flour bread (9,71)
Med GL	Apple juice (11,40) Bananas (12,52) Fettucine (18,40) Orange juice (12,50) Sourdough wheat bread (15,54)	Life Cereal (16,66) New potatoes (12,57) Wild rice (18,57)	Cheerios (15,74) Shredded wheat (15,75)
High GL	Linguine (23,52) Macaroni (23,47) Spaghetti (20,42)	Couscous (23,65) White rice (23,64)	Baked Russet potatoes (26,85) Cornflakes (21,81)

Source: Revised International Table of Glycemic Index (GI) and Glycemic Load (GL), *The American Journal of Clinical Nutrition*, July 2002

A. GLUCOSE

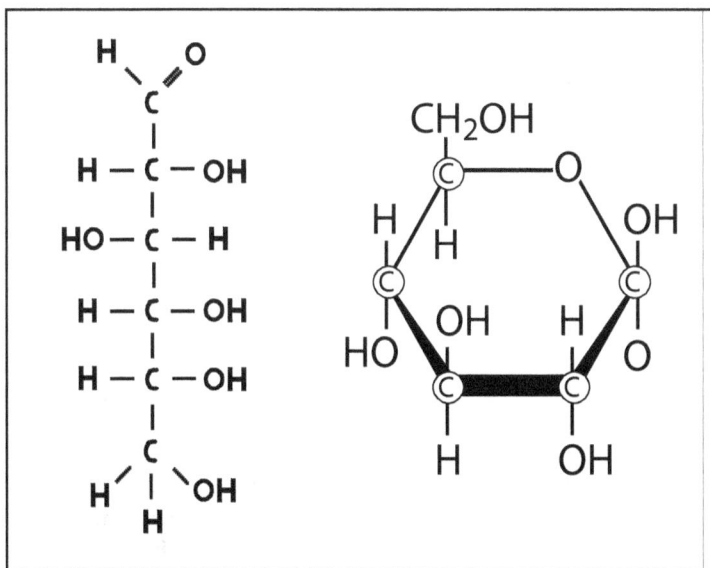

Glucose can be obtained from carbohydrates, but can also be synthesized from amino acids, and from the *glycerol* (alcohol) backbone of *triglycerides* (fat). This is your brain's and body's primary energy source, so you need a constant supply. In your body, it's used in *aerobic respiration*, where, along with oxygen, it extracts the ATP energy that drives metabolic and motor processes underlying everything you do physically and mentally. As you've seen, the twin signalling hormones insulin and glucagon are secreted by your pancreas to regulate glucose concentration in your blood.

As your brain's primary energy source, glucose profoundly affects your cognition, perception, focus and emotions. Low glucose – being hungry – can severely impair mental processes such as self-control, decision-making, and the ability to engage in complex logic.

The name "glucose" comes from the Greek word *glukus*, meaning "sweet", and in chemistry, the suffix "-ose" denotes a sugar. Glucose is made of six carbon, six oxygen and 12 hydrogen atoms, typically five *hydroxyl* (OH) groups arranged along a six-carbon "backbone". It takes either a chain or a ring form, with several different structures. *D-glucose,* often called *dextrose,* is "plant sugar"; removing water from dextrose molecules, so they bond (dehydration synthesis) creates the polymers starch and cellulose.

Breaking down carbohydrates with enzymes yields monosaccharides and disaccharides, primarily glucose. Through *glycolysis* and the *citric acid cycle,* (see the end of this chapter) glucose itself is further broken down, releasing energy using the ATP molecule, as well as the byproducts CO_2 and water.

In addition to obtaining glucose by digesting carbohydrates, your body can create it by breaking down glycogen; glucose is easily transported through your bloodstream, but its chemical structure makes it difficult to store long-term. Because of this, glucose is stored primarily in your liver and muscles as glycogen, then broken down for distribution and use by your tissues as glucose.

B. GLYCOGEN

Glucose molecules can be bonded by the thousands to form glycogen, stored for long-term energy reserve supplies in your muscles, liver and red blood cells. Your entire supply, however, is not a large amount, and can be depleted in a few short hours.

Glycogen is distributed as tiny granules in your cellular cytoplasm. It constitutes an energy reserve which can be quickly mobilized to meet sudden needs for glucose, but is less compact than your more-highly concentrated triglyceride (fat) energy reserves.

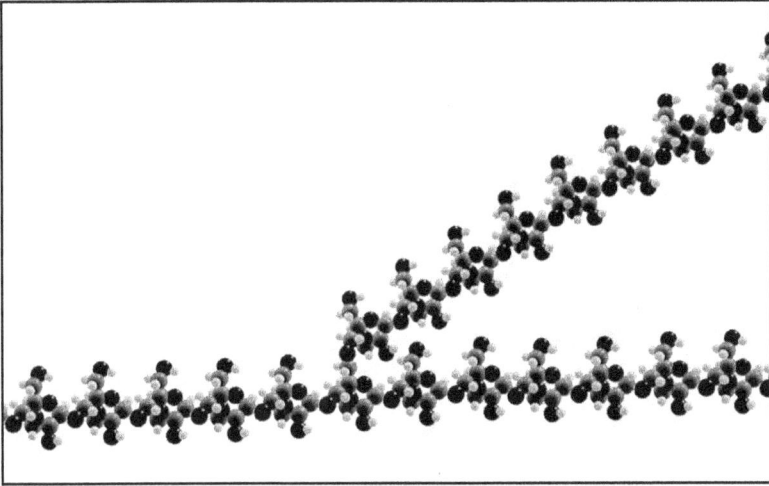

Glycogen, Wikipedia, 2011, public domain

When you digest carbohydrates, your blood glucose levels rise. In response, your pancreas secretes insulin, a signalling hormone. Glucose is absorbed by *hepatocytes* – your liver cells; insulin stimulates enzymes within these cells to bond glucose into glycogen. If insulin and glucose levels are high, glucose will continue to be added to glycogen chains for later slow release, providing between-meal energy as it's broken down again into glucose.

After you finish digestion, glucose levels start to fall, and insulin secretion drops in response. This triggers the end of glycogen production. Over the following 8–12 hours, this glycogen becomes your primary source of glucose, an energy reserve in your muscles and elsewhere. Marathon runners and other endurance athletes often reach a point of *glycogen debt*, where nearly all the body's glycogen stores have been depleted from prolonged exertion without replenishment; a state commonly called *hitting the wall*. Glycogen debt – hitting the wall – is a state of extreme exhaustion, to the point where movement becomes exceedingly difficult.

Among marathon runners, this typically occurs at about the 20-mile mark, but it can be delayed through *carb loading* before an event. Interestingly, a 2008 study conducted by the Royal Melbourne Institute of Technology University has also shown that adding caffeine (the equivalent of 5 to 6 cups of coffee) to carbohydrates will very rapidly replenish glycogen stores after this kind of depletion.

II. FATS

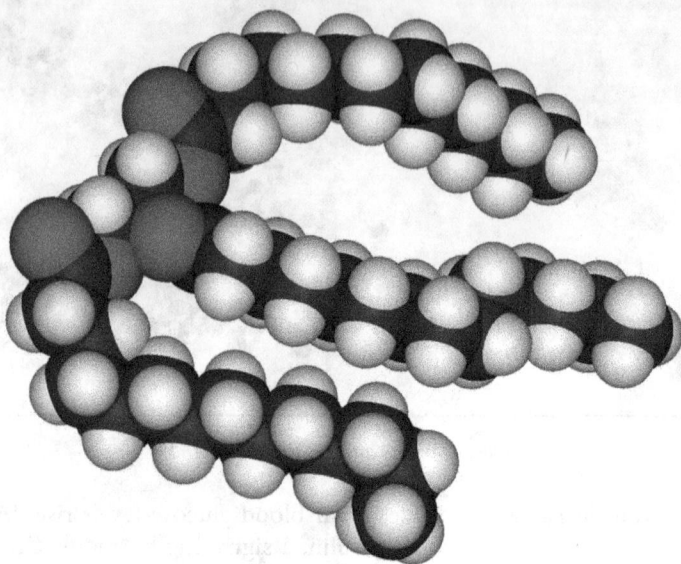

Triglyceride, Wikipedia, 2012, public domain.

Your body's longest-term energy storage molecule is *fat*. Fat is actually a vital nutrient, containing the most concentrated energy among the three macronutrients, at an average of nine calories per gram – over twice as much as proteins or carbohydrates. Body fat, called *adipose tissue*, is produced by your liver. It's how you and other animals most efficiently store long-term energy. This storage or use of fat is primarily controlled by insulin and glucagon.

Fat protects your body from cold and physical damage, acting as an insulating and protective layer around your vital organs. It also promotes healthy cell function, and maintains healthy hair and skin. *Fat soluble vitamins* (A, D, E, and K) require fat for digestion and absorption.

Fat even provides protection against toxins. When substances reach toxic levels in your bloodstream, your body can store them in fatty tissue as a safety measure – a means of both diluting them and removing them from general circulation. This protects your vital organs until the foreign substances can be metabolized or otherwise flushed out of your body by defecation, urination, sebum excretion, and even hair and nail growth.

274

Lastly, fat is a source of *essential fatty acids*, "essential" in your diet because your body cannot manufacture them on its own, so you have to obtain them from food. These fatty acids are used in the formation of cell membranes, and are necessary for a number of body functions, including sex hormone synthesis and metabolic regulation.

Fat molecules are *triglycerides*, made from three fatty acids attached to a glycerol molecule. They're insoluble, meaning they don't dissolve in your bloodstream, so special transportation systems are necessary.

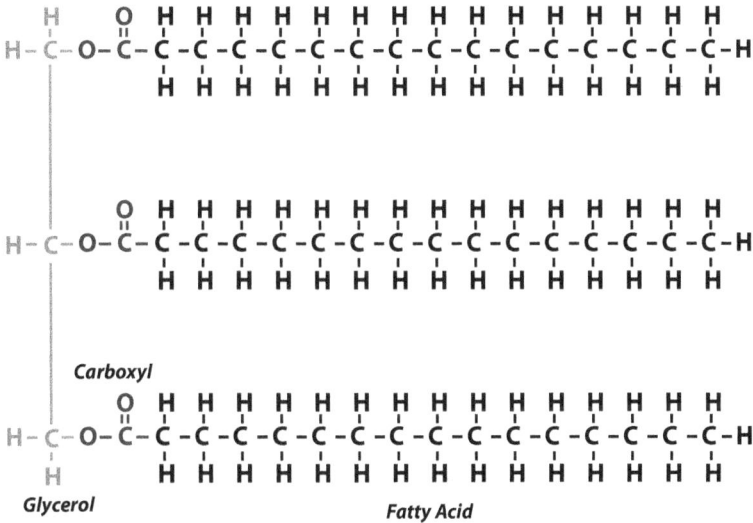

Glycerol   Fatty Acid

When needed, fat can be broken down by your digestive system into its constituents, glycerol and free fatty acids. *Glycerol*, a precursor of fat, is a thick, odorless and sweet syrup, widely used in the food industry as a filler, sugar substitute and preservative. In the pharmaceutical industry, it's used as a lubricant and smoothing agent. It's also an ingredient in many medicines, including anaesthetics, capsules, cough syrups, laxatives, skin care products and toothpaste. Glycerol can be converted by your liver into glucose when necessary.

Fatty Foods

A variety of fats are found in food, including: *monounsaturated, polyunsaturated, trans fats* and *omega fatty acids* (*saturated* and *interesterified fat*). Each of these is just a variation of the same molecular structure, consisting of fatty acids bonded to a (usually glycerol) backbone. As the diagram above shows, if the molecule were spread out, it would look like three horizontal lines (fatty acids) radiating out from the glycerol "backbone" like a capital letter E.

Each fat molecule's properties depend upon the fatty acid chains, which vary by number of carbon and hydrogen atoms. The more carbon atoms in a fatty acid, the longer the chain will be, and longer fatty acids hold more potential energy than shorter versions. The terms *lipid, oil*, and *fat* are all used interchangeably, but oils are liquid at room temperature, while fats are (usually) solid at room temperature. Oils are also generally substances with a greasy texture that don't mix with water.

Lipids are a much more general classification, of which liquid and solid fats are only one variety. Lipids also include waxes, cholesterol, phospholipids (cell membranes), myelin (nerve insulation), steroids (sex hormones) and more. Fats, oils and lipids don't dissolve in water, but are broken down by special enzymes produced by your pancreas called *lipases*.

Repellent – Lipids pull each other closer – thus repelling water molecules – because of a weak intermolecular attraction called the Van der Waals force – the same force allowing geckos to walk along walls. Opposite total charges between molecules create this attraction, which is much weaker than covalent bonds, where an electron is shared between atoms. The van der Waals force makes long-chained fatty acids more difficult to melt, meaning more energy (a higher temperature) is needed to turn them liquid.

Thus fats can be liquid or solid at room temperature, depending on the chemical composition. Animal fats include lard, fish oil, butter and ghee, derived from dairy, meat, or from under animal skin. Plant fats include coconut, olive, peanut, soya bean, sunflower, sesame, and vegetable oils, from which margarine and vegetable shortening are made. These fats can be categorized into *saturated* and *unsaturated* fats, which vary by melting point and energy content.

Fats are chained links of fatty acids, of which there are four types, categorized by *saturation* – how much hydrogen they contain. *Saturated fats* are "saturated" with hydrogen atoms, while *unsaturated fats* are not. Saturated fats solidify at room temperature and generally come from animals, while unsaturated fats are liquid and generally come from plants. Saturated fats are also considered to promote high blood cholesterol, while unsaturated fats can in some cases lower it.

Unsaturated *means a fatty acid's carbon chain is not* saturated *(filled) with hydrogen atoms.*

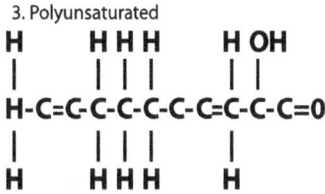

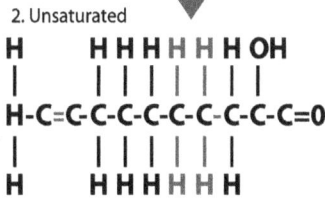

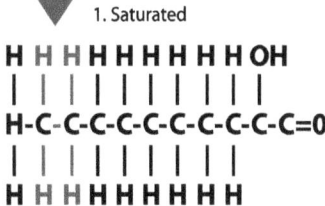

3. Polyunsaturated

```
H      H H H      H OH
|      | | |      | |
H-C=C-C-C-C-C-C=C-C-C=0
|      | | |      |
H      H H H      H
```

2. Unsaturated

```
H      H H H H H H OH
|      | | | | | | |
H-C=C-C-C-C-C-C-C-C-C=0
|      | | | | | |
H      H H H H H H
```

1. Saturated

```
H H H H H H H H H OH
| | | | | | | | | |
H-C-C-C-C-C-C-C-C-C=0
| | | | | | | | |
H H H H H H H H H
```

= *denotes a double-bond*

Unsaturated fats contain one or more double atomic bonds between carbon atoms in the fatty acid chain.

If the fatty acid contains one double bond, it's **monounsaturated**, and if it contains more than one, it's **polyunsaturated.**

Both monounsaturated and polyunsaturated fatty acids can be found in vegetable oils like olive and rapeseed oils, fish like sardines, mackerel and herrings, and nuts, seeds and grains such as flaxseed or quinoa. Fats, ranging from healthiest (top) to unhealthiest (bottom) are:

Unsaturated fats have fewer carbon-hydrogen bonds, providing less energy.

Polyunsaturated fats contain few hydrogen atoms, and help to lower blood cholesterol. This group of fats includes Omega 6 and Omega 3 Essential Fatty Acids, which are necessary for growth, and to protect the body and brain from disease.

Monounsaturated fats such as olive oil and canola contain a single region unsaturated with hydrogen, and they also help to lower blood cholesterol. Our bodies can create this acid by breaking down polyunsaturated fats. Among these is group, however, is omega fatty acid 9, which your body cannot naturally synthesize, so it must be eaten.

Saturated fats have slightly more energy; each carbon atom is bound to two hydrogen atoms, so the carbon is saturated with as many hydrogen bonds as possible.

Saturated fats stack into a densely-packed molecular configuration, so they freeze easily and are usually solid at room temperature. Animal proteins are usually high in saturated fats, which increase risks of heart disease, stroke, diabetes, and many varieties of cancer.

As well as in meat, saturated fats are found in dairy products such as cream, cheese, butter and lard. These can be unhealthy when eaten in excess, as they raise your blood cholesterol, and have been linked to increased risk of *atherosclerosis* (clogged arteries) and heart disease.

Trans fats are used in modern snack foods such as deep fried food, cakes, most margarines and butter, cookies, and cakes. One well-known example is Crisco.

Trans fats don't normally occur in nature, but are commercially produced through *hydrogenation*, the process of adding hydrogen to polyunsaturated fats. This straightens out the molecular twist in naturally-occurring fats, meaning they stack more efficiently, and the forces between molecules are stronger, making them solid at room temperatures and easier to freeze.

But because they are linked to an extremely high risk of heart disease, trans fats have been banned in a number of restaurants in the US and elsewhere.

The changes in the molecular configuration changes how these synthetic fats act upon human metabolism; some can become toxic, releasing tissue-disrupting free radical molecules, while others compete with healthy essential fatty acids.

This can disrupt production of hormones which help control inflammation (tissue swelling) and metabolism (energy consumption). Some trans fats can also increase blood cholesterol. Trans fats have also been implicated in cancer, immunodeficiency and cardiovascular diseases. They are considered unhealthy to the point of being extremely hazardous to your health.

Essential fatty acids (EFAs) include *Omega 3, 6* and *9*, found in monounsaturated and polyunsaturated fats. Omega 3, 6 and 9 fatty acids help maintain healthy skin, hormonal stability, and can also protect against a number of diseases such as diabetes. Olive oil is a particularly good source of these EFAs, which are used to produce the more complex long-chain fatty acids *EPA* and *DHA* (omega-3s), and *AA, GLA* and *DGLA* (omega-6s). Essential fatty acids are critical for a number of metabolic processes, and low levels or imbalances among them may contribute to several illnesses, including *osteoporosis* (bone brittleness) heart disease and depression.

While omega-6 essential fatty acids are plentiful in a variety of foods, including vegetable oils and meats, omega-3s are much more difficult to obtain, being found in oily cold-water fish like salmon, mackerel, and trout, and a few seeds and nuts, such as walnuts, flax and pumpkin seeds.

Sterols – A sterol is type of alcohol, found in both plants (*phytosterols*) and animals (*cholesterol*).

Cholesterol – This lipid is a soft, waxy substance found throughout your body, including in your heart, intestines, liver, muscles, nervous system and skin. Your body synthesizes it, but you also obtain it from eating animal products – meat or dairy. Your liver synthesizes cholesterol for a number of functions, such as producing hormones and bile (a digestive acid). It's transported via your bloodstream throughout your body.

Within the bloodstream, cholesterol can combine with fatty acids to form molecules called *low-density lipoproteins* (LDLs) and *high-density lipoproteins* (HDLs). LDLs are unhealthy – they're sticky and tend to clump together, forming dangerous *plaque deposits* that adhere to blood vessel walls, clogging the arteries. HDLs are thought to counteract the harmful effects of LDLs.

III. PROTEINS

Proteins are folded, twisted chains of linked amino acids. They're responsible for virtually every biological process in your body, and the specific geometric shapes and foldings are critical to each protein's proper function. Every living cell on Earth is comprised of proteins in one form or another, and they are used to build and repair tissue. They're also the basis of a number of critical biochemical processes, comprising enzymes, hormones and other regulatory chemicals.

Like fats and carbs, proteins are macronutrients, meaning they're required in relatively large amounts. But while fat and carbohydrates are stored by your body, protein isn't, so it must be constantly replenished through consumption.

Since proteins are long chains of linked amino acids (created by RNA translation), they're critical for your growth and repair. In other words, eating proteins supplies the amino acids your body uses to synthesize its own proteins. Thus, protein *consumption* supports protein *synthesis*.

Your organs, muscles, and other tissues are all built upon protein, as are your body's *enzymes*, chemicals which initiate and regulate most of your biochemical reactions, as well as synthesis of macromolecules, including other proteins.

Proteins also act as transporters, carrying biological molecules from one body region to another, through the bloodstream or across cellular membranes. *Albumin* is one such major transporting protein in your blood, to which a number of biological molecules and medicines bind. Some proteins also function as hormones, signalling between cells and regulating organs throughout your body; and as receptors, antibodies, and glands.

Too Much Of A Good Thing

Some evidence exists that high-protein diets induce significant fat loss, according to Dr. Frank Hu of the Harvard University School of Public Health; high-protein diets increase satiety (feelings of fullness) compared with other diets, and six month high-protein diets resulted in an average weight loss about 4.5 lbs. greater than that of other diets. After six months, however, these diets begin to lose their effectiveness, possibly because the body adjusts to it. The long-term effects of high-protein diets are still not completely clear.

However, the American Heart Association warns that concentrating on protein sources at the expense of dietary carbohydrates may raise sodium levels, and provide inadequate calcium, potassium, and magnesium, typically found in fruits, vegetables, and grains.

Studies also suggest that a high-protein diet results in excess calcium excretion. Eventually, calcium depletion may result in osteoporosis – the bone brittleness found in the elderly. According to University of California osteoporosis specialist Dr. Deborah Sellmeyer, excess protein consumption increases your blood's acidity. Calcium restores blood pH by neutralizing acid, so your body draws upon its internal calcium stores, releasing it into your blood to counter the acid increase.

Another danger of long-term high-protein low-carb diets is that your body can enter a state known as *ketosis* – switching from burning carbohydrates for fuel to burning fat stores. While this sounds ideal, and may be beneficial in the short term, as fat breaks down, it releases small carbon molecules called *ketones* into your bloodstream.

This state also occurs in diabetes, and while it can suppress appetite, it leads to excessive urination and fluid loss, and can build up excruciatingly painful deposits called kidney stones. Additionally, according to Stanford University's Dr. Christopher D. Gardner, high-protein diets like the Atkins Diet carry long-term risks such as higher levels of waste ammonia as protein is broken down; long-term effects of such elevated ammonia levels are still unknown. Animal proteins are also usually high in saturated fats, which increases risks of heart disease, stroke, diabetes, and many varieties of cancer.

Finally, cutting back on carbohydrates such as fruits and vegetables means you lack vital vitamins, minerals fiber, and antioxidants, which are critical for energy extraction and your immune system.

Essential Amino Acids – These are the building blocks of protein. There are many different known amino acids, but only 22 are *proteinogenic* – used by animals to manufacture proteins. Among these 22 are nine amino acids which cannot naturally be made by your body, and so must be included in the foods you eat. Proteins which contain all nine of these essential amino acids are called *complete proteins*.

---

*Protein **quality** varies, not just according to completeness but also digestibility, so that sufficient quantities of amino acids actually reach your body's cells for protein synthesis. Nutritionists suggest that egg protein is the highest quality, both for its completeness and digestibility. Because of this, it has been designated as the reference point for measuring protein quality. Whey protein from milk is also considered exceptional.*

The United Nations Food and Agricultural Organization (FAO) has devised protein quality standards which specify the amount of essential amino acids per gram of protein. 100 or above is a high-quality or complete protein, while lower scores indicate lower-quality proteins.

Because of the tremendous importance of proteins, for vegetarians, careful dietary planning is necessary to acquire all the essential amino acids. All of these nine essential amino acids must be present to synthesize protein, which means you need to consume foods which provide them all, or you inhibit your body's ability to produce the proteins it needs for growth, maintenance, function and repair.

While meat, fish, poultry, eggs, and milk can typically contain all nine amino acids (a complete source of protein), plants may not, and must be combined to provide the necessary nutrients. If two plants which contain complementary amino acids are eaten at the same time, they can make up a complete protein.

Along with proteins, you need to consume sufficient energy from complex carbohydrates, allowing the amino acids to be used to build and repair tissue rather than metabolized in your liver to provide energy in place of carbohydrates. Proteins also need to be accompanied by vitamins and minerals which facilitate their use.

Quality Over Quantity

The type of protein you consume plays a key role in your health. Processed meats like hot dogs, sausages, and deli meats, all high in sodium and nitrates, have been linked to heightened risks of diabetes, cardiovascular disease, and colorectal cancer, according to Dr. Frank Hu of the Harvard University School of Public Health. Dr. Hu recommends the following alternative healthy protein sources:

- *Fish* – high in omega-3 fatty acids and generally less fatty than animal meat.

- *Poultry* – Most saturated fat can by eliminated by removing the skin.

- *Beans* – Beans have the highest protein content of any vegetable, and are high in healthy, filling fiber.

- *Nuts* – An ounce of nuts contains nearly the same amount of protein as an ounce of rib eye steak.

- *Whole grains* – Whole wheat bread contains 3 grams of protein per slice in addition to fiber.

MICRONUTRIENTS – VITAMINS, MINERALS, ETC.

Because your body cannot produce (most of) its own vitamins and minerals, you obtain them from a varied, plant-rich diet. Vitamins contain chemicals your body uses for constant, essential processes, so you need to regularly replenish them. Neither vitamins nor minerals provide energy, and thus, these micronutrients in themselves contain no calories. However, you require them in trace amounts for a number of chemical processes related to growth, reproduction, fighting infectious diseases and promoting general health. Below are complete listings of all the essential micronutrients and their most highly-concentrated sources, in descending order.

Vitamins – Your body requires 13 vitamins to function. They're classified as either *water soluble* (B-complex and C) or *fat soluble* (A, D, E and K). This means they require either water or fat for your tissues to absorb and use them.

Water Soluble Vitamins

Water-soluble vitamins B and C are not stored in your body, unlike fat-soluble vitamins, and therefore you have to consume them daily. Any unused amounts are filtered out of your system by your kidneys and excreted in your urine.

B Vitamins – This vitamin group performs a range of functions, but all are central to nutritional absorption.

Vitamin B1 (Thiamin) – Needed to metabolize carbohydrates, fat, and protein. Every cell in your body needs B1 (thiamin) to form adenosine triphosphate (ATP), the molecular basis of energy production in most living creatures. It's also critical for proper neural function. The best sources of thiamin are:

- wheat germ
- sunflower seeds
- tuna
- macadamia nuts
- oats
- barley
- soy, pink, navy, black beans

Vitamin B2 (Riboflavin) – This vitamin helps you process amino acids and fats, to convert carbohydrates to adenosine triphosphate (ATP), and activates vitamins B6 and B9. It also functions as an antioxidant in some circumstances. The best sources of B2 (riboflavin) are:

- beef liver
- yoghurt
- soy milk
- portabella mushrooms
- spirulina
- passion fruit
- soybeans
- almonds

Vitamin B3 (Niacin) – Niacin is required for cell respiration, for freeing stored molecular energy from carbohydrates, fats, and proteins. It's also used to maintain healthy skin, to synthesize hormones. and to support healthy circulation, nerve function, and the secretion of digestive fluids.

A lack of niacin can result in a host of maladies such as depression, dizziness, fatigue, headaches and insomnia, as well physical ones – canker sores, diarrhea, *halitosis* (bad breath), indigestion, inflammation, limb pains, loss of appetite, low blood-sugar, muscular weakness, and skin eruptions. The best sources of niacin are:

- chicken breast
- tuna
- salmon
- liver
- turkey
- halibut
- peanut butter
- portabella mushrooms

Vitamin B5 (Pantothenic Acid) – This vitamin participates in the *Citric Acid Cycle* (see chapter end) for energy production, and is used to produce the neurotransmitter acetylcholine. Among its other functions, vitamin B5 is also vital for triggering the adrenal glands, and for transporting and releasing fat energy, enabling cholesterol, vitamin D, and steroid production. Its byproduct *pantethine* lowers blood cholesterol and triglycerides. The best sources of pantothenic acid are:

- liver
- shiitake mushrooms
- sunflower seeds
- yoghurt
- corn
- broccoli
- soymilk
- portabella mushrooms

Vitamin B6 – This is a water-soluble part of the vitamin B complex used to help produce antibodies, maintain normal neural function and form red blood cells. It's also required for digesting proteins – the greater your protein intake, the greater your need for vitamin B6. While a deficiency of vitamin B6 causes confusion, depression, irritability, and oral sores, such deficiencies are rare in North Americans. The best sources of vitamin B6 are:

- tuna
- bananas
- chicken breast
- turkey
- liver
- salmon, cod, snapper, halibut
- beef
- potatoes

Vitamin B9 (Folate) – Also called *folic acid*, this B vitamin is vital to cell growth and replication, helping form the nucleic acids needed for RNA synthesis. It's most critical for rapidly growing tissue, such as for babies, and for cells which need rapid replenishment, like red and white blood cells.

Vitamin B9 is particularly necessary during pregnancy, and most health-care professionals recommend women of childbearing age take a daily supplement which includes 400 mcg of folic acid, to protect against neural tube defects between conception and pregnancy. The best sources of folic acid are:

- liver
- lentils
- most beans (mung, pinto, pink, lima, navy, kidney)
- chick peas
- asparagus
- spinach, turnip and mustard greens, collards, broccoli

Vitamin B12 (Cobalamine) – This water-soluble vitamin is necessary for proper neural function, DNA synthesis and replication, and red blood cell production. It also works in concert with vitamins B6 and B9 to break down homocysteine, a sulphuric amino acid in the blood. High levels of homocysteine are thought to scar, harden and narrow arteries, increasing the risks of heart disease, stroke, Alzheimer's disease, and osteoporosis. The best sources of Vitamin B12 are:

- beef liver
- caviar/roe
- octopus
- cold water fish – mackerel, herring, salmon, tuna, cod and sardines
- crab and lobster

Vitamin C (Ascorbic Acid) – A critical water-soluble vitamin used in a wide range of functions. Vitamin C is used to develop and maintain healthy bones, cartilage, gums and teeth. It also strengthens your immune system and helps with iron absorption, necessary for cardiovascular health.

Vitamin C is used to form the digestive liquid *bile* in your liver, which also helps detoxify potentially dangerous substances like alcohol. Vitamin C levels in the eyes also decline with age, so vitamin C supplementation helps counteract this effect, defending against cataracts, a clouding of the lenses which is the cause of 48% of the world's blindness. It may also reduce *aldose reductase enzyme activity*, which is thought to benefit diabetes sufferers. It also protects your body against accumulation or retention of toxic lead.

Vitamin C is a potent antioxidant, protecting LDL cholesterol against oxidative damage, believed to lead to heart disease. Vitamin C also seems to protect against heart disease by reducing arterial stiffness and blood platelet *coagulation* (clumping) in your veins.

Its antioxidant properties also protect smokers from free radical destruction. Small amounts of vitamin C ingested by nonsmokers prior to smoke exposure reduces LDL cholesterol oxidation and free radical damage linked to cigarette smoke exposure.

Vitamin C is used to produce *collagen,* a substance which strengthens a number of tissues like muscles and blood vessels. It also helps in healing and has antihistamine properties.

The best sources of vitamin C include fruits and vegetables such as papayas, red bell peppers, broccoli, Brussels sprouts, strawberries, oranges, cantaloupe, kiwi, cauliflower, and kale.

Fat Soluble Vitamins

Fat-soluble vitamins are stored in your liver and *adipose* (fat) tissue until needed. These are vitamins A, D, E and K. These vitamins are best consumed in the presence of fat, so that nutrients can be properly catabolized and used by your body. However, they're stored long-term in your liver and body fat, so you need to replenish them less frequently than water-soluble vitamins. This also means that, unlike with water-soluble vitamins, megadoses of fat-soluble vitamins pose a toxicity risk, so **megadose supplements of vitamins A, D, E and K should be used with caution and only under the advisement of your doctor.**

Vitamin A – This fat-soluble vitamin serves multiple functions, such as helping in cell differentiation. Cells which cannot fully differentiate run the risk of undergoing precancerous changes. Additionally, vitamin A is critical for healthy vision, nourishing various cells in your eyes and used by your retinas to transduce light into neural impulses.

Vitamin A is critical during pregnancy, genetically stimulating normal fetal growth and development. It also influences the development and function of ovaries, placenta, sperm, and is critical throughout the reproductive process. The best sources of vitamin A are:

- carrot
- liver
- spinach
- sweet potato

- kale
- turnip and collard greens
- squash

Vitamin D – This fat-soluble vitamin helps you maintain blood insulin and calcium balance, increasing calcium absorption from food and reducing its loss from urination. Maintaining sufficient calcium stores ensures the strength and long-term health of your bones and teeth. Vitamin D is also critical to cell differentiation, and plays a part in your immune system and blood cell formation. Some evidence exists that vitamin D may also offer protection from juvenile diabetes , from *multiple sclerosis (*a degeneration of nerve cell myelin sheathing), and *autoimmune arthritis,* where the immune system attacks your body, causing crippling pain and a loss of mobility.

Receptors for vitamin D have been discovered within the pancreas, and there is evidence that suggests vitamin D supplementation may help increase insulin secretion for some diabetes sufferers. This is one of the only micronutrients produced by your body, during sunlight exposure, but the best dietary sources of vitamin D are:

- salmon
- sardines
- shrimp
- milk

- cod
- shitake mushrooms
- eggs

Vitamin E – This is an *antioxidant* (free radical scavenger) which protects your cell membranes and other fatty tissues from damage. It also protects your skin against ultraviolet damage. A number of studies report natural vitamin E supplementation also appears to reduce heart attack risk.

Vitamin E is involved in glucose conversion, and may be helpful in preventing and treating diabetes. Within the last ten years, it's also been shown to help control inflammation, genetic regulation of mitosis (cell division), blood cell regulation, and connective tissue growth. Sources of vitamin E:

- nuts and seeds (sunflower seeds, almonds, hazelnuts, pine nuts, peanuts and brazil nuts)
- olives
- spinach
- papaya
- mustard, turnip and collard greens
- peanut butter
- blueberries

Vitamin K – This micronutrient is critical for blood *coagulation* (clotting to stop bleeding) and proper bone development, by assisting calcium transport throughout your body. Almost all green, leafy vegetables are excellent sources of vitamin K, including kale, spinach, collards, beet, mustard and turnip greens, brussels sprouts, lettuce, cabbage, etc.

Minerals

Calcium – Calcium is well-known for its role in building and maintaining bone and tooth strength, but it is also necessary for blood clotting, muscle contracting (including in the heart) and in neural signal transmission. The best sources of calcium are:

- nonfat or low-fat yogurt and cheese
- low-fat or skim milk
- fish and seafood like sardines, salmon and perch
- beans like soy, white beans
- spinach
- oatmeal

Copper – This trace element is part of a number of enzymes, and is vital for absorption and use of iron. It reduces tissue damage from free radicals, and is vital for bone and connective tissue health, as well as proper thyroid gland function, and preservation of myelin sheathing. Copper's found in:

- beef liver
- seeds – sesame, sunflower, pumpkin and squash
- spirulina
- nuts – cashews, hazelnuts, filberts, walnuts, pine nuts
- barley
- garbanzo and navy beans

Iron – Iron is critical to proper health. It's part of the hemoglobin molecule, which transports oxygen to your cells. A lack of iron in your blood causes fatigue, as your body becomes oxygen-starved. Iron is also present in myoglobin, a molecule which allows your muscles to store oxygen. Without sufficient iron, adenosine triphosphate (ATP; your body's energy source) cannot be synthesized. Iron also helps to build red blood cells. The best sources of iron are:

- soybeans
- lentils
- spinach
- tofu
- sesame seeds
- kidney, garbanzo and navy beans

Magnesium – Magnesium is necessary for bone, cell, protein and fatty acid production. It's also critical for activating B complex vitamins, for muscle relaxation, blood clotting, the production and use of insulin, and the formation of adenosine triphosphate (ATP). Magnesium has also been found to help lower blood pressure. The best sources of magnesium are:

- pumpkin, sunflower and sesame seeds
- spinach
- soy, white, black, navy, northern, lima & kidney beans
- salmon, halibut
- Brazil nuts, almonds, cashews and peanuts

Manganese – This trace element is required to produce enzymes which synthesize fatty acids and cholesterol, and that regulate protein and fat metabolism. It also supports your immune system, cellular energy, bone growth and health, thyroid function, reproduction, and blood sugar regulation. Manganese works with vitamin K in supporting blood clotting, and with B vitamins in promoting calm in the face of anxiety, frustration, and other forms of stress. In addition, manganese helps your body use many vital nutrients, ensures nerve health, and protects cells against damage from oxidative stress – free radical damage. The best sources of manganese are:

- pineapple
- brown rice
- garbanzo beans
- spinach
- rye
- soybeans
- cloves
- Greens like mustard and collard greens, kale and romaine lettuce

Phosphorus – This mineral is found in every cell of your body. It assists in transporting nutrients into and out of cells, and plays a central role in the health of your bones and teeth. Phosphorus is the most plentiful mineral in the human body after calcium. Both nutrients work in concert to produce strong bones and teeth, where about 85% of phosphorus is concentrated.

Phosphorous is usually bound to oxygen as phosphate, and is present in bones, cell membranes (phospholipids) and cholesterol (lipoproteins). Phosphorus also helps to regulate your body's acid-base balance (pH), acting as a chemical buffer (acid-diluting agent). Phosphorus is also used by hemoglobin in red blood cells for oxygen delivery to every cell in your body. Finally, phosphorus is central to the balance and use of other mineral and vitamins.

Phosphorus is used by your kidneys to filter waste, and is central to ATP-ADP energy production cycles. It's used for growth, repair and maintenance of all cells and tissue, and is central to DNA and RNA, as well as phosphorylation, which regulates gene expression and activates a number of enzymes and hormones that trigger cell activity. Most people get sufficient dietary phosphorus from milk, grains, and proteins in common foods. The best sources of phosphorous are:

- wheat bran and bran cereals
- sesame and sunflower seeds
- dairy products such as milk, yoghurt and cheese
- eggs

- beef
- chicken
- turkey
- halibut, salmon
- almonds

Potassium – Potassium helps regulate your heart, blood pressure, and neuromuscular activity. It's also necessary for metabolizing carbohydrates and proteins, and for maintaining proper pH. Potassium can help you maintain healthy blood pressure, while low blood potassium levels increase the risk of *heart arrhythmia* (irregular heartbeat). Excessive sodium (extremely common in modern diets) can increase your potassium needs. The best sources of potassium are:

- white, soy, lima, kidney and pinto beans
- yams
- squash

- avocados
- spinach
- papaya
- lentils

Selenium – This trace mineral activates an antioxidant called *glutathione peroxidase*, which research indicates may protect against cancer. Selenium manufactured from yeast induces *apoptosis* (cell death) of cancerous cells in the laboratory. It's also been reported that men with the highest levels of dietary selenium developed 65% fewer prostate cancers than men with low levels of dietary selenium.

Selenium is central to a healthy immune system, stimulating beneficial white blood cell activity and protecting cells against oxidative damage. It's also needed to activate thyroid hormones, and has been found to improve sperm cell motility and increase the odds of conception. The best sources of selenium are:

- liver
- seafoods such as snapper, cod, halibut, tuna, salmon, sardines, shrimp
- crimini mushrooms
- turkey
- lamb
- chicken
- sunflower seeds

Sodium – Although sodium is a vital nutrient, modern diets tend to include far too much. A single teaspoon of table salt has about 2,300 mg, over 400% the daily required amount. Additionally, drinking water and a number of foods and medications naturally contain sodium, in addition to the salt you add to foods for flavor. In America, about 25% of adults suffer from high blood pressure, of which sodium intake is one contributory factor, though sensitivity varies between individuals, and usually increases with age. Sodium helps maintain blood volume, regulate cellular water balance, and neural function. Your kidneys control sodium balance by increasing or decreasing the amount you expel in your urine.

Zinc – Zinc has a number of critical functions. It's part of over 300 enzymes used to produce protein, assist cell mitosis, repair wounds, maintain growth, fertility and vision, boost immune function, balance blood sugar, stabilize your metabolism, maintain healthy olfactory and gustatory senses, and protect against oxidative stress, among other things. Zinc has also been found by some experiments to shorten cold recovery in adults, possibly due to zinc's antiviral activities in the throat.

A 2011 collaborative study between Duke University and MIT has also found that zinc helps regulate communication between hippocampus neurons, central to learning and memory, and disruptions in this hippocampal communication may play a part in epilepsy, according to Duke neurobiology chair Dr. James McNamara. High concentrations of zinc are found in synaptic vesicles, with the highest concentrations in hippocampus neurons. The best sources of zinc are:

- liver
- beef
- lamb
- venison

- sesame and pumpkin seeds
- yoghurt
- turkey
- green peas

Miscellaneous Terms

Adenosine Triphosphate (ATP) – This molecule is the universal source of energy for virtually all plants and animals. In the *mitochondria* – "energy factory" organelles of your cells – ATP sheds a phosphate group as it's broken down into *ADP (adenosine diphosphate),* releasing a significant amount of energy to power cellular activities.

During inactivity, the reverse chemical reaction occurs, as a smaller amount of energy is expended to reattach the phosphate group to the ADP molecule. Thus, ATP is continuously recycled by all your body's cells. The chemical processes are rather complex, so you don't have to learn them, but if you're curious, the process is explained at the end of this chapter.

Antioxidants – Antioxidants, also known as *free radical scavengers,* are naturally-occurring chemicals which include vitamins A, B2, C, E, grape seed extract, carotenoids, flavonoids and the minerals selenium and zinc. They bond to and thus stabilize and deactivate free radical molecules, unstable, naturally-occurring molecules linked to cellular damage, cancer, heart disease and the adverse effects of aging.

As you breathe and eat, oxygen is transported to all your body's cells through your bloodstream. An excess of oxygen, however, causes *oxidative stress,* with the potential to damage your cells and even your DNA. Oxidative stress is believed to be major factor in the onset and progression of a number of chronic illnesses, such as arthritis, cancer, cataracts, diabetes, heart disease and stroke.

Fresh fruits and vegetables are the best source of antioxidants, though research seems to suggest that obtaining sufficient levels from a normal modern diet is difficult, due to varying levels of quality and freshness of available produce. Thus, supplementation is often recommended.

Carotenoids – Carotenoids are natural plant-derived, fat-soluble pigments, which give certain fruits and vegetables their bright reds, oranges, and yellows. They act as antioxidants, and are often an excellent source of vitamins A and C.

Fiber – Fiber is vital to your health for a number of reasons. It assists in stabilizing blood sugar, lowering cholesterol, maintaining digestive function and possibly reducing cancer risk. Two types of fiber exist: *soluble fiber* dissolves in water, forming gels that help stabilize blood sugar and lower cholesterol. This type of fiber is in barley, oats, citrus fruit and vegetables like apples, oranges and potatoes. *Insoluble fiber* doesn't break down in the presence of water, and thus requires more time to digest. Foods with large amounts of insoluble fiber include seeds, whole grains and cereals, and fruit and vegetable skins.

Flavonoids – These naturally-occurring plant compounds act as antioxidants, protecting your cells from permanent damage in the presence of free radicals (see below). Flavonoids, like carotenoids, give flowers, fruits and vegetables rich hues, including apples, berries, broccoli, cabbage and onions. Flavonoids are also present in some teas, red wine and dark chocolate. Research shows they have both anti-cancer and anti-inflammatory properties.

Free Radicals – These unstable oxygen molecules can be very destructive to human cells. Atoms and molecules are stable when the electrons are in pairs and the *net charge* of the atoms is zero (electrons are matched by an equal number of protons), but when electrons are single or less than the number of protons, it creates an overall positive charge.

Positively-charged free radicals need to "steal" electrons from nearby molecules, often from the fatty acids of a cellular membrane. This electron loss then converts the damaged atoms into *secondary free radicals*, with the potential to initiate a chain reaction called *oxidation* (the mass electron loss which causes metal rusting, or the browning of a cut apple).

Such oxidation results in cellular damage, and is believed to underlie a number of diseases. While free radical development can have the positive effects of controlling bacteria, disposing of toxins and recycling cells, when the process is out of control, it results in health problems.

This kind of *runaway oxidation* occurs as a result of alcohol consumption, cosmic rays, emotional stress, heavy metal exposure, physical trauma, pollution, radiation, consuming rancid fats and oils, ultraviolet light, highly strenuous exercise, and even the cellular energy production cycle itself. Limiting exposure to these effects and eating a diet high in antioxidants can protect against adverse effects upon your health.

Omega-3 fatty acids – These essential unsaturated fatty acids are not naturally produced by your body, but are vital for metabolism, so they must be obtained from food or supplements. Omega-3 oils are plentiful in fatty fish like albacore, salmon, tuna, etc., as well as in algae, krill and some nuts. Recent studies at Oxford and elsewhere strongly indicate that Omega-3s boost cognition, stabilize behavior, and significantly reduce risks of developing several chronic illnesses.

Organic – Foods grown or raised without synthetic pesticides, and livestock raised without antibiotics or growth hormones, generally able to roam freely and raised on organic feed.

Phytochemicals – Naturally-occurring plant chemicals with beneficial, health-guarding properties, such as the ability to help prevent some carcinogens from leading to cancer. Not all of these substances are considered essential for human nutrition, though a number are held to boost health. Antioxidants are one variety of *phytochemicals*, as are carotenoids and flavonoids.

Normally, phytochemicals serve to protect plants from harmful elements, and such protective properties are passed on to you when you eat these plant-based foods. Phytochemicals also provide vivid colors, and rich aromas and flavors to fruits, vegetables and plant products. They also protect your cells from damage, boost immunity, improve vision and cardiovascular health, slow aging, promote *apoptosis* (programmed death of malformed cells), detoxify some carcinogens, and repair DNA.

Many plants store noxious chemicals in *inert* forms, meaning they are only activated in defense, by enzymes stored in nearby cell *vacuoles* (chemical sacs). These activating enzymes are released by cell damage: one example is garlic; when its cell walls are ruptured, the cells release an enzyme called *alliinase* which *catalyzes* (initiates) a reaction converting alliin into *allicin*. Allicin is garlic's natural defense against pests, and provides strong antibacterial, anti-fungal and antioxidant protection.

Phytoestrogen – Literally "plant estrogen", it mimics human estrogen. It's found primarily in soy products, and is believed to be healthy for women (although less so for men), as it seems to reduce cancer risks.

Digestion

Your digestive system is primarily comprised of your *digestive tract*, a 5-meter-long series of organs joined in a long, twisting tube from your mouth to your anus, which breaks down food and absorbs nutrients. The digestive tract includes your mouth, esophagus, stomach, duodenum, large intestine (colon), rectum, and anus.

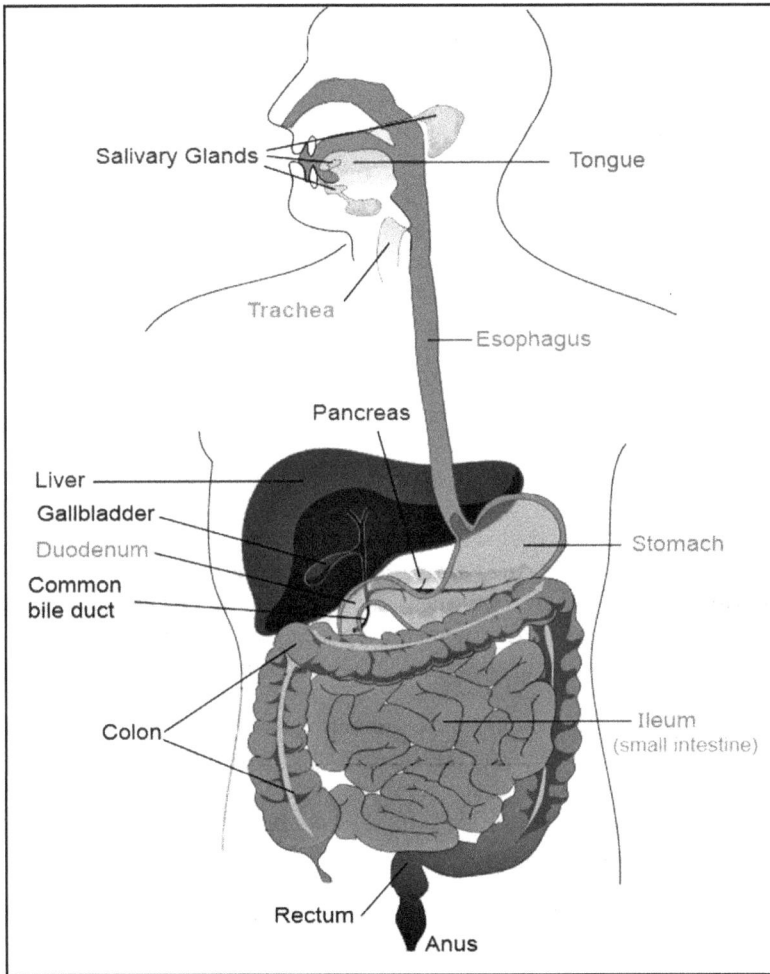

Digestive system, Wikipedia, 2011, public domain

Inside your mouth, stomach, and small intestine, a slimy lining called a *mucous membrane* protects, absorbs and glands in the system secrete digestive juices to *hydrolyze* (break down) food into nutrients your intestines can absorb. Layers of smooth muscle along your digestive tract churn food and digestive juices, and move this semi-digested "chyme" through your digestive tract. Digestion breaks down food and drink into the smallest nutritive components, to build and nourish your cells and provide them with energy: food and drink must be converted into smaller nutrients before they can be absorbed by your bloodstream and transported to your body's cells.

The final products of digestion are monosaccharides, amino acids and lipids. Carbohydrates digest most quickly, followed by proteins, while fats take the longest. These nutrients will either be stored as glycogen and adipose tissue, or catabolized (and thus expended) for protein synthesis, muscle contraction or enzyme activity.

Digestion begins when you chew and swallow, and digestive juices break food down into progressively smaller particles as it moves through your digestive tract. The process is completed in your intestines, where the extracted nutrients are fed through *capillaries* (the tiniest blood vessels) into your bloodstream to be transported throughout your body.

After you push food into your throat with your tongue (swallowing), the process becomes involuntary, proceeding under control of your parasympathetic nervous system. Salivary glands in your mouth produce saliva, which contains enzymes that begin to digest starch and fat into smaller molecules.

Food is automatically passed from one organ to the next through progressive muscle contraction and relaxation called *peristalsis,* like rippling waves moving through the muscles. The muscles contract to narrow and propel this narrowed region further along the digestive tract's length. This narrowing pushes food and fluid ahead and through each organ.

Your *epiglottis* closes in your throat, preventing food from passing into your *trachea* (windpipe) and lungs. Food then travels down your esophagus, passed along by twin layers of contracting muscles, which squeeze food downward toward your stomach. A ring like muscle called the *esophageal sphincter* then relaxes to allow food to enter your stomach, reclosing afterward.

A thick layer of mucus lines your stomach, protecting it from being dissolved by its own juices, as glands in your stomach produce *gastric juices* such as *hydrochloric acid*, mixing it with an enzyme to form *pepsin*, which digests proteins.

Your stomach churns swallowed food and liquid, mixing it with gastric juices through kneading contractions of three layers of muscles. It then slowly empties the contents into your *duodenum*, the entrance to your small intestine.

Your gall bladder stores digestive bile from your liver until food enters your duodenum. Here, bile and pancreatic enzymes are squeezed through small ducts into your small intestine. In the *ileum*, the longest region of your small intestine, protein is catabolized by *protease enzymes*, so you can use it to build and repair body tissues. Amino acids are small enough to pass through your small intestine into your bloodstream, to be distributed throughout your body for protein synthesis and tissue repair.

Most digested nutrients are now absorbed by your *small intestine.* Your small intestine is lined by numerous folds covered with tiny hairlike projections called *villi.* These structures allow absorbed nutrients to cross mucous membranes into your body's circulatory systems, to be transported for storage or further modification.

The villi absorb monosaccharides and amino acids, which diffuse across the cell membranes and are transported into your capillaries. From there, the nutrients travel through your bloodstream to your liver, which neutralizes toxins such as alcohol, drugs, and spent hormones. When these toxins have been rendered safe, they're transported to your kidneys, to be excreted when you urinate.

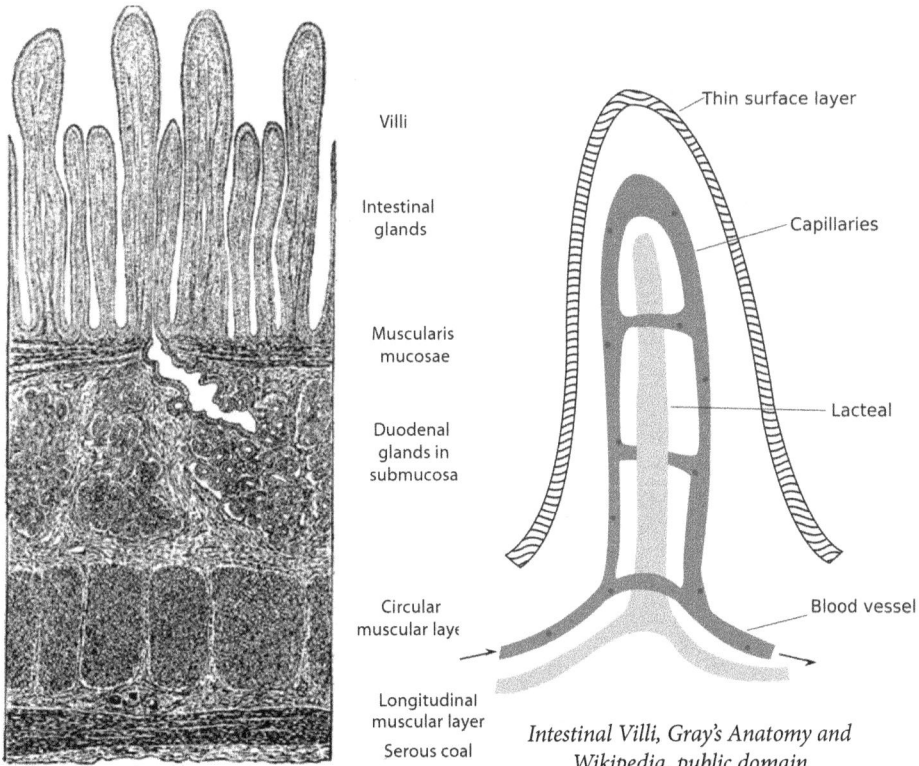

Villi

Intestinal glands

Muscularis mucosae

Duodenal glands in submucosa

Circular muscular layer

Longitudinal muscular layer

Serous coal

Thin surface layer

Capillaries

Lacteal

Blood vessel

Intestinal Villi, Gray's Anatomy and Wikipedia, public domain

The *microvilli* are where digestible carbohydrates—starch and sugar—are hydrolyzed (split) into simpler molecules by enzymes. Starch is digested first by an enzyme in your saliva and pancreatic juice, which breaks it into a disaccharide called *maltose,* the same sugar in fermenting barley when

297

beer is brewed. The enzyme *maltase* then splits maltose into two glucose molecules. Meanwhile, the disaccharides sucrose (table sugar) and lactose (milk sugar) are hydrolyzed into the monosaccharides glucose and fructose, to be passed through your small intestine and into your blood, so it can be transported via your bloodstream to your liver. Your liver will then create glycogen stores or release free glucose in your bloodstream to provide you with energy.

Vitamins are also absorbed through your small intestine. Fat-soluble vitamins (A, D, E, and K) are stored in your liver and fatty tissue, while water-soluble vitamins (B and C) are not easily stored, and excess amounts are flushed out in your urine.

Indigestible plant fiber moves through your digestive tract without being broken down. Indigestible matter – plant fiber and dead cells shed from the mucosa lining of your digestive tract, is pushed into your colon, where it remains until you expel it during a bowel movement.

Most nutrients absorbed by your small intestine are passed on to your liver for processing, but fats (lipids) are passed on to your lymphatic system, for use in your immune system before being transported into your bloodstream via your heart. As your blood circulates, it feeds your body tissues, removing waste and carrying food to your cells. These nutrients are then processed by your liver, after having circulated.

Bile acids from your liver dissolve lipids into fatty acids, an action similar to detergents dissolving grease from a frying pan. After it's been dissolved, fat's further broken down by enzymes from your pancreas and intestinal lining, which dissolve fat into tiny droplets, and the large molecules are broken down into smaller ones, providing fatty acids, glycerol and cholesterol.

Fatty acids and glycerol cannot directly enter your bloodstream, so they are reprocessed to form tiny fatty droplets called *chylomicrons*. These are absorbed by your villi into a second circulatory system, your lymphatic system (see below). After filtering and usage by your immune system, chylomicrons are pumped by your heart into your blood stream.

Your pancreas secretes pancreatic lipase, which breaks down triglycerides into two fatty acids and a monoglyceride. These fatty acids and monoglyceride molecules are absorbed by your small intestine, reassembled into triglycerides, and packaged into tiny particles called chylomicrons, which are released into your lymphatic system, for circulation in your bloodstream.

Chylomicrons are a type of molecule called *lipoproteins*. The outer layer acts as a water barrier, and within the core are triglycerides and cholesterol. A double layer of such lipoproteins makes up the protective membranes of cells in your body, allowing the interior to hold water. Some cell receptors also are specialized to recognize lipoproteins and allow their absorption for biosynthesis.

When chylomicrons reach adipose and muscle tissues, they're broken down by another enzyme (lipoprotein lipase) so they can be absorbed. Fat absorbed by adipose tissue gets stored; fat absorbed by muscle tissue can be burned for energy.

As triglycerides are extracted from chylomicrons, the circulating fatty droplets shrink in size. The remnants in your bloodstream are absorbed by your liver, your body's main lipid processor. You can see the process in an animation here: http://www.hhmi.org/biointeractive/obesity/obesity_processing_fat/13-vid.html

Lipoproteins And Fat Transportation

Your liver regulates fat circulating in your bloodstream, absorbing and releasing fat and cholesterol, converting fats to sugars and vice versa, and synthesizing a number of essential biochemicals, such as glycogen and various proteins.

During and after eating, your liver takes up and converts glucose into triglycerides and glycogen. The fat is released as *VLDLs (Very Low-Density Lipoproteins)*, which are stripped of fatty acids, added to your adipose tissue fat stores, and the remainder circulates as *LDLs (Low-Density Lipoproteins)*, used by your body as a source of cholesterol for hormonal manufacture and other purposes.

Fatty tissues take up circulating blood glucose and fatty acids from VLDL to make more triglycerides for long-term fat storage. Between meals, this adipose tissue can release fatty acids and glycerol for breakdown by your liver into glucose.

Lipoproteins are classified by size – from largest to smallest and least to greatest density:

Chylomicrons carry triglycerides (fat) from your intestines to your liver, muscles, and adipose tissue.

VLDLs (Very Low-Density Lipoproteins) carry newly synthesized fat from your liver to your adipose tissue.

LDLs (Low-Density Lipoproteins) carry cholesterol from your liver to your body's cells. These are sometimes called "bad cholesterol", because they contain a higher ratio of fat to protein.

HDLs (High-Density Lipoproteins) collect cholesterol from your body's tissues, and bring it back to your liver. HDLs are sometimes called "good cholesterol".

These molecules all transport fat and cholesterol throughout your body, between your intestines and liver. Your liver releases VLDL to deliver fat throughout your body. As these VLDLs are broken down, they become LDLs, used by your body as a source of cholesterol. Excess cholesterol is absorbed into HDLs and returned to your liver.

An imbalance – high LDL and low HDL – is associated with heart disease. So while cholesterol in itself is simply another potentially useful biomolecule, the specific ratio of high LDL/low HDL is unhealthy.

Neural Control

Two types of nerves help control your digestive system:

Extrinsic (outer) nerves enervate your digestive organs, using acetylcholine and epinephrine. Acetylcholine stimulates digestive muscle contractions, increasing the force of food and juices travelling through your digestive tract. It also triggers the production of more digestive juice from your stomach and pancreas. Epinephrine exerts the opposite effect, relaxing your stomach and intestinal muscles and decreasing blood flow to these organs, which slows or stops digestion.

Intrinsic (inner) nerves comprise an extremely dense network in the walls of your esophagus, stomach, small intestine, and colon. They're activated when the walls of your digestive system organs are stretched by the presence of food; in response, they release a variety of substances which speed up or delay food passage and digestive juice production. Working in concert, your circulatory system, nerves, hormones, and digestive organs conduct the complex tasks of digesting and absorbing the nutrients from food and liquid you consume every day.

Hormonal Control

The major hormones controlling digestion are produced and released by cells in your stomach and small intestine. These hormones are released into your bloodstream, where they circulate and return to your digestive system, stimulating digestive juices and organ muscle contraction. The primary hormones controlling digestion are *gastrin, secretin*, and *cholecystokinin (CCK)*:

Gastrin prompts your stomach to produce acid which dissolves and digests; it also aids stomach lining, small intestine, and colon cell growth.

Secretin makes your pancreas excrete a digestive juice which contains bicarbonate, to neutralize acidic, partially-digested food as it exits your stomach and enters your small intestine. Secretin also prompts your stomach to produce pepsin – a protein-digesting enzyme, and your liver to produce bile.

CCK makes your pancreas produce pancreatic juice enzymes, stimulates emptying of your gallbladder, and promotes pancreatic cell growth.

Additional hormones regulate appetite: *ghrelin* is produced by your stomach and upper intestine when your digestive system is empty, stimulating your appetite. *Peptide YY* is produced by your digestive tract when food is being processed, inhibiting your appetite. *Leptin* is produced by adipose tissue, signalling *satiety* – a feeling of fullness. These and other hormones signal neurons in your hypothalamus, helping regulate your food intake. Additional hormones are currently under study that may also be involved in appetite.

Your Lymphatic System

Your lymphatic system is part of your immune system, a network of channels called *lymphatic vessels,* which carry the clear fluid *lymph* (Latin for "water") through *lymphoid tissue* to your heart. Lymphoid tissue is contained in a number of your organs, and is chiefly involved in the immune response, consisting of *lymphocytes* (T cells and B cells) and six other types of white blood cells, which defend your body against infections and the spreading of tumors.

The lymphatic system consists of connective tissue, with various types of white blood cells enmeshed in it, most numerous being the lymphocytes, produced by your bone marrow and *thymus gland*. A *lymph node* is a collection of lymphoid tissue, through which lymph fluid passes on its way to returning to your blood stream. Lymph nodes are numerous in your chest, neck, pelvis, armpits, groin, and the blood vessels of your intestines.

The lymphatic system also comprises all the structures dedicated to producing and circulating pathogen-fighting lymphocyte cells: your *spleen,* thymus, bone marrow and the lymphoid tissue associated with your digestive system. They are circulated through your blood and lymphoid organs until they encounter a specific *antigen* – a foreign or altered native molecule.

Your lymphatic system carries lymph through tubular vessels including capillaries, lymph vessels, and thoracic (chest) ducts. Lymph is propelled through these lymphatic vessels by contractions, emptying lymphatic ducts, which drain into your bloodstream via your veins.

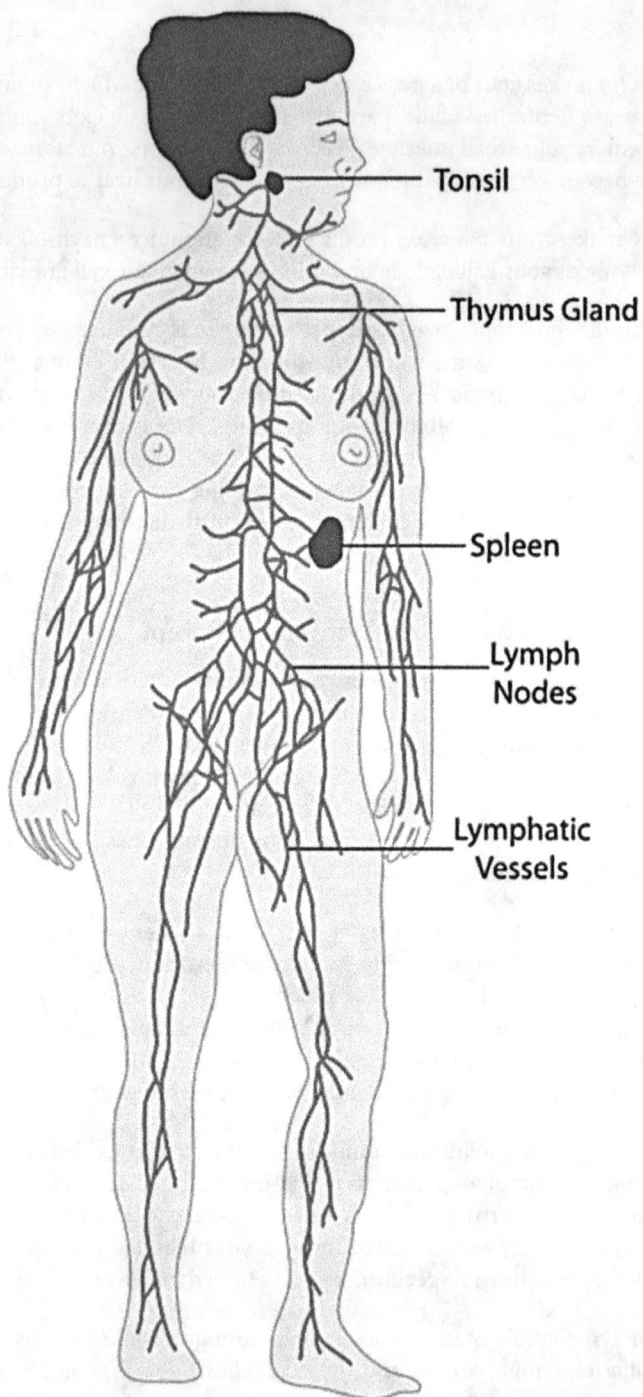

Lymphatic System, Wikipedia, 2012, public domain

The lymphatic system has multiple functions:

- removing fluid from tissues

- absorbing and transporting fatty acids from your digestive system

- transporting white blood cells to and from your lymph nodes and into your bones

- transporting cells to the lymph nodes to stimulate your immune responses

Lymphatic drainage of your body's tissues carries cancerous cells between various body parts, where lymph nodes can then trap cancer cells and attempt to destroy them.

Transforming Food Into Energy – How Your Cells Use Nutrients

Aerobic respiration is the catabolism (breakdown) of nutrients in the presence of oxygen to create carbon dioxide, water, and energy. This cellular energy production takes place in your *mitochondria*, sausage-shaped organelles which serve as your cell's energy factories. This is the chemical cycle using food and oxygen to chemically trap energy into ATP molecules, which can then be used to power virtually all the chemical processes sustaining life. Enzymes power each of the steps, one reason for your body's constant need for proteins and other nutrients to maintain the energy-production necessary for life.

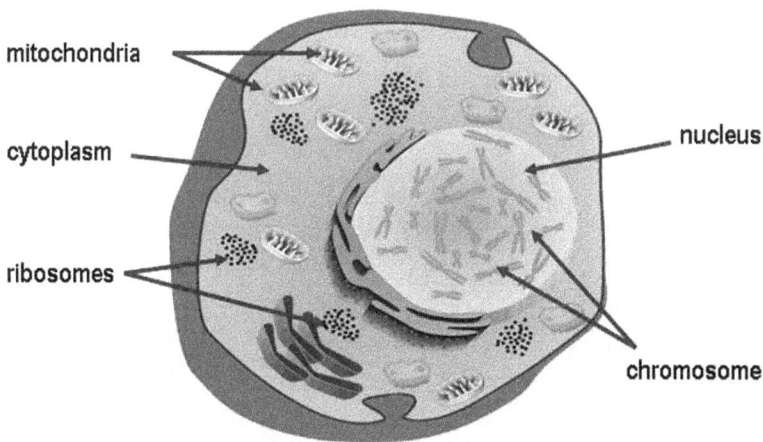

Cell with Labels, Government of Australia, 2011, Creative Commons

303

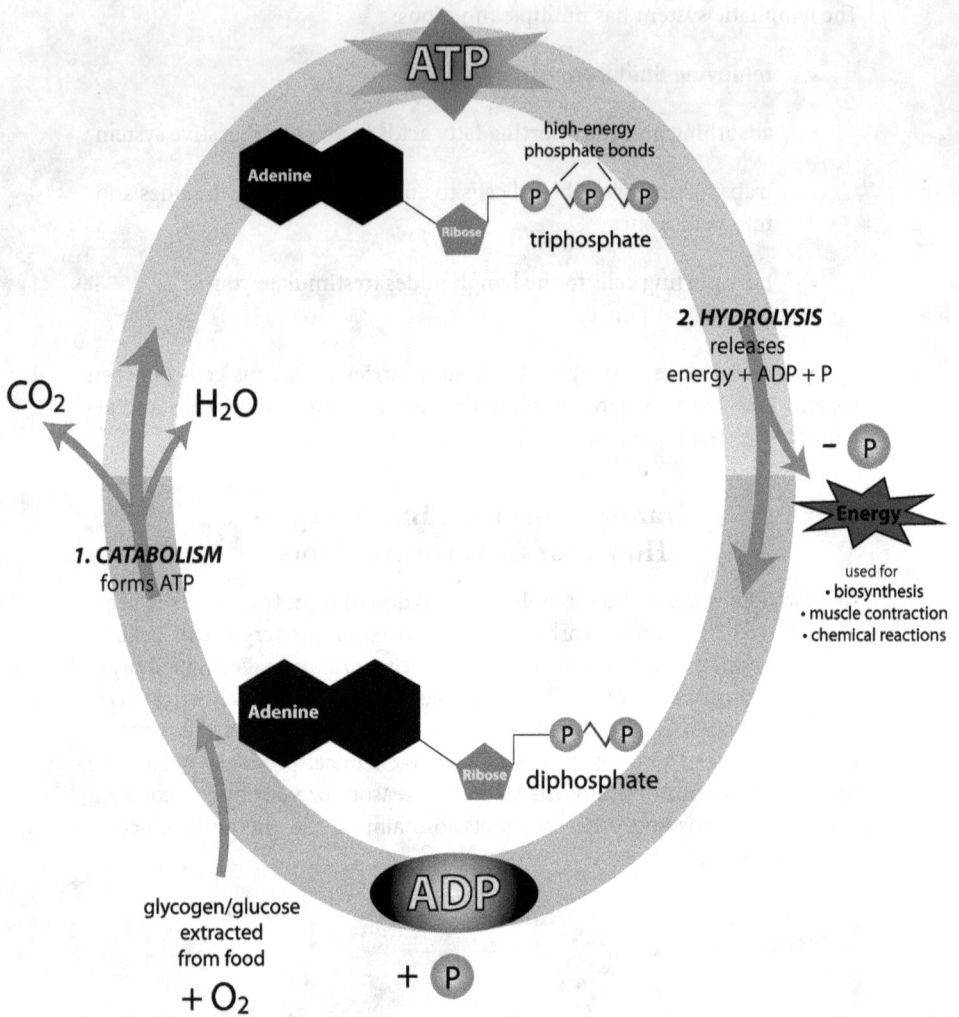

In aerobic respiration, *your mitochondria use glucose and oxygen to generate energy. The Citric Acid Cycle, 2011, Polyglot Studios*

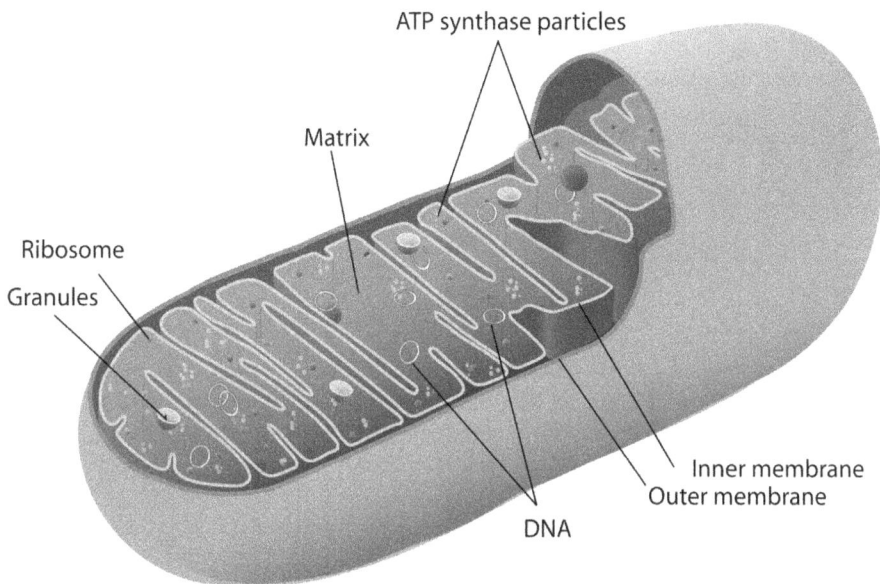

ATP synthase particles

Matrix

Ribosome

Granules

Inner membrane
Outer membrane

DNA

Mitochondrion, Wikipedia, 2011, public domain

One Page of Very Optional Biochemistry

If chemistry makes your eyes glaze over, feel free to skip the following one-page summary. The *citric acid cycle* is a series of seven chemical transformations, breaking down ATP molecules to release energy trapped in phosphate bonds. This also releases positively-charged hydrogen ions, which are pumped into the outer area of the mitochondrion, for reuse in forming more ATP:

1. Glycolysis – Glucose passes from your bloodstream across the microscopic blood vessels called capillaries into the cell cytoplasm. In the cytoplasm, enzymes split six-carbon glucose into two triple-carbon *pyruvate* molecules, casting off high-energy fuel molecules NADH and ATP.

2. Decarboxylation – Pyruvate is brought into the inner chambers (matrix) of your mitochondria by a *transport protein*. Inhaled oxygen combines with one of pyruvate's carbon atoms, forming waste carbon dioxide and more of the energy-dense NADH. This loss of a carbon atom changes pyruvate into *acetyl co-A*, a two-carbon compound.

3. Acetylation – Oxaloacetic acid (a four-carbon chain compound) merges with the acetyl co-A (a two-carbon compound). This forms the six-carbon molecule *citric acid*, the same substance found in oranges and other citric fruits.

4. Oxidation – Oxygen you've inhaled combines with two of the citric acid molecules, pulling them away as waste carbon dioxide. The six-carbon citric acid is again reduced to the four-carbon oxaloacetic acid. In the process, more energy-dense NADH and $FADH_2$ molecules are formed.

The results of metabolizing one glucose molecule at this point are

- 10 x NADH

- 2 x $FADH_2$

- 4 x ATP

5. Electron Transport – Within the mitochondria, high-energy electrons shed from NADH and $FADH_2$ molecules are used to pump positively-charged hydrogen ions out of the mitochondrial matrix, where they can be packed and stored.

Each NADH molecule produces three ATP molecules (10x3), and each $FADH_2$ molecule produces two ATP molecules (2x2), so a single citric acid cycle produces 38 ATP molecules, used to power various cellular processes.

The hydrogen ions combine with oxygen atoms you've breathed to form water molecules, and the NADH and $FADH_2$, which have shed their hydrogen ions, are recycled as NAD+ and FAD, to be used again by the citric acid cycle.

6. Phosphorylation – Stored hydrogen ions are pulled back into the mitochondrial matrix, combining another phosphate group with ADP (adenosine *di*phosphate) to reform ATP (adenosine *tri*phosphate).

7. Hydrolysis – When needed, ATP energy is released by hydrolysis (the third phosphate group's bond breaks using water to release one phosphor group. When the chemical bond is broken, high-energy electrons release energy, dropping into a lower, more stable energy state), resulting in ADP, which is recycled in the mitochondria.

Metabolizing glucose results in waste carbon dioxide production – six CO_2 molecules are created and discarded for every glucose molecule used in energy production. These carbon dioxide molecules are carried on hemoglobin in the red blood cells across the membrane and into microscopic capillaries, then pumped through your veins to your heart and then out to the alveoli (sacs) of your lungs for exhaling. The above process describes the conversion of glucose into ATP, but both fats and proteins can also be catabolized into ATP.

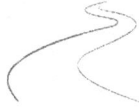

Carbohydrates, Proteins, and Fats, November 10, 2010, The Merck Manuals

Carbohydrates – Monosaccharides, author unattributed, 1996, Chem 102, College of Sciences, Department of Chemistry, Washington State University; http://dwb.unl.edu/Teacher/NSF/C10/C10Links/www.chem.wsu.edu/chem102/102-GlucStr.html

High Rates Of Muscle Glycogen Resynthesis After Exhaustive Exercise When Carbohydrate Is Coingested With Caffeine, David J. Pedersen, Sarah J. Lessard, Vernon G. Coffey, Emmanuel G. Churchley, Andrew M. Wootton, They Ng, Matthew J. Watt, and John A. Hawley, 2007, Journal of Applied Physiology, vol. 105 no. 1 7-13 doi: 10.?1152/?japplphysiol.?01121.?2007; http://jap.physiology.org/content/105/1/7.full

Why Excess Glucose Is Toxic, Science Signalling, 2006, DOI: 10.1126/stke.3202006tw40; http://stke.sciencemag.org/cgi/content/abstract/sigtrans;2006/320/tw40

Essential Fatty Acids, Wikipedia, 2011

Biochemistry of Amino Acids, November 10, 2010, The Medical Biochemistry Page

Protein in Diet, November 10, 2010, University of Maryland Medical Center

How Your Body Uses Protein, Jacob Seykans, Nov 10, 2010; http://www.suite101.com/content/how-the-body-uses-protein-a307059#ixzz1PH7LJ6Tq;

Protein Synthesis: How does the Body Use and Break Down Protein?, A to Z Fitness.com

Post-exercise Caffeine Helps Muscles Refuel, Press Release, 7/1/2008, American Physiological Society (APS) http://newswise.com/articles/view/542216/

How the Body Uses Fat, Dr. Satoshi Amagai, 2010, Howard Hughes Medical Institute; http://www.hhmi.org/biointeractive/obesity/obesity_processing_fat/27.html

Is All Saturated Fat The Same? Dr. David Katz, 06/14/11, The Huffington Post; http://www.davidkatzmd.com/articles.aspx

XIV. Appendix F: Calculate the Percent Daily Value for the Appropriate Nutrients, November 10, 2010, The Food and Drug Administration

A High Antioxidant Spice Blend Attenuates Postprandial Insulin and Triglyceride Responses and Increases Some Plasma Measures of Antioxidant Activity in Healthy, Overweight Men, Ann C. Skulas-Ray, Penny M. Kris-Etherton, Danette L. Teeter, C-Y. Oliver Chen, John P. Vanden Heuvel, and Sheila G. West, June 22, 2011, Journal of Nutrition, doi: 10.3945/?jn.111.138966; http://jn.nutrition.org/content/141/8/1451

Dietary Supplement Fact Sheets, 2003, Office of Dietary Supplements, US National Institutes of Health; http://ods.od.nih.gov/factsheets/list-all/

Vitamin and Mineral Supplement Fact Sheets, National Institutes of Health, 2010; http://www.cdc.gov/nutrition/everyone/basics/vitamins/index.html

Vitamins and Minerals: How to Get What You Need, 2011, American Academy of Family Physicians; http://familydoctor.org/online/famdocen/home/healthy/food/general-nutrition/914.printerview.html

The World's Healthiest Foods, George Mateljan, et al, 2011, The George Mateljan Foundation; http://www.whfoods.com/

Nutrition Glossary, 2011 Condé Nast Digital; http://nutritiondata.self.com/topics/glycemic-index#ixzz1SkvZgKV5

New Naturally Occurring Amino Acids, Ingrid Wagner, Dr. Hans Musso, 2003, DOI: 10.1002/anie.198308161; http://onlinelibrary.wiley.com/doi/10.1002/anie.198308161/abstract

Vesicular Zinc Promotes Presynaptic and Inhibits Postsynaptic Long-Term Potentiation of Mossy Fiber-CA3 Synapse, Enhui Pan, Xiao-an Zhang, Zhen Huang, Artur Krezel, Min Zhao, Christine E. Tinberg, Stephen J. Lippard, James O. McNamara, 2011, Neuron; 71 (6): 1116 DOI: 10.1016/j.neuron.2011.07.019

Carbohydrates, 1996, Chem 102, College of Sciences, Department of Chemistry, Washington State University; http://dwb.unl.edu/Teacher/NSF/C10/C10Links/www.chem.wsu.edu/chem102/102-GlucStr.html

Your Digestive System and How It Works 2008, National Institutes of Health; http://www.digestive.niddk.nih.gov

NIH Publication No. 08–2681, National Digestive Diseases Information Clearinghouse (NDDIC), 2008, National Institutes of Health (NIH) http://www2.niddk.nih.gov/

Integrative Biology 131: General Human Anatomy, Fall 2005, Dr. Marian Diamond, University of California Berkeley; http://science-documentaries.com/?p=760

The Digestive System, 2011, Edd Turtle, Biology Innovation; http://www.biology-innovation.co.uk/pages/human-biology/the-digestive-system/

Lymphoid System, Wikipedia, 2011

Krebs / Citric Acid Cycle, Sal Khan, Khan Academy; http://www.youtube.com/user/khanacademy#p/c/7A9646BC5110CF64/24/juM2ROSLWfw

The Krebs Cycle, animation, John Kyrk, 2011 http://www.johnkyrk.com/krebs.html

Citric Acid Cycle Reactions, Virtual Chembook, Elmhurst College, Charles E. Ophardt, 2003 http://www.elmhurst.edu/~chm/vchembook/index.html

Superfood

Certain foods have been found just as effective as medicine in the long term for keeping you young, strong and healthy. However, it is important to eat them in a raw state as often as possible. As a close second, flash-frozen foods are often still quite high in nutrients.

Dangerous Radicals

Biologists believe a major cause of aging and disease, including cancer, is *reactive oxygen species*, more commonly known as "free radicals". These ions tear apart biological molecules like DNA, RNA, proteins and lipids, mutating or weakening them, and this appears to play a major role in aging and diseases such as Alzheimer's, heart disease and cancer. However, certain fruits such as blueberries and other plant products, particularly green tea, red wine and grape juice, contain *phyto-* (plant) chemicals which stimulate the body to fight free radicals and make them pass harmlessly out of your system.

Superfoods For You

Here are the world's top superfoods, according to the latest research:

Apples – Apples contain high levels of antioxidants, vitamin C, fiber, and potassium, with only 47 calories on average. The skin contains two to six times the antioxidants of the apple's flesh. Natural compounds in apple peels have also been found to help prevent muscle atrophy (weakening) in mice. These compounds are currently being explored for drug development to combat illness- and age-related muscle atrophy.

Dr. Christopher Adams of The University of Iowa discovered *ursolic acid* counteracts genetic changes associated with atrophy. Ursolic acid is part of a normal diet, commonly found in apple peels. His team found in addition to protecting against atrophy, it helps add muscle mass. The effects are apparently derived from enhanced insulin signalling and in correcting altered gene expression linked to muscle wasting. Mice fed ursolic acid also grew leaner, with lower glucose, cholesterol and triglyceride blood levels.

309

In 2007, Cornell university professors Drs. Rui Hai Liu and Xiangjiu He also isolated 13 cancer-fighting compounds called *triterpenoids* in apple peels, which either kill or inhibit growth of cancer cells in the human liver, breast and colon. They say in addition, apple consumption is linked with reduced risks of lung cancer, heart disease, and stroke.

Apple antioxidants have also been shown to extend the average lifespan of test animals by 10 percent. Chinese University of Hong Kong's Food and Nutritional Scientist Dr. Zhen-Yu Chen and his colleagues found apple polyphenols are particularly potent antioxidants, even reversing levels of age-indicative *biochemical markers*. Dr. Chen adds that women who regularly consume apples were found to have a 13-22 percent decrease in heart disease risk.

2006 research indicates apple juice also increases acetylcholine production, with memory benefits comparable to current medications. Because of these findings, Dr. Thomas Shea, director of the UML Center for Cellular Neurobiology and Neurodegeneration Research, believes apples and apple products will one day be recommended alongside popular Alzheimer's medications.

Increasing acetylcholine has been found to help slow mental decline from Alzheimer's. Alzheimer's medications inhibit the production of enzymes which break down acetylcholine in the brain. Inhibiting these enzymes – and thus stabilizing acetylcholine levels – enhances memory. The results came from moderate amounts of juice consumption, the equivalent of 2-3 apples or two 8 oz. glasses of apple juice per day. Human clinical studies are currently underway.

A series of studies showed apple juice enhances maze navigation, and prevents age-related mental decline in mice given the human equivalent of two glasses of apple juice a day for a month. These mice also produced fewer of the *beta-amyloid* protein fragments thought to lead to the neural-killing plaques commonly found in the brains of Alzheimer's patients. Apples also contain a unique mix of antioxidants which improve cognition and memory by inhibiting oxidation in the brain.

Avocados – Recent research has shown that avocados are high in fiber, folate, potassium, vitamin E, and magnesium. They also contain a monounsaturated fat called *oleic acid*, which helps lower cholesterol. Exercise burns this kind of monounsaturated fat more quickly than saturated fat, so even though avocadoes are "fatty", the calories are burned more quickly than those from the saturated fat found in meat and dairy foods.

Beans – Beans are considered the world over to be the "poor man's meat". Since there are many diseases that come from eating large amounts of saturated fat found in meat, beans provide an excellent low-fat, high-protein alternative. Beans are also an excellent source of fiber, B vitamins, iron, folate, potassium, magnesium, and many phytonutrients, and should be consumed on a regular basis to promote optimal health.

Blueberries – New research shows that blueberries are just as strong as drugs in reducing cholesterol, without the negative side effects. Blueberries are packed with phytochemicals that prevent cell damage. They're also an excellent source of vitamin C and E, manganese and fiber, but are very low in calories. Researchers at Tufts University recently measured the antioxidant capacity of 60 fruits and vegetables, and found blueberries rated the highest in the ability to destroy free radicals.

While red wine is said to protect the arteries and heart, a recent study found that blueberries contain 38% more of the same phytochemicals. Berries and red wine also contain flavonoids which boost brain-derived neurotrophic factor (BDNF), stimulating axon growth and enhancing circulation. In 2011, Harvard School of Public Health researchers also found flavonoids in berries and brightly-colored fruits like apples and oranges appear to be highly neuroprotective, lowering Parkinson's risk as much as 40% among men.

Broccoli sprouts – Broccoli sprouts have a spicy taste derived from an antioxidant that protects your body against disease, primarily cancer. In 1992, Johns Hopkins University scientists found the cytoplasm of broccoli sprout cells contains a special phytochemical called *glucoraphanin*, which combines with an enzyme found in the plant cell walls and in specialized cells called *myrosinase*.

Chewing ruptures broccoli cell walls, and the two chemicals combine to form *sulforaphane*, a natural plant defense against herbivorous insects. In humans, sulforaphane stimulates production of an enzyme that deactivates free radicals. In 1997 it was found that this chemical is at least 20 times more concentrated in sprouts than in full-grown broccoli. Since then, more than 700 studies have confirmed the powerful anticancer effects of sulforaphane, which is found in lower concentrations among other *cruciferous* (Latin meaning cross-shaped) vegetables, like cauliflower, cabbage, horseradish, kale, collard greens, mustard and wasabi, and radishes.

Dark Chocolate – Although you shouldn't gorge yourself on milk chocolate because of its high calories and fat content, dark chocolate helps lower blood pressure, increase blood flow, and promote cardiovascular health. Additionally, although some worry about the amount of caffeine in chocolate, it's actually quite low – one chocolate bar contains from 1 to 11 mg of caffeine, while a regular cup of coffee has about 137 mg. As long as you limit your daily consumption to about 100 calories, and eat only dark chocolate, it will give you a significant health boost.

Eating small portions of dark chocolate daily has been shown to lower cortisol, reduce blood pressure and free radical damage, boost metabolism, thin the blood (providing the same anti-clotting effects as aspirin), and promote positive gut microbial activity.

But you need to be choosey – overly sweetened, processed chocolate is made with butterfat and raises cholesterol and causes significant blood sugar spikes. Dark chocolate, on the other hand, has four times the concentration of flavonoids as milk chocolate, while white chocolate contains no flavonoids. Cocoa solids or cocoa mass should be listed as the first ingredient and not sugar. You can choose chocolate with high cocoa content, such as 70 per cent or higher "bitter" varieties.

The same heart-disease preventing antioxidant substances found in red wine are also found in chocolate to a similar degree. These polyphenols inhibit blood platelet aggregation (clumping), reduce cellular and arterial damage from free radicals, and inhibit LDL cholesterol oxidation – the process that makes cholesterol stick in fatty deposits to arterial walls, increasing risk of heart attacks and strokes. According to the American Journal of Clinical Nutrition, only half an ounce of dark chocolate daily increases antioxidant capacity 4 percent, and lessens LDL cholesterol oxidation.

Cocoa also temporarily lifts mood with a mild stimulant called *theobromine,* a chemical similar to caffeine. It also contains a mild sedative called *anandamide,* a fatty substance discovered in 1992 that appears to ease pain, alleviate depression, curb appetite, and assist memory and fertility. Anandamide is naturally synthesized in the cortex and other brain regions central to memory, cognition, and motor control, suggesting it has other important functions in addition to sedation and elation.

Anandamide acts as a chemical messenger between a mother and embryo at the point of implantation, in effect providing one of the first biological communications between a mother and child. It binds to the same neural receptors as *cannabinoids* – marijuana's euphoria-inducing chemicals. The USDA is also currently studying anandamide as a natural animal sedative, because it lowers body temperature and slows respiration. It may one day become the basis of a new class of therapeutic drugs.

Chocolate also contains other substances with mood-elevating effects. One is *phenethylamine,* which triggers the release of endorphins and dopamine. This is the same substance released in the brain when someone falls in love. Finally, dark chocolate has been shown to boost serotonin levels, stabilizing mood and creating a sense of calm and well-being. Because women experience lower serotonin levels during PMS and menstruation, chocolate may be helpful. It also appears to have a positive effect on people with depression.

Elderberries – These berries may help prevent heart disease and cancer because of their high concentration of the antioxidant *anthocyanin.* A 2007 study has also suggested other compounds in elderberries may boost eye health, neural and cognitive function, and protect against DNA mutations. Elderberry juice has been recommended as an excellent alternative to more common fruit juices.

Green Tea – It's widely believed that green tea and/or soy may be the reasons Japanese live longer than anyone else on the planet. Research from the UK, Spain and Japan shows that two to three cups a day protects against heart disease and certain types of cancer, as well as making bones and teeth healthier and improving brain function. There is also substantial evidence green tea speeds up the metabolism, helping to burn calories and stored body fat. Powdered green tea has a much more powerful effect than tea bags.

In a recent Israeli study, it was found that polyphenols in green tea extract help to protect and even repair brain cells of mice suffering from Parkinson's and Alzheimer's disease, a process called *neurorestoration.*

A compound in green tea has been found to increase regulatory T cells, which are central to immune function and suppression of autoimmune diseases, according to a 2011 study at Oregon State University. This might account for green tea's abilities to help control inflammation, improve immunity and help stave off cancer. According to Dr. Emily Ho of the OSU Department of Nutrition and Exercise Sciences, a variety of cells play different roles in the immune system, which must balance the role of fending off disease and avoiding damage to normal cells. Autoimmune diseases, from allergies to diabetes or terminal conditions like Lou Gehrig's disease, arise when this protective system is faulty and the body begins to mistakenly fight itself.

Certain cells, such as regulatory T cells, exist to help control this problem and "dial down" or shut off the immune system. Proper function and number of regulatory T cells is in turn controlled by other biological systems such as methylation of DNA and transcription factors.

Dr. Ho's team discovered that the polyphenol *EGCG* triggers this increased regulatory T cell production. While this increase is not as high as with prescription drugs, there are no risks associated with toxicity or with long-term use. Dr. Ho believes EGCG operates through *epigenetics* – rather than changing genetic code, it controls what proteins get expressed, and therefore what kinds of tissues are produced.

Studies upon mice have showed that EGCG significantly increases regulatory T cells in the spleen and lymph nodes, thereby helping regulate the immune response. Medicines can perform similar functions, but often have toxic side effects, so natural products may be a long-term, sustainable alternative to achieving these ends without the toxicity.

Kale – Kale is considered an anti-cancer food because of its high amounts of organosulfur compounds, which allow the body to detoxify *carcinogens,* cancer-causing agents. It also contains the phytochemicals *lutein* and *zeaxanthin,* proven to prevent cataracts, the most common eye disease among those over 55.

Kale also contains significant amounts of vitamins A, C, E, and B, as well as manganese, copper, calcium, and iron. The Japanese drink powdered kale, called "aojiru". While it admittedly tastes foul, because of its tremendous health benefits, it's highly recommended, and now is sold in a much more palatable fruit flavor.

Kiwi – A single kiwi fruit contains 100 percent of the daily recommended amount of vitamin C; more than an orange. The peel can also be eaten. Regular consumption has also been shown to help promote eye and cardiac health.

Omega 3 Fish – Omega 3 oils found in salmon, herring, sardines, and mackerel lower heart disease risk, help ease arthritis, and appear to help alleviate memory loss, Alzheimer's, and depression. Two to three servings a week are recommended. Omega 3s are also found in flax seed and walnuts.

In 2002, British researchers found a 35 percent reduction in violent offenses among prisoners taking recommended daily amounts of vitamins, minerals, and healthy omega-3 fatty acids (as fish oil supplements). Studies have also found links between national depression and murder rates, and per capita Omega 3 consumption. Says nutritional advocate and bestselling author Dr. Mark Hyman, omega-3 fatty acids have a profound effect, helping determine brain, eye, heart, and immune system function:

That's because omega-3s affect every cell in your body. They help form the cell membranes of all of your trillions of cells and regulate hormones and inflammation throughout your system.

He adds that the effect upon cognition is particularly profound: children with attention deficit disorder, the reading disability *dyslexia*, the writing disability *dyspraxia*, and other learning disabilities, tend to be deficient in omega-3 fatty acids. Studies have demonstrated that fish oil supplements improve these children's reading, spelling, and behavior.

The American National Institutes of Health has information on your body's omega-3 content here: http://efaeducation.nih.gov

Pumpkin – Pumpkin is one of the most nutritious foods known. It's actually a fruit, rather than a vegetable, related to melons and gourds.

Seaweed – Seaweed contains significant amounts of vitamin B, magnesium, iron, folate, and calcium. It also contains more minerals than any vegetable, and has anti-inflammatory and stress-relieving nutrients. It is also shown to lower the risk of heart disease. Some varieties of seaweed, such as kelp, also contain large amounts of iodine, used by the thyroid to regulate most growth and many other bodily functions.

Soy – Soy contains an inexpensive, high-quality, vitamin- and mineral-rich plant protein with lots of fiber, and plant-based omega-3 fatty acids. It's the richest known dietary source of powerful health-promoting *phytoestrogens*. Soy has been found to help prevent cardiovascular disease, cancer, and osteoporosis as well as helping to relieve menopausal and menstrual symptoms.

Spinach – Spinach appears to lessen the risk of cardiovascular disease such as stroke and coronary artery disease; cancer, including colon, lung, skin, oral, stomach, ovarian, prostate and breast cancer; age-related tooth degeneration and cataracts. The latest research also suggests spinach may assist in preventing or delaying cognitive decline in the elderly. Spinach contains an impressive number of healthy compounds, including iron, carotenoids, antioxidants, vitamin K, coenzyme Q10, B vitamins, minerals, polyphenols, and plant-derived omega-3 fatty acids.

Tomatoes – It was once believed that tomatoes were dangerous, possibly even poisonous (at one time they were called "wolf peaches" in the mistaken belief they were toxic). Originally grown and enjoyed by the Aztecs in Mexico, tomatoes were imported to Europe by Spanish missionaries. It's now known that tomatoes are one of the healthiest of fruits, full of cancer-fighting polyphenols such as *lycopene*.

Turkey – Turkey is low in fat, one of the leanest meat protein sources available, with a powerful variety of nutrients, notably niacin, selenium, vitamins B6 and B12, and zinc. These nutrients promote cardiovascular health and help lower cancer risk.

Walnuts – Many people believe nuts are too high in calories, but the phytonutrients in nuts significantly reduce the risk of coronary heart disease, diabetes, cancer, and many other illnesses. Eating ten to twenty grams of unsalted nuts five times a week reduces the risk of heart attacks by 25 to an astounding 51 percent, according to the latest research.

Ancient Japanese Dietary Superstars

According to Dr. Mark Hyman:

> *Medicine doesn't always come in a pill. In fact, some of the most powerful medicines are delicious and can be found at your local supermarket or 'farmacy.' Healing foods have been used for centuries in Asia as part of the cuisine. In Asia food and medicine are often the same thing.*

The following foods can be found in most Asian markets:

Arame – Arame is a type of kelp, one of a number of seaweeds used in Japanese dishes. Usually sold dried, it can by rehydrated in five minutes. It's dark brown, with a mild, salty-sweet flavor, and a firm texture. It's served among other seaweeds, in salads, and in marinated dishes. It can also be added to appetizers, casseroles, pilafs, soups, and a variety of other dishes. This amazing seaweed is extremely dense in minerals – calcium, iodine, iron, magnesium, and vitamins A and K, as well as *eisenin*, which boosts the immune system. It also contains *lignans*, phytoestrogens which act as antioxidants.

Burdock – Greater burdock root has been used since the Middle Ages as a vegetable. The Japanese call it *gobo*. The long slender roots, which are soaked in water or miso stock, can reach up to a meter in length and 2 cm in diameter. Burdock is low-calorie and contains a fair amount of fiber, calcium, potassium, amino acids, and unique polyphenols. It is usually julienned or shredded and added to miso soup or *kinpira gobo*, a delicious, sweet, tart burdock-carrot salad, lightly cooked in soy sauce, sugar, sake, and sesame oil.

Daikon – This is a large white root vegetable which resembles a carrot. Daikon are said to be "radishes", but are much milder in flavor than the western radish. Rich in vitamin C and folate, with only 6 calories per ounce (23 calories per 100 grams), daikon contains enzymes which aid digestion, and the enzyme myrosinase, which helps detoxify hazardous chemicals in the body. Daikon is usually grated, used as a garnish, or in salads. A 100-gram serving contains 34 percent of the government's recommended daily allowance of vitamin C.

Konnyaku – This chewy Japanese jelly is made from "Devil's tongue", the konnyaku potato. It's been used in Japanese cuisine for over 1,500 years. The fiber, called *glucomannan*, is remarkable for its absorbency, retaining up to 17 times its weight in water. It thus expands in the digestive system, absorbing fat, accelerating waste elimination, and reducing cholesterol. Because it contains almost no calories, and blunts sugar absorption and increases feelings of satiety, konnyaku is often used for weight loss.

Miso – Miso is a thick paste used for seasoning. It's made from fermented soybeans and sometimes barley, rice or other grains, with salt and the yeast called *kojikin*. The Japanese use miso in *misoshiru* soup, and add it to a number of sauces and spreads. Miso is a very protein- and mineral-dense food, which has been used since at least the 6th century AD. It's generally salty with a rich, zesty, meaty flavor, although there are many regional varieties. I personally use it in place of salt in sauces, and it's delicious atop steamed broccoli.

Natural miso contains a number of healthy microorganisms, like *Tetragenococcus halophilus,* but these microorganisms are extremely heat-sensitive and die if overcooked. Because of this, miso should be eaten either uncooked, or added to food just before removal from the heat source. Miso is high in sodium, however, so those on sodium-restricted diets should eat it sparingly.

Shiitake Mushrooms – Also called Chinese black mushrooms, these are originally native to Korea, China and Japan, where they've been cultivated since prehistory. The highest grade is called *donko* by the Japanese. Drying these mushrooms breaks down their proteins into amino acids, and transforms their fungal sterols into vitamin D.

They're also high in minerals, particularly iron, and appear to help prevent immune cells from adhering to arterial walls, thus helping prevent atherosclerosis. Recent research indicates shiitake mushrooms reduce blood platelet aggregation, stimulate immunity, and boost antiviral *proteinase inhibitors*; in Japan, shitake-derived *AHCC (Active Hexose Correlated Compound)* is a popular alternative medicine for cancer patients. It appears to increase resistance to pathogens such as viruses and bacteria, and to enhance immunity. Shiitake also contain *lentinan*, a compound which appears to have antitumor properties.

Umeboshi – These are extremely sour, salty pickled apricots. They're made by pickling *ume*, which are then dried in the open air, packed in sea salt and *shiso leaves*, pressed, and aged for approximately six months. Modern Japanese generally eat umeboshi in *onigiri*, rice balls wrapped in seaweed, but they have an ancient history in Asian cuisine. They're reputed to have originated in China as far back as 4,000 years ago, and in Japan, the elite samurai warriors used umeboshi as their primary field ration, adding flavor to foods, and using the highly antibacterial acidity to purify water and to ward off battle fatigue.

Umeboshi are moderately high in potassium, necessary for cardiac and digestive health, and in iron, which promotes red blood cell production. They also are said to help stimulate digestion, and promote toxin elimination. However, each umeboshi contains from 690 to 839.8 mg of sodium, about half your daily allowance, so for those on sodium-restricted diets, caution should be exercised.

Spice Up Your Life

A diet full of turmeric, cinnamon, black pepper and other spices reduces your body's negative responses to high-fat meals, according to 2011 Penn State research. According to Dr. Sheila West, high-fat meals increase blood triglycerides, and chronic high levels increase your heart disease risk, but adding spices to fatty meals reduces triglyceride responses about 30 percent, compared to meals without added spices.

Dr. West's team found rosemary, oregano, cinnamon, turmeric, black pepper, cloves, garlic and paprika all demonstrate high antioxidant activity. A single meal with about two tablespoons of mixed spices raises blood antioxidant activity by 13 percent and decreases insulin response by about 20 percent.

An additional 2011 study at the University of Illinois shows the enzyme myrosinase, found in broccoli sprouts, mustard, horseradish, and wasabi, significantly enhances broccoli's anticancer properties, and ensures maximum absorption in your upper digestive tract, where you derive the greatest health benefits.

The spicier the better, according to nutrition professor Dr. Elizabeth Jeffery. Myrosinase is an enzyme necessary for synthesizing *sulforaphane*, broccoli's super cancer-fighting substance. When myrosinase is present, sulforaphane can be released in your ileum, the entry to your digestive system. This gives the fastest and greatest nutrient absorption. As few as three to five servings of broccoli a week provide potent cancer-protective benefits. Broccoli sprouts are one of the richest sources of antioxidants, and their myrosinase content can be easily obtained by adding them to sandwiches or atop pizza, according to the study's authors.

Bitter cumin – This member of the daisy family is a major ingredient in Indian curries, used for centuries in folk remedies for a wide range of diseases. It has both antiparasitic and antimicrobial properties, and research has shown its additional fever-reducing and pain reduction properties. Recent studies have also shown it is a rich source of antioxidants. Free radicals are naturally produced during the metabolic processes that maintain life, however, when free radicals are over-produced or under-removed, it results in oxidative stress, a destructive process implicated in aging, atherosclerosis, cancer and neural degeneration.

Antioxidants are believed to clean up free radicals, reducing oxidative stress, and helping to prevent diseases. Plant phenolic compounds are antioxidants. Researchers from Mysore, India, have demonstrated that bitter cumin seeds are a potent source of these phenolic antioxidants. Cumin contains strong antioxidants for scavenging free radical molecules, inhibiting the oxidation of liposomes (which, when attacked by free radicals can rupture cell membranes) and offering protection from DNA damage.

Cilantro – Cilantro, also called *coriander,* appears to reduce cholesterol and blood sugar levels, to kill harmful bacteria, and to help in shedding toxic metals by chemically binding to them, allowing your body to expel them. Although dried cilantro contains less antioxidants than fresh, there is still a significant amount of antioxidants in both forms.

Cinnamon – One of the oldest spices used in human society, and even in traditional medicine, cinnamon comes from the bark of evergreen trees grown in China, Vietnam, and Ceylon. Cinnamon has recently been found to lessen the symptoms of type II diabetes and to significantly extend test animal life.

Garlic – this member of the allium vegetable group, which includes chives, leeks and onions, has been proven to boost immunity, helping your body fight nasty tumors, thus helping reduce stomach, colon and prostate cancer risks.

Oregano Oil – Oregano oil contains carvacrol, an antimicrobial agent.

Parsley – these garnishes are rich in anti-inflammatory polyphenols and carotenoids. Parsley raises blood antioxidants more than almost any vegetable, and contains nearly twice the carotenoids of carrots (which are named after carotenoids); only red peppers and kale contain as much. The main polyphenol in parsley, *apigenin*, is a flavonoid.

In a 2011 study, University of Missouri researchers discovered apigenin, also found in fruits and nuts, has the power to stop breast cancer tumor cells from multiplying and growing. Dr. Salman Hyder found apigenin led to fewer tumor developments and significant delays in tumor formation compared to those unexposed to apigenin. He believes this could help women taking hormone replacement therapies. Some HRTs contain synthetic hormones that accelerate the development of breast tumors, such as the *progestin* MPA – a synthetic hormone which accelerates breast tumor development.

When breast tumor cells develop in response to MPA, blood vessels form within the tumors, supplying nutrients for tumors to grow and multiply. Apigenin blocks formation of these new blood vessels, delaying and sometimes halting tumor development. The compound also reduces overall tumor numbers, but cannot prevent the initial formation of breast cancer cells.

Apigenin is most prevalent in parsley and celery, but can also be found in apples, oranges, nuts and other plant products. No specific dosage has been yet been determined for humans, but a little parsley and some daily fruit consumption can confer benefits.

Rosemary – *Heterocyclic Amines* (HCAs) form when beef and pork are exposed to high heat and open flames, as when barbecued. The substances have been linked to several forms of cancer; however, a 2008 study showed adding rosemary to meat before cooking appears to lower HCAs. The result was linked to the high antioxidant levels of rosemary.

Turmeric – The spice turmeric, one of the chief ingredients in Indian curries and American mustard, has also been used for centuries as a medicinal herb. According to the American National Institutes of Health, two dozen current studies being conducted worldwide on turmeric's effects (and that of its principle active component, curcumin), indicate curcumin and turmeric:

- offset liver damage

- weaken cancer cells

- may have a tremendous impact on arthritis treatment

- may prevent or significantly reduce the onset of Alzheimer's disease

- inhibit growth and spread of melanoma, skin and breast cancers

- reduce levels of heterocyclic amines (carcinogens formed when cooking meat) by up to 40 percent

Curcumin has been shown to exhibit antioxidant, anti-inflammatory, antiviral, antibacterial, antifungal, and anticancer activities and thus has a potential against various malignant diseases, diabetes, allergies, arthritis, Alzheimer's disease and other chronic illnesses.

Because of its bitterness, only one or two teaspoons should be added to soups or stews. Although both turmeric and curcumin supplements are now widely available, absorption by the digestive system is enhanced by black pepper.

Extra Credit

Chamomile Tea – reduces gastro-intestinal muscle spasms, indigestion, and menstrual cramps. This tea has also been proven to have a moderate calming effect on those with General Anxiety Disorder.

Grape Seed Extract – research shows it helps with wound healing and fights tooth decay, osteoporosis, skin and breast cancers, Alzheimer's and heart disease.

Ginseng and Cinnamon Bark – a recent study found these two supplements appear to have "significant" lifespan-extending effects. Ginseng has also been found to have anticancer properties, and has been used for thousands of years as an energy tonic and libido booster in traditional Chinese medicine.

Mixed Essential Oils – a 1- to 2-gram mixture of gamma linolenic acid, oleic acid, linoleic acid, polyunsaturated acids and vitamin E all but eliminates PMS symptoms with no notable side effects, according to a 2010 study conducted at the University of Brazil.

Propolis – A resin made by bees, it's one of the most broad-spectrum antimicrobial compounds known, and is also a rich source of caffeic acid and apigenin, two compounds that boost immunity and even help ward off cancer.

Supplements With Proven Effects

Studies are inconclusive about the effectiveness of several supplements, but I've taken daily multivitamins/multiminerals since the age of 16, always opting for organically-based rather than petroleum derivative supplements. Although the jury's still out, Nobel prizewinning biochemist Linus Pauling – the "father of molecular biology" – wrote a book recommending multivitamin supplementation. As he lived to be 93, I plan to continue following his advice.

In 2006, the Lewin Group (an ISO 9001 certified independent medical-industry consultant) conducted a massive survey of modern medical research on supplementation, and concluded the health benefits of vitamin and Omega-3 fatty acid supplementation are incontrovertible and, at pennies a day, well worth the cost.

Functional medicine expert Dr. Mark Hyman also points out that many of us are deficient in B-complex vitamins, needed for methylation. Methylation, if you recall, is essential for proper body functions, occurring billions of times every second, helping to regulate and repair your DNA among other critical processes. Methylation breakdown, notes Dr. Hyman, increases the risk of diabetes and various cancers, as well as depression, dementia, stroke, and mood and behavior disorders in children.

In addition to a vitamin/mineral supplement, Dr. Hyman recommends eating generous daily amounts of fresh, dark, leafy greens. In particular, he recommends at least one cup a day of the most nutrient-dense vegetables: bok choy, escarole, Swiss chard, kale, watercress, spinach, or dandelion, mustard, collard, or beet greens. He also warns against methylation-impairing habits like consuming excessive animal protein, sugar, saturated fat, processed and canned foods, coffee, and alcohol.

Roughing It

A nine-year study of 388,000 adults Americans aged 50 to 71 by the National Institutes of Health found that fiber helps lower risks of death not just from heart disease, but even from infectious and respiratory illnesses. The government study says sufficient fiber lowers the risk of death from diabetes, heart disease, and cancer, and even helps prevent pneumonia and flu. It also improves cholesterol levels, blood pressure, inflammation and blood sugar levels. Researchers believe fiber binds to toxins and quickly flushes them out of the body.

In the study, men and women who ate the recommended amount of daily fiber were 22 percent less likely to die over the nine-year course of the study, according to the National Cancer Institute's Dr. Yikyung Park, who led the research. Fiber from grains seems to have the greatest effect, although fruits, vegetables and beans also contain it. They suggest substituting whole wheat for white bread to increase daily fiber intake.

Most Americans don't get enough daily fiber, on average eating only about 15 grams a day, much less than the daily recommended 25 (for women) and 38 (for men). To give you an idea of how much fiber that means, a woman needs to eat one-third of a cup of bran cereal, a half a cup of cooked beans, a small apple and a half a cup of mixed vegetables. A man needs to eat the same, adding 23 almonds, one baked potato, an oat bran muffin and an orange.

Fat Up Your Salad For Better Health

Fatty dressings get a bad rap. While you definitely want less fat from dairy and meats, it turns out the opposite is true with salad dressings – recent findings show that the single most critical part of a salad lies in the dressing – and the fattier, the better. Although it may seem counterintuitive to switch from low-fat or fat-free to oil-based dressings, the small number of calories you save come at a significant cost.

While lettuce is almost entirely water, it also contains abundant phytochemicals, not to mention vitamins A and C, potassium, fiber, lycopene, lutein, and, in the case of dark varieties, beta carotene, linked to reduced cancer risks.

These nutrients are called fat-soluble because the presence of fat is necessary to absorb them, so if you're topping salads with fat-free dressing, you're just throwing away nutritive benefits. According to research, fatty acids make a huge difference in the amount of phytochemicals your body absorbs.

Scientists at the University of Iowa measured and compared nutrients absorbed into the blood after subjects ate salads with three different categories of dressings: fat free, reduced fat, or conventional full fat. They found subjects who used fat-free dressings absorbed almost no phytonutrients. Reduced-fat dressing provided a minimal improvement, but full-fat dressing allowed maximal nutrient intake.

Monounsaturated fats in vegetable oils, such as olive, grape seed, almond or canola oils, protect against heart disease and other cardiovascular illnesses and provide fatty alpha-linolenic acid and vitamin E.

The topping champion is avocado – adding it to salad provides a staggering 1500% times more beta-carotene, 700% more alpha-carotene and 500% more lutein than a plain salad. Nuts also greatly enhance the absorption of phytonutrients from raw vegetables. So to really benefit from your veggies, make sure you add avocados, nuts, cheese and/or oils – just don't overdo it.

You're Hosting Alien Life!

The bacteria in your body outnumber your own cells by a factor of ten – 100 trillion, mostly in your digestive system. While this sounds scary, in truth, the relationship is symbiotic – both you and your gut bugs benefit – usually.

Your potential to host both beneficial and detrimental intestinal flora can be profoundly influenced by your diet. Many anaerobic bacteria, fungi, and yeast feed on simple carbohydrates (sugar and fruit juices), and can impair immunological and neurological function.

Microbes in the digestive systems of carnivores are adapted to breaking down amino acids which predominate their hosts' diets, while bacteria in the guts of herbivores are specialized in building new amino acids from constituent parts.

Fermented foods – cultured and grown with beneficial bacteria – are very good for your digestive system, however, promoting healthy and combatting unhealthy gut flora. Among the most powerful fermented foods you can eat are yoghurt, miso, kim chee, sauerkraut, and pickles, although you may want to watch for high sodium levels.

Remember too, the majority of your serotonin is produced in your intestine, not your brain. Your digestion has a profound effect upon your moods and your immune system.

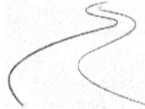

Prescription for Nutritional Healing, 4th Edition, Phyllis A. Balch, CNC, 2004

Biomarkers of Dairy Intake and the Risk of Heart Disease, S. Aslibekyan, H. Campos, and A. Baylin, 2011, Nutrition, Metabolism and Cardiovascular Diseases, 2011; DOI: 10.1016/j.numecd.2011.02.003

Catecholamines Inhibit Ca (2+)-Dependent Proteolysis in Rat Skeletal Muscle Through Beta(2)-Adrenoceptors and cAMP, Navegantes LC, Resano NM, Migliorini RH, Kettelhut IC, 2001, American Journal of Physiology – Endocrinology and Metabolism;281(3):E449-54.

Melanocortin Activity in the Amygdala Controls Appetite for Dietary Fat, Stéphane Boghossian, MieJung Park and David A. York, American Journal of Physiology, 2010 Feb;298(2):R385-93)

Carotenoid Bioavailability is Higher from Salads Ingested with Full-Fat Than With Fat-Reduced Salad Dressings as Measured with Electrochemical Detection, Melody J Brown, Mario G Ferruzzi, Minhthy L Nguyen, Dale A Cooper, Alison L Eldridge, Steven J Schwartz and Wendy S White, 2004, American Journal of Clinical Nutrition, Vol. 80, No. 2, 396-403; http://www.

ajcn.org/content/80/2/396.full.pdf

Salad and Raw Vegetable Consumption and Nutritional Status in the Adult US Population: Results from the Third National Health and Nutrition Examination Survey, Dr. L. Joseph Su, PhD, MPH; Dr. Lenore Arab, PhD, MS, 2006, Journal of the American Dietetic Association, Vol. 106, No. 9, 1394-404 http://www.ncbi.nlm.nih.gov/pubmed/16963344)

Superfoods To The Rescue, Mallika Marshall, 2008

Superfoods to the Rescue! Deana Embury, 2010

Turmeric Health Benefits, Dr. Andrew Weil, 2010

An Evidence Based Study of the Role of Dietary Supplements in Helping Seniors Maintain their Independence, The Lewin Group Inc., 2006; http://www.lewin.com/content/publications/3393.pdf

Maximizing Methylation: The Key to Healthy Aging, Dr. Mark Hyman, 2011 http://drhyman.com/maximizing-methylation-the-key-to-healthy-aging-3012/

mRNA Expression Signatures of Human Skeletal Muscle Atrophy Identify a Natural Compound that Increases Muscle Mass, Steven D. Kunkel, Manish Suneja, Scott M. Ebert, et al, 2011, Cell Metabolism; 13 (6): 627-638 DOI: 10.1016/j.cmet.2011.03.020

Apple Polyphenols Extend the Mean Lifespan of Drosophila Melanogaster, Cheng Peng, Ho Yin Edwin Chan, Yu Huang, et al, 2011, Journal of Agricultural and Food Chemistry; 110214164435048 DOI: 10.1021/jf1046267; http://www.j-alz.com/issues/9/vol9-3.html

Metabolic Effects of Dark Chocolate Consumption on Energy, Gut Microbiota, and Stress-Related Metabolism in Free-Living Subjects, Francois-Pierre J. Martin, Serge Rezzi, et al, 2009, Journal of Proteome Research; 091007113151065 DOI: 10.1021/pr900607v; http://pubs.acs.org/doi/abs/10.1021/pr900607v

The Bliss Molecule, Fred Senese, 2010, General Chemistry Online; http://antoine.frostburg.edu/chem/senese/101/features/anandamide.shtml

Chocolate's Startling Health Benefits, John Robbins, February 22, 2011 The Huffington Post; http://www.huffingtonpost.com/john-robbins/chocolates-startling-heal_b_825978.html

Induction of Regulatory T Cells by Green Tea Polyphenol EGCG, Carmen P. Wong, Linda P. Nguyen, Sang K. Noh, Tammy M. Bray, Richard S. Bruno, Emily Ho, Immunology Letters, 2011; DOI: 10.1016/j.imlet.2011.04.009

Apigenin Prevents Development Of Medroxyprogesterone Acetate-Accelerated 7, 12-Dimethylbenz (A) Anthracene-Induced Mammary Tumors In Sprague-Dawley Rats, B. Mafuvadze, I. Benakanakere, F. Lopez, C. L. Besch-Williford, M. Ellersieck, S. M. Hyder. Cancer Prevention Research, 2011; DOI: 10.1158/1940-6207.CAPR-10-0382

Triterpenoids isolated from Apple Peels Have Potent Antiproliferative Activity and May be Partially Responsible for Apple's Anticancer Activity, Xiangjiu He and Rui Hai Liu, Journal of Agricultural Food Chemistry, 2007; http://pubs.acs.org/doi/abs/10.1021/jf063563o

325

Dietary Supplementation with Apple Juice Decreases Endogenous Amyloid-B2 Levels in Murine Brain, Amy Chan and Thomas B. Shea, 2009, Journal of Alzheimer's Disease, 16:1

Antioxidant Potential Of Bitter Cumin (Centratherum Anthelminticum (L. Kuntze) Seeds In In Vitro Models, V Ani email and Kamatham A Naidu, 2011, BMC Complementary and Alternative Medicine, doi: 10.1186/1472-6882-11-40; http://www.biomedcentral.com/1472-6882/11/40/abstract

Dinner Is A Date With The Doctor: 5 Asian Superfoods, Dr. Mark Hyman, October 29, 2011, The Huffington Post; http://www.huffingtonpost.com/dr-mark-hyman/asian-superfoods_b_1033903.html

Dietary Fiber Intake and Mortality in the NIH-AARP Diet and Health Study, Yikyung Park, Amy F. Subar, Albert Hollenbeck, Arthur Schatzkin; February 14, 2011, Archives of Internal Medicine, doi:10.1001/archinternmed.2011.18;

Healthy Herbs: Springtime Picks, Leo Galland, M.D., 05/ 7/11, The Huffington Post; http://www.huffingtonpost.com/leo-galland-md/healthy-herbs_b_853597.html

In Vitro Antimicrobial Activity of Ten Medicinal Plants Against Clinical Isolates of Oral Cancer Cases, Manju Panghal, Vivek Kaushal and Jaya Parkash Yadav, 2011, Annals of Clinical Microbiology and Antimicrobials, 10:21 doi:10.1186/1476-0711-10-21; http://www.ann-clinmicrob.com/content/10/1/21/abstract

What Criminals and Fish Have to Do With Your Health, Dr. Mark Hyman, MD On June 18, 2010; http://drhyman.com/what-criminals-and-fish-have-to-do-with-your-health-3531/

Routine Periodic Fasting is Good for your Health, and Your Heart, Study Suggests, 2011, Intermountain Medical Center (the body is always trying to achieve recovery from stress – releasing hormones or neurotransmitters in response)

Effects Of Botanical Dietary Supplements On Cardiovascular, Cognitive, And Metabolic Function In Males And Females, S. Carlson, N. Peng, J. K. Prasain, et al, Gender Medicine, April 2008;

Grape-Derived Polyphenolics Prevent Aß Oligomerization and Attenuate Cognitive Deterioration in a Mouse Model of Alzheimer's Disease, J. Wang, L. Ho, W. Zhao, et al, The Journal of Neuroscience. June 18, 2008;

Essential Fatty Acids for Premenstrual Syndrome and their Effect on Prolactin and Total Cholesterol Levels: a Randomized, Double Blind, Placebo-Controlled Study, YB Yu, L. Dosanjh, L. Lao L, et al.

Cinnamomum Cassia Bark In Two Herbal Formulas Increases Life Span In Caenorhabditis Elegans Via Insulin Signalling And Stress Response Pathways, Edilberto A Rocha Filho, José C Lima, João S Pinho Neto and Ulisses Montarroyos, 2011, Reproductive Health 8:2;

Probiotics, Dr. Joseph Mercola, video, 2011; http://probiotics.mercola.com/probiotics.html?e_cid=20110804_DNL_art_1

Your Gut Microbes are What You Eat – Diet Strongly Influences Intestinal Bacteria Populations, Daniel Strain, 2011, Science News

Diet

"My ability to tolerate shame, to compartmentalize it, to swallow it, increased right along with my belt size. It came with the territory of being heavy. Obese people have a lifetime of experience with shame."
– Edward Ugel, I'm With Fatty: Losing Fifty Pounds in Fifty Miserable Weeks, 2010

The Secret To Fitness: 80% Of The Equation Is Diet

If weight loss is your aim, nutrition expert Dr. Joseph Mercol says 80% of the equation rests in your dietary habits, rather than exercise. Eating healthier probably means you need to make permanent changes to your eating patterns. You undoubtedly already know about calorie counting and which foods are low in fat, sugar and salt. But what follows are additional secrets cutting-edge research has recently discovered to help keep you trim, energized and mentally and physically healthy for the rest of your life:

If you're unsure about specifically how many fruits and vegetables you're supposed to be eating, the US CDC has a website with a calculator based on your age and sex, as well as a great deal of other informative data online here: http://www.fruitsandveggiesmatter.gov/

Most people believe that drinking fruit juice is healthy, but, in fact, it contains a significant amount of fructose, which is chemically similar to refined white sugar. The calories from fruit juice can add up quite quickly. Additionally, after being processing, sitting in your refrigerator and opened, half the beneficial nutrients disappear within a day. You're always better off choosing fresh or frozen fruits or vegetables.

Habit-Forming

Modern research is beginning to show how the brain controls eating habits. Your hypothalamus maintains homeostasis, reducing your drive to eat (appetite) when with the hormone leptin signals your brain that your stomach is full. Specialized cells in the hypothalamus respond to hormones and fatty acids circulating in the blood, in this way controlling appetite. But chronically high levels of fatty acids in the blood, from eating a high-fat diet, are thought to alter hypothalamic function, "setting up a vicious cycle of overfeeding and altered energy balance."

A lack of awareness may lead you to establish destructive habits which sabotage your best efforts at weight management. Simple deprivation – spending long periods of time without food, slows your metabolism and makes your body go into starvation mode – so your body begins to conserve calories.

Other forms of dieting are a short-term solution leading to long-term health problems – including eventually making you fatter. Some people believe low-carbohydrate diets are an effective means of losing weight, but over the long term they may be extremely unhealthy, possibly even dangerous. Such diets are low in fiber, and restrict grains, fruits, and vegetables, which protect against disease and provide critical nutrition.

Training Your Hunger Clock

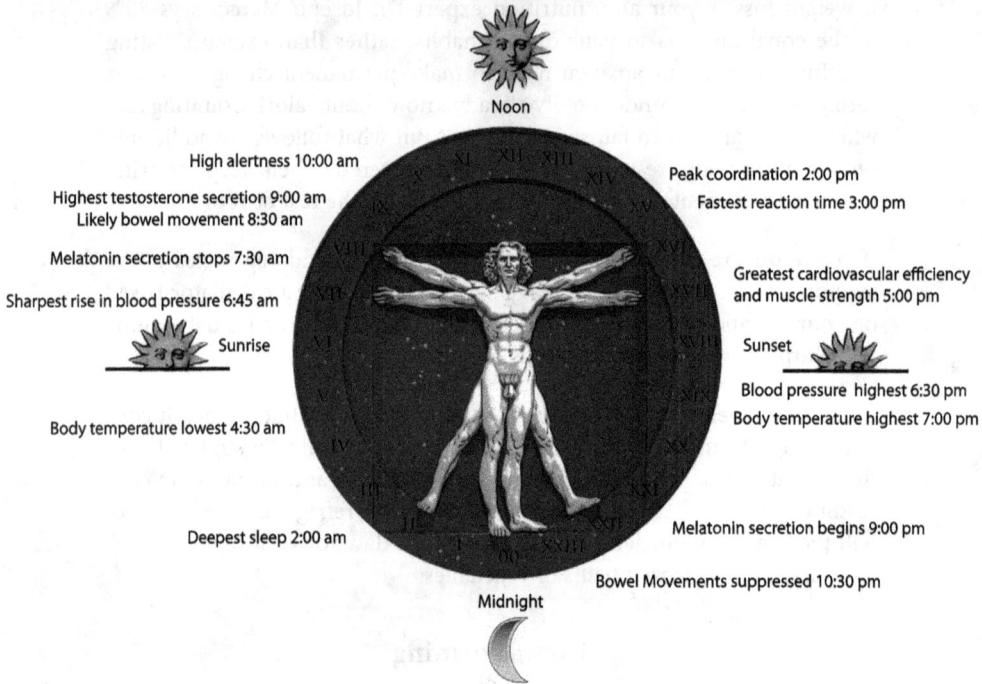

High alertness 10:00 am

Highest testosterone secretion 9:00 am
Likely bowel movement 8:30 am

Melatonin secretion stops 7:30 am

Sharpest rise in blood pressure 6:45 am

Sunrise

Body temperature lowest 4:30 am

Deepest sleep 2:00 am

Noon

Peak coordination 2:00 pm
Fastest reaction time 3:00 pm

Greatest cardiovascular efficiency
and muscle strength 5:00 pm

Sunset

Blood pressure highest 6:30 pm
Body temperature highest 7:00 pm

Melatonin secretion begins 9:00 pm

Bowel Movements suppressed 10:30 pm

Midnight

Circadian Rhythms, 2011, Polyglot Studios

Humans evolved to eat an omnivorous diet. You have the digestive system of a predator, which means you're designed to eat large amounts of food at a time, and then digest it slowly, while engaging in other activities, such as hunting. Conversely, prey animals are designed to eat and digest constantly. Their systems require constant caloric intake. You have the advantage of being able to wait between meals, necessary because hunting is much more difficult and time-consuming than gathering plant-based food.

However, to avoid *insulin spikes* (sudden increases in insulin responses to blood sugar), you should ideally spread your meals throughout the day, with the largest immediately after waking, and the quantity of food tapering off throughout the day, an "inverted pyramid" plan – starting with a solid breakfast, then gradually less throughout your day. In fact, to supercharge your body's fat-burning capabilities, professional bodybuilders and other athletes recommend "grazing", eating six or seven regularly-spaced, scheduled small meals every day, in portions that fit in the palm of one hand.

At night, when your metabolism is at its slowest, you should stop eating after 7 pm. If you do eat, carbohydrates are best limited after 7 pm, unless you're having difficulty sleeping, in which case a small carbohydrate-rich snack can help you nod off.

The Hunger Hormone

In 2009, collaborators at Columbia and Rockefeller Universities identified stomach cells which time release of ghrelin, a hormone which makes animals eat even when they're not hungry. This is a significant milestone in the decades-long search for biological hunger clocks.

Dr. Rae Silver of Columbia University, along with Drs. Joseph LeSauter, Helene L. Kaplan and Mark N. Kaplan of Barnard College, and Donald W. Pfaff of Rockefeller University demonstrated how the cells operate. A circadian clock, set by eating schedule patterns, controls their ghrelin release. Stomach cells release ghrelin into circulation prior to mealtimes, and the hormone stimulates appetite, spurring active searching for food and its consumption, even if creatures aren't hungry.

> Circadian clocks allow animals to anticipate daily events rather than just react to them. The cells that produce ghrelin have circadian clocks that presumably synchronize the anticipation of food with metabolic cycles.

Daily fluctuations in CNS arousal and behavior expend energy, creating your needs for regular, cyclical food intake. Special cells in your stomach secrete ghrelin before regularly-scheduled mealtimes, and this rhythmic timed release pattern is set by your prior eating schedules.

Ghrelin activates GHSR receptors in the vagus nerve and hypothalamus, thus controlling food-seeking and eating behavior. In this way, ghrelin increases CNS arousal (wakefulness), metabolic rate and food-seeking activity, and prompts the synthesis and secretion of digestive enzymes prior to mealtimes.

A Salty Tale – *A study on hypernatremia (elevated salt levels) in rats shows salt also reduces stress. Researchers found reduced stress hormone responses in restrained animals with higher salt levels. But HPA suppression isn't the only reason salt makes you feel good; hypernatremic rats also had increased oxytocin; oxytocin triggers stress reduction when you're in love or experiencing other positive social interactions.*

The researchers believe there is a connection between social "watering hole" drinking and high salt, says TIME magazine. They reason that elevated salt drives dehydration, compelling animals to find a good water source, and the same elevated salt levels lead to stress decreases, allowing communal interaction.

But it's not all good news. Salty foods have been found to significantly and immediately affect the arteries, severely impeding blood flow within 30 minutes of consumption: Dr. Kacie M. Dickinson of the Commonwealth Scientific and Industrial Research Organization in Adelaide, Australia measured differences in the arteries between healthy volunteers fed low-salt tomato soup and volunteers who ate the same soup with 10 times as much added salt. The diets were then switched between groups.

After volunteers ate the soup, Dr. Dickinson's team used ultrasound to measure their arteries. The arteries of volunteers who ate saltier soup widened only half as much as in those who ate low-sodium soup. This severely restricted blood flow wore off after two hours, but the effects seem to be cumulative over time. In other words, eating a high-sodium diet leads to permanently impaired blood vessel function, over time, contributing to atherosclerosis, a fatty clogging. This in turn can cause blockages, resulting in heart attacks and strokes.

When pumping blood, the heart creates nitric oxide gas to relax artery walls. Dr. Dickinson's team believes salt somehow blocks this nitric oxide production, temporarily hardening artery walls. Because of this effect, two grams of sodium a day or less is recommended, although those who exercise and lose sodium through sweat every day may safely consume slightly higher amounts.

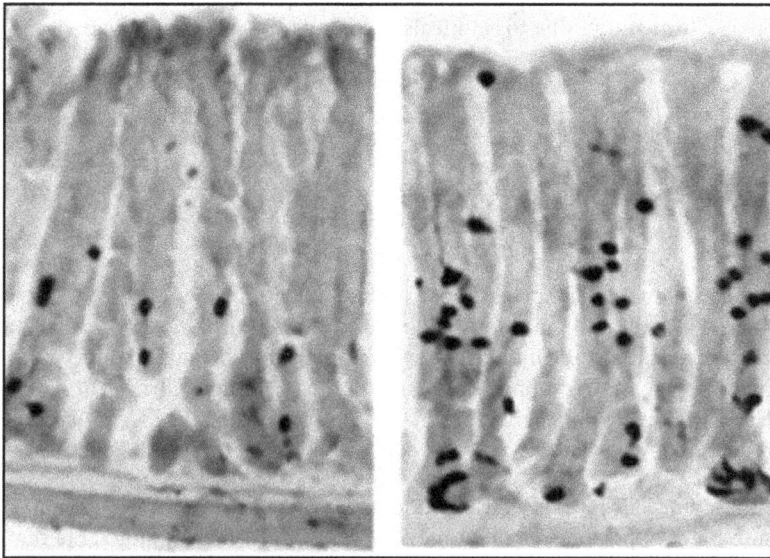

A photomicrograph of the stomach wall. The black dots are ghrelin, a hormone associated with appetite. Dr. Rae Silver, Joseph LeSauter and Donald Pfaff, 2009. Used with permission.

The photosensitive *suprachiasmatic nucleus*, which sets your body's circadian rhythms based on available light, can be removed without affecting this rhythmic feeding schedule, indicating timed ghrelin release is independent of your hypothalamus' master clock, but is instead "entrained" by your eating habits.

In its "default" state, ghrelin synthesis peaks during the day and falls at night, the cells which produce it receiving input from the suprachiasmatic nucleus. But this "default" release schedule can be overridden by your eating habits, and the schedule appears to take root within as little as four days.

Ghrelin, released from your stomach's *oxyntic glands*, circulates via your bloodstream to your brain, where it influences cortical decision-making. Your cortex is constantly evaluating whether or not to eat and, as mealtime approaches, ghrelin increases the number of "yes" signals.

People injected with ghrelin become voraciously hungry and eat more than normal. This new research thus points to your stomach as the main site for regulating the timing of meals, promoting food anticipation, and compelling you to eat. Your stomach tells your brain when to eat, and training yourself with a regular eating schedule allows you to regulate your stomach's ghrelin release. Thus, while you should eat several meals throughout the day to keep your metabolism high, you need to schedule it for specific times:

"If you eat all the time, ghrelin secretion will not be well controlled," says Silver. "It's a good thing to eat meals at a regularly scheduled time of day."

This research also suggests ghrelin, the only natural appetite stimulant synthesized outside the brain, is a promising target for drug development. Drugs which suppress ghrelin production could help curb appetite before dieters even begin to eat.

Pleasure And Stress

Pleasurable activities such as food, sex and activities you love provide more than just agreeable sensations (dopamine and endorphins). According to 2010 research at the University of Cincinnati, they actually reduce stress, inhibiting anxiety responses in your brain. Drs. Yvonne Ulrich-Lai, James Herman, director of the Laboratory of Stress Neurobiology say this stress reduction lasts at least seven days, conveying long-term health benefits:

"These findings give us a clearer understanding of the motivation for consuming 'comfort food' during times of stress. But it's important to note that, based on our findings, even small amounts of pleasurable foods can reduce the effects of stress," says Dr. Ulrich-Lai.

The team provided rats twice daily access to a sugar solution for two weeks, then tested their stress responses. Compared with controls, rats with access to sugar had lower heart rate and stress hormone levels when placed under restraint, and when freed, they were more willing to explore unfamiliar environments and interact socially with other rats.

Rats fed a saccharin-sweetened solution instead of sucrose showed similar reductions in stress responses, the researchers say, as did rats given access to sexually responsive partners. But sucrose supplied directly to the stomach did not blunt stress, the researchers say. "This indicates that the pleasurable properties of tasty foods, not the caloric properties, were sufficient for stress reduction," says Dr. Ulrich-Lai.

Physiological responses to stress include activation of the hypothalamic-pituitary-adrenocortical (HPA) axis, regulated by the basolateral amygdala (BLA). Rats exposed to pleasurable activities, such as tasty foods and sex, had reduced HPA axis stress responses. Deactivating the BLA prevented the stress reduction, suggesting BLA neural activity is necessary for the effect.

"Our research identifies key neural circuits underlying the comfort food effect," notes Ulrich-Lai. "Further research is needed, but identification of these circuits could provide potential strategies for intervening to prevent or curtail increasing rates of obesity and other metabolic disorders."

Food As Drugs

You need to get in the habit of asking yourself a single question before putting anything in your mouth: *"Will this benefit me or harm me?"*

According to the US Department of Agriculture, in the year 2000, the average American ate an astounding 52 teaspoons (nearly half a **pound** per **day!)** of refined sugar – 152 pounds per year, mostly in soft drinks, table sugar, and jams or jellies. But you need to start looking at refined sugar as a mildly poisonous, addictive drug, because of its biochemical effects.

If you picture a bag of refined sugar as a bag of pure, uncut heroin or cocaine, you won't be far off the mark, and you might think twice about putting things that contain large amounts of it into your body – or feeding it to your children. Extend this thought to white flour and fruit juices as "watered down" or "cut" versions of the same deadly, addictive drugs, and you'll be doing yourself and your loved ones a tremendous service – extending lives, strengthening immunity against disease, and promoting significantly greater mental, physical and emotional health.

Eating sugar affects opioid receptor synthesis in your brain, and, over time, lowers dopamine sensitivity – exactly the same neurological process that "hooks" addicts on crack, heroin and other life-destroying drugs. And, of course, the more often you eat foods with sugar and/or high fructose corn syrup, the more you substantially raise the chance you'll contract diabetes, heart disease, cancer and/or Alzheimer's disease. If you start to think of sugar as crack cocaine, you'll have a much more responsible attitude toward its consumption.

Dr. Joseph Mercola, author of the *New York Times* best-seller *The No Grain Diet*, is a four-decade-long marathon runner and considered a foremost authority on natural health, appearing on the Today Show, CNN, ABC's World News Tonight, *Time* and *Forbes* Magazines. He says an additional reason to limit total fructose intake is because it raises *uric acid*, which is hard on the joints. He recommends no more than 25 grams per day; most Americans, he says, consume much more than this 25 daily grams, with 25% consuming as much as 134 grams of fructose daily.

Toxic Industrial Food-Like Substances

According to Dr. Mark Hyman, author of *The Ultrasimple Diet*, high fructose corn syrup is a "toxic industrial food product" that kills. If "high fructose corn syrup" is written on the label, he warns,

...it's not whole, real, fresh food full of fiber, vitamins, minerals, phytonutrients and antioxidants. Stay away if you want to stay healthy.... this one simple dietary change can radically reduce your health risks and improve your health.

In *Five Reasons High Fructose Corn Syrup Will Kill You* he notes that typical Americans consume over 60 pounds a year of their sugar intake in the form of HFCS, usually in sweetened drinks and processed foods. At these doses, he notes, "...we are conducting a largely uncontrolled experiment on the human species".

One 20-ounce HFCS-sweetened soda, sports drink or tea has 17 teaspoons of sugar – nearly *a full year's supply* of what our ancient hunter-gather ancestors used to consume, about 20 teaspoons a year.

In just moderate doses, he says, HFCS is a major cause of cancer, dementia, heart disease, obesity, liver failure, tooth decay and more. But in the "pharmacologic" doses westerners eat, it can punch holes in your intestine, trigger body-wide inflammation and obesity, and may eventually kill you.

HCFS is cheaper to produce than cane sugar because the American government subsidizes corporate corn production. HFCS is also sweeter, but it's nearly always an indicator of nutrient-poor, disease-inducing "industrial food products" or, as Dr. Harman puts it, "food-like substances".

In contrast, naturally-occurring fructose comes with a complex of nutrients and fiber, making it biologically quite different from the free-floating, rapidly-absorbed high fructose doses of HFCS. High fructose corn syrup is, he points out, an industrial chemical product, far different from any naturally-occurring substance. Synthesized from corn stalks in a highly-secretive laboratory process, HFCS is extracted by enzymes to create a chemical compound not found in the environment.

HFCS contains double-sugar molecules, equal amounts of glucose and fructose. These sugars are rapidly absorbed into your bloodstream with little digestion required. From this point, fructose travels straight to your liver, where it triggers lipogenesis – fatty triglyceride and cholesterol synthesis.

This makes it a major cause of liver damage. The rapidly-absorbed glucose also triggers insulin spikes, leading to metabolic disturbances, driving appetite increases, cancer, dementia, diabetes, heart disease, weight gain, and more. Says Hyman, HFCS may also well be the underlying cause of the modern explosion in obesity rates.

334

Food And Mood

What you eat impacts not just your risk for disease but also your mood – nutrition profoundly affects your state of mind. An estimated 21 million American adults suffer from mood disorders, and 40 million from anxiety disorders. The breakdown of the family and other support systems certainly plays a significant role, but nutritional deficiencies may well play just as great a role.

Maureen Nagle, a licensed nutritionist at St. Joan of Arc's Mental Illness Ministry points out that woman are twice as likely as men to have depression, and attributes this to the fact woman are also twice as likely to try fad dieting, cutting protein and fat intake to try and lose weight. This primary focus on calorie-cutting leads to malnutrition, depleted brain chemistry and blood sugar imbalances, she believes.

> *I believe food is the most powerful drug we come in contact with several times a day. Do we need more prescription medication or is it possible that we need to address our nutrient deficiencies?*

Mood disorders stem from biochemical imbalances; Nagle cites amazing changes when people choose to incorporate a balanced nutrition plan that restores these balances. Key to this is maintaining stability. Blood sugar levels can be kept stable by eating every 3-4 hours daily, with every meal consisting of healthy protein, fat and carbohydrate. This will rev up the metabolism and supply the brain with its critical glucose supply.

What you eat influences and regulates the neurotransmitters your brain produces every moment, significantly affecting your behavior and general emotional health. Proteins from fish, poultry, eggs, beef, and nuts supply the vital amino acids used to synthesize neurotransmitters. Those with the greatest impact on your mood, behavior and cognitive function are serotonin, dopamine, norepinephrine, and GABA:

Serotonin, a neuromodulator derived from the amino acid L-Tryptophan, supplies feelings of optimism, calm, and the ability to focus and sleep well.

Dopamine, derived from the amino acid *L-Tyrosine*, is one of the most important neuromodulators. It provides feelings of empowerment and motivates. It's produced in abundance during the state of romantic love, and when appreciating art and things of beauty. People with adequate dopamine have high self-esteem, pain tolerance, and an ability to assume responsibility for their actions.

Norepinephrine is synthesized from dopamine, acting as an energy booster, generating alertness and allowing focus.

GABA is synthesized from the amino acid *L-Glutamine*, and helps your brain in filtering information, suppressing and inhibiting, and promoting calm, essentially functioning as your body's natural Valium.

Magnesium, zinc and the b-complex vitamins are used to convert these amino acids into these mood-controlling neurotransmitters, and Omega-3 essential fatty acids are also vital to ensure post-synaptic receptor function.

Junk Food Addiction

A great deal of research conducted in the last decade has shown startling similarities between consuming energy-dense, fatty, sugary, and salty foods, and taking cocaine, heroin, and nicotine. Foods high in sugar, fat, and salt can be addictive in exactly the same manner as alcohol, cocaine, heroin, or nicotine.

People eat more because these foods trigger cravings and addiction. Like an alcoholic after the first drink, once people start eating processed food, the sugar, fat and salt trigger the brain's reward centers, and it becomes damned hard to stop. So despite the stigma and health consequences of being overweight, and despite an intense desire to lose weight, some people just cannot manage it, not because they WANT to be overweight, but because certain foods are highly addictive, highjacking their brain's core control centers.

In *The End of Overeating*, former head of the Food and Drug Administration Dr. David Kessler describes how food is made into drugs – hyperpalatable foods that lead to neurochemical addiction. Dr. Mark Hyman, in *The Science and Nature of Food Addiction*, contends that "Big Food" thrives on a kind of propaganda, pretending weight management is solely a matter of self-control, and encouraging more "personal responsibility". But he says the food industry has been researching ways to exploit the natural human biological wiring underlying fat, sugar and salt cravings, and is using the information to create specifically more addictive, "drug-like" food substances.

Thus, food addictions are not driven by a lack of willpower or character deficiency: "Nobody chooses to be a heroin addict, cokehead, or drunk. Nobody chooses to be fat either. The behaviours arise out of primitive neurochemical reward centers in the brain that override normal will power and overwhelm our ordinary biological signals that control hunger."

This is why cigarette smokers continue smoking when they know it leads to cancer and heart disease, why fewer than 20 percent of alcoholics successfully quit drinking, and why most addicts continue using cocaine and heroin even as it tears their lives apart.

Mental health professionals, government agencies and the worldwide medical industry refer to the *Diagnostic and Statistical Manual of Mental Disorders (DSM)* to classify such disorders as addictions. A diagnosis of addiction is based upon the following criteria:

- A substance is taken in greater amounts and for longer periods than usual

- There is a persistent desire to quit or repeated unsuccessful attempts at quitting

- A great deal of time and energy is spent in obtaining, using, or recovering from use

- Important social, occupational, and/or recreational activities are given up or reduced

- Use of the substance continues despite knowledge of its adverse effects, such as health dangers or an inability to meet life obligations

- A gradual buildup of tolerance – the need to take more and a decline in its effectiveness with repeated use

- Withdrawal – unpleasant physical and mental effects as a result of not using the substance

Fatty and sweet foods stimulate the release of endogenous opioids (the body's natural morphine), so consumers build up a tolerance to sugar, needing ever greater amounts for satisfaction, just as with alcohol or heroin. And, just as with these drugs, after the initial high, these foods no longer bring enjoyment, but become necessary just to feel normal.

Just like a heroin addict in a rehabilitation center detoxifying his body, a sugar addict will experience symptoms of "withdrawal" when cut off from sugar. And constant environmental cues in the form of advertising can trigger relapses of junk food binge-eating, just like an alcoholic "falling off the wagon".

The Crash

Activating the D2 receptor with dopamine creates a chemical cascade that gives feelings of pleasure. Addictive substances increase dopamine release. But these rushes of dopamine trigger neural self-protection systems, which "downregulate", reducing receptors, so dopamine sensitivity decreases with repeated exposures to massive artificial dopamine surges.

This drop in dopamine response results in feeling terrible (withdrawal), so addicts chase their drug of choice in ever greater quantities, eventually just to feel "normal" again. Unfortunately, some people are born with fewer D2 dopamine receptors, making them more susceptible to addictions, and needing greater amounts of stimulation to activate dopamine in their brains.

The Yale University Rudd Center for Food Policy and Obesity has created a "food addiction" scale; 25 questions that can be used to test yourself for food addictions. You can download it online from here: http://www.yaleruddcenter.org/resources/upload/docs/what/addiction/FoodAddiction-Scale09.pdf

Born That Way

Obesity is the number one public health problem in the United States.

It's estimated that 75 percent of Americans will be overweight or obese by 2019, a massive future policy challenge that threatens to derail the US economy. Dr. David Katz of Yale University recently reported the shocking fact that even children are beginning to suffer strokes, a stunning result of America's obesity epidemic.

Obesity isn't just a lifestyle issue; it's a chronic, relapsing, neurochemical disorder with a genetic cause. Because of this, telling someone who's overweight to simply eat fewer calories and do more exercise is ineffective and doesn't touch upon the core reasons for obesity's occurrence. Diet and exercise are indeed critical to obesity treatment, but because it's a chronic medical disorder, bioregulatory mechanisms undermine an individual's efforts and sustain the condition. Because of this, many obesity sufferers need long-term medical intervention to really overcome the problem.

In other words, obese people don't simply overeat because they lack willpower, and obesity isn't a character deficit; it's a chronic neurochemical disorder. But biased public attitudes, fomented by advertising, compound the problem.

In the guidebook *From Fat to Fit: Turn Yourself into a Weapon of Mass Re-duction*, Carole Carson relates how she shed 62 pounds. In an interview with Dr. Jennifer Lovejoy, president of the Obesity Society, she describes three myths about obesity. These myths, she asserts, are dangerous because they perpetuate stigma suffered by the obese, and prevent research into critically important medication for treating a serious medical disorder: only one FDA-approved drug is available for long-term obesity treatment.

But because obesity is seen as a lack of willpower rather than a chronic illness, the FDA and the pharmaceutical industry lack incentive to create and approve appropriate medications, despite obesity's status as the most pervasive health issue in America.

You Say "Tomato", I Say "Blech!" – How Food Preferences Develop

Whether you love to munch on celery or prefer to gobble cheese doodles by the pound largely depends on what you were fed as a baby, according to researchers at Monell Chemical Senses Center in Philadelphia. Feeding experiences during a baby's first seven months contribute strongly to food preferences, long before solid food has been introduced.

In 2004, Dr. Julie Mennella and a team of researchers looked at flavor pref-erences of infants raised over the course of seven months with two types of infant formula. The first group was raised on milk-based formulas, which have a bland taste, and the second group was given a *protein hydrolysate* formula, 'pre-digested' proteins that are easier for babies to absorb, but taste bitter and sour. Both formulas have similar nutritive content.

Control groups were given three months of hydrolysate formula followed by four months of standard formula. After seven months had elapsed, all the babies were given a choice of formula. Babies who had never been given hydrolysate-protein formulas rejected it strongly, but those who had grown used to it drank it readily, and appeared content, showing how food prefer-ences are formed at the very start of life.

But, according to Dr. Mennella, early feeding patterns aren't the whole story. Genetics, age and culture also play a part in shaping food preferences. Children tend to eat what they prefer based on flavors, and, because many vegetables are bitter, many children opt for sweets or other unhealthy foods.

A follow-up study in 2005 looked at how the *TAS2R38 gene*, which encodes bitter taste receptors, influences eating behaviours. Three groups of mothers and children aged 5 to 10 with varying genetic bitter sensitivities were given a harmless but bitter compound of varying strength. The most genetically bitter-sensitive children and mothers found even the weakest solution to taste bitter, while those whose DNA made them less bitter-sensitive thought the same concentration tasted like water.

Co-author Dr. Danielle Reed says this means children aren't simply being defiant or rebellious in rejecting food, but that they have an inborn difference in taste sensitivities. The sensitivity appears to fade with age, however, with a 21% drop in sensitivity between adults and children in the most genetically bitter-sensitive group. Children with the highest bitter-sensitivity also preferred sugary cereals and sodas over milk and water. In adults, however, Dr. Mennella's team found that the bitter receptor genotype lost its influence. Culture and experience seemed to have overridden the tendency for bitter receptor genes to be linked to a preference for sweets.

The Regulators: Ghrelin, Leptin, Insulin

Your hypothalamus "reads" your body's condition from moment to moment through hormonal and other blood chemistry signals, using these cues to regulate your body functions and maintain biological balance through hormonal and neurotransmitter release. Thus your hypothalamus is central to regulating body mass, via controlling both appetite and calorie expenditure. Several hormones help regulate appetite, particularly *leptin* and ghrelin.

Leptin is the hormone which reports satiety – the psychological state of having had enough to eat and drink – to the hypothalamus. It's produced by white adipose (fat) cells, and causes changes in brain function to control appetite. Leptin is involved in the emotional state of satiety, inhibiting cells which stimulate appetite, and exciting cells which suppress appetite, according to Howard Hughes Medical Institute's Dr. Jeffrey Friedman, who discovered the hormone in 1994. Mice engineered without leptin have uncontrollable appetites and grow extremely obese.

In response to leptin, the hypothalamus releases hormones controlling bodily functions like reproduction, growth hormone, sexual behavior and appetite.

Conversely, hunger is triggered by the hormone ghrelin, produced in the stomach. Discovered in 1999 by Japanese researchers and named after the Hindi word for "growth", ghrelin was first discovered in 1999. It's a hormone produced in the stomach that was previously associated with a wide range of functions including appetite, learning, memory and growth hormone release. Ghrelin increases before meals and subsides after eating. A 2010 Swedish study found rats can be induced to seek out sweets or to lose interest in them, depending on ghrelin levels in their bloodstream.

Ghrelin moderates not just appetite, but acts on the mesolimbic pathways, the brain's reward and pleasure centers, the same areas activated by addictive drugs and sex. Thus, the same mechanisms in alcohol and drug addiction appear to be at work in food addiction. Given ghrelin, rats will work twice as hard to press a level for sugar rewards, as if they had not eaten. But when ghrelin is blocked in hungry rats, they are less motivated to work for sugar rewards, acting as if they were full.

Some people eat even when they're not hungry due to ghrelin's apparent activation of the pleasure response to food instead of hunger, according to Dr. Karolina Skibicka, of the University of Gothenburg in Sweden. Ghrelin receptors (GHSR) are present in both the hypothalamus, where the hormone helps control energy metabolism, and in the VTA, a region involved in motivation. Since the VTA is known to be involved in reward expectations, ghrelin stimulation of the VTA is likely central to overeating, inducing food cravings and other reward-associated behavior just like drug addictions. By activating dopamine release, ghrelin can indirectly control reward-associated behavior, promoting interest in food as a reward. Ghrelin receptors on VTA neurons trigger dopamine secretion in the mesolimbic pathway in response to the sight, smell and taste of food.

A 2006 study at Yale has shown that ghrelin injections to the VTA increase food intake in laboratory animals, while inhibiting ghrelin receptors in the VTA decreases food intake. These findings also suggest ghrelin may affect a wide variety of behavior. Says Dr. Horvath, "Anything associated with rewards is probably affected by ghrelin, be it your family or your girlfriend".

Drugs that target ghrelin pathways appear to suppress feeding and the desire to seek out food, and may even be able to help treat drug addictions.

Yale School of Medicine studies have also linked high estrogen levels to weight loss, indicating that estrogen appears to curb hunger. While leptin is the main weight-controlling hormone, affecting fat storage and long-term body weight, estrogen is now known to act in a similar manner. This is why, as women enter menopause and estrogen levels drop, they put on weight.

Hunger Heightens Your Senses, Sharpens Your Thinking, Protects Your Brain And Enhances Your Fertility

Mammals rely upon smell to locate food and discriminate food quality and safety. In 2011, experiments at the University of Cincinnati show how ghrelin secretion heightens this olfactory sensitivity. In other words, when you're hungry, your sense of smell improves.

Yale scientists have also discovered that ghrelin profoundly influences cognition, a surprising development. The project's leader, Dr. Tamas Horvath, chair of comparative medicine at Yale Medical School, says, "Ghrelin binds to brain regions that regulate food intake, as well as the cortex and hippocampus. This means not overeating at breakfast will likely result in better learning".

Yale researcher Tamas Horvath has found that ghrelin also protects dopamine neurons, impacting degenerative brain diseases; it's been found that ghrelin deprivation accelerates die-off of dopamine-producing neurons in the substantia nigra, producing the impaired motor control of Parkinson's disease in mice.

Obesity, which lowers ghrelin output, and insulin resistance have both been linked to the onset of Parkinson's and Alzheimer's diseases, but adequate exercise, proper diet and a high metabolism boost ghrelin production. Ghrelin directly stimulates VTA and substantia nigra dopamine cells, boosting resistance to neurodegenerative diseases like Parkinson's. Low ghrelin levels have also been linked to infertility, affecting the *HOXA 10* gene, important for healthy development of the uterus in the embryo. Mice deficient in ghrelin produce offspring with decreased fertility and smaller litters.

In adults, HOXA 10 maintains the uterine environment for proper embryonic development. The effects are also apparently hereditary – their offspring also have suppressed HOXA 10 gene expression. "People know that it's not healthy to be obese, but they didn't necessarily know it was affecting their children and their children's fertility," says Yale obstetrics and gynecology professor Hugh Taylor.

Due to abnormal uterine gene expression, healthy embryos don't implant as well, reducing the ability to reproduce. Maternal obesity thus affects the well-being of future generations, with the full effects showing up as late as 20 to 30 years later. This ghrelin-related fertility reduction is preventable, says Dr. Taylor, as only those women who are obese during pregnancy are affected. Women who are obese at a young age – but later recover – produce fertile offspring with normal ghrelin levels.

Junk Food Makes You Weak, Sick, And Stupid

The very brain cells capable of protecting you from weight gain may be injured by eating fatty foods, according to research by Dr. Joshua Thaler at Seattle's Diabetes and Obesity Center of Excellence. Brain injury from overconsumption of the typical western diet is probably the reason weight loss is so difficult for the obese, he maintains.

Studying high-fat dietary effects upon rodents over varying periods, Dr. Thaler's team was able to compile detailed biochemical and imaging data. Within just three days of consuming a fatty diet like that of the typical modern American, Dr. Thaler's rodents had taken in nearly double their usual daily calories. Over time, in addition to gaining weight, the animals developed inflammation in the hypothalamus, which controls metabolism and appetite. Simultaneously, glia (support) and microglia (scavenger) cells multiplied in the hypothalamus and appeared to activate, a collective response to brain inflammation called *gliosis*. The condition subsided within days, but returned after a month.

This, explained Dr. Thaler, is the brain's equivalent to wound healing, typically found in response to neural injuries like stroke and MS (multiple sclerosis, a disease caused by degeneration of neural myelin insulating sheaths). Dr. Thaler believes gliosis to be a protective response which gradually fails after repeated activation.

His team also found damage and eventual loss of vital *POMC (pro-opiomelanocortin)* weight-regulating neurons, which were significantly reduced among the fat-consuming animals within 8 months, while remaining intact among those which ate normal, non-fatty diets. The team is not yet certain whether or not this neuronal injury is permanent, but Dr. Thaler believes it may lie at the heart of weight gain and an inability to lose weight.

Poor diets also appear to lower intelligence in young children: high fat, sugar and processed food diets lower IQ in developing children, according to a British study of 14,000 mothers and children that has been ongoing since 1991.

A child's brain develops at its fastest rate from birth to age three, at which point the brain's capacity has largely become set for life. A diet highest in processed food at the age of three has been directly linked with lower IQ as children reach maturity, while a vitamin- and nutrient-rich diet markedly boosted mental performance over the same period.

For each point of increase in the dietary score – which recorded consumption of processed fat – there was a 1.67-point IQ drop, indicating that good nutrition during this critical period is essential to brain development.

Extended fat consumption also weakens the immune response. Coupled with the fact that obesity increases the risk of infections, it's doubly dangerous. White blood cells can lose the ability to stave off blood-borne bacteria, even contributing to the deadly condition known as *sepsis*.

Sepsis, also known as blood poisoning, is a potentially deadly medical condition in which the entire body enters an inflammatory response by the immune system typically triggered by microbes in blood, urine, lungs, skin, or other tissues.

A joint 2006 study between Ohio State, Duke and Ohio Universities indicates that the obese have a lower tolerance for pain than non-obese people, although musical relaxation exercises lowered pain response in both groups. Researchers used mild electric shocks to the volunteers' *sural nerves*, which extend along the ankle and up into the calf.

By measuring lower leg muscle reflex contractions to escape pain, they could objectively measure pain tolerance, and found consistently that obese volunteers did not tolerate pain as well as non-obese participants.

Obese patients with diabetes also often have problems with long-term memory. 2011 Saint Louis University research may have uncovered the reason. According to Dr. Susan A. Farr, who led the study:

> *Leptin is a hormone secreted by fat cells that tells us to stop eating. In obese people, it doesn't cross into the brain to help regulate appetite. We've now found leptin affects the brain in other ways, compromising learning and memory.*

Farr's team tested leptin's role in learning and memory using laboratory mice, and found that leptin improved their navigation.

Obesity also impairs normal muscle function, according to 2011 Penn State research. Dr. Rudolf J. Schilder says obesity is more than just a simple accumulation of excess fat or constantly carrying excess weight. During the onset of the condition, muscles fail to appropriately adjust their molecular composition in response to increasing body weight and become improperly adapted to the higher bodyweight they're forced to carry.

This means obese animals begin to suffer from reduced muscle function and mobility. As animals gain weight, expression of the *troponin T* gene drops. Troponin T encodes a protein critical for muscle function, but obesity impairs its appropriate expression for a given body weight. Troponin T expression is adjusted within a matter of days to match body weight during normal growth, but in obese animals, troponin T expression does not adjust appropriately. This is believed to be one of the reasons it becomes tremendously difficult to recover from the condition.

Sugar's Neural Destruction

Dr. Zane Andrews, a neuroendocrinologist at Monash University, says key appetite-suppressing neurons are attacked by free radicals after meals and slowly degenerate, causing increased hunger and weight-gain as we age.

The degeneration, he says, is greater after meals high in carbohydrates and sugars; and the more carbs and sugars that are eaten, the more destruction there is to these appetite-controlling neurons, creating a spiralling tendency to overeat.

People between the age of 25 to 50 are at the greatest risk, he says, as these neurons which signal when to stop eating are destroyed: an empty stomach triggers the hormone *ghrelin*, sending hunger signals to the brain. When full, the hormone *leptin* triggers hypothalamus *POMC* neurons. POMC neuron signals control both eating and energy use, in this way maintaining *homeostasis* – the body's energy balance.

But free radicals naturally occurring in the body gradually degrade these POMC neurons, affecting a person's ability to judge satiety – the state of having eaten a sufficient amount. This reduction in appetite-suppression neurons could explain adult-onset obesity.

Fat's Neural Destruction

It's patently obvious that fatty foods make you fat, but underlying the simple truism are complex processes your brain uses to control your energy balance. The upshot is that eating fatty foods shuts down your ability to sense when you're full.

The Max Planck Institute and University of Cologne have brought into focus insulin's role in the process, as it acts upon the hypothalamus. Blood glucose from food consumption triggers insulin release. This insulin binds to receptors, prompting glucose uptake, where it's then available for energy.

Consuming fatty foods prompts increased insulin release, not just in the body, but also in the brain. Here, insulin stimulates special hypothalamus *SF-1 cells*, which impede POMC cell signalling – feelings of satiation and slow down energy use, promoting weight gain. When animals consume fatty foods, insulin-stimulated SF-1 cells secrete the enzyme P13-kinase, which suppresses POMC neurotransmission of satiety signals.

To discover how insulin acts upon the brain, the team compared mice without insulin receptors on their SF-1 neurons with mice whose insulin receptors were normal. When the mice ate normal, healthy food, there was no difference between the two groups, indicating that insulin does not influence the activity of these cells in animals of normal weight.

But when the same mice ate fatty foods, those lacking hypothalamus insulin receptors stayed slim, while those with normal receptors quickly gained weight. This weight increase was due to both their increased appetite and their reduced caloric expenditure. This insulin activity is thought to be an evolutionary adaptation to irregular food supplies and extended bouts of deprivation: if an excess of energy-dense food becomes temporarily available, the body can store energy reserves very efficiently through this mechanism.

How Exercise Can Help

According to researchers at Brazil's University of Campinas, aside from simply burning calories, exercise also restores the sensitivity of these leptin- and insulin-sensing neurons. This results in reduced appetite and food con-sumption, leading to weight loss.

An estimated 40% of people worldwide suffer from obesity and weight problems. In fact, obesity is now considered a worldwide epidemic, and is thus a target of intense study worldwide. Both poor dietary habits and a sedentary lifestyle play a part in the onset of obesity and other diseases related to being overweight.

Dr. José Barreto C. Carvalheira led a 2010 study which demonstrates that when rodents exercise, functionality returns to satiety-responsive neurons in the hypothalamus, and, as a result, animals eat less. He says exercise specifically increases IL-6 and IL-10 proteins in the hypothalami of obese animals, and these proteins increase sensitivity to insulin and leptin, which signal satiety to regulate eating.

Hunger is suppressed during and immediately after vigorous exercise like running and, to a lesser degree, weight lifting. The appetite suppression lasts about two hours, including the time spent exercising.

Dr. David J. Stensel of the UK's Loughborough University led the 2008 study, in which 11 male university students did three eight-hour training sessions. During one session, the volunteers ran for 60 minutes on a treadmill, and then rested for seven hours. During another session, they did 90 minutes of weight lifting, and then rested for six hours and 30 minutes. During another session, the participants did not exercise at all.

60 minutes of vigorous aerobic exercise affects the release of two key ap-petite hormones, ghrelin and peptide YY, while 90 minutes of weight lifting affects only ghrelin levels, showing aerobic exercise is better at suppressing appetite than anaerobic exercise.

A Powerful Dieting Success Secret

If you're dieting, you can make things a lot easier on yourself by making simple changes to your surroundings, changes which can result in effortlessly healthier eating, according to consumer psychologist Dr. Brian Wansink of Cornell University's Food and Brand Lab:

> *Our homes are filled with hidden eating traps. Most of us have too much chaos going on in our lives to consciously focus on every bite we eat, and then ask ourselves if we're full. The secret is to change your environment so it works for you rather than against you.... People don't think that something as simple as the size of a bowl would influence how much an informed person eats.*

Several studies demonstrate they do, however. Dr. Wansink's own study looked at 168 movie attendees eating either fresh or stale popcorn from different-sized containers. His subjects ate 45 percent more fresh popcorn from extra-large buckets than from large ones, and those who eating stale popcorn consumed 34 percent more from extra-large containers than people who were eating fresh popcorn.

The size of children's cereal bowls can play just as large a part. Children of a range of bodyweights will pour twice as much cereal into a 16-ounce bowl than children given an 8-ounce bowl. His studies also show people pour about 37 percent more liquid into wide, short glasses than into tall, skinny ones that contain the same volume.

"They just don't realize they're doing it," says Dr. Wansink; people don't necessarily know when they're full and when to stop before overeating. His team tested this theory with a "bottomless bowl":

60 people were offered a free lunch in the study. Half were given 22-ounce bowls of soup, while the other half received 22-ounce bowls which were secretly pressure-fed from under the table, to slowly refill. The subjects with "bottomless bowls" ended up eating 73 percent more than those with normal bowls, but had no idea they'd eaten more. "The lesson is, don't rely on your stomach to tell you when you're full. It can lie," says Dr. Wansink.

Just being aware of these findings can help you make healthier eating decisions, he adds. A follow-up study showed subjects losing up to two pounds a month after making just a few simple changes to their environments, such as:

- eating from salad plates in place of larger dinner plates.

- placing unhealthy foods out of the immediate line of sight, replacing them with healthier foods at eye-level in cupboards and refrigerators.

- avoiding eating in front of the television, opting instead for the kitchen or dining room.

"These simple strategies are far more likely to succeed than willpower alone. It's easier to change your environment than to change your mind," Wansink advises.

How Not To Diet: Skipping Breakfast Makes You Fat

If you're planning on skipping breakfast to lose weight, you're making a serious mistake. Skipping breakfast slows your metabolism so your body can conserve energy, preserving fat storage. The drop in blood sugar also impairs brain function, energy levels, insulin balance, serotonin levels and mood. Breakfast is the most important meal of all – in fact, to really rev up your metabolism, eat within 30 minutes of waking, starting with a tall glass of ice water, with freshly-squeezed lemon in it.

Additionally, you want to stick to whole grains – not bleached white flour, or bleached white flour that has been dyed brown and had a few grains of wheat sprinkled into it. Bran cereal, oatmeal, rye toast and the like burn more slowly, fill you up faster and act like a scrubbing brush in your digestive system. Protein from low-fat milk, yogurt, and eggs is also important.

Instead of juice, which contains high amounts of fructose (making it not much better than sugary snacks), eat fruit for the fiber it contains. You can also add fruit to cereal, oatmeal or yogurt. Berries in particular are extremely good for you, with blueberries and strawberries ranking at the top in terms of antioxidants and minerals. Adding vegetables like tomatoes or spinach to scrambled eggs is another extremely healthy strategy.

You want to avoid pastry, doughnuts and sugary cereals; they'll give you sugar spikes that later make you "crash" and feel hungry again sooner. Most breakfast bars also have a large amount of corn syrup, dextrose or sugar in them. If sugar or syrup is listed among the top five ingredients, it's junk food. Coffee is a temporary energy booster with polyphenols, but you might want to consider green tea instead – particularly powdered green tea. The Japanese have a drink called "macha" – milk with powdered green tea – that is both delicious and incredibly good for you.

Skipping breakfast also appears to make you crave high-calorie foods over low-calorie alternatives, according to Dr. Tony Goldstone of the Imperial College of London. Changes in ghrelin levels help regulate your caloric intake, and the increase in ghrelin released from the stomach into the bloodstream thus explains why skipping breakfast leads to cravings for high-calorie foods.

With fMRI scans to measure mesolimbic activity, Dr. Goldstone used ghrelin injections to discover that volunteers who had skipped meals crave high-calorie foods like chocolate, cake and pizza over low-calorie foods like salads, vegetables and fish.

When you fast, the mesolimbic reward pathways become more active at the sight of high-calorie foods. After eating breakfast, however, the preference for high-calorie foods disappears. Skipping meals, and breakfast in particular, changes brain reward center responses to specific foods, which have a significant impact on weight maintenance.

How Not To Diet II: Yo Yo Diets

Junk foods cause addiction using the same chemistry as other drugs. When rats binge on sugary snacks for just two days, and are then switched to normal food, their amygdalae secrete five times the normal amount of the protein *CRF* (corticotropin-releasing-factor), the stress hormone that punishes addicts with withdrawal when they try to quit using.

The elevated CRF release is in response to the stress of being denied the junk foods, just like withdrawal from drug addiction. CRF is a neurotransmitter and hormone which activates the adrenal cortex in response to stress. It's central to negative reinforcement, the aversive motivation which drives avoidance behavior – the drive to escape pain or other stressful circumstances. In the case of the sugar-addicted lab rats, whenever they're switched to normal foods, their anxiety levels skyrocket and they lose all interest in normal foods.

"This (CRF) punishment, this negative reinforcement, is causing anxiety and is increasing the probability that bad behavior is performed in the future to relieve anxiety", says Dr. Pietro Cottone, of Boston University's Laboratory of Addictive Disorders.

CRF is central to withdrawal from every major drug of abuse, including alcohol, nicotine, cocaine, opiates and amphetamines. The same neuroadaptations in the amygdala-adrenal gland CRF system seem to help drive compulsive consumption of energy-dense "junk" foods, the underconsumption of healthy alternatives, and the negative emotional states of withdrawal when access to preferred junk foods is denied.

Just as intermittent drug abuse progressively leads to *dependence* – the need for ever greater quantities of an addictive drug to maintain a normal emotional state and to avoid feelings of anxiety when the drug is unavailable, the same mechanism kicks in with yo-yo dieting. CRF stress systems drive the transition from recreational use to dependence, as addicts become increasingly less motivated by the need to experience positive feelings, and increasingly more motivated to avoid negative ones.

This is the same mechanism at work when you eat "comfort foods" like cake and ice cream – eating junk foods to relieve your anxiety. Just like humans engaged in "yo-yo dieting" with repeated bouts of junk-food binging, rats cycled between sugary or normal edible foods compulsively binge on sweets, stop eating regular food, and show withdrawal behaviours associated with drug addiction. And just as with addiction to drugs or alcohol, alterations to the brain's stress system helps drive each of these behavioral changes.

> Our research suggests that this eating pattern leads to a vicious circle. The more you cycle this way, the more likely it is you cycle again. Having a 'free day' in your diet schedule is a risky habit.

Unlike most research in the field, which focuses on the positive motivation derived from eating pleasurable food, Dr. Cottone's team focused instead on whether the same negative reinforcement which drives compulsive drug use might play a similar role in overeating, and whether the stress response was involved in the process.

> For example, I can be motivated to work hard because I get praise from my boss – that's positive reinforcement. Conversely, I can work hard to avoid being fired – that's negative reinforcement. Similarly, I can either eat a lot for the pleasure of eating, or I can eat a lot to relieve the stress of not having certain foods. We wanted to know if negative factors were involved.

Zeroing in on the mechanics of the stress system – previously found to contribute to drug and alcohol binging and withdrawal behavior – his team measured levels of the stress neurohormone CRF, as well as mRNA and peptide synthesis by the central amygdala, involved in fear, anxiety, and stress responses.

The results were stark: the diet-cycled group of rats had five times the control group's CRF levels when forced to eat normal food. Only when they were fed sweet food did their CRF expression return to normal levels. "In observing the activation of the amygdaloidal CRF system during abstinence from sweet foods, we understood the causes of recurrent dieting failures," said Cottone. This increase in stress was due specifically to food withdrawal, rather than to outside factors.

Said Scripps Research's Dr. Eric Zorrilla:

> *People will often say they are eating bad foods or fail a diet because they 'are stressed'. Our findings suggest that intermittently eating sweet food changes the brain's stress system so that you might feel stressed, even though nothing that terrible has happened. In other words, you might be self-medicating stress-like symptoms of abstinence with that piece of pie. Or, the adaptations in your brain stress system might make you more reactive to otherwise minor stressors.*

Just as with alcoholics, the brain makes adaptations in response to intermittent junk food consumption. This helps explain how yo-yo dieting can establish unhealthy patterns and neuroadaptations, and why it is largely so ineffective for weight loss. It also underscores the health risks of such eating patterns – chronic stress is linked with both emotional disorders and conditions like heart disease. Says Dr. Cottone, "The findings suggest that frequent dieting with frequent relapse is worse than dieting by itself".

Using a CRF antagonist (blocker), Dr. Cottone's team was able to restore normal dietary habits in his lab rats – they once again began to eat normal food, and their taste for sweet foods diminished considerably. The pharmaceutical industry is currently involved in research to use CRF agonists for addiction treatment.

Dieting - What REALLY Works...

In November 2011, *U.S. News and World Reports* asked a panel of 22 professional nutritionists to rank the top 20 modern diets according to effectiveness, flexibility and difficulty, long and short-term potential weight loss, safety and nutritional completeness.

All the healthiest diets emphasized adequate calories supplied primarily by vegetables, fruits, and whole grains, modest amounts of lean protein, nonfat dairy, healthy fats, and occasional luxuries. Minimal processing and an emphasis on plant-based foods were central to all the highest-ranking diets.

The *Paleo*, *Raw Food*, and *Atkins* diets were found to be too restrictive: The Paleo diet bans grains and dairy and is too meat-heavy, delivering inadequate calcium and vitamin D. The Atkins diet severely cuts carbs, and allows excessive fats, and the Raw Food Diet may expose practitioners to shortages of calcium and vitamins B-12 and D.

According to Madelyn Fernstrom, founding director of the University of Pittsburgh Medical Center's Weight Management Center, you need to listen carefully to how your body reacts. Fatigue, sleeplessness, dizziness and aches are all red flags warning you to reassess what you're doing.

The most and least highly recommended of modern diets:

1. DASH Diet (3.9 out of 5.0 stars) – The American National Heart, Lung, and Blood Institute (NHLBI), helped develop DASH, *Dietary Approaches to Stop Hypertension*, specifically to manage high blood pressure, but as an overall diet, it ranked highest among those chosen by the panel of experts, for nutritional completeness, safety, ability to prevent or control diabetes, and heart health support. The panel rated it as balanced, "heart healthy" and "nutritionally sound", but said it required a lot of effort and was a little expensive.

The program consists of determining caloric need for your age and activity level, then recommending specific foods. You design your own eating plan, and can lose weight if you follow the rules you set and design a plan with a "calorie deficit." DASH lowers blood pressure, increases HDL cholesterol and decreases LDL cholesterol and triglycerides, reflecting the medical community's accepted definition of "heart-healthy" eating.

DASH doesn't restrict entire food groups, which increases its long-term appeal. It emphasizes fiber and lean protein, to increase feelings of satiety, even when lowering caloric intake. Eventually taste preferences adjust to the lower salt intake levels if you use a variety of other spices. The free online PDF guides are here (basic): http://www.nhlbi.nih.gov/health/public/heart/hbp/dash/dash_brief.pdf

and here (advanced): http://www.nhlbi.nih.gov/health/public/heart/hbp/dash/new_dash.pdf

2. Mediterranean Diet (3.8 out of 5.0 stars) – This strategy is based on findings that citizens of Mediterranean countries live longer, healthier lives than most Americans. In addition to an active lifestyle, this diet is low in red meat, sugar, and saturated fat and high in produce, nuts, and other healthy foods. Oldways, a Boston-based nonprofit nutrition group, co-developed this diet with the Harvard School of Public Health. The food pyramid emphasizes limiting animal proteins, only allowing sweets and red meat on special occasions.

This diet has been linked with decreased heart disease risk, and shown to reduce blood pressure and LDL cholesterol. You prepare all the dishes yourself, and while certain food groups are restricted, none are completely forbidden. You can download the free guidelines and recipes here: http://oldwayspt.org/mediterranean-diet-pyramid

3. TLC Diet (3.8 out of 5.0 stars) – The National Institutes of Health created the *Therapeutic Lifestyle Changes*, or TLC diet, with a particular emphasis on cardiovascular health. It's a "very healthful, complete, safe diet", but requires a "do-it-yourself" approach, rather than having everything prepared for you, as with commercial diets. The TLC diet emphasizes sharply cutting saturated fat and cholesterol intake and increasing fiber. In this way, say its advocates, heart health and high cholesterol can be managed, often without medication.

A study by the *Journal of Atherosclerosis and Thrombosis* found TLC significantly lowered fasting insulin levels among high-cholesterol participants – elevated insulin levels are a predictor of type 2 diabetes. Experts call this style of eating "the gold standard of diabetes prevention", emphasizing the right foods and discouraging the wrong ones. You can get the free guideline manual here: http://www.nhlbi.nih.gov/health/public/heart/chol/chol_tlc.pdf

4. Weight Watchers Diet (3.8 out of 5.0 stars) – The panel of nutrition experts found Weight Watchers to be "smart and effective", claiming it was the best among commercial diets, particularly regarding short- and long-term weight loss, safety, and ease of adherence. There is an emphasis upon group support, and it allows occasional indulgence.

The monthly, fee-based PointsPlus program claims 2 pounds average weekly weight loss. It assigns points to over 40,000 foods, based upon protein, carbohydrate, fat, fiber, calories, and how much work is required to burn it off. You're allowed to eat whatever you wish, as long as it's within your daily allotted points, a number based upon gender, weight, height, and age. The website database quickly helps you choose from among foods, based upon sugar, sodium, protein, fiber, and fat. There are no food restrictions, but you control your portions and adjust recipes to make meals as healthy as possible.

5. Mayo Clinic Diet (3.7 out of 5.0 stars) – This diet is the Mayo Clinic's recommendations on healthy lifelong eating, which ranked highly due to its safety and nutrition and effectiveness against diabetes. It was said to be moderately effective for weight loss.

... and What Doesn't

Raw Food Diet (2.4 out of 5.0 stars) – The raw food diet delivered "impressive" weight loss, but raised concerns about its nutrition, safety, and ease of adherence, because it requires significant commitment, effort, knowledge, and sacrifice, according to the panel.

Atkins Diet (2.3 out of 5.0 stars) – The team said the Atkins diet jumped ahead in short-term weight loss, but was poor at delivering long-term weight loss, nutrition, safety, and heart health.

Dukan Diet (2.0 out of 5.0 stars) US New and World Report's experts listed the Dukan diet among the bottom, one expert even describing it as "idiotic". The team assessed it as "too restrictive, with lots of rules, and there's no evidence it works."

Paleo Diet (2.0 out of 5.0 stars) – The panel rated the Paleo diet lowest in all aspects, including weight loss, heart health, and ease.

Fasting

As opposed to "yo-yo dieting", which involves binging on addictive unhealthy foods followed by anxiety-triggering deprivation, fasting has been used throughout history, for religion, dieting and health. Researchers at America's Intermountain Medical Center Heart Institute now say it's for a good reason: periodic fasting on a routine basis is good for your health, particularly your heart.

The researchers conducted a pair of studies on more than 200 volunteers from among their patients and other healthy participants who had been recruited through the Center. A later follow-up study in 2011 tracked 30 patients as they only drank water for 24 hours, and ate normally for 24 hours afterward.

Fasting lowers the risk of diabetes and coronary heart disease (the number one preventable American killer) and makes significant changes to blood cholesterol levels. It has also been shown to lower weight and reduce other cardiac risk factors like levels of triglycerides and blood sugar.

The team recorded physiological changes as volunteers fasted, and were surprised to find an increase in both "bad" cholesterol (LDL-C, or low-density lipoproteins, which increased by 14 percent) and "good" cholesterol (HDL-C, or high-density lipoprotein cholesterol, which increased 6 percent) raising their total cholesterol.

It appears the body releases cholesterol in response to hunger, which is a kind of stress. In this way, the body is using stored fat for fuel in place of glucose. And, as the number of fat cells in the body decreases, the likelihood of contracting diabetes (insulin resistance) decreases.

In addition, fasting for 24 hours has been shown to trigger an increase in Human Growth Hormone (HGH) by an astounding 1,300 percent in women, and almost 2,000 percent in men on average. Human growth hormone is a protein that promotes lean muscle tissue and metabolic balance, and the process is massively accelerated by fasting.

Dr. Benjamin D. Horne, who led the study, says it's not yet entirely clear if fasting itself specifically reduces health risks, or if fasting is just an indicator of someone with a healthy lifestyle, but he believes that fasting may one day be prescribed as part of a program for diabetes prevention and heart health.

Radical New Findings About Eating Disorders

At the extreme end of the dieting spectrum are eating disorders like *anorexia nervosa* and *bulimia*. The behavior is puzzling; while most people have extreme difficulty in dieting and losing weight, anorexia nervosa sufferers can literally starve themselves to death, and very frequently do.

According to Dr. Daniel Goleman, the main cause of these eating disorders are feelings of a lack of control in life, an inability to soothe anxiety, and an inability to properly identify and express emotions.

A 2011 study at the University of California, San Diego may have uncovered the underlying neural pathology behind this dangerous coping strategy: while most people derive pleasure from eating, it makes anorexics anxious, while refusing food calms them. In other words, a normally *appetitive association* is an *aversive* one.

Dr. Walter Kaye used PET scans to study dopamine function in the brain of women with and without eating disorders. Normally, pleasurable sensations arise from the mesolimbic dopamine pathways in response to eating, but the same striatal dopamine release appears to trigger anxiety in women with anorexia nervosa, causing greater activation of the caudate and putamen. This region primarily processes worry over consequences, and is the same region central to obsessive compulsive disorders.

As a result of this activation, says Dr. Kaye, "Food generates intensely uncomfortable feelings of anxiety." His study says anorexic tendencies and temperament traits like anxiety, harm avoidance, perfectionism and obsessiveness appear to be heritable, making some more susceptible to these illnesses. Evidence points to altered D2 receptor genes as the probable source of this susceptibility.

The Heartbreak Of Bulimia

My girlfriend in university had bulimia to such a degree she had been repeatedly hospitalized. Her plight was incredibly frustrating and heartbreaking. No amount of pleading, reasoning or threatening had any effect; her pathology ruled her, and everything else – love, friendship, family, academics – was incidental.

Bulimics force themselves to vomit, an extremely dangerous practice. The greatest risk of the behavior is of tearing the esophagus, the tube down which food passes on its way to the stomach. This is one of the few organs in the body with limited protective lining, making it incredibly difficult to stitch or staple in emergency surgery. If vomiting causes it to tear or rip free from the stomach, a huge gout of blood fills the mouth, and profuse bleeding follows. Freed, partially-digested food particles can then be loosed into the bloodstream, with a major risk of infection and death.

Additionally, in advanced starvation, the human body engages in *autophagy*, the process of eating itself to generate energy for survival. This occurs not just in body tissues, but in the brain – the brain begins to eat itself to survive, and those (hypothalamic) neurons can never be regenerated. The gruesome process occurs throughout the body, permanently damaging everything from the heart, liver and kidneys to the immune system.

If you or someone you know has an eating disorder, please seek the help of a professional immediately. This slow (or occasionally, accidently fast) suicide is an extremely cruel punishment on those who care. Inflicting it on those who are important to you may leave them emotionally crippled for the rest of their lives.

By now, I hope you're convinced of how important sensible eating is to your health. If not, I want to leave you with just one last sobering finding:

In 2009, both the American Institute for Cancer Research and World Cancer Research Fund said up to 45 percent of cancers around the world could be completely avoided by the combined habits of maintaining a healthy weight, regular exercise and a healthy diet. According to Dr. Michael Marmot, who led the study, cancer is mostly preventable.

A study by the same group two years earlier had shown that fast weight gain and an unhealthy diet were both major causes of cancer. They echo the advice of the World Health Organization in recommending a diet based primarily on fruit, fresh or frozen vegetables and whole grains, with light consumption of red meat, dairy and fats.

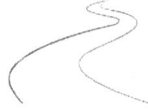

Stomach Ghrelin-Secreting Cells As Food-Entrainable Circadian Clocks, LeSauter et al, 2009, Proceedings of the National Academy of Sciences; 106 (32): 13582 DOI: 10.1073/pnas.0906426106

Why Diets Don't Work: Starved Brain Cells Eat Themselves, Study Finds, Cell Press, 2011

How Eating Breakfast Can Keep You Thin: Healthy Breakfast Ideas, Kristin Kirkpatrick, the Huffington Post, 2011; http://www.huffingtonpost.com/kristin-kirkpatrick-ms-rd-ld/healthy-breakfast-ideas_b_830387.html

Short-Term Weight Loss and Hepatic Triglyceride Reduction: Evidence of a Metabolic Advantage With Dietary Carbohydrate Restriction, Jeffrey D Browning, Jonathan A Baker, Thomas Rogers, Jeannie Davis, Santhosh Satapati, and Shawn C Burgess, 2011, American Journal of Clinical Nutrition, doi: 10.3945/?ajcn.110.007674; http://www.ajcn.org/content/early/2011/03/02/ajcn.110.007674

CRF System Recruitment Mediates Dark Side of Compulsive Eating, 2009, Zorrilla et al, PNAS

Autophagy in Hypothalamic AgRP Neurons Regulates Food Intake and Energy Balance, Susmita Kaushik, Jose Antonio Rodriguez-Navarro, Esperanza Arias, Roberta Kiffin, Srabani Sahu, Gary J. Schwartz, Ana Maria Cuervo, Rajat Singh, 2011, Cell Metabolism, Volume 14, Issue 2, 173-183, 3 August 2011 DOI: 10.1016/j.cmet.2011.06.008

Does Eating Give You Pleasure, Or Make You Anxious? Debra Kain, News Release, May 19, 2011, UC San Diego; http://health.ucsd.edu/news/2011/05-19-anorexia-nervosa-dopamine.htm

Amphetamine Induced Dopamine Release Increases Anxiety In Individuals Recovered From Anorexia Nervosa, Ursula F. Bailer, Rajesh Narendran, W. Gordon Frankle, et al, 2001, International Journal of Eating Disorders; http://eatingdisorders.ucsd.edu/documents/Bailer-AMPHDAanxietyIJED2011epub.pdf

Obesity: Character Flaw or Neurochemical Disease? Carole Carson, March 10, 2011 The Huffington Post; http://www.huffingtonpost.com/carole-carson/is-obesity-a-character-fl_b_831143.html

The Skinny on Fitness Trends in 2011, Carole Carson, January 6, 2011 The Huffington Post; http://www.huffingtonpost.com/carole-carson/the-skinny-on-fitness-tre_b_804383.html

Protein Tyrosine Phosphatase Epsilon Affects Body Weight by Downregulating Leptin Signalling

in a Phosphorylation-Dependent Manner, Liat Rousso-Noori, Hilla Knobler, Einat Levy-Apter, et al, 2011, Cell Metabolism; 13 (5): 562-572 DOI: 10.1016/j.cmet.2011.02.017

Protein Active In Small Part Of Brain Contributes To Obesity, Researchers Discover, Weizmann Institute of Science, 2011, May 9; http://www.sciencedaily.com /releases/2011/05/110504091840.htm

Flavor Programming During Infancy, Julie A. Mennella, Cara E. Griffin, and Gary K. Beauchamp, 2004, Pediatrics, 2004 http://www.monell.org/images/uploads/mennella_pr_web.pdf

Genetic and Environmental Determinants of Bitter Perception and Sweet Preferences, Julie A. Mennella, M. Yanina Pepino, and Danielle R. Reed. Pediatrics, 2005, 115 (2), e216-e222.; http://www.monell.org/images/uploads/pediatric_gene_website.pdf

High-Fat Feeding Promotes Obesity Via Insulin Receptor/PI3K-Dependent Inhibition Of SF-1 VMH Neurons, Tim Klöckener, et al, 2011, Max-Planck-Gesellschaft, Nature Neuroscience, doi:10.1038/nn.2847; http://www.nature.com/neuro/journal/vaop/ncurrent/full/nn.2847.html

Brain Enzyme May Play Key Role In Controlling Appetite And Weight Gain, Albert Einstein College of Medicine (2008, December 16). Brain Enzyme May Play Key Role In Controlling Appetite And Weight Gain. ScienceDaily. Retrieved June 7, 2011, from http://www.sciencedaily.com /releases/2008/12/081212141845.htm

Ghrelin Modulates the Activity and Synaptic Input Organization of Midbrain Dopamine Neurons, Alfonso Abizaid, Zhong-Wu Liu, Zane B. Andrews, et al, 2006, Journal of Clinical Investigation, 116(12):3229–3239. Doi: 10.1172/JCI29867;

Salt Addiction? Why French Fries Are So Good, Dean Praetorius, 04/ 9/11 The Huffington Post

Eating Salty Snacks Damages Arteries Within 30 Minutes, Deborah Huso, Jan 31st 2011 AOL News; http://www.aolhealth.com/2011/01/31/eating-salty-snacks-damages-arteries-within-30-minutes/

Fatty Food Can Weaken the Immune System, thesis, Louise Strandberg, 2009, University of Gothenburg; http://www.sahlgrenska.gu.se/english/news_and_events/news/News_Detail//fatty-food-can-weaken-the-immune-system.cid906630

Body Weight-Dependent Troponin T Alternative Splicing Is Evolutionarily Conserved, R. J. Schilder, S. R. Kimball, J. H. Marden, L. S. Jefferson, Journal of Experimental Biology, 2011; 214 (9): 1523 DOI: 10.1242/jeb.051763

Obese People Are More Sensitive to Pain, Suggests Study, Charles Emery, 2006, Ohio State University: http://researchnews.osu.edu/archive/obespain.htm

Eating a High-Fat Diet May Rapidly Injure Brain Cells That Control Body Weight, The Endocrine Society, 2011, June 9

Ghrelin Increases the Rewarding Value of High-Fat Diet in an Orexin-Dependent Manner, Mario Perello, Ichiro Sakata, Shari Birnbaum, et al, 2009, Biological Psychiatry; DOI: 10.1016/j.biopsych.2009.10.030

Pleasurable Behaviours Reduce Stress Via Brain Reward Pathways, Y. M. Ulrich-Lai, A. M.

Christiansen, M. M. Ostrander, et al, 2010, Proceedings of the National Academy of Sciences; DOI: 10.1073/pnas.1007740107

Killer Carbs: Scientist Finds Key To Overeating As We Age, Monash University, 2008; http://www.sciencedaily.com /releases/2008/08/080821110113.htm

Ghrelin Linked to Addictive Behavior, Ashish Bakshi, 2006, Yale Daily News; *Study Links Obesity, Infertility,* Hugh S. Taylor, Amy Tetrault, Sarah Lieber, Marya Shanabrough and Tamas Horvath, 2011, Yale Daily News; http://www.yaledailynews.com/news/2011/mar/30/study-links-obesity-infertility/

Fatty Foods – Not Empty Stomach – Fire Up Hunger Hormone, University of Cincinnati Academic Health Center, 2009; http://www.sciencedaily.com /releases/2009/06/090605151351.htm

Fasting Biases Brain Reward Systems Toward High-Calorie Foods, Arlyn G. Riskind and Aaron Lohr, 2009, press release, Endocrine Society; http://www.endo-society.org/media/ENDO-09/Research/Fasting-biases-brain-reward-systems-toward-high-calorie-foods.cfm

Ghrelin Enhances Olfactory Sensitivity and Exploratory Sniffing in Rodents and Humans, J. Tong, E. Mannea, P. Aime, P. T. Pfluger, et al, 2011, Journal of Neuroscience, 2011; 31 (15): 5841 DOI: 10.1523/JNEUROSCI.5680-10.2011

Obesity Study Finds New Link, Della Fok, Yale Daily News, 2007; http://www.yaledailynews.com/news/2007/jan/17/obesity-study-finds-new-link/?print

Hormone May Fight Parkinson's, Christian Eubank, 2009, Yale Daily News, http://www.yaledailynews.com/news/2009/dec/02/hormone-may-fight-parkinsons/?print

The Influence Of Resistance And Aerobic Exercise On Hunger, Circulating Levels Of Acylated Ghrelin And Peptide YY, Broom et al., 2008, AJP; DOI: 10.1152/ajpregu.90706.2008; http://ajpregu.physiology.org/content/296/1/R29

CRF System Recruitment Mediates Dark Side Of Compulsive Eating, Pietro Cottone, Valentina Sabino, Marisa Robertoet al, 2009 November 24, Proceedings of the National Academy of Sciences; doi: 10.1073/pnas.0908789106; http://www.ncbi.nlm.nih.gov/pmc/articles/PMC2785284/?tool=pubmed

Nourishing Your Mind, Body and Soul, Maureen Nagle M.S., L.N., 2010; http://old.stjoan.com/feature7/food/food.htm

5 Reasons High Fructose Corn Syrup Will Kill You, Dr. Mark Hyman, May 13, 2011,UltraWellness Library; http://drhyman.com/5-reasons-high-fructose-corn-syrup-will-kill-you-5050/

USDA Agriculture Factbook 2001-2002, http://www.usda.gov/factbook/

Processed Food Diet in Early Childhood May Lower IQ, 2011, Avon Longitudinal Study of Parents and Children; http://www.bristol.ac.uk/alspac/documents/pr-junk-food-and-iq-jan-11.pdf

Intake of Sucrose-sweetened Water Induces Insulin Resistance and Exacerbates Memory Deficits and Amyloidosis in a Transgenic Mouse Model of Alzheimer Disease, Dongfeng Cao,

Hailin Lu, Terry L. Lewis, and Ling Li, 2007, Journal of Biological Chemistry; http://www.jbc.org/content/282/50/36275.abstract

Does Sugar Feed Cancer? – New Research Sheds Light on Old Saying, press release, 2009, Huntsman Cancer Institute (HCI) at the University of Utah; http://www.huntsmancancer.org/publicweb/content/pressreleases/2009_8_17.html

Ten Studies Showing the Link Between Sugar and Increased Cancer Risk, Reuben Chow, 2008, Natural News; http://www.naturalnews.com/024827_cancer_sugar_women.html

Sugar and Cardiovascular Disease, Barbara V. Howard, Judith Wylie-Rosett, 2002, American Heart Association; http://circ.ahajournals.org/cgi/content/full/106/4/523

Higher Amounts of Added Sugars Increase Heart Disease Risk Factors, Ashante Dobbs, 2010, Emory University; http://shared.web.emory.edu/emory/news/releases/2010/04/higher-amounts-of-added-sugars-increase-heart-disease-risk-factors.html

Dopamine-Based Reward Circuitry Responsivity, Genetics, And Overeating. Stice, E., Yokum, S., Zald, D., and A. Dagher. 2011, Current Topics in Behavioral Neuroscience. 6: 81–93.

Preliminary Validation of Yale Food Addiction, Gearhardt, A.N., Corbin, W.R., and K.D. 2009, Appetite 52(2): 430–436.

Excessive Sugar Intake Alters Binding to Dopamine and Mu-Opioid Receptors in the Brain. Neuroreport. 12(16): 3549–3552, Colantuoni, C., Schwenker, J., McCarthy, P., et al. 2001.

"Nonhedonic" Food Motivation in Humans Involves Dopamine in the Dorsal Striatum and Methylphenidate Amplifies This Effect, Volkow, N.D., Wang, G.J., Fowler, J.S., et al. 2002, Synapse. 44(3): 175–180.

Mindless Eating: Losing Weight Without Thinking, Dr. Brian Wansink, August 5, 2011, The American Psychological Association; http://www.apa.org/news/press/releases/2011/08/losing-weight.aspx

IL-6 and IL-10 Anti-Inflammatory Activity Links Exercise to Hypothalamic Insulin and Leptin Sensitivity, Ropelle ER, Flores MB, Cintra DE, et al. 2010, Public LIbrary of Science Biology, 8(8): e1000465 DOI: 10.1371/journal.pbio.1000465

U.S. News Ranking Of Best Diets For Healthy Eating, Kurtis Hiatt, November 3, 2011, U.S. News; http://health.usnews.com/best-diet/best-overall-diets

Clean Living Could Cut Third of Many Cancers, Michael Kahn, 2009, Reuters; http://www.reuters.com/article/2009/02/26/us-cancer-risks-idUSTRE51P2P920090226

Energize

Metabolic Control

To recap: when you digest food, it's chemically broken down and glucose (blood sugar) is secreted by your small intestine into your bloodstream, where it constitutes your primary source of fuel. Responding to the presence of blood glucose, your pancreas manufactures the hormone insulin. Insulin binds to cell receptors, opening channels in the membranes that allow glucose to enter and be used to extract energy to power your body's functions.

Insulin's second function is to trigger glucose absorption from the bloodstream into adipose and liver cells, to be converted into glycogen (long repeating chains of glucose) or fat (much larger molecules that store glucose and other molecules) for future energy needs. In this way, insulin regulates carbohydrate and fat metabolism – conversion and consumption for energy – allowing your muscles to use blood glucose for immediate energy, or for storage as glycogen or fat. This also removes excess blood sugar which would otherwise be toxic

Countering the effects of insulin is the hormone glucagon, which is released by your pancreas when glucose levels drop too far. Glucagon prompts your liver to convert stored glycogen into glucose, releasing it into your bloodstream to raise your blood glucose. Glucagon also triggers the use of fat as an energy source, converting triglycerides into free fatty acids for diffusion through your bloodstream for your liver and muscles to use. Glucagon and insulin thus form a feedback system maintaining stable blood glucose levels.

One of the most common endocrine system diseases is *diabetes*, in which blood sugar levels cannot be regulated by insulin. There are three major types, with *Type 2 Diabetes* (90% of cases) developing over time, often as a result of a lack of exercise or obesity. *Type 1 Diabetes*, on the other hand, is not fully understood, but is thought to arise from a combination of genetics, viral infection and immune system problems.

Diabetics either cannot manufacture enough insulin or their muscles, fat, and liver cells don't respond normally to insulin. If your pancreas creates too little insulin, or your body is resistant to insulin, high levels of glucose will circulate in your blood, with potentially fatal results. Over 20 million Americans have diabetes, with twice as many in the early stages of developing the disease.

Maximizing Metabolism

Endocrine glands, such as your pituitary, thyroid, and adrenal glands produce, store and secrete the chemical messengers called hormones into your blood to regulate your body's homeostasis. Exercise stimulates significant beneficial hormonal release.

Hormones can be either anabolic or catabolic, depending on which metabolic process they stimulate. *Anabolic steroids* stimulate protein synthesis and tissue growth, while catabolic hormones stimulate molecule breakdown to release energy. This anabolic-catabolic balance is to some degree regulated by your circadian rhythms, with glucose metabolism fluctuating throughout the day to match your activity levels.

Resistance training (weightlifting) is ultimately designed to promote tissue growth, increasing the anabolic hormones which promote it. Such anabolic hormones include testosterone, insulin, *somatotropin* (growth hormone) and *IGF* (Insulin-Like Growth Factors).

Catabolic hormones reduce the effectiveness of resistance training. These catabolic hormones include the stress hormone *cortisol*, as well as *glucagon* and *progesterone*, which can contribute to muscle protein breakdown. Your body can be reshaped – *tissue remodelling* – by these hormonal secretions, ideally of the anabolic variety. This is a dual process, with catabolism initiating energy *release* during exercise, and anabolism leading to *growth and repair* during recovery. In other words, both catabolic and anabolic hormones are central to the process of tissue remodelling.

Anabolic hormone production increases after 15–30 minutes of high-volume, moderate-to-high-intensity resistance training. Exercise programs that stress large muscle groups with short rest intervals produce the greatest elevations in testosterone, growth hormones, cortisol and other hormones, compared with low-volume, high-intensity programs that include long rest intervals.

Motor Unit Recruitment

Motor unit recruitment is a measure of how many motor neurons-muscle fiber groups are activated by an exercise. The greater the recruitment, the stronger the muscle contraction will be. *Progressive overload* (gradually increasing weight), increases motor unit recruitment, as increasing power is needed to perform the exercises.

A single motor unit consists of one motor neuron and all the muscle fibers to which it connects. Muscle fibers from one motor unit can be spread throughout a given muscle group. When the motor neuron is activated, all the muscle fibers it innervates are stimulated and will contract.

Activating a single motor neuron results in a weak, distributed muscle contraction, whereas stimulating a greater number of motor neurons results in more muscle fibers activating, and a stronger muscle contraction. This increased recruitment results in increased beneficial hormonal release.

Here are the main hormones involved in resistance training and how you can increase anabolic effects while limiting catabolic effects:

Testosterone (Anabolic) – This is the primary hormone needed for muscular development. While concentrations of testosterone in women are 15-20 times lower than in men, the same general principles apply.

Your circadian rhythms dictate that your testosterone levels are highest in the morning, gradually dropping as the day progresses. Because of this, anabolic activation from morning exercise is easiest to trigger, but training in the afternoon – when your energy levels peak – will raise total testosterone levels at other periods of the day, because resistance training increases testosterone production.

To maximize testosterone production, concentrate on *compound exercises* like the bench press, squats, deadlift, and chin-ups. Maximal testosterone synthesis is triggered by a) high intensity, heavy resistance exercises at 85% to 95% of your *one-rep max* (the maximum weight you can move in a single repetition); or b) high-repetition, multiple exercises with rest periods of one minute or less.

Resistance training results in a much greater testosterone increase than endurance exercises (such as long-distance running or swimming), and bodybuilding with moderate loads at high volume (many reps) with shorter rest periods also creates a greater testosterone increase than high-load, low-volume training with long (3-minute) rest periods. Many trainers also advocate switching exercise programs between heavy/low-rep and light/high-rep training sessions to offset body adaptation suggesting it's important to "shock" your body to achieve maximum fat catabolism and protein anabolism.

Somatotropin (Anabolic) – Somatotropin (growth hormone), secreted by your pituitary gland, is vital to normal childhood growth as well as to adapting your muscles to resistance training. Its production is triggered by resistance training, resulting in a number of desirable effects, including *hypertrophy* (muscle growth), an increase in fat breakdown and the use of fat for energy, an increase in protein production and enhanced immune function.

Training programs that are moderate- to high-intensity, high-volume, which use compound exercises and relatively short rest intervals tend to produce the largest growth hormone releases.

The greatest GH elevations were found to result from two different programs:

a) 3 sets of 8 exercises, 10 repetitions, with a 1-minute rest between each exercise; or b) 3 sets of 8 exercises, 1 repetition at 90% maximum weight, with a 3-minute rest between each exercise, FOLLOWED BY a final set of high repetitions at 50% of one repetition max at the very end.

Insulin (Anabolic) – Insulin can significantly affect muscle protein production. It's essentially an energy-storage hormone, promoting fat and glycogen storage. Because insulin is affected by blood glucose levels, ingesting a combination of amino acids and carbohydrates before, during, and immediately after resistance training raises insulin levels and maximizes its anabolic effects. Supplementing before and during exercise particularly helps to maximize protein synthesis, because it allows efficient amino acid delivery to the tissues during the large exercise-induced increase in muscle blood flow. Without this supplementation, insulin levels will decrease during exercise.

Additionally, your body's insulin sensitivity can be heightened to take advantage of its growth-promoting potential. Both aerobic and anaerobic exercise greatly increase insulin sensitivity, as do Omega-3 fatty acids, alpha-lipoic acid, and fiber-rich, moderate carbohydrate diets. Conversely, low-carb, high-fat diets can decrease insulin sensitivity.

Post-workout insulin spikes can be good, but at night before bedtime, they are detrimental to your aims, as insulin sensitivity declines at night.

Insulin-Like Growth Factors, IGFs (Anabolic) – Out of these, *IGF-1* appears to be the most important, playing a central role in protein synthesis. The immediate physical responses of IGF-1 to exercise are still unclear; most studies show no change in IGF-1 during or just after resistance exercise, though a few studies show acute elevations during and following resistance exercise. It's been suggested that IGF-1 secretion takes anywhere from 3–9 hours, as it's synthesized and secreted by the liver.

Weightlifters have higher resting IGF-1 concentrations than non-weightlifters, and it seems to increase genetic expression of IGF *isoforms* (proteins varying slightly in structure) in the muscles, substantially increasing protein synthesis. This increased gene expression seems to result from stretching and tension of the muscles. High-weight/low-rep resistance training produces significant IGF-1 increases, which fosters cellular repair, particularly in the brain, heart and muscles, plays a role in cellular division, and inhibits *apoptosis* (cellular suicide).

Epinephrine (Anabolic) – Epinephrine is one of the first hormones to be released by the endocrine system in response to exercise, secreted by the adrenal glands to stimulate the motor system and decrease the genetic expression of enzymes which break down muscle protein. Maximal effort increases epinephrine release during exercise.

Cortisol (Catabolic) – A significant amount of cortisol is released by the adrenal glands in response to the stress of exercise. It stimulates *lipolysis* (the breakdown of fatty deposits), increases protein degradation and decreases protein synthesis. It's released in greater levels in response to resistance training than endurance training. Generally, levels increase with workload – the more and harder you train, the greater the cortisol release will be. And while *chronic* (long-term) high levels of cortisol are bad for your health, exercise-induced *acute* (short-term, high) levels may just be a normal response to the stress of exercise, without negative consequences.

Overtraining – too much exercise with insufficient rest – can result in chronically high cortisol levels and, as a result, chronic catabolic responses; greater amounts of protein and sufficient rest between training can reduce these chronically high cortisol levels, however.

Prepare And Replenish

Recent studies show consuming protein both before and after strength training promotes greater muscle hypertrophy (growth) and adaptation (strength gains). Protein, or a combination of protein and carbohydrates immediately before and after exercise enhances both growth and strength gains. For convenience, beverage forms are recommended and whey protein (a derivative of milk) is the most rapidly absorbed, which is why it's favored by professional athletes.

You can tailor this replenishment to suit the type of sport you engage in; if you want gains in strength or power, place a greater emphasis upon protein intake rather than carbohydrates, to enhance muscle growth; if you want gains in endurance, place a greater emphasis upon carbohydrate intake with your protein, to promote replenishment of muscle glycogen stores.

Over a 10-week course, researchers compared the effects on hypertrophy, strength, and body composition of supplementation directly before and after resistance training vs. supplementation in the morning and late evening. Two groups of randomly-selected, strength-matched male subjects all consumed the same supplement, a combination of protein, creatine, and glucose, at one gram per kilogram of bodyweight. Their supervised training course was identical.

Assessments conducted the week before and after the 10-week course showed significantly greater gains in lean body mass and one-rep-max strength among those who supplemented directly before and after training. This study seems to confirm that timing of nutritional intake has a major impact upon your body's response to exercise. But it also seems to have other health benefits:

In a related study, six platoons of healthy male US Marines were randomly assigned to three different supplement programs during their 54 days of basic training. Their immediate post-workout supplements were either a placebo (0g carbohydrate, 0g protein, 0g fat), control (8g carbohydrate, 0g protein, 3g fat), or protein supplement (8g carbohydrate, 10g protein, 3g fat). The protein-supplementing volunteers had 33% fewer total medical visits, 28% fewer visits due to bacterial/viral infections, 37% fewer visits due to muscle/joint problems, and 83% fewer visits due to heat exhaustion. Post-exercise muscle pain was also reduced by protein supplementation.

Homework: Watch *Dragon: The Bruce Lee Story.*

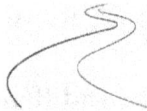

How Does Insulin Trigger the Uptake of Glucose by Cells? Dr. Adam Cloe, 2010, Livestrong.com; http://www.livestrong.com/article/84740-insulin-trigger-uptake-glucose-cells/#ixzz1Svn4t8kZ

Optimizing Your Hormone Levels – NATURALLY – Analysis of Anabolic and Catabolic Hormones, Dr. Mark Kovacs, 2003 Authentic Health Fitness Australia; http://healthfitness.com.au/articles/highperformancetraining/hormones-exercise-anabolic-catabolic.htm

The Role of Nutrient Timing in the Adaptive Response to Heavy Resistance Training, Dr. Jose Antonio, Dr. Tim Ziegenfuss, 2008, National Strength and Conditioning Association; http://www.nsca-lift.org/HotTopic/download/Nutrient%20Timing.pdf

Cellular Respiration, Dr. Michael J. Gregory, 2006, The Biology Web, Clinton Community College; http://faculty.clintoncc.suny.edu/faculty/michael.gregory/files/bio%20101/bio%20101%20lectures/cellular%20respiration/cellular.htm

Hormonal Responses and Adaptations to Resistance Exercise and Training, William J. Kraemer and Nicholas A. Ratamess, 2005, Sports Medicine; 35 (4): 339-361; http://www.exerciciofisi-coesaude.com.br/PDF/artigos/andrericardo2010/3.pdf

Alpha-Lipoic Acid Increases Insulin Sensitivity by Activating AMPK in Skeletal Muscle, Woo Je Lee, Kee-Ho Song, Eun Hee Koh, Jong Chul Won, Hyoun Sik Kim, Hye-Sun Park, Min-Seon Kim, Seung-Whan Kim, Ki-Up Lee and Joong-Yeol Park, 2005, Biochemical and Biophysical Research Communications, Volume 332, Issue 3, Pages 885-891; doi:10.1016/j.bbrc.2005.05.035; http://www.sciencedirect.com/science/article/pii/S0006291X05010120

High Omega-3 Fat Intake Improves Insulin Sensitivity and Reduces CRP and IL6, but does not Affect Other Endocrine Axes in Healthy Older Adults, P. D. Tsitouras, et al, 2008, Hormone and Metabolic Research, DOI: 10.1055/s-2008-1046759; http://www.kronoslaboratory.com/dotnetnuke/Portals/1/TsitourasPD1.pdf

Move!

"Idleness is to the human mind like rust to iron." – Ezra Cornell

Sitting On Your Ass Is Killing You

On a late 2011 May afternoon, 20-year-old UK student Chris Staniforth was standing outside a job center complaining to his friend about chest pains. A tad stout, he otherwise had a clear record of health. Moments later, however, after begging his friend to call an ambulance, he dropped to the sidewalk, spasming in wordless agony.

Within minutes, an ambulance arrived to rush him to the hospital, where he was pronounced dead of a *pulmonary embolism* – a blood clot had travelled through his bloodstream from his leg vein to lodge in one of his lungs, cutting off part of its blood supply. The condition that led to his death is called *deep vein thrombosis* (DVT); a *thrombus* is a blood clot, occurring in a vein within the calf or thigh. Narrowed or blocked veins lead to this clumping of the blood, and the cause is usually poor circulation due to prolonged inactivity, or injury to a vein.

In Chris's case, his love of video games was rather extreme. His father noted in an interview with the UK Sun that Chris liked to sit and play games for up to 12 hours a day nonstop. But this could just as easily have been extended television watching or a desk job.

The evidence has been mounting: too much sitting on your ass will kill you.

In fact, even if you're lean and exercise regularly, sitting too much every day is extremely hazardous to your health. Dozens of studies within the last five years have linked extended sitting with obesity, heart disease, diabetes, and even cancer. A 2011 UK study found the risk is highest for women. Those who sit every day for extended lengths of time are 200 to 300% more likely to develop fatal blood clots than women who are physically active. Fatal blood clots are rare – only about one out of every 1,400 person years, but the potential is serious, particularly when the additional effects on blood glucose and increased risks of cancer are also considered.

In the UK, Dr. Christopher Kabrhel's research team monitored the habits of 69,950 female nurses over 18 years, and discovered the risk of developing pulmonary embolisms is over 200% greater for women who spend most of their time sitting (over 41 hours weekly outside of work), when compared to those who spend the least time sitting (less than 10 hours a week outside of work). The study took into account other risk factors such as age, BMI and smoking, contributing to the growing body of evidence that shows physical inactivity is a major cause of pulmonary embolism. The findings also demonstrated how physical inactivity is linked to heart disease and hypertension.

Sitting shuts off circulation of the fat-metabolizing enzyme *lipase*, while standing engages the muscles and promotes lipase distribution. This triggers the processing of fat and cholesterol, even without exercise. Because standing also burns glucose, it may also help reduce the likelihood of contracting diabetes.

> *Type I Diabetes is an autoimmune disease, where the body destroys its own insulin-producing pancreatic cells. When all these cells have been destroyed, Type I diabetes symptoms appear, including unexplained weight loss; vision problems; frequent urination; and extreme hunger, thirst or fatigue. In the long run, Type I diabetes increases the chance of kidney failure, heart disease, neural damage, and even blindness.*

When lipase functions normally, fat is reabsorbed by muscles, but when you sit, this function shuts down, and fat just circulates throughout the bloodstream, being stored as fatty deposits, or clogging arteries, causing dangerous cardiovascular disease. The amount of circulating fat is quite substantial as well, as shown by blood samples from volunteers after eating.

Sitting also reduces HDL ("healthy cholesterol") levels as much as 22 percent, and diabetes, heart disease, and obesity rates double and triple among those who sit the most. Circulating fat leads to plaque formation inside the blood vessels carrying blood and oxygen to your heart, brain and other body parts. Arteries have an inner muscle layer, which, if damaged, inflames (bulges) the arterial walls. These bulges can eventually rupture, and the body responds by sending clotting fibers to the damaged tissue.

Minerals like calcium, and fats like cholesterol, can become trapped in the clotting fibers, building up over time, and constricting or clogging the arteries. This means blood flow to the heart, brain and other vital organs can be reduced or even completely blocked, possibly leading to organ failures and death.

Researchers describe these body chemistry changes as "extremely rapid" and "dramatic" – after just six hours (a typical school or work day) there's a 35% reduction in food-energy use (*muscle triglyceride uptake*) and a 50% increase in insulin resistance. LDL (harmful) cholesterol, fat and blood sugar levels also increase significantly, in both fit and obese subjects.

Dr. Marc Hamilton of the University of Missouri says that most people have no idea how dangerous to their health sitting is. He contends that our sitting habits are at the heart of widespread *metabolic syndrome*, a condition from which over 47 million American adults suffer. He takes his own findings seriously enough that he has substituted a treadmill for his chair and now recommends standing for every possible activity. Standing while you talk on the phone or watch television, and taking frequent walk- and stretch breaks at work is recommended at a minimum. Simply by standing, you can burn an extra 60 calories an hour.

Your Television Is Killing You

Doctors have recently begun to find that excessive television viewing is extremely hazardous to your health – and the more you watch, the greater your risks of contracting serious diseases and dying prematurely. Data from eight separate studies was combined to show that every two hours people spend in front of a screen increases the risk of developing type 2 diabetes by 20% and heart disease by 15% (four hours equating to a 40% and 30% increase in risk, etc.. For every additional three hours people spend watching a screen, the risk of death from any cause jumps an average of 13%.

The combined findings are "remarkably consistent" among the various studies and populations, according to Harvard School of Public Health's Dr. Frank Hu, who co-wrote the meta-analysis. This increase in disease risk factors from television viewing is on a par with high cholesterol, high blood pressure or chronic smoking. Worldwide, with the exception of when working and sleeping, people spend more time in this unhealthy activity than in any pastime, with Americans leading the pack by far – it's been estimated that the average American spends at least five hours a day sitting and watching a television screen, more than anywhere else in the world.

The hazards stem from more than merely neglecting exercise, or simultaneously consuming a lot of salty, sugary high-fat snack foods. Prolonged sitting seems to result in metabolic changes that lead to unhealthy cholesterol levels and weight gain. Couch-potato syndrome, as Dr. Hu puts it, consists of extremely sedentary people spending many hours at a time sitting and passively staring at a screen. Their energy expenditure is quite low, even when compared to similar sedentary behaviours such as sitting and reading or driving.

His meta analysis drew upon data collected from more than 175,000 people worldwide, examining studies lasting from 6 to 10 years on average. Based on their findings, Hu and his coauthor estimate that, out of every 100,000 people, 176 will be newly diagnosed with diabetes, 38 will die from heart disease, and 104 will die from other television-viewing related causes per year for every two hours spent watching daily television. Over the long term, it's expected to have a major impact on public health in the near future.

But Not Just Americans

In 2009, Canadian researchers came to some stunning conclusions. After a massive, multi-year study of the daily sitting habits and the death rates of 17,000 Canadians, they were shocked to learn that it didn't matter how old the subjects were, how much they exercised, or even if they smoked – those who spent the most time sitting had as much as a 50% greater likelihood of dying prematurely.

In fact, according to the study, each hour spent in front of a television or computer monitor equals an 11% increase in the risk of death regardless of age, sex, weight, and/or other physical activity.

It's the same story around the globe. A second major study in Australia also shows every two-hour-a-day increase in TV viewing time means a 20% increase in the risk of contracting diabetes. And Spanish researchers published a 2008 study that showed those spending more than 42 hours a week watching TV compared with those watching less than 10.5 hours a week were 31% more likely to suffer from mental disorders.

Last year, a similar study in the Netherlands found strong links between mental disorders such as anxiety and depression, and extended sitting coupled with computer or television use. While correlation doesn't necessarily mean causation, the findings are sobering.

Unfortunately, modern civilization is built around sitting – during a typical school or workday, we tend to sit six to eight hours, more during our commute, and still more when relaxing at home. What this means is, if you're a typical worker or student, you have to start minimizing your daily sitting, standing whenever possible, and constantly interrupting sitting with breaks, even if that means only stretching or walking to the bathroom – studies show that even short, slow walks may be sufficient to quickly undo the metabolic damage from extended sitting.

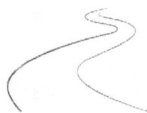

Gamer Chris Staniforth's Death Blamed on DVT, news staff, BBC, July 30, 2011; http://www.bbc.co.uk/news/uk-england-south-yorkshire-14350216

Stand Up for Your Health: Physiologists and Microbiologists Find Link Between Sitting and Poor Health, Jacqueline London, press release, May 1, 2008 American Institute of Physics; http://www.aip.org/dbis/stories/2008/18067.html

Physical Inactivity and Idiopathic Pulmonary Embolism in Women: Prospective Study, Christopher Kabrhel, Raphaëlle Varraso, Samuel Z Goldhaber, Eric Rimm, Carlos A Camargo Jr, British Medical Journal, , 2011; 343 (jul04 1): d3867 DOI: 10.1136/bmj.d3867

TV Watching Raises Risk of Health Problems, Dying Young, By Amanda Gardner, CNN, June 14, 2011; http://edition.cnn.com/2011/HEALTH/06/14/tv.watching.unhealthy/index.html?iref=obinsite

Physiological and Health Implications of a Sedentary Lifestyle, Mark Stephen Tremblay, Rachel Christine Colley, Travis John Saunders, Geneviève Nissa Healy, Neville Owen, January 2011, Scientific American; 121:384-391;

Television Viewing Time and Mortality – The Australian Diabetes, Obesity and Lifestyle Study, D.W. Dunstan, PhD, et al, Heart and Diabetes Institute, Melbourne, Australia et al;

Physical Activity, Sedentary Index, and Mental Disorders in the SUN Cohort Study, Almindena Sanchez-Villegas, et al, 2008, Medicine & Science in Sports & Exercise, Vol. 40, Issue 5 – pp 827-834;

Are Sedentary Television Watching and Computer Use Behaviours Associated with Anxiety and Depressive Disorders? Leonore de Wita, Annemieke van Stratena, Femke Lamersb, Pim Cuijpersa and Brenda Penninxb, 2010, Psychiatry Research

Safety

"Every one of you sitting here today is carrying at least 500 measurable chemicals in your body that were never in anybody's body before the 1920s... We have dusted the globe with man-made chemicals that can undermine the development of the brain and behavior, and the endocrine, immune and reproductive systems, vital systems that assure perpetuity... Everyone is exposed. You are not exposed to one chemical at a time, but a complex mixture of chemicals that changes day by day, hour by hour, depending on where you are and the environment you are in... In the United States alone it is estimated that over 72,000 different chemicals are used regularly. Two thousand five hundred new chemicals are introduced annually—and of these, only 15 are partially tested for their safety. Not one of the chemicals in use today has been adequately tested for these inter-generational effects that are initiated in the womb. "
– Theo Colburn, Speech, State of the Word Forum, San Francisco, 1996

"There are no passengers on Spaceship Earth. We are all crew."
– Marshall McLuhan, public statement, 1965

"If sunbeams were weapons of war, we would have had solar energy centuries ago."
– Sir George Porter, The Observer, 1973

Home Health Hazards

Recent research has discovered more than 400 toxic chemicals in the typical American's blood and fatty tissue. Many of these toxins are common in household products and even foods. Indoor air pollution in particular is a major health risk. Because indoor pollutants are not as easily dispersed or diluted as outdoor pollutants, concentrations of toxic chemicals can be much greater indoors. At least 20 toxic chemicals are common in western homes, at concentrations 200 to 500 times higher than outdoors. Many of these are known carcinogens, or have been linked to lung disease and birth defects.

Approximately 70,000 chemicals are now in commercial production, many for use in household products. Many have not been thoroughly safety tested, and are known to accumulate in the bloodstream and fatty tissue, causing cancer and other diseases. Second-hand cigarette smoke, gas stoves, wood-burning stoves and fireplaces are major sources of indoor air pollution, but home products like cleaning agents, aerosols, air fresheners, and disinfectants also contribute to the problem. These products often contain carcinogenic or otherwise hazardous ingredients.

Common reactions to indoor air pollution include symptoms such as a runny nose, itchy eyes, a scratchy throat, headaches, fatigue, dizziness, skin rash, and

373

respiratory infections. Long-term exposure to these pollutants can cause lung cancer or damage the liver, kidney and central nervous system. Children are particularly at risk of contracting respiratory and other illnesses.

Please choose your products carefully by reading the labels, and use organic products whenever possible. Check product labels to avoid these, the most toxic of common chemicals:

Cleaners, Cat Litter

- Formaldehyde – highly carcinogenic

- Crystalline Silica – eye, skin and lung irritant, highly carcinogenic

- Butyl Cellosolve, irritant, toxic to developing cells, neurotoxic, toxic to kidney and liver

- Perchloroethylene, irritant, neurotoxic, carcinogenic

Deodorants, Air Fresheners

- Isopar (deodorized kerosene), manufacturers admit to a wide range of toxic effects

- Paradichlorobenzene, toxic to liver and kidneys, carcinogenic

Cosmetics

Typically, women expose themselves every day to a number of known carcinogens and other poisons through their beauty-care products. When diluted sufficiently, single doses no longer kill or cripple the (millions of) animals used in lab tests, but people apply dozens of these products – each containing the same toxins – to their bodies every day for decades. These substances are "resistive", meaning they linger in your body and the environment for a long time, so toxic buildup can be extensive, and the combined effects are completely unknown. Toxic ingredients include:

- Siloxanes – directly linked to uterine and reproductive tumors, found in about 15% of household products such as lipstick, body lotions, hair-care products, soaps, cookware and cleaners

- 1,4 Dioxane – carcinogen found in 22 percent of personal care and children's products

- Mercury

- Nanosilvers – used to kill bacteria

- Cow placenta – full of hormones linked to precocious puberty

- Phthalates – endocrine disrupters, found in body lotions

- Methylparaben – antifungal preservatives found in many cosmetics and lotions

- Toluene – used in nail polish, reproductive/developmental toxin

- Stearalkonium Chloride – used in hairsprays, carcinogenic

- Mercury – carcinogenic

- Lead Acetate – carcinogenic

- Formaldehyde – carcinogenic

- Dibutyl Phthalate – reproductive/developmental toxin

- Cosmetic talc – carcinogenic

- 2-Bromo-2-Nitropropane-1,3-Diol – can form carcinogens if mixed with nitrosating agents

After years of consumer pressure, nail polish manufacturers have begun to market "three-free" products, which are free of the known carcinogens *toluene, dibutyl phthalate (DHB)* and *formaldehyde*. But in America, the FDA has comparatively lax policies regarding cosmetics (testing is completely voluntary, for example), so two ways to protect yourself are to look for labels that say "European Union Cosmetics Directive Compliant" and to replace personal care products with nontoxic versions

Pesticides

- Carbaryl and Diazinon – four- to seven-fold risk of leukemia and increased risk of brain cancer in children

Aerosols (Spray paints and Paint Strippers)

- Methylene Chloride – carcinogenic

Black and Dark Brown Hair Dye

- Coal Tar – extremely carcinogenic (long-term use is said to double the risk of blood cancers)

Skincare Products

- TEA (triethanolamine) – can combine with other chemicals to form highly carcinogenic nitrosamine.

- DEA (diethanolamine) – can combine with other chemicals to form highly carcinogenic nitrosamine.

- lauramide DEA – can combine with other chemicals to form highly carcinogenic nitrosamine.

Detergents

- Dioxane – can combine with other chemicals to form highly carcinogenic nitrosamine.

- DEA – can combine with other chemicals to form highly carcinogenic nitrosamine.

Plastic Containers, Bags, Some Plastic Toys and Some Capsule Medicines

- Phthalates (DBP, BBP, MBP, DEHP) – linked to hormonal disruption, birth defects and possibly autism, obesity and ADHD.

Handling Chemical Toxins Indoors

Many common houseplants can help filter contaminants from indoor air. Spider plants and golden pothos, Chinese evergreen, English ivy, peace lily, Marginata, potted mum, and Warneckii have been proven to absorb significant amounts of household pollutants.

Rooms should be well-ventilated and the windows kept open, to maintain low levels of indoor air pollution. An electric air filter/ionizer may also be a good idea. Never mix chemical products unless they contain instructions to do so. Mixing may cause explosive or poisonous chemical reactions. Even mixing different brands of the same product may be dangerous.

Use chemicals in well-ventilated areas to avoid fume inhalation. Open windows and use fans to disperse air outside. Use skin, eye, and respirator protection. Don't eat or drink when using hazardous products; trace amounts of chemicals can be carried from hand to mouth.

Antibiotics In Commercial Meat

Currently, more Americans die from antibiotic-resistant bacterial infections than from car accidents, prostate cancer and AIDS combined. A great number of these deaths could have been prevented, if the standard treatments still worked.

In 2011 the FDA reported that a staggering 80 percent of all the antibiotics used in America go into feeding livestock. This is despite the fact the FDA itself has officially stated the non-therapeutic use of antibiotics in livestock feed is dangerous to human health, because it creates antibacterial resistance.

This massive overuse of antibiotics is meant to prevent the spread of disease in "factory farms", where animals are so densely packed into cages and pens it can cripple them and diseases are otherwise rampant. Unfortunately, this quick fix for the problems factory farms have created in the quest for squeezing out greater profits is creating what scientists call an "army" of drug-resistant bacteria. What's worse, the drugs are often used not specifically to prevent disease, but because they have the side effect of spurring weight gain in livestock, making them more profitable.

Of course, when we eat this antibiotic-tainted meat, we absorb the antibiotics ourselves, and develop a cumulative resistance to the healing properties of the antibiotics. This is one of the causes of modern "superbugs" that are resistant to antibiotics, and often kill patients.

What this means for you is that if you eat meat, you should try to buy organic and, whenever possible, try to help change this intolerable system, through the ballot box and the power of your voice.

The Toxin You've Never Heard of That May be Slowly Killing You

A chemical called *isocyanic acid*, found in wildfire and cigarette smoke and in urban air, has been linked to health hazards ranging from cataracts to cardiovascular disease. Chronic exposure to lower-level amounts of this toxin can occur near wildfires or when coal, wood or other biomass is burned for heating and cooking in the home. Cigarette smoke also contains very high levels of isocyanic acid, although the substance is not currently listed as among the "potentially harmful" constituents of tobacco.

A new National Oceanic and Atmospheric Administration spectrometer study has collected atmospheric readings of isocyanic acid for the first time. Head researcher Jim Roberts, a chemist at the Boulder, Colorado

NOAA, says the group has detected isocyanic acid in a number of settings, and found it easily dissolves in water, meaning it can easily enter the body through the eyes and lungs.

Isocyanic acid (HNCO) is part of a chemical cascade that can lead to cataracts and inflammation, known to trigger cardiovascular disease and rheumatoid arthritis. With billions of people worldwide burning vegetation and other biomasses for cooking and heating, the pollutant is widespread.

At 1 ppb (parts per billion), the NOAA estimated enough HNCO would dissolve into exposed tissues in the lungs and eyes to make them vulnerable to *carbamylation,* the chemical alteration of proteins that triggers inflammation and cataract formation.

Noise Pollution And Your Body

Like the frog in a pot of water that cannot feel the slow temperature change until the water boils, we are generally oblivious to the slow buildup of stress-inducing noise creeping into our daily lives, says Reverend Susan Sparks, author of *Laugh Your Way to Grace: Reclaiming the Spiritual Power of Humor.*

Everything from the steady hum of machinery all around us, to our iPods, cellphones, car engines, and the blare of our home entertainment systems is washing over us in a steady flood of noise that we have become gradually accustomed to.

This constant cacophony, which we believe to be harmless, says Sparks, is a very real health hazard; she says the Occupational Safety and Health Administration has reported that excessive noise causes a loss of concentration and a buildup of stress, muscle tension, ulcers, increased blood pressure and hypertension. Additional studies show human noise also wreaks havoc on our ecosystems, disrupting core wildlife biological functions like mating, foraging, and tending to the young.

Because of this, the National Park Service (NPS) has taken steps to restore quiet in some major parks such as Muir Woods, the great Californian redwood forest, installing sound meters and moving parking spaces farther from the trees.

Sparks urges us to consider taking *sound breaks* – unplugging appliances, all the beepers, buzzers, tweeters and woofers. "Even if only for half an hour a day, our blood pressure and stress levels might lower for those few precious moments."

The Nasties – Common Household Pathogens

The most common harmful bacteria found in households are

- Bacillus – carried by insects such as houseflies and cockroaches

- Corynaebacterium – found in soil brought from outside on shoes, or in plants

- E. Coli – Sometimes found around toilets

- Salmonella – Found in sinks and on cutting boards and faucets

- Staphylococcus – Forms in tubs, showers, on faucets and carpets – infects skin and mucous membranes

- Streptococcus – Easily transferred by touch, inhabits the mucous membranes of the mouth and nose

Bleach is your most effective antibacterial cleaner, but take particular care regarding the following:

- Bath & Shower – should be cleaned regularly, including shower curtain

- Carpets – regular vacuuming eliminates airborne pathogens like dust, skin and pet dander (dead skin cells)

- Cutting Boards – One should be for meat and one for produce. Clean with dishes; replace when grooved

- Dishtowels – wash in bleach and hot water and machine dry

- Kitchen sink – clean with bleach or a detergent that contains bleach

- Sponges – Replace regularly

- Telephones, computer keyboards, door knobs and remote controllers – Clean with bleach to destroy bacteria transferred by hands and mouths

- Toilet – Be aware that flushing ejects an aerosol spray of microscopic fecal matter and bacteria, including e. coli and staphylococcus bacteria. Close the lid when flushing, keep toothbrushes at least 10 ft. (3 meters) away, and clean inside and out, along with the surrounding floor

- Toothbrushes – wash and store in a dry cabinet after every use

Household Mold

Molds and their spores are found everywhere, including in home and office dust. A mildewy or moldy smell is a good indicator you have a problem. Yellow, brown, green or black discoloration on carpeting or other surfaces is another.

Adverse reactions to mold can include itchy, red eyes, runny nose, breathing difficulty, headaches, asthma attacks, dizziness and/or fatigue, coughing, memory loss and fatigue. In the worst circumstances, mold toxicity can even cause infertility, nerve and organ damage and even death.

Mold thrives in dampness, and can grow on walls, ceilings, floors, and even furniture and clothing, if there is a mild temperature, a little light and enough moisture. It can even grow in air conditioning systems, so filters should be regularly cleaned and/or replaced. The greatest concentration of mold is usually in bathrooms, so be sure to carefully clean your tiles, curtains and fixtures.

The key to preventing mold is in controlling moisture – fix any leaks and make sure to regularly ventilate your home, opening doors and windows to allow outside air circulation. You might also consider installing air purifier/humidifiers in each room. Certain commercial household paints also prevent mold.

Although *borax* is an effective mold killer, much safer alternatives include tea tree oil or a mixture of baking soda and white vinegar. Shake a quarter tablespoon of baking soda with one cup of distilled white vinegar in a spray bottle and spray it over the infected area before scrubbing. For tea tree oil, mix one teaspoon of oil with one cup of water in a spray bottle.

Are Your Teeth Killing You?

According to the Centers for Disease Control and Prevention, the number one killer in America is heart disease. More than 50% of Americans die from heart attacks. Following closely, at number three, are strokes.

The latest research has shown a significant link between oral hygiene and both heart attack and stroke risk. Research conducted by state health agencies and the CDC on over 40,000 adults across America between 1999 to 2002 discovered details of a disease called *subacute bacterial endocarditis*, a condition where the heart's lining is severely damaged by bacteria. A similar 21-year study of nearly 10,000 US adults by the State University of New York at Buffalo found a similar strong link between gum disease and strokes, where a blood vessel in the brain ruptures or becomes blocked by a clot.

It's been estimated that 75-95 percent of adults have gum disease. The first stage is *gingivitis,* which includes swollen, easily bleeding gums and bad breath. This condition is easily reversible. But before getting it, you can easily prevent it with regular dental visits, brushing and flossing, and drinking water.

Gums, the tissues that hold your teeth in place, provide the perfect environment for bacterial growth – warm, moist and full of micronutrients. Between the base of your teeth and your gums there is a tiny gap, a trench where bacteria can lodge and multiply. Over time, this trench can deepen into a "pocket" shape, which teems with bacteria. Beginning with gingivitis, if unchecked, gum disease eventually advances into severe inflammation, swelling from infection, a condition called *periodontitis*.

Blood is normally a sterile environment, but when your gums have become this infected, bacteria can enter your bloodstream, a condition called *bacteremia*. Through a process not yet fully understood, these bacteria then stimulate the clumping of plaque deposits within blood vessels, while simultaneously attacking and weakening the vessel walls. If untreated, this can lead to heart failure or stroke, with often fatal results.

The upshot of this is that, if you don't want to kill yourself through sheer laziness, you need to be taking good care of your teeth. This means brushing soon as you can after eating, thoroughly for two to three minutes. If you don't have the opportunity to brush, vigorously swirling water in your mouth and straining it through your teeth (with your mouth closed!) is a temporary solution.

At a bare minimum, brushing is necessary immediately after you awaken and in the evening before you sleep. If you're not flossing at least once a day, consider this: floss is designed to remove tiny particles of food that get lodged between your teeth where brushing can't reach. If those food particles remain, they begin to decay within a matter of minutes, becoming covered with bacteria. In essence, when you don't floss, you're leaving chunks of rotting food, teeming with bacteria, to slowly decay in your mouth. After days, weeks or (ick) MONTHS without flossing....

Many studies have also shown the key role diet plays in dental health; a 2010 Harvard Medical School study showed a 20% reduction in gum disease from eating polyunsaturated fats – the DHA and EHA found in fish oil and nuts. Strawberries are also great for your teeth because they contain bacteria-cleaning fiber and *malic acid*, the same ingredient used in many whitening toothpastes.

Hydrogen peroxide mixed with equal parts water is also recommended as an antiseptic twice a month that's superior to commercial mouthwashes. It prevents infections and bacterial growth. As a bonus, it also whitens your teeth and combats bad breath. You should mix one tablespoon of water and one tablespoon of hydrogen peroxide, then swish it around your teeth for a minute and spit it out. Leave the residue on your teeth for another two minutes and then rinse with water for maximum effect.

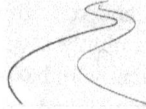

Your Personal Grooming Products Could Be Making You Sick, Estelle Hayes, March 11, 2011 The Huffington Post

Database of safe cosmetics: http://www.ewg.org/skindeep/

Today's Food System: All Drugged Up, Laurie David, March 2, 2011, Huffington Post;

The Antibiotics Crisis, Dan Rather January 12, 2011, Huffington Post

Smoke-related Chemical Discovered in the Atmosphere Could Have Health Implications, Patrick R. Veres, Anthony K. Cochran, Carsten Warneke, et al, 2011, press release, National Oceanic and Atmospheric Administration, Proceedings of the National Academy of Sciences, 2011; DOI: 10.1073/pnas.1103352108

Unplug and Recharge: Taking a Silence Siesta, Rev. Susan Sparks, March 5, 2011, The Huffington Post

National Report on Human Exposure to Environmental Chemicals, US Centers for Disease Control and Prevention, 1999-2010

The Six Common Household Items with the Most Germs, Joseph M. Mercola, MD, 2003

Tooth Loss and Heart Disease: Findings from the Behavioral Risk Factor Surveillance System, Catherine A. Okoro, MS; Lina S. Balluz, ScD: Paul I. Eke, PhD et al, The American Journal of Preventative Medicine, 2005 vol. 29, issue 5

N-3 Fatty Acids and Periodontitis in US Adults, Naqvi AZ, Buettner C, Phillips RS, et al., 2010, Journal of American Dietetic Association

Hollywood Beauty Secrets: Remedies to the Rescue, Louisa Maccan-Graves, 2003

Periodontal Disease and Risk of Cerebrovascular Disease, Tiejian Wu, MD, PhD; Maurizio Trevisan, MD, MS; Robert J. Genco, DDS, PhD; Joan P. Dorn, PhD; Karen L. Falkner, PhD; Christopher T. Sempos, PhD, 2010, Archives of Internal Medicine;160:2749-2755

Sleep

"Death, so called, is a thing which makes men weep.
And yet a third of life is passed in sleep."
– Lord Byron, Don Juan, 1875

A Scientific Mystery

One of the most puzzling of animal behaviours is sleep. You'll spend over 200,000 hours in sleep during your lifetime – more than 8,000 days. For such a large part of human existence, sleep's precise purposes aren't yet fully understood. We know that wound healing and growth are optimized by sleep, and it appears to help maintain the immune system, as measured in white blood cell counts and human growth hormone levels. HGH and your immune system go into high production during sleep, and your body's immobilized during most sleep, suggesting it's primarily meant to restore and repair. In fact, it's vital; five days without sleep is almost certainly fatal.

Sleep is a state of reduced consciousness, lowered sensory awareness, and immobility of most voluntary muscles, observed in all mammals, birds, and many amphibians, reptiles, fish and even insects. It's characterized by a decreased ability to react to stimuli. During sleep, the immune, nervous, skeletal and muscular systems undergo accelerated repair and growth.

Sleep has a marked impact on your mood, cognition, memory, focus and coordination, keeping neuromodulators such as serotonin and dopamine in balance. A regular sleep routine, in which you go to bed and awaken at the same time every day will keep you healthy, calm, cheerful, energized and focused.

In terms of your appearance, skin is also very sensitive to sleep patterns, as your body uses sleep time to regenerate skin cells. If you lack sufficient sleep, your skin will begin to look pale or even grey, and you'll eventually get dark circles under your eyes. To avoid all of these unpleasant effects, make sure your sleep patterns are consistent. Aside from cellular repair, one of the many functions of sleep is to flush out the stress hormone cortisol, which can slow metabolism. Getting regular high-quality sleep reduces cortisol and thus helps you maintain weight loss.

Sleep cycles are a balance of sleeping and waking states controlled by your circadian clock. (Circadian is Latin for "approximately a day"). Your circadian clock lowers body temperature during sleep and raises it again upon waking; the neurotransmitter *adenosine*, which builds over the course of the day, helps promote sleep by inhibiting many natural body processes that normally occur while you're awake. High adenosine levels create sleepiness.

As night falls, the decrease in light affects photosensitive cells of your *suprachiasmatic nucleus*, which triggers pineal gland release of the hormone *melatonin*, also used as an ingredient in some commercial sleep aids. Melatonin is a sleep-inducing hormone naturally produced by the pineal gland in the brain, which converts serotonin into melatonin.

Many people have a temporary drop in alertness in the early afternoon, commonly known as the "post-lunch dip." While a large meal can make a person feel sleepy, the post-lunch dip is mostly an effect of the biological clock. The circadian rhythm naturally makes people sleepiest at 2:00 am and 2:00 pm, leading to the custom of *siestas* (afternoon naps) in some countries.

Interestingly, however, even while you sleep, your brain is still monitoring the outside world; for example, your auditory cortex can still respond to danger signals, and your amygdala will awaken you if there is a sudden, unfamiliar noise.

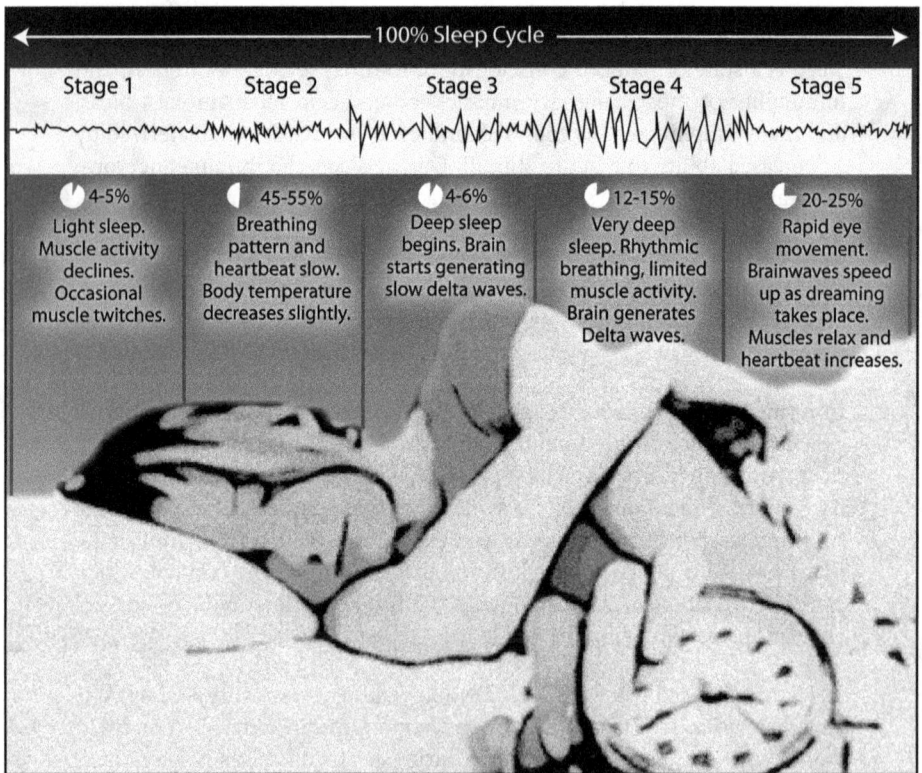

100% Sleep Cycle				
Stage 1	Stage 2	Stage 3	Stage 4	Stage 5
4-5%	45-55%	4-6%	12-15%	20-25%
Light sleep. Muscle activity declines. Occasional muscle twitches.	Breathing pattern and heartbeat slow. Body temperature decreases slightly.	Deep sleep begins. Brain starts generating slow delta waves.	Very deep sleep. Rhythmic breathing, limited muscle activity. Brain generates Delta waves.	Rapid eye movement. Brainwaves speed up as dreaming takes place. Muscles relax and heartbeat increases.

Sleep Cycles, Polyglot Studios, 2011

Sleep Cycles

Mammals and birds share two types of sleep – *rapid eye movement (REM)* and *non-rapid eye movement (NREM)*. Non-REM sleep is made up of three stages, with little dreaming. The last NREM stage is deepest – slow- or delta-wave sleep. Sleep progresses through these REM and NREM cycles, and each cycle lasts about 90 minutes for humans. Most sleep is deep, early in the cycle, with REM sleep increasing later at night and just prior to awakening. Depending on the amount and types of sleep experienced, some of its benefits may not be achieved, making it possible to still be tired after a full night's sleep.

The best sleepers transition fall into deeper stage 1 sleep within ten minutes. The brain then transitions into slower *theta-frequency* activity, muscles relax, and the heart rate drops. This is the state of "drifting off" or "dozing". After a few minutes of theta-activity stage-1 sleep, most sleepers pass into stage 2, where bursts of activity called *sleep spindles* occur. Some 30 to 45 minutes later, they enter stages 3 and 4 – recently consolidated into a single stage by researchers.

In this deepest phase of sleep, the brain produces the slowest of brain waves, the *delta wave pattern*. Deep sleep lasts for about 45 minutes, during which the body is at its quietest in terms of respiration, heart rate, blood flow and neurological activity.

From deep sleep, you cycle briefly through stage 2 sleep and then transition into *REM* sleep, when dreaming begins. Dream sleep includes vivid imagery and intense physiological and emotional activity. Although the muscles are kept in a state of paralysis (theoretically to keep you from injuring yourself while dreaming), breathing, heart rate, and blood pressure are just as high or higher than when you're awake, and brain wave activity resembles that of your waking state.

A number of brain regions are extremely active during REM sleep, particularly the limbic system and other emotion- and stress-related areas. In contrast, the logic and self-awareness centers of the brain in the frontal lobes deactivate during dream sleep. Although most people can't recall their dreams in detail, everyone has them.

A single night's sleep cycles through stages one to three, followed by REM sleep, at generally 90 minutes per cycle. Six hours of sleep thus results in four one and one-half hour cycles, while eight hours results in five cycles. Although the cycles progressively vary through the night, the breakdown is on average:

385

- Stage 1: 5%

- Stage 2: 50%

- Stage 3 and 4: 20%

- REM: 25%

You obtain the deepest sleep over the first half of the night, and the most dream sleep over the second. Because sleep is shallower in the second half of the night, it's easier to awaken at that time.

NON-REM

Stage 1 involves the brain's transition from alpha waves (a state of wakefulness) to theta waves, the state of "drowsy sleep". Twitches and jerking, called hypnic myoclonia, can occur during this stage – sleep starts which give a sensation of falling. At this point, awareness of the external environment starts to fade.

*In **Stage 2**, muscle activity decreases further, and all conscious awareness of the external environment fades away. This stage comprises about half of total sleep time. During this period, special spikes of neural activity called sleep spindles occur, a process thought to be the consolidation of long-term memories.*

Stage 3 is the first stage of deep sleep, consisting of long, slow delta waves (from 0.5–2 Hertz – cycles per second) combines with faster waves.

Stage 4 is the second stage of deep sleep, characterized by nearly total delta wave activity. At this point, it becomes very difficult to rouse the sleeper. Both stages of deep sleep are necessary to awaken refreshed and well-rested.

REM

70 to 90 minutes after you fall asleep, you enter the REM phase. This sleep stage occurs during about 25% of an adult's sleep cycle, and is when the most memorable dreaming takes place. In EEG scans, REM activity looks like wakeful brain activity. During REM sleep, the muscles are kept in a state of paralysis, probably to protect the body against thrashing about, as the mind enacts vivid dreams.

386

Gotta Have It

Required sleep duration varies, depending upon the person and his or her age, but if you don't feel any daytime sleepiness, you're probably getting enough. Some people require less sleep than others; it's believed to be genetically based, probably due to a mutation in the DEC2 gene. The recommended minimum sleep time decreases as you age – newborns sleep as much as 18 hours; 3-5 year olds about 12 hours; children and teens about 10, and adults, seven to eight. For most adults, seven hours a night is optimal for health. A University of California, San Diego study of more than a million adults discovered that those who sleep six or seven hours a night live the longest – if they awaken naturally. But those who force themselves awake with insufficient sleep don't show such benefits.

Too little and too much are both detrimental to your health: studies have shown that too little or too much sleep more than doubles the risk of early death. Over time, consistently insufficient sleep, called "sleep debt", results in mental, emotional and physical fatigue, as well as impaired cognitive functionality. On the other hand, sleeping more than 7 or 8 hours a night has been linked consistently with increased mortality, although it's believed the cause is probably a separate issue such as depression or low socioeconomic status.

Sleep quality is just as important as sleep length. If you have recurring nightmares or still feel tired after a full night's sleep, try meditation, a warm bath or soothing music before bed. If none of these help, you may have serious health issues or excessive stress, and should seek medical help. Sleep difficulties are associated with psychiatric maladies like depression, alcoholism, and bipolar disorder. It's also important when you sleep; sleeping outside your natural rhythm cycle doesn't provide the same rejuvenation benefits. You need to sleep at least six hours before your lowest daily body temperature and highest concentration of melatonin.

Sleep And Memory

Research within the last two decades has shown that sleep is when memories are reorganized, and physically solidified in the neurochemical process called consolidation. According to Harvard researchers, an essential part of learning and memory formation is the signalling of dendrites to create new connections. The process can proceed optimally when there is a temporary blocking of incoming information, which may be why, during sleep, as the senses "tune out", memories and knowledge are organized and solidified. Sleep moves your day's memories from short-term into long-term storage.

Slow wave sleep is a period of review, in which your hippocampus reactivates new experiences and synchronizes with the neocortex, which receives these memories and integrates them with existing, relevant knowledge. The cortex upgrades these synapses in the process called long-term potentiation (LTP). Such "upgraded" and reinforced neurons hold memories for long-term storage and easier retrieval.

Memory is affected differently within the various sleep phases, but in general, sleep assists the neuroplastic changes underlying consolidation of recently-learned knowledge. The same neural circuits reactivate or "replay" during sleep, strengthening recent experiences as memories. Experiments have shown that deep, slow-wave sleep assists with consolidating declarative semantic and episodic (conscious, factual and life events) memory, and after spatial exploration, neurons in the hippocampus reactivate in the same patterns during SWS, suggesting it is central to consolidating navigational memory.

A Memory-Boosting Trick – *If you tell yourself you'll need certain information in the future, studies have shown your brain will build stronger memories for you in your sleep. Scientists at the University of Lübeck in Germany tested memory with subjects memorizing 40 word pairs, the location of 15 cards, and a finger-tapping sequence. Only those who had been told in advance that they'd be tested improved in retention after sleeping.*

Those who were given a surprise quiz did not see the significant benefits. Said Jan Born, who directed the study, just telling yourself that you will need to memorize data determines whether or not your brain solidifies it in your memory during sleep.

EEG measurements showed the group who knew they needed to remember for a test spent more time in deep, slow-wave sleep than the group who were unaware of the upcoming test. A greater number of sleep spindles" (short spikes of heightened electrical activity which prime cortical circuits for memory storage) were also seen in the group that knew of the upcoming test.

In humans, there are three levels of nervous system arousal: 1) waking, 2) non-REM, and dreaming (REM) sleep. Slow-wave sleep also consists of four separate stages, during which activity within the brain and body are at very low levels.

Every 90 minutes, the highly-activated state of REM sleep follows slow-wave sleep stages. At this point, the cortex is even more activated than during wakefulness, and the sleeper's eyes will shift back and forth in rapid eye movement (REM). This is the point at which the most vivid dreams appear, and the sleeper's limbs will be held in the state of paralysis called *atonia,* the body's natural method of preventing possible injuries from thrashing about during sleep.

Carl Sagan theorized that sleeping occurs in 90 minute cycles, returning us to shallow sleep states regularly throughout the night because that is the time we most needed to be alert in the past – the night was when predators or rivals were most likely to attack. We have evolved a built-in vigilance system to compensate for this.

Although slow-wave sleep is thought to be the period during which the body undergoes cellular repair, it is also when "sleep spindles" are seen – spikes of EEG activity in which data is being exchanged between the hippocampus and cortex. This, experiments have shown, is the first phase of the conversion of short-term memories into long-term memories (consolidation).

REM sleep however, appears to be a "sorting" phase for memory, during which creatures "rehearse" (repeat motor patterns that have been learned during the day) and reorganize associations between new and existing memory traces. The hippocampi enter highly synchronized theta wave rhythm patterns resembling those of animals exploring their surroundings and indicative of information encoding (translating recent experiences into long-term memories).

This REM portion of sleep is the most beneficial for creative problem-solving. It also appears to be when LTP occurs at a cellular level – acetylcholine levels are high, triggering the *labile state* (temporary structural flexibility) during which neural structures can change, growing new receptors and dendrites to enhance synaptic conductivity and create new connections between neurons.

Norepinephrine and serotonin, which help generate arousal, are at their peak during states of wakefulness, but decline during slow-wave sleep and completely cease during REM sleep – meaning they are inactive as you dream. The logic centers in the prefrontal lobes also shut down throughout sleep, which probably explains why the content of dreams defies normal logic. The limbic system is also highly active, particularly the amygdala. Dopamine neurons fire at generally steady levels throughout the night and day, except during firing bursts that occur as creatures seek rewards while awake.

When you're sleeping, studies indicate you appear to be reliving the day's events. During the REM state, the cortical logic centers have been shut down, so thinking becomes more free-flowing, and less restricted by the laws of physics your logical mind automatically applies to your perception. Time, space, gravity are all highly plastic in this mental state.

All-Nighters Are The Worst Study Method

"Sleep spindles predict learning refreshment," according to Dr. Matthew Walker, director of the Sleep and Neuroimaging Laboratory at the University of California, Berkeley. His study found that spindle activity was most likely during Stage 2 non-Rapid Eye Movement (NREM) sleep, before slow-wave sleep and dreaming (REM) sleep. The shallow dreamless, stage 2 sleep is half of the entire sleep process, occurring most during the second half of the night.

"A lot of that spindle-rich sleep is occurring the second half of the night, so if you sleep six hours or less, you are shortchanging yourself. You will have fewer spindles, and you might not be able to learn as much," says colleague Dr. Bryce Mander. These sleep spindles are thought to clear your hippocampus of short-term memory to make room for new data. Fact-based memories (*declarative memories*) get stored temporarily in your hippocampus before being relayed and consolidated in various regions of the cortex. The hippocampus is a much smaller physical region, limiting the amount it can hold in short-term memory. Sleep clears it out for the next day's information by moving what's important into cortical long-term memory storage.

The longer you stay awake, the more sluggish your brain will become. Pulling an all-nighter decreases your memory by almost 40 percent, and sleep-deprived brain centers will begin to shut down.

The Secret To Boosting Your Creativity And Problem-Solving Skills

REM sleep appears to boost spatial-navigational and *procedural memory* - skills like riding a bicycle, which you perform without requiring deliberate conscious thought. It's been demonstrated that people practice and solidify these procedural motor skills while sleeping. fMRI scans show the replay of neural activity patterns controlling recently-practiced physical movements, as sleepers reenact new motor skills they've learned during the day.

During REM sleep, norepinephrine, serotonin and histamine shut down, resulting in REM *atonia*, in which the motor neurons shut down, preventing thrashing about. Nerves in the brain stem called *REM sleep-on cells* begin major activity, and are thus thought to control the REM state.

Vivid dreams appear, which are thought to perform multiple functions: acting as mental wish fulfillment, an opportunity to confront and find solutions to fear-inducing stressors, and a sort of "free association" period which enhances creativity, creating new associations between information, these associations physically manifested as neural connections. Integration of disparate pieces of information significantly improves after even a short REM sleep session; says UCAL Dr. Denise Cai, this period of sleep allows the brain to make new connections between unrelated information.

To test her theory, she gave 77 volunteers a list of three words and asked them to come up with a fourth which was linked to the three. "Heart" "cookie", and "sixteen", for example, can be associated with the word "sweet". The relationship between the three supplied words and the missing fourth varied. The volunteers were tested at 9 am and 5 pm in a single day and were monitored in a lab at 1 pm. Some rested quietly to classical music, or slept a maximum of 90 minutes. 28 of the 40 who slept underwent REM sleep.

All the volunteers improved at the word games during the second session, which is logical – having had time to consider the problems, they naturally did better. However, a portion of the recruits did an additional set of tests after the morning puzzles, filling in a missing word in an analogy (e.g. HARD is to EASY as FAST is to S…). They were not told these were the same words used as answers to the earlier word puzzles.

Volunteers who experienced REM sleep showed dramatic improvements in subsequent tests, while those who underwent non-REM or no sleep showed no improvement. It was found that *quality* of sleep (getting REM-state sleep) mattered more than *quantity* in improving performance – those who had experienced REM sleep were better able to link the hidden clues in the additional tasks.

A siesta – afternoon nap –improves a range of cognitive operations from alertness to creativity, she says. A 90-minute (full cycle) nap in the afternoon significantly increases learning capacity, appearing to clear out the hippocampus for fresh input in the same way as a full night's sleep.

REM-sleepers weren't better than others in remembering morning test answers – all groups scored about 90%, but only those who underwent REM sleep improved in the additional tests. REM sleepers also scored the same as others when given *new* words – they only showed sleep-enhanced improvements on information they had studied previously. This demonstrated that REM sleep specifically boosted their ability to create associations between ideas they had already assimilated. This ability to create associations is believed to be the fundamental basis of creativity.

A 2004 study by Ullrich Wagner also showed subjects are twice as likely to find new solutions to mathematical problems after mulling over them in their sleep. He says this is evidence that sleep improves "cognitive flexibility". He believes REM sleep helps people incorporate new data into existing mental information, creating a richer neural network for future use, and providing the groundwork for the flashes of insight we call *epiphanies*.

To Sleep, Perchance to Dream

Why you dream is not yet fully understood, but it seems to be a mental review and information reorganization – sorting, discarding, linking and strengthening. This also seems to lead to a lot of creative thinking, and some of history's most famous discoveries (Einstein's theory of relativity and Mendeleyev's periodic table of elements, for example) and artistic creations arose from dreams. Dreams seem to be a replaying of images, sensations and information you've collected throughout the day. In addition to helping with mental "filing and sorting" though, they also appear to help you overcome anxiety and live out your desires.

Dreams have common themes, according to dream reports collected by psychologists and sociologists. Dreambank.net lists the results of 50,000 dream reports, from which some generalizations can be made.

According to Yale Professor Paul Bloom, most dreams are bad. Not nightmares or catastrophic in content, but generally negative, dealing with misfortunes. In tribal societies, dreams tend to be more physically aggressive than those of people from industrialized societies, and men tend to experience more aggressive dreams than women. Americans also tend to have more aggressive dreams than Europeans.

The most common theme is of being chased. Other common themes include falling, flying, public speaking, and being naked in public. Says Bloom, the primary purpose of sleep appears to be memory consolidation and tissue repair, and some psychologists believe dreams are just a side effect:

> One theory which is popular is that dreams are a side effect of memory consolidation so your body, sort of below the neck, rebuilds itself while you're sleeping, but also what happens while you're sleeping is your memories get played over and over again to consolidate them into different parts of the brain. Almost – the best analogy here is backing up a computer. Your brain backs itself up. In the course of backing itself up, there are sort of random events which flash to consciousness and get put together in a coherent story. From this perspective, dreams serve no adaptive function at all but rather they're epiphenomena; they're the byproducts of another system.

Dream Management

Everybody dreams three to four times a night, but most people normally don't remember their dreams. However, you can train yourself to remember them with a *dream diary*. Dream diaries are said to be very beneficial to creativity and problem-solving skills; because dreams fade quickly, writing them into a dream diary as soon as you awaken is the key.

Some people, such as Salvador Dali and physicist Neils Bohr, have also practiced *dream management* techniques to help with creativity and problem-solving. Techniques such as *lucid dreaming* teach people how to become aware within their dreams that they're dreaming, and how to guide their dreams. Usually lucid (self-aware) dreaming is triggered when the sleeper notices some impossible circumstances in the dream, such as having the ability to fly or speak with the dead.

Dr. Steven LaBerge, the world's expert in lucid dreaming, believes lucid dreaming may be a powerful aid in self-actualization – in helping discover meaning and purpose in life. He has invented a mask that flashes light at the commencement of REM movements, a trigger that alerts the sleeper she's dreaming, without awakening her.

> *...being in a lucid dream clearly demonstrates the astonishing fact that the world we see is a construct of our minds. This concept, so elusive when sought in waking life, is the cornerstone of spiritual teachings. It forces us to look beyond everyday experience and ask, 'If this is not real, what is?'*

Sleep Your Way to the Top – Improving Athletic Performance
According to a 2007 study, athletes who get extra sleep tend to show improved game performance. Cheri Mah of Stanford University studied members of the Stanford men's basketball team while they got as much extra sleep time as possible. Measuring sprint times and shooting percentages, she found significant improvements in speed and free-throws. The volunteers also reported increased energy, improved mood, and decreased fatigue during games and practice.

Studies have consistently shown that sleep time affects physical, mental and emotional health, productivity and performance. Insufficient sleep has been linked to major health problems like depression, diabetes, cardiovascular disease and obesity.

Sleep Control Mechanisms

University of Texas professor Michael Smolensky is considered a pioneer in the emerging field of *chronotherapy*, and, together with co-author Lynne Lamberg, he explains in *The Body Clock* how to use these rhythms to maximize health, weight loss, sleep, sex, exercise, and recovery from injuries and illness.

Two systems control sleep – the *wake system* and the *sleep system*. The wake system fosters daytime alertness, and is generally dominant about sixteen hours, while the sleep system fosters nighttime sleeping, dominating the remaining eight hours of the day. Directly behind each eye and linked via your optic nerve to your retinas are two clusters of neurons called the *suprachiasmatic nuclei* (SCN). Based upon the amount of light in your environment, these light-sensitive structures regulate your sleep-wake cycles, controlling your circadian rhythms through pineal gland release of your body's natural "sleep aid", the hormone melatonin. The suprachiasmatic nuclei also output to *locus coeruleus* neurons in your *pons* which produce norepinephrine, used to regulate arousal.

Your brain's internal 24-hour clock is regulated by your SCN, which is attuned to both daily and seasonal light cycles. Both these light cycles trigger several instinctive behaviours in mammals, including sleeping, eating, weight gain and breeding. In humans, the SCN regulates sleep cycles and appears to control seasonal mood changes.

Bright light, even in brief pulses once a day, can synchronize circadian rhythms, although caffeine and melatonin production can also influence SCN function. SCN neurotransmitter control can cause particularly sensitive people to suffer from winter depression, a syndrome called *Seasonal Affective Disorder (SAD)*.

Melatonin is produced by the *pineal gland*, a pea-sized organ in the center of your brain, which induces drowsiness and lowers your body temperature. Interestingly, melatonin production decreases with age, which explains to a degree why the elderly sleep less.

Pineal gland melatonin production is inhibited by light and encouraged by darkness. In early evening, production starts with Dim-Light Melatonin Onset (DLMO). This melatonin production peaks in the middle of the night, gradually decreasing as morning approaches. Primarily blue light of 460 to 480 nanometer wavelength suppresses melatonin, and the more intense the light and longer the exposure, the greater the reduction. This is one of the reasons people watching television, computer monitors, and other light-emitting portable devices sometimes suffer from insomnia.

Melatonin was also recently discovered to act as a powerful antioxidant, scavenging free radicals and thus theoretically preventing DNA damage from carcinogens. It may also reduce Parkinson's disease damage, protect against cardiac arrhythmia, and even increase longevity – the average mouse lifespan has been shown to increase as much as 20% in some studies of melatonin administration. Melatonin also appears to have a positive effect on the immune system, and may be useful in fighting infectious bacteria, viruses, and even cancer.

Melatonin is sometimes sold as a supplement, and, together with light therapy, is used to restore normal circadian rhythms to insomniacs.

A Vital Rhythm

Your circadian rhythm, which controls your energy, metabolic and alertness levels during the day, serves a much wider role than that of a simple ticking clock, says Stanford biologist Dr. Norman Ruby – it also appears to be crucial for memories of your daily learning.

Like any animal, Siberian hamsters have a canny survival sense that allows them to learn and remember critical aspects of their environment. But disrupting their circadian rhythm makes it impossible for them to remember their environmental at all, and they fail to recognize objects in the environment they had previously investigated. Prior to this 2008 study, the link between the circadian system and memory had not been known. But the finding has deep potential meaning for learning- and memory-related disorders like Down syndrome and Alzheimer's disease.

According to Dr. Ruby, GABA causes this memory decline. GABA is the brain's most plentiful inhibitory neurotransmitter. Circadian rhythms partly control animal sleep-wake cycles by inhibiting different brain regions with GABA release. An overabundance of GABA in the hippocampus—critical for memory formation—inhibits the normal function of circuits which govern memory storage. These circuits need to be in an excited state to encode and strengthen memories on a molecular level, according to Dr. Ruby.

Using bright light exposure late at night, Dr. Ruby's team was able to quickly and completely disable lab animal circadian systems. With their circadian rhythms malfunctioning, the Siberian hamsters had chronically high GABA levels. Instead of a rhythmic release of GABA, it was being constantly output.

His team next used a GABA *antagonist* (blocker) called *PTZ,* which prevents GABA from binding to synaptic receptors. As a result, the hamsters' hippocampal synapses continued firing, keeping the brain in an excited state, and allowing the formerly learning-impaired animals to catch up to their fellow (non-circadian-disrupted) hamsters in learning ability. In the same way, Down syndrome sufferers have been found to perform poorly on cognitive tests because they have overly-inhibited brains. Mice with Down syndrome and Alzheimer's symptoms respond to PTZ just as Dr. Ruby's hamsters, improving significantly in learning and memory.

Because GABA antagonists improve Alzheimer's symptoms, there may be a link to the circadian system: degradation of the sleep-wake cycle is common among aging humans, and if circadian regulation of GABA levels is indeed a major component of memory function, it may underlie short-term memory impairment. This also suggests that losing your circadian timing may have serious negative consequences, triggering excessive inhibitory GABA levels, which impede your ability to learn.

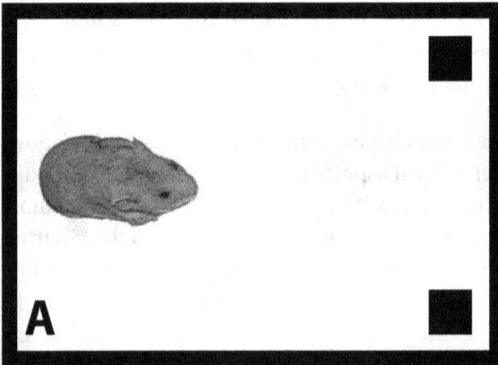

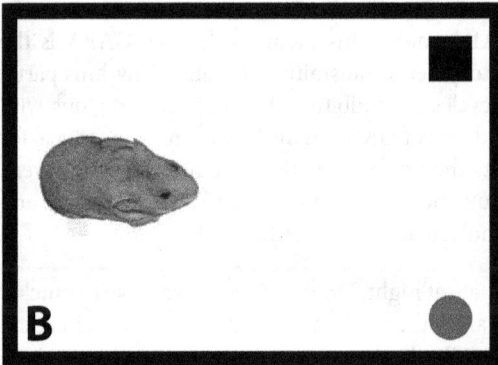

Two steps of the novel object recognition test: hamsters with disrupted circadian rhythms have elevated GABA in their hippocampi, inhibiting memory retention. Illustration, Polyglot Studios, 2011

While laboratory animals with disabled circadian systems tend to live long, healthy lives, they can become completely incapable of remembering. To measure these effects, Dr. Ruby's research team ran the animals through a novel *object recognition task* which uses hamsters' innate exploratory natures.

Two identical objects like saltshakers were placed in adjacent corners of a 2-foot square box, and each hamster was placed opposite them in the box. The hamsters spent roughly the same amount of time investigating each object, and were taken out of the box after 5 minutes, and one of the objects replaced with a different object, such as a shot glass.

20 minutes to an hour later, the hamsters were returned to the box. Most animals will spend twice as much time concentrating on investigating the new object, because they understand they've seen the other previously, but every time Dr. Ruby's circadian-rhythm-disabled hamsters were returned to their boxes, they acted as if both objects were completely new, spending an equal amount of time upon each object. In other words, they were unable to remember having encountered one of the objects previously.

__Keeping Time__ – Biological clocks regulate several biochemical processes, including cell division and the sleep/wake cycle, irrespective of external time. This is the basis of jet lag: when you've spent a lifetime waking and sleeping on Pacific Standard Time, then take a flight across the globe, while it's nighttime during your visit to Paris, your body still "knows" it's midmorning in Seattle. This internal timer needs to be reset like your wrist watch when you change time zones or work in shifts, according to Dr. Ralf Stanewsky of the University of London.

In 2011, Dr. Stanewsky discovered how light synchronizes internal biological clocks. The proteins he calls quasimodo (QSM) and cryptochrome (CRY) use fluctuations in light to control biological clocks. QSM and CRY increase dramatically in response to light. This increase breaks down a timing protein called timeless (TIM). Conversely, as QSM and CRY levels decrease, TIM protein stabilizes. These fluctuating levels of TIM protein are what trigger alertness and rest states in fruit flies, and, he says, in humans.

One Amino Acid to Rule Them All

Paolo Sassone-Corsi, Distinguished Professor and Chair of Pharmacology at the University of California, has found a single amino acid which functions as a genetic switch controlling your circadian rhythms. Circadian rhythms adapt your metabolic, arousal and endocrine states based upon the time of day. As many as 10 to 15 percent of all human genes are regulated by such circadian rhythms, and disrupting them can profoundly impact health, with the potential for depression, heart disease, cancer and neurodegenerative disorders.

Dr. Sassone-Corsi's team has discovered that changes to this single amino acid trigger the genetic production involved in regulating circadian rhythms. The *CLOCK gene* expresses an enzyme which modifies *chromatin*, the protein-DNA-packaging in the nucleus of your cells. If this amino-acid modification is impaired, it can alter the genetic basis of circadian-rhythm protein production, and may thus be at the bottom of a great range of sleep-cycle disorders.

Sleep Deprivation

It's possible to force yourself to stay awake for extended periods, but after approximately 48 hours, your prefrontal function begins to significantly decline. 24 hours later, your PFC effectively shuts down, dropping your performance to the level of someone who is legally defined as drunk. After 88 hours with no sleep, you'll start to experience hallucinations. At this point (luckily) your brain will automatically shut down, rendering you unconscious.

Sleep deprivation impairs working memory, and, because of this, higher-level cognitive functionality in terms of decision-making, reasoning, and semantic and episodic memory. After four days of sleep deprivation, working memory functionality drops by 38%.

But even losing half a night's sleep has a major impact on the ability to think and form memories, according to 2011 research at MIT, Penn and Tufts Universities. Sleep deprivation elevates adenosine in the hippocampus, the brain region responsible for memory consolidation and spatial navigation. Adenosine binds to receptors which inhibit synaptic plasticity, making memory formation much more difficult to achieve. As a result, there is significant impairment to memory and attention.

Adenosine triphosphate (ATP) is the chemical basis for energy transfer between cells. When an animal has insufficient sleep, glial support cells release adenosine from the ATP molecule, and this adenosine binds to A1 receptors in the hippocampus, receptors which inhibit memory formation.

Less than seven hours of sleep per night also decreases blood flow to the brain. At the same time, the sleep-deprived brain produces more dopamine, presumably to maintain attention and wakefulness despite the need and/ or urge to sleep; this is the same mechanism at work with drugs like amphetamines (speed). The increased attentiveness does not compensate for the memory and cognitive impairment of sleep deprivation, however.

According to Dr. Nora Volkow, director of the National Institute on Drug Abuse, sleep deprivation increases dopamine in the striatum, which plays a central role in motivation. It also boosts dopamine release in the thalamus, central to alertness. The dopamine increase is enough for minimal functionality, but not enough to overcome the cognitive and memory impairment of sleep deprivation, and the excess dopamine may contribute to sleep-deprived cognitive decline.

The long-term effects of chronic sleep deprivation on dopamine pathways in the brain are not yet known, but *sleep apnea* is known to cause serious brain problems over time – dramatically impairing parietal lobe activity, for example.

Breakdown Of Self-Control And Judgment

On a personal level, sleep deprivation's effects on judgment can have extreme negative consequences. Healthy adults use the prefrontal cortex to inhibit impulsive behavior, but a lack of sleep can reduce PFC functionality.

Dysfunctional emotional processing can lead to dangerous, risky behaviours such as addictions and to mood disorders. Your prefrontal cortex is key to inhibiting undesirable behavior. Sleep deprivation impairs PFC emotional regulation, creating exaggerated limbic system reactions to both positive and negative experiences.

Using fMRI scans, researchers found sleep deprivation amplifies reactivity to pleasure-evoking stimuli in the mesolimbic system. This amplified reactivity is accompanied by enhanced visual and limbic processing, and with a reduction in medial frontal and orbitofrontal inhibitory and judgmental processing. This increases emotional reactions to potential rewards, and enhances reactivity toward negative stimuli. In other words, the less sleep you've had, the more appealing temptations and risky behavior look to you.

2011 research at the Walter Reed Army Institute of Research shows that daytime sleepiness also impairs self-control in particular. fMRI scans show greater sleepiness during the day correlates with decreased PFC activity as subjects look at temptations like high-calorie food.

Harvard Medical School's Dr. William Killgor says this study demonstrates how even normal fluctuations in sleepiness alter brain activity that regulates willpower-related behavior such as caloric consumption. In his experiment, 12 healthy 19- to 45-year-olds of both sexes received fMRI scans while looking at pictures of high-calorie foods, low-calorie foods, and non-food-related control images.

In modern industrialized societies, sleep deprivation is at "chronic levels", with profound implications, according to Dr. Kilgore. His previous studies have shown that women's PFCs respond significantly more to such images than men's.

Sleep deprivation also impairs the integration of cognition and emotion when making moral decisions. Dr. Killgore had 26 subjects choose appropriate solutions to three kinds of moral dilemmas. Each subject was tested twice – once in a normal state, and again after 53 hours without sleep. Sleep deprivation resulted in significantly longer times to decide upon a course of action. Says Dr. Kilgore, the state detracts from the ability to integrate emotion as a guide to judgments and decision-making, an ability controlled mainly by the ventromedial (bottom and center) prefrontal cortex. People with damage to this region have major deficits in their ability for emotional responses, and react quite differently to moral questions.

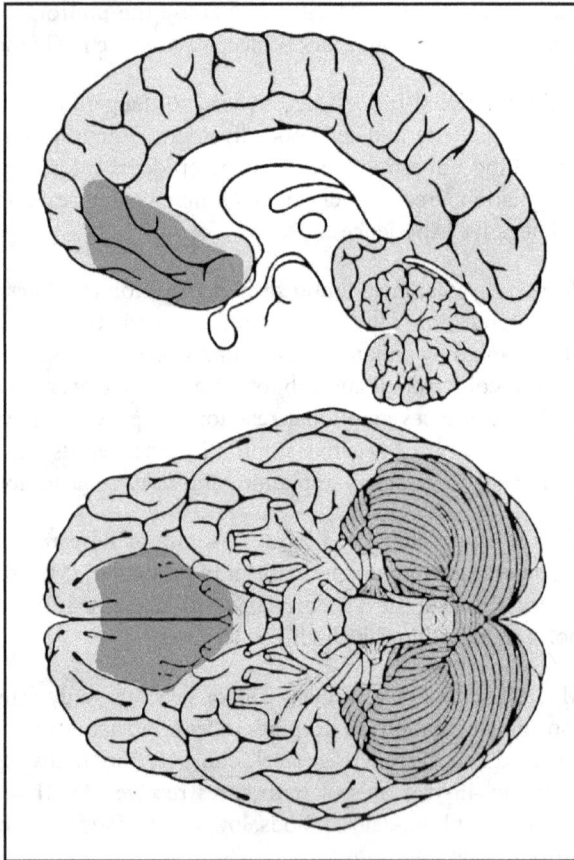

Ventromedial prefrontal cortex, Wikipedia, 2011, public domain

Minor to major moral dilemmas affect everyone on a daily basis, says Dr. Killgore. And as sleep declines, it slows the ability to respond to such dilemmas, and leads to greater moral tolerance. His findings are particularly significant to people who deal with real-world moral dilemmas in chronic sleep-deprived states – doctors, emergency response teams, police and military personnel.

Gadgets Are Ruining Your Sleep - *95% of respondents surveyed by the National Sleep Foundation said they watched television, used smartphones or computers or played videogames within an hour of turning in for the night.*

Heavy use of these light-emitting screens within an hour before bed-time enhances alertness and suppresses the release of melatonin, the body's natural sleep hormone, leading to sleep problems, according to Harvard Medical School director Dr. Charles Czeisler.

Particularly among the young, increasing exposure to these sleep-disrupting technologies can lead to a deterioration of physical health and mental function over time. To combat the effects of a lack of sleep, many people then turn to excessive amounts of caffeine, which only serves to compound the problem.

A number of things can contribute to poor sleep. Within the last 75 years, we have become progressively more exposed to bright artificial lights at night, which have been shown to reduce melatonin secretion, and older people tend to be more sensitive to such environmental sleep disturbances. Deliberately resisting sleep can also lead to a *second wind*, making it difficult to return to sleep afterwards. Clinical disorders, including excessive worry, sleep apnea, narcolepsy and circadian rhythm disorders are generally treatable, however.

Exercise appears to improve sleep for most, even insomniacs. Although any time of day is beneficial, the best time for exercise is thought to be four to eight hours before bedtime. However, immediately before bedtime, exercise may disrupt sleep.

The Super-Easy Weight Loss Secret

In 2009, *Glamour* magazine conducted a fascinating experiment: a pair of doctors had said it was possible to drop weight through just changing sleep-ing routines. With the magazine's go-ahead, Drs. Michael Breus and Steven Lamm wrote a 10-week plan for seven women of varying weights.

The only change to their lifestyles was to get a minimum of seven and a half hours of sleep every night. They were specifically instructed to continue eating the way they normally did, and to exercise the same amount, trying to determine if sleep alone could make a difference. All but one of the seven subjects lost weight, between six and 15 pounds.

A number of studies within the last decade have shown strong links between sleep deprivation and weight gain. Sleeping under seven hours increases obesity risk about 30 percent. A 2005 multi-year study of 8,000 adults in the National Health and Nutrition Examination Survey found that sleeping less than seven hours nightly increases the risk of obesity, the risk increasing for every hour of lost sleep.

Since human sleep cycles are synchronized to the Earth's daily rotation, when the sun sets, the body is programmed to sleep, rather than eat. Sleeping and eating habits which are out of alignment with the body's natural circadian rhythms lead to substantial changes in appetite and metabolism.

According to Case Western Reserve University's Dr. Sanjay Patel, 24 separate studies have shown that people tend to weigh more when they get less sleep. Dr. Patel and his colleagues studied nearly 70,000 women over the course of 16 years and found those getting five hours or less sleep per night had a 30 percent greater likelihood of gaining 30 pounds or more than those who slept better.

Short sleepers have a 27-percent increased risk of becoming obese, whether or not they're active, and irrespective of diet. This is likely due to sleep's role in regulating a number of metabolic- and appetite-controlling signalling molecules like human growth hormone, leptin, and ghrelin.

Clinical psychologist Dr. Michael J. Breus, known as "The Sleep Doctor", also says too little sleep unquestionably leads to weight gain, and that working out and dieting alone cannot be completely effective for weight maintenance with insufficient sleep. Sleep deprivation causes significant imbalances in the hormones controlling appetite, cravings and fat metabolism, so people tend to eat more the less sleep they get. Sleep deprivation specifically triggers an increase in the appetite-stimulating hormone ghrelin, accompanied by a drop in leptin, the hormone which signals satiety.

To add icing to the proverbial cake, tiredness also prompts cravings specifically for the quick energy boost of simple carbohydrates, so when you don't sleep, you're driven to eat white flours, pastries, ice cream, candy, and the like.

Subjects with only five and a half hours of sleep take in dramatically more carbohydrate-based calories than after sleeping for eight and a half hours.

Late sleepers eat more and worse calories at night, tending to weigh more, and to eat too little produce and too much fast food, according to a 2011 study conducted at Northwestern University. While most people are asleep, late sleepers tend to consume up to an additional 248 calories a day, 200% as much fast food and 50% of the fruits and vegetables as regular sleepers, most of those extra calories during dinnertime or later, when the brain's natural circadian rhythms slow energy consumption. These extra calories can add up to an extra two pounds of weight per month if there is no regular exercise to offset the calorie boost.

A similar study conducted at the University of Chicago showed subjects ate 221 more calories on average when they were tired. Over the course of just two weeks, that translates into a pound of extra fat – 26 pounds a year. And in 2010, the American Journal of Clinical Nutrition found that men who only slept four hours took in over 500 extra calories (about 22 percent more) than when they slept for eight hours. 500 calories a day for just one week results in one pound of fat gain.

Your brain secretes a large amount of human growth hormone during slow wave sleep, which assists in the metabolism of fat. When you don't get enough slow-wave sleep, excess calories consumed during the day get stored as fat. Conversely, sufficient sleep restores energy levels, providing the motivation to exercise and the perception that the exercises are easier.

The effects are reciprocal: a 2010 Australian study of over 300 obese individuals who received surgery for weight loss showed a tremendous reduction of sleep problems after their weight loss:

- Habitual Snoring (82 percent) reduced to 14 percent

- Observed sleep apnea (33 percent) reduced to two percent

- Abnormal daytime sleepiness (39 percent) reduced to four percent

- Poor sleep quality (39 percent) reduced to two percent

Sleep Deprivation and Health

For poor sleepers, the news gets worse: in 2011, the University of Toronto's Dr. John Peever discovered a major link between a sleep disorder, Parkinson's and other diseases. 60 to 80 percent of those diagnosed with human REM sleep behavior disorder (RBD) eventually develop Parkinson's and other neurodegenerative diseases later in life, according to Dr. Peever. RBD is characterized by violent movements during REM sleep. Its sufferers don't undergo REM *atonia*, the typical muscle paralysis that prevents thrashing about in dreams; some RBD sufferers need to be tied to their beds as a safety precaution. *Clonazepam* is currently used to treat human RBD patients.

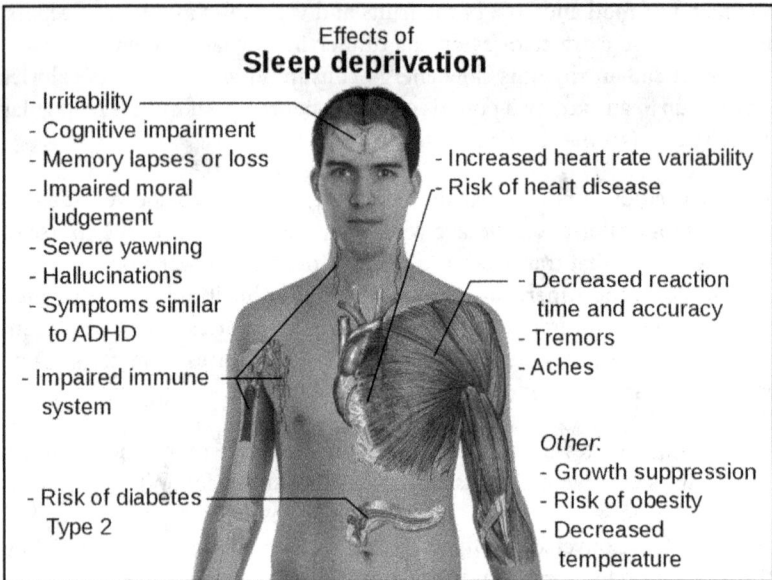

Effects of
Sleep deprivation

- Irritability
- Cognitive impairment
- Memory lapses or loss
- Impaired moral judgement
- Severe yawning
- Hallucinations
- Symptoms similar to ADHD
- Impaired immune system
- Risk of diabetes Type 2

- Increased heart rate variability
- Risk of heart disease
- Decreased reaction time and accuracy
- Tremors
- Aches

Other:
- Growth suppression
- Risk of obesity
- Decreased temperature

Effects Of Sleep Deprivation, Michael Haggstrom, 2009, public domain

Sleep Deprivation And Cancer

A study at the University of Barcelona has linked *sleep apnea* (recurrent awakening due to interrupted breathing) to the spread of aggressive cancer and increases in tumor growth in mice. This is the first experiment showing *hypoxia* (high-rate intermittent lack of oxygen) enhances tumor growth.

The condition affects 5 percent of Americans, and is associated with a heightened risk of cardiovascular disease, high blood pressure, daytime sleepiness and lower quality of life. Says lead author Dr. Ramon Farre, hypoxia is known to promote cancer growth, though it's not yet known whether it specifically triggers tumor formation or promotes *metastasis*, the spread of tumors between organs. Sleep apnea is linked to obesity as well as cancer promotion, so it's not yet clear to what extent hypoxia and obesity interact to promote cancer.

Master Regulators

Sleep and wakefulness need to occur at the most appropriate times to help you avoid danger and find food. These two survival activities are controlled by internal and external conditions – your emotions, your energy needs, and the presence of potential rewards. Both avoiding danger and finding food require vigilance, and therefore a state of wakefulness.

The *orexin* hormonal system is remarkably efficient at helping creatures meet their homeostatic needs: when faced with a reduction in available food, animals adapt a longer waking period, disrupting circadian rhythms. On the other hand, during REM sleep, where recuperation and memory consolidation are a priority, orexin activation stops.

Your hypothalamus is sent hormonal and neurotransmitter signals indicating your internal and external states, and it responds by releasing the hormones *orexin A* and *orexin B*. The neurons which release these hormones interact with systems regulating emotion (the limbic system), reward (the VTA-NA dopamine circuit) and energy homeostasis (blood glucose, ghrelin and leptin levels).

Orexin neurons promote wakefulness and are inhibited to allow sleep. These orexin neurons project throughout the CNS, particularly exciting the thalamus, VTA, brain stem and midbrain, where they increase arousal and attention by triggering dopamine, norepinephrine, serotonin (monamines), acetylcholine, and histamine release, exciting the cortex and thalamus.

Hunger (low blood glucose and stomach release of ghrelin), emotional excitement (excitation from the limbic system, primarily the amygdala), sensory stimulation, and sleep deprivation all increase orexin release, thus increasing arousal.

To promote sleep, another set of neurons in the hypothalamus called the *preoptic nucleus* releases inhibitory GABA and *galanin* to shut down orexin and brain stem monoamine activity.

In addition to regulating sleep/wake cycles, orexins amplify chemical sensitivity, with a major impact upon metabolism, feeding behaviours, and reward responses, helping increase dopamine release in the NA-VTA dopamine circuit, for example.

Orexin And Cancer

Now the role of orexins in the spread of cancer is also coming to light. Southwestern Medical Center researchers studying orexin effects on sleep and hunger discovered it primarily activates the *HIF-1 gene*, well-known to stimulate glucose catabolism – and to promote cancerous tumor growth.

Dr. Thomas Kodadek, a senior author of the study, says "HIF-1 is very big in the cancer community." Your body revs up orexin production when blood sugar gets low, and this increase activates HIF-1 expression, encouraging your body to extract energy from available glucose supplies in the most efficient manner possible: at the coaxing of orexin, HIF-1 makes cells use oxygen to burn sugar, (aerobic metabolism), processing and consuming glucose more quickly and efficiently. This strategy makes evolutionary sense, says lead author Dr. Devanjan Sikder:

> *You need to be active and energetic, especially when you're hungry, so you can search for a meal. This orexin pathway we found is basically an overdrive function. Even though blood sugar levels are low, you're not only awake, but you're also energetic because of the action of HIF-1.*

But HIF-1 acts differently upon tumors than upon normal cells, altering cellular metabolism to allow sugar to be burned for energy in the *absence* of oxygen (*anaerobic metabolism*), and thus promoting the survival of malignant cells.

Orexin And Alzheimer's

A 2009 Washington University study discovered links between sleep deprivation, orexin, and the production of *amyloid beta protein fragments,* associated with Alzheimer's disease. The study strongly suggests the development of Alzheimer's may be linked to chronic or acute sleep deprivation.

Amyloid betas are secreted by neurons into the fluid between brain cells, called *interstitial fluid* or *ISF.* These amyloid betas can degrade into tangled protein strands called *fibrils*, which clump into *plaques*, thought to cause the neural die-off of Alzheimer's. The disease starts in the hippocampus, which leads to *dementia* – permanent memory loss and disorientation.

Sleep-restricted laboratory mice have much greater plaque deposits and hippocampal damage when compared with litter mates allowed to sleep normally. Orexin neurons project to the hippocampus, where orexin receptors are expressed, so this is the location chosen to monitor Aß production.

Amyloid beta production increases when orexin is administered or with wakefulness, particularly during acute sleep deprivation. Production of these amyloid beta fragments decreases when orexin is blocked or when sleep cycles are normal. Synaptic activity has been found to influence amyloid beta production, with greater activity during wakefulness, so differences in synaptic activity between sleep and wake states, via orexin signalling, apparently underlie fluctuations in Aß levels.

According to the study's authors,

Sleep disturbances, in addition to being prominent in neurodegenerative diseases, could exacerbate a fundamental process leading to neurodegeneration, and optimization of sleep time could potentially inhibit aggregation of toxic proteins and slow the progression of AD.

The long and short of it is that researchers are finding unhealthy sleep habits have a much more significant impact upon your health than simply making you feel tired. The benefits of a good night's rest, on a regular basis, cannot be overstated.

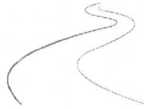

The Mind and Body During Sleep, Dr. Gregg D. Jacobs, 2011; http://www.talkaboutsleep.com/sleep-disorders/archives/insomnia_drjacobs_mindandbodyduringsleep.htm

QUASIMODO, a Novel GPI-Anchored Zona Pellucida Protein Involved in Light Input to the Drosophila Circadian Clock, Ko Fan Chen, Nicolai Peschel, Radka Zavodska, Hana Sehadova, Ralf Stanewsky, 2011 Current Biology; 21 (9): 719 DOI: 10.1016/j.cub.2011.03.049;

The ELF4–ELF3–LUX Complex Links the Circadian Clock to Diurnal Control of Hypocotyl Growth, Dmitri A. Nusinow, Anne Helfer, Elizabeth E. Hamilton, Jasmine J. King, Takato Imaizumi, Thomas F. Schultz, Eva M. Farré, Steve A. Kay, 2011, Nature; DOI: 10.1038/nature10182; http://www.nature.com/nature/journal/vaop/ncurrent/full/nature10182.html

Circadian Clock may be Critical to Learning and Memory, press release, Louis Bergeron, Stanford Report, October 8, 2008;

Extra Sleep Improves Athletes' Performance. American Academy of Sleep Medicine, 2007, June 14, ScienceDaily, February 23, 2011

The Memory Function of Sleep, Jan Born, Christian Benedict, Sonja Binder, Gordon Feld, Susanne Diekelmann, Stoyan Dimitrov, Spyridos Drosopoulos, Stephan Fischer, Steffen Gais, Manfred Hallschmid, Rosi Krug, Tanja Lange, Lisa Marshall, Matthias Mölle, Barbara Ölke, Volker Ott, Christiane Otten, Anja Otterbein, Björn Rasch, Ullrich Wagner, Ines Wilhelm, Trends in Cognitive Science 2007;11:442-50

Sleep's Role in the Consolidation of Emotional Episodic Memories, Elizabeth A. Kensinger and Jessica D. Payne, 2010, Current Directions in Psychological Science, doi: 10.1177/0963721410383978 vol. 19 no. 5 290-295;

Sleep Selectively Enhances Memory Expected to Be of Future Relevance, Ines Wilhelm, Susanne Diekelmann, Ina Molzow, Amr Ayoub, Matthias Mölle, and Jan Born, 2011, The Journal of Neuroscience, 31(5): 1563-1569; doi: 10.1523/JNEUROSCI.3575-10.2011;

The Body Clock Guide to Better Health: How to Use your Body's Natural Clock to Fight Illness and Achieve Maximum Health, Michael Smolensky and Lynne Lamberg, 2000

Sleep And Weight-Loss: They Are More Connected Than You Think, Jacob Teitelbaum, M.D., February 19, 2011, The Huffington Post

As We Sleep, Speedy Brain Waves Boost Learning Ability, Yasmin Anwar, 2011, University of California Berkeley press release; http://www.universityofcalifornia.edu/news/article/25099

Afternoon Nap Boosts Brain's Learning Capacity, Yasmin Anwar, 2011, University of California Berkeley press release; http://www.universityofcalifornia.edu/news/article/22872

REM, not Incubation, Improves Creativity by Priming Associative Networks, Denise Cai, D., Mednick, S., Harrison, E., Kanady, J., & Mednick, S., 2009. Proceedings of the National Academy of Sciences DOI: 10.1073/pnas.0900271106

Sleep Your Way to an A, Sharon Begley, 2011, Newsweek; http://www.newsweek.com/2011/02/13/sleep-your-way-to-an-a.html

New Regulator of Circadian Clock Identified: Dopamine Study May Have Impact on Activity and Sleep Rhythms in Parkinson's Disease, Sylvain-Jacques Desjardins, October 18, 2010, Concordia University

Endogenous Dopamine Regulates the Rhythm of Expression of the Clock Protein PER2 in the Rat Dorsal Striatum via Daily Activation of D2 Dopamine Receptors, Suzanne Hood, Pamela Cassidy, Marie-Pierre Cossette, Yuval Weigl, Michael Verwey, Barry Robinson, Jane Stewart, and Shimon Amir. Journal of Neuroscience, 2010; DOI: 10.1523/JNEUROSCI.2128-10.2010

Genetic Switch For Circadian Rhythms Discovered, press release, Dec. 12, 2007, UC Irvine

Hippocampal Synaptic Plasticity and Memory in Mice, Cédrick Florian, Christopher G. Vecsey, Michael M. Halassa, Philip G. Haydon, and Ted Abel, 2011, . Journal of Neuroscience, 2011; 31 (19): 6956 DOI: 10.1523/JNEUROSCI.5761-10.2011; http://www.jneurosci.org/content/31/19/6956.abstract

Astrocyte-Derived Adenosine and A1 Receptor Activity Contribute to Sleep Loss-Induced Deficits in Hippocampal Synaptic Plasticity And Memory In Mice, Florian C, Vecsey CG, Halassa MM, Haydon PG, Abel T., J Neurosci. 2011 May 11;31(19):6956-62.

Evidence for the Re-Enactment of a Recently Learned Behavior during Sleepwalking, Delphine Oudiette, Irina Constantinescu, Laurène Leclair-Visonneau, Marie Vidailhet, Sophie Schwartz,Isabelle Arnulf, PLoS ONE, 2011; http://www.plosone.org/article/info%3Adoi%2F10.1371%2Fjournal.pone.0018056

One Sleepless Night Increases Dopamine In The Human Brain, press release, Sarah Bates and Kat Snodgrass, 2008, Society for Neuroscience;

Sleep Deprivation Amplifies Reactivity of Brain Reward Networks, Biasing the Appraisal of Positive Emotional Experiences, Ninad Gujar, Seung-Schik Yoo, Peter Hu, and Matthew P. Walker,

2011; The Journal of Neuroscience, 23 March 2011, 31(12): 4466-4474; doi: 10.1523/?JNEU-ROSCI.3220-10

Improved Academic Success, Kelly Wagner, June 02, 2009, American Academy of Sleep Medicine; http://www.aasmnet.org/articles.aspx?id=1328

Lucid Dreaming FAQ, Stephen LaBerge, 2004; http://lucidity.com/LucidDreamingFAQ.html

Not Getting Enough Sleep? Turn Off the Technology, Patricia Reaney, Reuters, Mar 7, 2011

Sleep More. Weigh Less. Sleepiness May Impair The Brain's Inhibitory Control When Viewing High-Calorie Foods, Emilee McStay, 2011 Media Relations, American Academy of Sleep Medicine; http://www.aasmnet.org/articles.aspx?id=2308

Sleep Deprivation Affects Moral Judgment, Study Finds, American Academy of Sleep Medicine March 2, 2007

Obstructive Sleep Apnea Linked To Cancer Growth In Mice, ScienceDaily, May 18, 2011, from http://www.sciencedaily.com/releases/2011/05/110517141448.htm

The Link Between Sleep and Weight Loss, Dr. Michael J. Breus, May 24, 2010, Huffington Post;

Hormone Links Sleep, Hunger And Metabolism, UT Southwestern Medical Center, ScienceDaily. Retrieved June 4, 2011, from http://www.sciencedaily.com /releases/2007/11/071114183255.htm

Human Growth Hormone Release: Relation to Slow-Wave Sleep and Sleep-Waking Cycles, J. F. Sassin, D. C. Parker, et al, 1969, Science 1 August:Vol. 165 no. 3892 pp. 513-515; DOI: 10.1126/science.165.3892.513; http://www.sciencemag.org/content/165/3892/513.short

Role of Sleep Timing in Caloric Intake and BMI, Kelly G. Baron, Kathryn J. Reid, Andrew S. Kern, Phyllis C. Zee, 2011 Obesity; DOI: 10.1038/oby.2011.100; http://www.ncbi.nlm.nih.gov/pubmed/21527892

Role of Sleep and Sleep Loss in Hormonal Release and Metabolism, Rachel Leproult and Eve Van Cauter, Pediatric Neuroendocrinology, 2010; 17: 11–21 doi: 10.1159/000262524; http://www.ncbi.nlm.nih.gov/pmc/articles/PMC3065172/

Lose Weight While You Sleep! Jenny Stamos Kovacs, Glamour Magazine, February 2, 2009; http://www.glamour.com/magazine/2009/02/lose-weight-while-you-sleep?mbid=huffposleep

Going To Bed Late May Affect The Health, Academic Performance Of College Students, American Academy of Sleep Medicine (2007, June 14)

The Neural Circuit Of Orexin (Hypocretin): Maintaining Sleep And Wakefulness, Takeshi Sakurai, 2007, Nature Reviews Neuroscience 8, 171-181; doi:10.1038/nrn2092; http://www.nature.com/nrn/journal/v8/n3/full/nrn2092.html#B15

Amyloid-ß Dynamics are Regulated by Orexin and the Sleep-Wake Cycle, Jae-Eun Kang,1 Miranda M. Lim,1 Randall J. Bateman,et al, 2009, Science; 326(5955): 1005–1007; doi: 10.1126/science.1180962;

409

Live

"Age is strictly a case of mind over matter. If you don't mind, it doesn't matter."
– Jack Benny, US comedian, NY Times, Feb. 15, 1974

"This is real science.... It's going to happen. It's no longer an 'if', but a 'when' now."
– Dr. David Sinclair, Harvard Medical School, speaking about life extension, 2009

The Genes Of 800-Year-Olds

By repressing two genes, the University of Southern California's Dr. Valter Longo extended the normal lifespan of baker's yeast from 6 days to 10 weeks – equivalent to 800 human years. A human with this benefit would have been born when Genghis Khan's Mongol hordes invaded central China, between the fourth and fifth Crusades.

Dr. Longo has been studying metabolic regulatory pathways since 1997. His research team had first tripled the lifespan of yeast by inhibiting a growth stimulant – deleting the single *SCH-9 gene*. Seven years later, his lab discovered life could be extended a staggering tenfold by removing a second (*RAS2*) gene, along with restricting calories. Along with the *Insulin-Growth Factor-1* chemical pathway, these pathways are at work in most multicellular life, including humans.

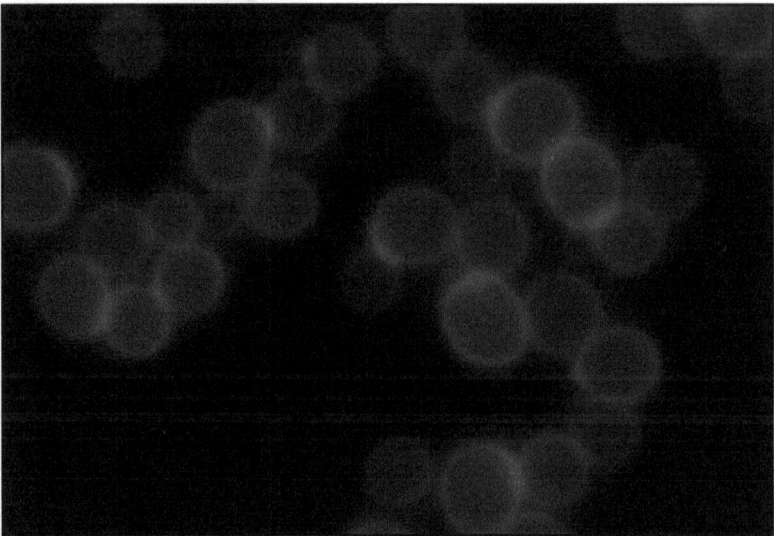

Methuselah yeast. By knocking out two genes, Dr. Longo created baker's yeast capable of living the equivalent of 800 human years. Valter Longo, 2008. Used with permission.

The two genes control twin metabolic pathways at the heart of caloric restriction and its life-extending benefits. Many scientists believe mito-chondria breakdown is the source of age-related diseases like cancer, heart disease, and Alzheimer's.

Caloric restriction triggers the production of enzymes which protect and restore mitochondria, cellular energy factories. In other words, a shortage of nutrients pushes cells into "maintenance mode", redirecting energy from growth and reproduction into protective and restorative anti-aging processes.

Cracking Cancer

In related research, Dr. Longo announced in 2008 that 48-hour fasting helps protect cells against the chemotherapy toxicity, without reducing its ability to kill cancer cells:

> A few years ago, I realized, the same genes that are controlling aging are sort of stuck in "on mode" in the majority of cancers. If in fact these genes that are stuck in the on mode are present in all cancer cells, then those cells would be the ones that do not respond to the order to be protected.
>
> And that's in fact what we saw; that you starve the cells and the or-ganism goes into high protection mode, but the cancer cells fail to enter this high-protection mode. And so they continue to be in a pro cell-division mode but also a mode that makes them... sensitive to chemotherapy.

With an $11.5 million-dollar award from the National Institutes of Health providing momentum, Dr. Longo's pioneering studies are continuing.

The Age "On-Off" Switch

The announcement was electrifying:

"What we have identified is a binary switch that turns the aging process on and off," said Salk Institute's Dr. Andrew Dillin in 2011.

That year, he and colleague Dr. Reuben Shaw found a protein "on-off switch" for aging in a wide range of species. Deactivating this single pro-tein in roundworms increased their lifespan 40%, apparently through the same pathways activated by calorie restriction. The enzyme *AMPK* acts as a sensor when food is scarce, switching cells into a state of low energy. This in turn appears to directly extend life.

Said Dr. Dillin, "We knew AMPK was a major energy sensor, but didn't know what it was talking to. Our goal was to understand the genetic circuitry."

The AMPK-boosting effects of dietary restriction are a powerful means of combatting age-related diseases like cancer, diabetes and Alzheimer's in a wide swath of life, from the simplest of yeasts to roundworms, labrador retrievers and rhesus monkeys. *Metformin*, a medication for diabetes, and *resveratrol*, a lifespan-extending antifungal enzyme produced by grapes, both have functions activated by the AMPK enzyme.

AMPK is a *kinase*, an enzyme which deactivates proteins. Kinases bind phosphate "locks" to proteins, changing their molecular form and rendering them inactive. A second enzyme called *calcineurin* can later remove these phosphate locks.

AMPK deactivates a special growth-promoting protein called CRTC1, and this extends a roundworm's lifespan by an incredible 40% – from three weeks to over a month. Suppressing calcineurin's "lock removal" keeps these CRTC1 proteins locked into a nonfunctioning state. Together, this AMPK-calcineurin "push-pull switch" extends roundworm's lives by regulating CRTC1.

The same molecular switch exists in a variety of species, and learning to control it may soon significantly reduce the effects of a number of age-related diseases. The entire pathway – AMPK, calcineurin, and CRTC1 – appears to function in humans just as with roundworms. A well-known version of CRTC1 in humans is the gene regulator *CREB*, and worms without the worm form of CREB live longer, just like worms deficient in CRTC1.

Skin Returned To Newborn State In Two Weeks

Suppressing a single gene, Stanford University researchers returned aged mouse skin to newborn condition. Genetically engineering mice to inhibit skin *NF-kappa-B* proteins returned the cells to the same appearance and genetic status as in newborns after just two weeks.

As you age, the gene which produces NF-kappa-B protein becomes progressively more active. Stanford professor Dr. Howard Chang says this gene doesn't specifically cause aging, but is involved in a number of processes related to immunity and inflammation. It has several functions, including some involved in cancer's onset, so potential side effects have to be carefully studied before the process can be used with human patients. The expression of a number of genes changes as you age, some becoming more and some less active over time. So far scientists have discovered about 60 genes involved in aging. Many of these are regulated by the NF-kappa-B protein.

The team engineered mice which aged normally, but with a single patch of skin which returned to youth. This, says Dr. Chang, shows it's possible to selectively target specific body regions, and by manipulating a single gene, to turn back the clock. This also seems to add strength to the theory that aging comes not so much from life's wear-and-tear as from specific, age-related genetic changes; changes that can (at least temporarily) be halted.

Because NF-kappa-B participates in so many varied biochemical processes, however, scientists are proceeding with caution; long-term risks of blocking aging through this gene therapy are still unknown; nor does the team know if the youthful tissue will rapidly age after stopping treatment (mice don't live long enough for us to find out).

A Roundworm's Secrets

While lifestyle factors such as diet, stress and physical activity have a marked influence on lifespan, genetics appear to play an even bigger part.

Dr. Dillin uses the tiny roundworm Ceanorhabditis elegans to study the genetics of aging. He says there are presently three known genetic networks which can be manipulated to extend life. The first centers on insulin and the related hormone insulin growth factor-1, which regulates metabolism and growth; the second regulates mitochondria function; and the third centers on caloric restriction.

Among Dr. Dillin's studies is one focusing on insulin, a hormone mostly known for its role in diabetes. The insulin signalling pathway in worms is almost identical to that of humans, helping control many biological processes in worms, including reproduction and larval development – growth. For humans, insulin/IGF-1 signalling control may eventually not only boost longevity, but also lead to cures for diabetes and cancer.

Because the insulin pathway influences multiple processes, manipulating it is tricky. But Dillin's research has led to a means of genetically manipulating one element of the pathway without disrupting additional functions; recently, his team found a protein which extends lifespan and youthfulness without disrupting development and fertility processes, all controlled by the same insulin signalling pathway.

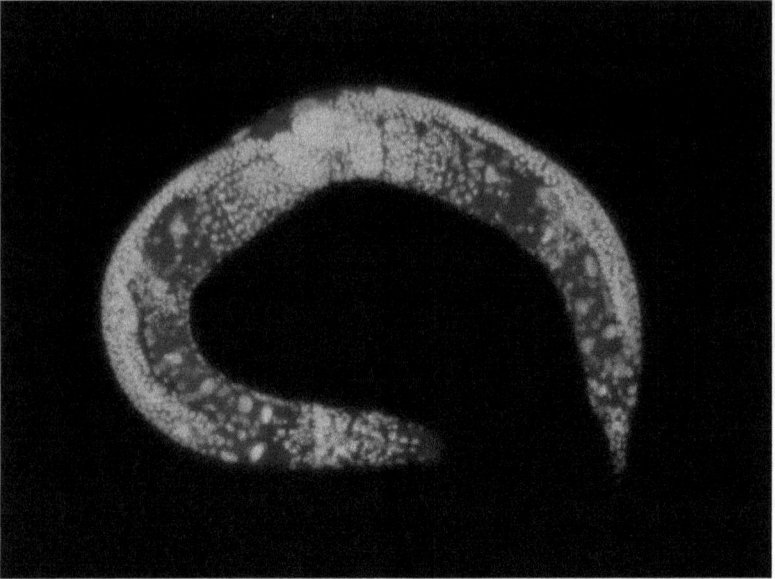

Although it's only about the size of a comma, the tiny roundworm known by the scientific name Caenorhabditis elegans made a huge splash in 1998, when it became the first animal to have its entire 97 million-base genome decoded by a joint US-UK team, a project which took eight years to complete. Like humans, c. elegans has a nervous system, digests food and has sex. Several features make C. elegans ideal for studying gene regulation and function:

1. RNA interference can be used to reduce or eliminate a single gene's function in roundworms, to immediately see how the gene's suppression affects roundworm development.

2. It's a eukaryote, sharing the same cellular and molecular structures and control pathways as more complex creatures, with membrane-enclosed organelles and DNA packed into chromatin and chromosomes. It's also multicellular, so it undergoes complex development as it matures into adulthood. Because of this, information from C. elegans is often directly applicable to humans and other creatures.

3. About 35% of C. elegans genes have human homologs – shared DNA or protein sequences because of common ancestry.

4. The C. elegans genome is comparatively small – 9.7 million base pairs or 97 Megabases compared with the 3-billion-base-pair human genome. The entire C. elegans genome has been mapped out, and several techniques for manipulating its genes are routinely used and well understood.

5. C. elegans is easy to keep alive in laboratory petri dishes, and has a conveniently rapid life cycle: embryogenesis occurs in about 12 hours, maturation to adulthood occurs in 2.5 days, and its full lifespan is 2-3 weeks.

6. Its 1mm long body is transparent, and the development of every one of its 959 cells has been recorded.

General Biology of C. elegans, Human Genome Project, public domain. Summary: C. elegans as a Model System, Andrey Revyakin, Rutgers University

414

The Hunt For One Receptor

Dr. Dillin says a single undiscovered receptor is responsible for triggering cellular longevity. Two enzymes are necessary for activating this receptor; lacking either enzyme cancels out the effects of caloric restriction in round-worms. Finding this receptor may allow scientists to trigger it with drugs that mimic the calorie-restriction signal, leading to radical new treatments for age-related degenerative illnesses. You could then enjoy the life-extension of caloric restriction without unpleasant dieting.

The two regulating enzymes *WWP-1* and *UBC-18* work in tandem, attaching to other proteins, flagging them for destruction; WWP-1 also serves as a regulatory signal. Worms without the WWP-1 gene appear normal but are more susceptible to stress, and mutations related to stress are often involved in longevity.

Even well-fed roundworms engineered to overexpress WWP-1 lived 20 percent longer. The enzyme UBC-18 also plays a part: overexpressing UBC-18 doesn't extend life, but shutting it down negates dietary-restricted longevity. These life-extending effects are also stopped by suppressing PHA-4, the only gene known to be essential for calorie-restricted longevity.

Mitochondria

Dialing down metabolism has long been believed the key to longevity. According to numerous studies, specifically reducing mitochondria energy production extends life.

Researchers have found the mitochondrial *cco-1* gene synthesizes a protein used for ADP-ATP energy production. When the gene is disabled in the intestines and nerves, production of the necessary protein reduced, metabolism slows, and affected creatures live much longer. Because mitochondria are the cell's power generators, it's been proposed that leakage of the high-energy electrons produced by the ADP-ATP cycle may be the source of free radicals linked to disease and aging.

But mitochondria perform a wider range of functions than simple energy production – including helping prevent age-related cell death: Dr. Dillin's latest findings contradict previous beliefs that a simple slowing of metabolism is the sole specific route to extending life – he believes preserving the integrity of cellular protein is the key.

In early 2011, Dr. Dillin's team altered roundworm mitochondria, affecting the entire creature. He says "distressed" mitochondria produce signals to distant tissues, enhancing longevity. He calls these as-yet theoretical distress signals *mitokines*, and, although they have not yet been found, he believes they will someday be used to treat degenerative disorders.

For example, he predicts, we may be able to irritate liver mitochondria, triggering a mitokine signal to degenerating brain neurons, exploiting a natural cell rescue signal that could one day eliminate the need for many drugs.

The specific process enhancing longevity appears to be the *Unfolded Protein Response (UPR)*: When excessive proteins accumulate, they can begin to unravel, and this is toxic to living cells. To avoid cell death, the UPR response recruits molecular "assistants" which refold the unravelling proteins.

By blocking the response, Dr. Dillin's team cancelled its life extension effects, indicating the distress-signal triggered protein refolding – the UPR – the key to longevity.

Says Dr. Dillin, "… it all comes down to protein folding". There are limits, however – this gene manipulation had to take place within a critical window of time for maximal effect. He says that manipulating the mitochondria in a 30-year-old human in this manner might grant an extra 15 years of life, while doing it in an 80-year-old would only grant two or three extra years.

Calorie Restriction

Clinical evidence continues to mount, showing calorie restriction helps lengthen life. The Washington University School of Medicine reported in early 2011 that reducing calorie intake lowers core body temperatures in both animals and humans, to boost longevity.

Human body temperatures vary through life, ranging from 96 to almost 100 degrees, but optimal efficiency for all bodily functions is considered to be 98.6 degrees Fahrenheit (37.7 degrees Celsius). People eating calorie-restricted diets have lower core body temperatures by an average of about 0.2 degrees Celsius. Although this sounds trivial, it's comparable to the reduction found in calorie-restricted mice which far outlive their siblings.

In the simplest of organisms such as yeasts, caloric restriction can double and even triple lifespan, while calorie-restricted rodents live up to 50 percent longer. Human studies in the field are still in their infancy, however, as the link was only discovered within the last decade.

Calorie-restricted diets involve a caloric reduction of 25 percent or more, but vitamins and nutrients are carefully monitored to avoid malnutrition.

Dr. Luigi Fontana, who led the Washington University study, compared core body temperatures between 24 human volunteers in their 50s who had practiced six or more years of calorie restriction, and 24 subjects of the same age who had been eating a standard Western diet. The calorie-restricted participants were members of the CR Society, who like to refer to themselves as *CRONies* (Calorie Restriction with Optimal Nutrition).

Dr. Fontana also measured the core body temperatures of 24 endurance runners of the same age to discover if specifically being lean or calorie restriction is linked to lower body temperatures: lower core body temperature were not found among the endurance runners who were lean but not calorie-restricted.

Dr. Fontana is not sure whether the severe caloric restriction or something else is causing the lower body temperatures, but he is certain the lower temperatures are important to increased longevity. In other words, causality has not yet been proven, but experiments have consistently shown that creatures with lower core body temperatures tend to outlive their warmer fellows.

But it looks like there is more to the longevity equation than simply lowering body temperature. Rodents whose core body temperatures have been lowered by regularly swimming in cold water don't outlive their peers, so it seems that the *manner* in which these lower temperatures are achieved is important.

In the end, it may never be possible to live a wild lifestyle and just pop a single pill which lowers body temperature to extend life, says Dr. Fontana, but it may soon become possible to lengthen lifespan with mild calorie restriction, healthy eating, regular moderate exercise and taking a drug which provides the same benefits as severe calorie restriction.

Hungry Worms

Dr. Matthew Gill of the Scripps Research Department of Metabolism and Aging in Florida has discovered an additional chemical signalling pathway which guides metabolism and longevity. His 2011 study of roundworms uncovered special molecules which regulate metabolism and extend life; molecules which are also present in humans.

Dietary restriction has long been known to extend lifespan and to postpone age-related illnesses in a number of species, including yeast, worms, flies, and rodents, but until this decade, the chemical signals involved were little understood.

In animals, special *signalling molecules* control processes such as helping to maintain internal cell energy balance. These signalling molecules are released by one cell, and then cross over to another cell by *diffusion*, the natural process of moving from an area of higher concentration to one of lower concentration. On the receiving cell, signalling molecules bind to receptors, triggering internal enzyme processes within the cell. Signalling molecules called *N-acylethanolamines (NAEs)* decrease after dietary restriction; Dr. Gill believes this lowered NAE promotes longevity. Roundworms can live 40 to 50 percent longer by caloric restriction, but just adding back one of the NAE signalling molecules completely cancels out this dietary-restricting lifespan extension.

Dr. Gill's team also found a link between fat, NAE levels, and longevity; a lack of polyunsaturated fatty acids was linked to life-extending reduced NAE.

Genes And Life Expectancy

One of the most tragic of diseases is the process of premature aging called *progeria*. Progeria (Hutchinson-Gilford progeria syndrome), is an extremely rare genetic disorder, which causes its victims to age at 10 times the rate of healthy children, living at most to about 13 years of age. Symptoms begin to appear around a child's first birthday – hair loss, an unusually large head, visible veins, stiff joints and dislocated hips.

The disorder disrupts synthesis of the protein *lamin A,* which assists in shaping cellular nuclei. In place of lamin A, cells produce an excess of an abnormal protein called *progerin*, and the cell nuclei malform, blistering and buckling, disrupting synthesis of normal tissue.

According to Dr. Tom Misteli of the National Cancer Institute, low levels of progerin are also produced by healthy people – these faulty proteins build up within cells, and the aging body becomes gradually less able to repair them. This, he contends, is the basis of aging.

In 2011, researchers found a genetic switch to turn excess progerin production on and off, according to CBS News. Based upon their findings, three drugs which limit progerin synthesis are currently being tested on approximately 50 children, with the urgency of the disease spurring quick development. One is the immune-suppressant *rapamycin* (see below), which may clear cellular progerin and even delay aging, according to *Science* magazine; rapamycin is already known to extend life in mice.

The drug already shows promise: progeria-afflicted cells, treated with rapamycin in petri dishes, eliminate the abnormal progerin buildup and live longer, and their nuclei return to normal, ovoid shapes, according to Drs. Collins and Kan Cao of the National Human Genome Research Institute. Rapamycin promotes clearance of progerin from within cells by triggering *autophagy*, the destruction of abnormal proteins like progerin.

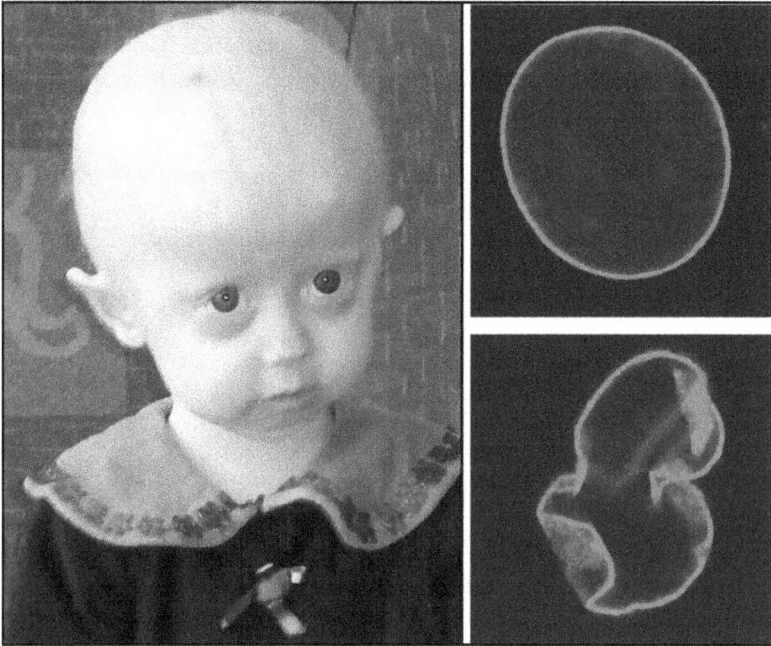

Progeria is a disease caused by a point mutation in the LMNA gene, which provides instructions for a protein called Lamin A. The gene replaces cytosine with thymine, creating unusable Lamin. The protein Lamin A is what holds the nucleus of cells together. Defective Lamin A (called progerin) ultimately leads to premature aging.

Progerin causes the cell to be unstable, gradually damaging the nucleus. This means cells die earlier, though the causes are still not fully understood. Approximately 13 people in the whole of the United States of America have Progeria, showing its rarity. The Cell Nucleus and Aging, public domain.

Telomerase

It was an stunning discovery, one that would lead all the way to a Nobel Prize: in 1984, Berkeley professor Elizabeth Blackburn and graduate student Carol Greider co-discovered *telomerase*, an enzyme which protects DNA.

Telomeres are protective caps on the ends of chromosomes. They're simple nucleotide repetitions, hundreds to thousands of times, of a 6-nucleotide DNA sequence (TTAGGG or AATCCC). Like plastic tips on the ends of shoelaces, telomeres protect chromosomes and their genetic information from unravelling.

Normal cell aging – called *senescence* – is the changes a cell undergoes as it makes a limited number of divisions during its lifetime. Every time a cell undergoes *mitosis* (divides and copies), between 50 to 200 of these repeated nucleotides are lost, gradually shortening the chromosome cap's overall length. After about 50 divisions, telomeres become depleted and a normal cell is no longer able to divide and dies. This maximum number of divisions before a cell reaches the end of its life is the *Hayflick Limit*; prior to its discovery in 1961, it was believed that cells were virtually immortal.

Upon reaching the Hayflick Limit, a cell's telomere loss appears to generate a signal that it can no longer divide. This "cellular clock" appears to predetermine each cell's lifespan.

High levels of stress appear also significantly linked to shortened telomeres, possibly shaving a decade or more from one's life, while exercise has been associated with longer telomeres.

However, in 1984, Blackburn and Greider zeroed in on a magical enzyme that rebuilds telomere nucleotides, adding repeat sequences to the ends. *Telomerase (hTERT)* "resets the clock", allowing cell division to continue much longer than normal and significantly extending cell life – without further telomere shortening.

Telomerase is only produced by our bodies intermittently and in minimal amounts, sufficient to give the longest lived among us about 120 years of life. After an organism's primary growth, telomerase production is switched off in all but immune, egg, sperm – or tumorous – cells.

Dr. Bill Andrews, an anti-aging specialist, thinks telomere shortening is the basis of aging itself, limiting the number of times cells can divide: By injecting telomerase into cells, researchers have been able to significantly reduce cellular aging. Among twins studied for extended periods, the one with longer telomeres has lived longer in 60 percent of recorded cases.

Reactivating the enzyme dramatically lengthens mouse life spans. This means it may soon be possible to slow normal human aging by reawakening telomerase in cells where it's stopped functioning.

In 2010, Harvard Medical School cancer geneticist Dr. Ronald DePinho genetically altered mice to produce telomerase, restoring their organs. Their atrophied sex organs returned to normal, as did their fertility. Additional vital organs, including the brain, spleen, liver, and intestines also returned to a youthful state. Oxford University's Dr. Lynne Cox says DePinho's study is proof that short-term telomerase reactivation can restore aged tissue and functionality. Mice genetically engineered to lack telomerase enzyme production prematurely age, but when the enzyme production is restored, the aging process actually reverses, revitalizing tissue.

Mice without telomerase have impaired fertility, age significantly faster than others, suffer from age-related conditions like osteoporosis, diabetes and neurodegeneration, and die prematurely. But after researchers switch telomerase production back on for only a month, these decrepit lab mice regain their fertility, and their internal organs return to normal. A one-month resurgence of telomerase also reverses neural degeneration in their brains.

These findings suggest a drug or gene therapy which can *upregulate* (increase production of) telomerase in humans might not just extend life, but reduce such major age-related illnesses as heart disease, diabetes, and Alzheimer's. Dr. DePinho believes we are only a decade away from such anti-aging cures.

On the downside, however, this kind of clock resetting is part of the mechanism underlying cancer – cells which continue to divide and multiply unchecked. Unlike normal cells, cancer cells continuously synthesize telomerase, exploiting its powers of chromosome protection. Thus, scientists like Dr. Blackburn suggest proceeding with caution – "magic pills", as she puts it, tend to have unpleasant consequences down the road.

The US Government Weighs In

In the summer of 2011, National Institutes of Health researchers identified a new pathway that promotes longevity, along with new insights: the team found that short or dysfunctional telomeres activate progerin synthesis, and as telomeres shorten, this progerin production escalates.

Progerin is a mutated version of the cell protein lamin A, which helps to maintain the normal structure of a cell's nucleus, the cellular repository of genetic information. In 2003, researchers had discovered a point mutation in the lamina A-producing LMNA gene causes the premature aging disease progeria.

NIH scientists had learned in 2007 that healthy cells also produce small amounts of progerin, even without the genetic mutation. The more often cells divide, the shorter telomeres become, and the more progerin production increases.

Their latest studies show the point mutation strongly promotes lamin A splicing, producing the toxic progerin protein that leads to premature aging. But modifications to the splicing of normal LMNA can also occur. The research indicates that telomere shortening during normal cell division triggers RNA splicing, which alters how cells process genetic information during protein translation.

When proteins are synthesized, RNA is transcribed from DNA, but the RNA doesn't contain all the information embedded in the DNA; instead, the cell splices together *exons*, RNA segments of genetic information which guide protein synthesis, removing intervening unused nucleotides, called *introns*.

Telomere shortening appears to alter RNA splicing, affecting production of a number of proteins important for *cytoskeleton* (cell structure) integrity, particularly the processing of LMNA *messenger RNA*, and this leads to a buildup of toxic progerin proteins.

"Telomere shortening during cellular senescence plays a causative role in activating progerin production and leads to extensive change in alternative splicing in multiple other genes," according to lead author Kan Cao, PhD., assistant professor of cell biology and molecular genetics at the University of Maryland, College Park. His study shows cells with a perpetual telomerase supply, called "immortalized cells", produce very little progerin RNA. Most cells like this are cancerous, never reaching a normal end of the cell cycle, instead replicating uncontrollably.

No matter their age, cells which had passed through several cell cycles produced progressively higher levels of progerin, and normal cells which produce higher progerin levels also displayed shortened, faulty telomeres, a tell-tale sign of numerous divisions.

Aside from the focus on progerin, the NIH team also conducted the first systematic analysis of alternative splicing during cellular aging, searching for additional protein effects from scrambled instructions resulting from RNA splicing. With investigatory techniques analyzing the order of RNA nucleotide units, the team discovered that shortened telomeres alter splicing, and this affects a number of other genes in addition to lamin A, including others which encode proteins playing a part in cell structure.

The "All-In" Bet: TA-65

In 2000, startup pharmaceutical company Geron created the first telomerase-activating compound from the dried root of *Astragalus membranaceus*, also called *huong qi (yellow leader)*, one of 50 herbs central to traditional Chinese herbal medicine, said for centuries to help boost immunity.

Geron was planning human trials in 2012; however, New York entrepreneur Noel Patton bought the production rights in 2002, allowing him to market the formula as a supplement (thus bypassing strict FDA testing regulations). Patton first began testing it on himself and then, in 2008, under medical supervision, upon a group of 100 clients, each of whom paid $25,000 a year for the privilege of being human guinea pigs with his "TA-65" Telomerase-Activating (65 being the year in which Patton began using it) formula. Its active ingredients are produced at very low levels by the astragalus plant, but TA Sciences purifies and concentrates it, asserting that their formula switches on telomerase production.

Large scale, long-term, controlled studies have not yet been conducted on humans, and small scale studies are thus far inconclusive, though some patients and doctors have reported beneficial effects. But within the four years since TA-65 first hit the market, none of the original group have contracted new cancers, so Patton has made TA-65 available to the general public at a slightly more affordable $2,400 to $8,000 a year, with the price based upon dosage. He currently has several thousand clients. Isagenix is Geron's first competitor, selling a TA supplement through private doctors, online, and door-to-door sales. Its formulation is a closely-guarded trade secret, created by a former Geron researcher.

TA proponents are hoping that telomerase activators won't just enable them to live up to 150 years, but will also keep them relatively youthful past the centenarian mark.

The Magic Of Omega 3s

In addition to their other powerful effects, Omega 3 oils also have been shown to preserve telomeres.

The Hayflick limit sets your potential lifespan at 120 years, after which it's believed your cells run out of the ability to split and divide, and to regenerate and repair themselves. The Hayflick limit is a mathematical calculation which depends upon the number of telomeres shed for each cell division. Under perfect conditions, cell division can continue for 120 years before telomere depletion ends your life. Telomere length is therefore considered a *marker* of biological age.

Unfortunately, however, it's all too easy to accelerate telomere shortening, thus speeding up your own aging and shortening your life, through exposure to damage from radical oxygen species, infections, stress, inflammation, and drug or alcohol abuse.

Nutrients or lifestyle changes which eliminate potential telomere damage can extend your potential lifespan, and this telomeric protection is thought to be one of the primary reasons antioxidants like carnosine, which deactivate free radicals, are thought to be anti-aging substances.

Trying to determine why heart patients taking fish oil live longer, cardiologist Ramin Farzaneh-Far led a team which measured omega-3 fatty acids (DHA and EPA) and telomeres in the leukocytes (white blood cells) of 608 patients with stable heart disease; they repeated the measurement five years later. They found patients with the lowest omega 3 levels also had the shortest telomeres, while those with the highest DHA and EPA concentration had the longest telomeres. Studies of twins have also found that those who exercise have longer telomeres; with cells that look decades younger. *(Bear in mind that these findings show correlation, but not necessarily causation. There may be other reasons.)*

Supergenes

Since 1998, the Albert Einstein College of Medicine's Longevity Genes Project has been studying over 2,000 seniors who have lived into their 90s and beyond. In one part of the study, director Nir Barzilai focused on 500 centenarians from New York's Ashkenazic Jewish population. An astoundingly high number of this small, concentrated population has lived past the century mark, through no particular effort on their parts: only *one* of the 500 had been an athlete, *none* were vegetarians, nor had any of them paid undue attention to preserving their health; in fact, says Dr. Barzilai, *30% were obese, 30% smoked two packs of cigarettes for over 40 years, and they generally exercised less than average Americans.*

Professor Barzilai is certain their longevity secret is genetic – he's found three "super genes" common to all of them. These genes are involved in raising HDL levels, in preventing diabetes, and in decreasing the likelihood of contracting Alzheimer's disease by 80%. According to BBC's *Horizon*, possessing these three super genes increases the likelihood of surviving to 100 years or more by 2000% – a factor 20 times the likelihood for anyone in the typical population.

He predicts drugs will be commercially available by 2013 that mimic the genes' HDL-raising effects. Currently, pharmaceutical giant Merck is developing a medication based upon this approach.

Switching On Cellular Repair

UCSF biochemist Dr. Cynthia Kenyon is also betting on gene manipulation as a means of extending life. At the Kenyon Lab she recently discovered mutations to a single gene can double the lifespan of C. Elegans. *daf-2* genes encode a hormone receptor regulating a cell's aging. By disrupting this receptor, aging slows.

Hormones, says Kenyon, control aging, and the daf-2 receptor is similar to the human insulin and IGF-1 receptors. Insulin triggers cell uptake of nutrients after you eat, while IGF promotes growth. They also appear to be responsible for aging, and for age-related diseases like cancer, heart disease, and Alzheimer's.

Suppressing genes encoding either insulin or IGF-1 receptors extends the lives of mice and flies, and studies have found that centenarians like the Ashkenazic Jewish population tend to carry mutations which reduce IGF-1 receptors.

Says Dr. Kenyon, in daf-2 mutants, the defective receptors don't function as well, and this unlocks the ability of a gene-regulating protein called *FOXO*. FOXO binds to DNA in the nucleus, switching on synthesis of protective and damage-repairing proteins – antioxidants, immune-system components, and "caregiver proteins", which repair or recycle faulty proteins. In normal worms, an active daf-2 hormone receptor prevents FOXO from entering the cell's nucleus, so it cannot work to switch on the genes.

Dr. Kenyon theorizes that Insulin and IGF hormones are at high levels in "good times", when food is abundant, promoting growth and nutrient uptake and storage. Under stressful conditions - such as when food is scarce – these hormones are produced at lower levels. She believes low levels of insulin and IGF-1 are a "danger signal" to animals, which then go into "self-protective and repair" mode. FOXO is activated, prompting cell protection and repair.

Armed with her discovery, she founded Elixir Pharmaceuticals, which is trying to create a pill that can slow aging by mimicking this gene manipulation. To do this, she's looking for molecules that can activate the FOXO3A protein in humans. Rapamycin already functions in this way, but suppresses the immune system, so is not appropriate for non-emergency use.

As a side note, because of her research, Dr. Kenyon has stopped eating high glycemic index carbohydrates, such as candies, rice, bread and pasta – adding sugar to the worm diet shortens their life spans.

Empowerment, Or Mind Over Matter

Harvard University psychology professor Dr. Ellen Langer says there's clinically-demonstrated truth to the phrase, "you're only as old as you think". For example, she says, your vision isn't just a matter of how well your eyes function – it also depends to a great degree upon your mindset.

Dr. Langer has studied the effects of mindset on the body for over 30 years, and says she has discovered some truly remarkable things. She contends – and says she has proof – that much of our personal limitations are simply due to our expectations, rather than our body's abilities. As a result of her studies, she advocates what she calls *the psychology of possibility*.

In a group of experiments, Dr. Langer explored the possibility that simply believing one's vision is better improves eyesight substantially. Expectations, she says, don't just increase alertness or motivation to focus the eyes, but measurably enhance visual clarity. To determine the extent to which belief affects eyesight, she devised an experiment:

20 volunteers with normal eyesight looked at an eye chart where the sizes had been arranged in reverse, so letters grew progressively larger further down the chart, ending in a giant "E". All subjects accurately reported a greater number of letters from the two smallest lines than when they were shown an eye chart progressing from largest to smallest letters. Dr. Langer and her team believe this is because people expect letters at the top will be easy to see, based on previous experience with normal eye charts. Interestingly, the biggest improvement in vision was among volunteers who had answered in a prior survey that they thought eyesight could improve with practice.

A follow-up group of her experiments used volunteers from MIT's Air Force ROTC cadets. Prior to the experiment, their vision was tested, and ranged from below average to excellent. None of them knew the experiment's true purpose.

From the volunteers, 22 randomly-selected cadets were dressed in flight suits and instructed to role-play being pilots in an Air Force flight simulator machine. During the exercise, they were asked to try to read letters on the wings of approaching planes they saw through the flight simulator's cockpit window – a sequence of letters taken directly from the bottom four lines of the eye chart they had been tested on earlier.

20 more cadets only sat in the simulator in normal clothes and were told the simulator was broken (with only the video functioning), but were asked to read the wing letters in the same way as the previous group.

40% (nine) of the 22 cadets who role-played being pilots in the flight simulator performed significantly better on the wing-spotting visual test; none of the second group improved. It's believed that the first group performed so much better because, in pretending, they had adopted the mind-set of "real" pilots (who they knew are legally required to have a minimum of 20/70 to 20/20 vision). Those flight simulator players with below-average vision made the greatest improvements. The results, says Dr. Langer, suggest that simply believing one's vision is superior has genuine, measurable effect.

A video of the experiment can be seen online at this URL (watch from the 20:40 mark): http://video.google.com/videoplay?docid=8673118115997325318#

It gets even more interesting. In 1981, Dr. Langer was attempting to discover how preconceptions and expectations affect the aging process. She arranged for two groups of 70- and 80-year-olds to stay in an isolated New Hampshire monastery, where the environment of 1959 was recreated. The first group was asked to pretend they were young men living once again in the 1950s for one week. A week later, a second group was brought into the 1950s environment and instructed simply to reminisce about the era, without pretending to be younger men.

The subjects were treated like able-bodied, independent younger men. No assumptions of incapacitation were placed upon them, nobody "babied" them, and they were expected to do their own chores, and to be independent, without caretakers to help them. From the moment they were dropped off at the site, for example, they were expected to carry their own luggage, no matter how long it took them. "They were being treated as if they were capable, autonomous individuals."

Mementos of the 1950s had been placed everywhere – a black-and-white television, vintage radio, and copies of *Life* magazine and the *Saturday Evening Post*, and the subjects discussed current events of the bygone era, from the first U.S. satellite launch to the rise of the Cold War, Fidel Castro, Nikita Khrushchev, and bomb shelters.

Entertainment took the form of 1959 films, famous radio broadcasts and group discussions about star athletes. The first group had been pretending to experience all of these events for the first time, while for the second, it brought back a rush of nostalgic memories. The results, says Dr. Langer, were astonishing. Both groups of men had grown physically stronger and more flexible. Their sight, hearing, weight, walking speed, posture and even height had changed. Intelligence test scores improved, and symptoms of arthritis faded.

427

But for the first group of 70- and 80-year-old men (those who had pretended to be younger), there was significantly greater improvement – their bodies had become physically younger as a result of the experience. How much? Dr. Langer reports that, by the end of the two weeks,

> *I was playing football—touch, but still football—with these men, some of whom gave up their canes.... It is not our physical state that limits us – it's our mindset about our own limits, our perceptions, that draws the lines in the sand.*

Previously, in studies with colleagues from Yale, Langer had demonstrated that age-related memory loss could be reversed by simply giving the elderly incentives to remember; personal ties were established between the researchers and their elder subjects, and small gifts were given as rewards for success. As a result, she says, their memory improved measurably.

Her classic follow-up study showed that giving nursing-home residents a degree of autonomy in their lives – such as letting them choose where to meet guests, what activities to engage in, and giving them houseplants to care for – improved their physical and mental health, and even increased their longevity.

In a related 2005 experiment, Langer and a Yale colleague gathered a group of 84 hotel workers, who claimed to never exercise, but spent every working day pushing carts and cleaning rooms. Half of the group was told their jobs provided the same exercise as attending a gym, while the other half were told nothing.

After a month – in which none of the subjects made any dietary, exercise or other changes – the first group had lost two pounds each on average, reduced their waist-to-hip ratios and lowered their blood pressure by 10 points; the second group had *gained* body fat.

In her book *Counterclockwise*, Dr. Langer says our "mindless" acceptance of doctors' opinions and even how we talk about our own illnesses can drastically affect our physical health, and she has the data to prove it. Her life story is said to be currently under production as a film starring Jennifer Aniston, who is a co-producer.

In 2010, Dr. Michael Mosley repeated Langer's experiments for the BBC, and reported similar results. The series is ongoing. More information is available at http://bbc.co.uk

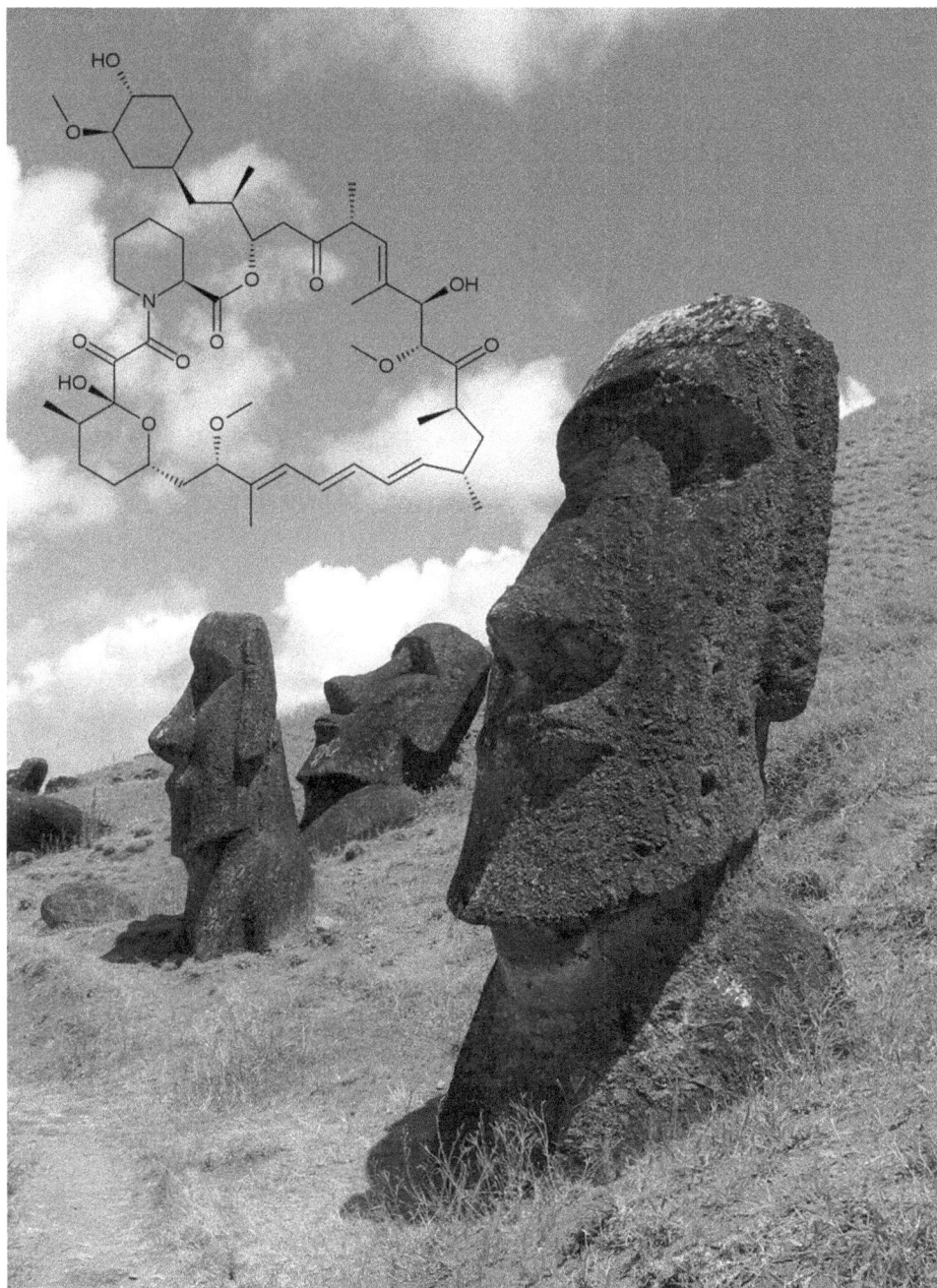

Rapamycin is produced by the bacterium Streptomyces Hygroscopicus.
It was first discovered in a soil sample from Easter Island.
Composite from public domain images, 2011, Polyglot Studios

Rapamycin

Among the mysteries of Easter Island is that of a special substance discovered in the soil called *rapamycin*. It was originally discovered in the 1970s, and has been used since then to suppress the immune system, so transplanted organs are less likely to be rejected. However, researchers at three separate institutes in Texas, Michigan and Maine discovered it extends the lifespan of mice up to 38%. When 20-month-old mice – the equivalent of 60-year-old humans – were given rapamycin, they lived another 8 months – the equivalent of 23 human years.

Barshop Institute's Dr. Arlan Richardson believes rapamycin constitutes the world's first true "anti-aging pill", the first he's seen in over 35 years of anti-aging research, and colleague Dr. Randy Strong of the University of Texas concurs, calling this the first real evidence that aging can be slowed and lifespan extended by drug therapy, even at an advanced age. Rapamycin is also being tested as a possible new cancer drug. And if rapamycin prevents and/or cures cancer and heart disease as well as extending life, the drug can be of tremendous benefit to humanity.

Rapamycin's effects seem close to those of caloric restriction, consistently demonstrated to boost longevity. It targets the cellular protein *mTOR*, which controls a number of metabolic and stress-response processes. However, since rapamycin suppresses immunity, some scientists are advising caution. Dr. Lynne Cox, an Oxford University aging expert, warns against casually experimenting with rapamycin to extend life at this point, because of its immunity-suppressing effects.

Hormone Therapies

Aging and diseases like HIV and cancer can lead to a loss of muscle mass. Sometimes anabolic steroids are used to reverse this muscle tissue loss, but they can have unpleasant side effects.

Nine human blood proteins, such as Insulin-like Growth Factor 1 (IGF-1) and *pro-collagen*, are linked to both muscle maintenance and immune system regulation, and alter with age. Some of these alterations, however, can be reversed with testosterone.

In 2008, researchers under Dr. Monty Montano at Boston and Texas Universities compared blood serum protein levels in two groups of healthy men, the first aged 18-35, and the second aged 60-75.

Pro-collagen and seven other proteins involved in growth and immunity were lower among the older men, while *monokine MIG* (also involved in the immune system), was elevated. Treatment with testosterone increased pro-collagen and IGF-1 in young men and a small number of the older men. Muscle mass and the appetite-suppressing hormone leptin also increased among both groups.

Later that same year, Virginia University's Dr. Michael O. Thorner found that mimicking the effects of ghrelin in stimulating growth hormone receptors and altering fat metabolism with the drug *MK-677* restores up to 20% of the muscle mass and bone density lost to aging in 60- to 81-year-old humans. After taking the drug, Growth Hormone and IGF-1 increased to levels typical of healthy young adults among the volunteers, and no side effects were observed.

Switching on Natural Regeneration

A Berkeley husband-and-wife bioengineering team has discovered the secret of reversing aging in living tissue, triggering innate cell regeneration using biochemical signals.

Drs. Irina and Michael Conboy of the Berkeley Stem Cell Center, along with Dr. Hanadie Yousef, have found that by activating specific receptors, muscle cells can be restored to a youthful state. Switching on *progenitor* (originating) cells builds and repairs muscles in the extremely aged – just as if these tissues had returned to their youth.

Stem cells are *pluripotent,* in a generic state of potential, capable of becoming a variety of different cell types, and of replicating indefinitely. They remain *undifferentiated* in tissue which they maintain and repair throughout adult life. They self-renew through *asymmetric cell division* – when a cell divides, one daughter cell differentiates – becomes one of several potential specific kinds of cells – while its twin remains a pluripotent stem cell.

Progenitor cells exist in a more intermediate, specific state, differentiating into specific "target" cells, and only replicating a finite number of times.

Functional stem cells and progenitor cells exist in animals throughout life, but cellular *damage* eventually overwhelms cellular *replacement*, leading to tissue breakdown and eventually, organ failure and death.

The regenerative capacity of these special cells declines with age, because aged tissue begins to actively inhibit stem cell regeneration, possibly as an adaptation to prevent cancer - runaway cellular production. Stem cell function degrades due to changes in biochemical pathways – genetic regulation of tissue repair. In other words, aging tissue begins to inhibit its own regeneration.

With age, as these repair processes decline, damage to DNA and proteins, protein misfolding, RNA misprocessing and mistargeting of key biomolecules increases. Old differentiated cells lose functionality, and the stem and progenitor cells which can generate *new* differentiated cells dial down their regenerative capacity. The combination of wear and tear, along with the decline in restorative function, causes organs to eventually fail, and organisms die of old age.

This aging seems to be unavoidable, because it comes from the normal use of signalling pathways necessary for survival, such as the *IGF/insulin pathway* and energy-generating *cellular respiration*, which produces destructive Reactive Oxygen Species (ROS).

Since stem cells reside in aged muscles for life and never completely lose their ability to repair tissue, they can be coaxed into performing as they had during the creature's youth, forestalling age-related tissue degeneration.

Their regeneration function is controlled by cell life-cycle "check point proteins" and *mitogens* (chemicals which induce cell division - triggering *mitosis*), but this control system changes as a creature ages. Dr. Conboy and her team have found that this protein control system can be manipulated to promote regeneration without forming cancerous tumors.

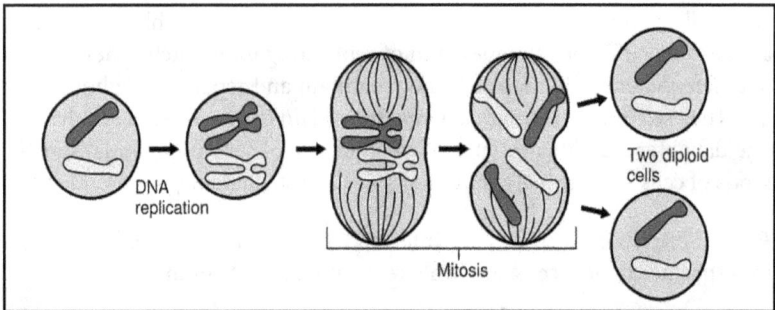

Mitosis is the division of cells into genetically identical pairs. Stem cells are an exception to this rule, with the "mother" cell remaining unchanged, and the "daughter" cell differentiating into a tissue-specific cell, e.g. bone, hair, blood, muscle, etc.

During mitosis, chromosomes in the cell nucleus split into two identical sets, in two separate nuclear centers. This is usually followed by cytokinesis, in which the nuclei, cytoplasm, organelles and cell membrane divide into two cells with approximately equal portions of these cellular components. Wikipedia, 2011, public domain.

In 2011, Dr. Conboy demonstrated aged stem cells can be revitalized in humans as well as in laboratory animals. In cooperation with Dr. Michael Kjaer of the University of Copenhagen, Dr. Conboy's team examined muscle tissue samples from 28 healthy men who volunteered for an exercise study. Young subjects were 21 to 24 years old, while older subjects ranged from 68 to 74.

Muscle *biopsies* (thin slices of tissue) were removed from the volunteers' quadriceps (thigh muscles) at the study's commencement. The legs from which tissue had been taken were then immobilized in casts for 14 days to trigger muscle atrophy. After their casts were removed, the subjects weight-lifted to rebuild muscle mass. Biopsies were again taken three days after, then again after four weeks.

Before subjects' legs were immobilized, adult stem cells governing muscle repair and regeneration were only half as prevalent in old muscle tissue as in young tissue. During the exercise phase, this age difference doubled, with younger tissue possessing four times the regenerative cells actively repairing tissue compared with older muscles, in which the stem cells were inactive.

Two weeks of immobilization had only minor effects upon young muscle tissue, but old muscle tissue had quickly begun to atrophy. Nor did the older muscle tissue recover as well from exercise, exhibiting signs of inflammation and scar formation while immobile, and again a month after the casts had been removed.

Dr. Conboy says this underscores the importance of exercise for the elderly, because extended inactivity may permanently impair stem cell regenerative power. However, to avoid injury or the replacement of functional muscle tissue with scar tissue or inflammation, easing into an exercise program is important, especially at an advanced age.

The team shut down molecular signals controlling stem cell responses, and the young muscle tissue deteriorated, just like the old tissue; conversely, in old muscles, *activating* these stem cell responses regenerated aged tissue. The team found similar rejuvenating effects with blood, brain and pancreas stem cells.

Notch receptors promote muscle cell regeneration, while TGF-beta proteins inhibit it, and age-related tissue degeneration results from a decline in Notch activation coupled with an increase in TGF-beta activity. Together, both eventually shut down stem cell tissue regeneration, leading to senescence – biological aging.

Dr. Conboy found Notch receptors necessary for muscle repair (normally inactive in old tissue) can be reactivated with *mitogen-activated protein kinase (MAPK)*, an enzyme important for organ formation in a wide range of species, from worms to mice to humans.

This MAPK pathway has been *conserved* throughout evolution (appearing unchanged throughout the evolution of advanced species), demonstrating its importance for life, according to Dr. Conboy. It is now known to play a central role in regulating regeneration and human tissue aging.

MAPK levels decline in older muscles, so Notch pathways are inactive and stem cells no longer regenerate tissue effectively. Artificially inhibiting MAPK shuts down young muscle regeneration, while enhancing MAPK in older muscles significantly enhances regenerative power.

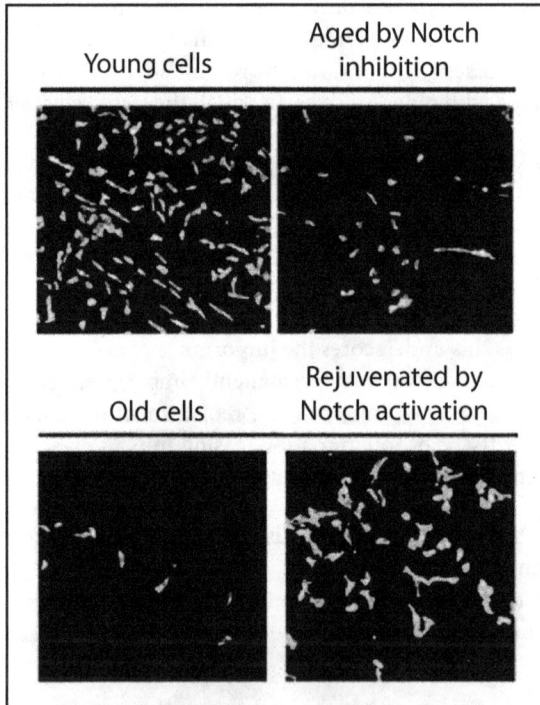

Human muscle stem cell regenerative activity is depicted in green and red. Stem cell responses were incapacitated when researchers inhibited the activation of key biochemical pathways, making the young muscle behave like old muscle. Old cells exhibited regenerative responses when properly triggered by experimental activation of biochemical signals. Morgan Carlson and Irina Conboy, UC Berkeley, 2011. Used with permission.

Walnuts

In 2009, researchers at the U.S. Department of Agriculture and Tufts University in Boston demonstrated that simply adding the human equivalent of seven to nine walnuts a day to the diet of aged rats could significantly improve their cognitive function and motor skills. The active ingredients underlying the improvement are essential fatty acids, as well as polyphenols and other antioxidants.

As animals age, a number of changes naturally occur in the brain, resulting in impaired or altered neural function, disruptions stemming from impaired synaptic plasticity and increased oxidative damage. These changes manifest in laboratory animals as impaired balance, coordination, and navigation.

In the USDA's study, weight-matched older rats were randomly assigned to each of four diets for eight weeks before undergoing a series of motor and memory tests. These diets contained either 0, 2, 6 or 9 percent walnuts. Interestingly, 2 or 6 percent of walnuts improved age-related motor and cognitive impairment, but a greater amount proved detrimental to memory. A moderate amount appears to be most beneficial for neural tissue in a number of ways, according to the researchers.

A Dissenting View – *The conventional wisdom has long held that aging and a number of diseases are due to oxidative stress – a theory from the 1950s that said it was the result of destructive oxygen byproducts from respiration – the use of oxygen in generating life-sustaining energy.*

Molecular oxygen ions (called free radicals or Reactive oxygen species (ROS)), are byproducts of aerobic metabolism, the breakdown of chemicals in the presence of oxygen to supply energy to fuel cellular processes. They cause oxidative damage, by leeching electrons, rupturing chemical bonds, breaking down life-sustaining molecules and cellular membranes. This process has been long and widely held to limit both lifespan and general health.

Dr. Arlan Richardson, Director of the Barshop Center for Longevity and Aging Studies, and Professor Rochelle Buffenstein of the University of Texas Graduate School of Biomedical Sciences say they have disproven the link between oxidative stress and longevity, however. Dr. Richardson bred mice genetically resistant to oxidative stress; his ten-year experiment found no difference in mice bred to resist oxidative stress and normal mice, appearing to disprove prevailing conventional wisdom on oxidative stress and aging and disease. It's possible, he says, to have high levels of oxidative stress and still live a long, healthy life. Because this is hardly welcome news to the multibillion-dollar annual antioxidant supplement market, these findings are getting a chilly reception, but should certainly be examined.

Resveratrol And Glaxo's SuperYouth Pill

Scientists everywhere are confident they're closing in on the secrets of significant life extension. Dr. David Sinclair is one of them. In 2003, he discovered the antioxidant *resveratrol*, a natural protective phytochemical grapes secrete to combat fungal infections. It's found in red wine and grape juice, and has been shown in some experiments to extend animal life spans from 24 to 59 percent.

Dr. Sinclair says resveratrol acts upon the *SIRT-1* gene, which plays a central role in regulating mammalian life spans. He says increasing the SIRT-1 gene's expression slows aging and age-related diseases. In the natural world, SIRT-1 gene production is amplified by calorie restriction. SIRT-I activates special proteins called *sirtuins,* believed to underlie these life-enhancing effects.

Scientists have known since the 1940s that mice live significantly longer when they eat a nutritious diet that has 30 to 40 percent fewer calories than normal. Sinclair suggests this is an evolutionary adaptation to starvation, the metabolism slowing to conserve available energy stores. He says resveratrol mimics this caloric restriction, but without the discomfort of food deprivation.

As of yet however, results of resveratrol studies have varied widely, and it remains largely untested on humans. That hasn't deterred Dr. Sinclair, who co-founded Sirtris Pharmaceuticals, since sold to international pharmaceutical giant GlaxoSmithKline for 720 million dollars (!)

Glaxo reports it has recently synthesized an improved formulation the company calls *SRT501*, and is at work developing sirtuin activators researchers claim are one thousand times as potent as SRT501. The first of these drugs are scheduled for commercial production by 2012 or 2013.

Concorde Grapes: The Fruits Of Exercise?

Both astronauts in low-gravity environments and workers chained to nine-to-five desk jobs may find it nearly impossible to get the exercise necessary for maintaining health. Their sedentary lifestyle results in muscle atrophy, loss in bone density, insulin resistance, and an unhealthy shift in the body's energy consumption from fats to carbohydrates.

In 2011, scientists discovered that with diets high resveratrol, laboratory animals in weightless environments didn't develop this insulin resistance or bone mineral density loss. But control animals not given resveratrol suffered a decrease in muscle mass and strength, developed dangerous resistance to insulin, and lost bone mineral density, their bones becoming more brittle.

Each one of these changes can lead to serious health issues in the long term, but treatment with resveratrol maintained the balance of protein, muscle mass, muscle force contraction, mitochondria capacity, and appeared to reduce oxidative wear on tissue. It also protected insulin sensitivity and lipid transport. This suggests that in the sedentary, resveratrol may slow muscle, bone and pancreas deterioration until it's possible to return to normal levels of activity.

Resveratrol can be obtained through supplements or red wine and red grape juice. It's naturally produced by grapes to protect against fungal infections, and is found primarily in the skin. The amount varies among varieties: white wine contains little resveratrol, because white wines are fermented and bottled after the skin has been removed. The highest levels of are reported to be found in dark purple concord grapes. Some foods, such as peanuts, cocoa and dark chocolate also contain trace amounts.

According to Mayo Clinic cardiologist Dr. Martha Grogan, red grape antioxidants are also thought to relax the blood vessels, aiding blood flow. Studies suggest that red and purple grape juice contain approximately the same protective properties of red wine, including:

- Reduction in blood clot risk and LDL (low-density lipoprotein) cholesterol

- Prevention of cardiac blood vessel damage

- Assistance in maintaining healthy blood pressure

Red wine contains approximately 2 to 7 mg of resveratrol per liter, depending upon the variety and fermentation process, while Spanish red grape juice contains approximately 1 to over 8.5 mg per liter, again depending upon the variety.

Uncertain About Sirtuins

Cutting calories 30 to 40 percent has long been known to boost lifespan and improve health. In 1996, MIT Professor Leonard Guarente first discovered the special proteins called *sirtuins,* which he initially believed underlay these calorie-reduction life-enhancing effects: mice genetically engineered without sirtuin receive no life-extending benefits from calorie restriction, which would seem to indicate sirtuins are critical to the process.

In theory, sirtuins keep cells alive and healthy in the presence of stress, regulating the central nervous system's *somatotropic signalling axis*, a key network of hormonal and regulatory proteins controlling growth and lifespan.

Decreasing calories makes the hypothalamus slow growth-hormone production, and animals are consequently smaller but longer-lived. In normal healthy mammals, calorie restriction boosts levels of *NAD*, a substance which activates sirtuins, lowering growth-hormone production and lengthening life spans.

Professor Guarente initially believed drugs would soon be marketed to boost sirtuin production, helping fight age-related diseases like diabetes and Alzheimer's, improving health in the elderly, and potentially extending life spans. Such sirtuin-promoting drugs are already undergoing clinical trials.

However, in September, 2011, David Gems of the Institute of Healthy Aging at the University College London announced solid evidence which he says disproves any cause-and-effect relationship between sirtuins and longevity. The last decade's research purporting to show that sirtuins increase lifespan by up to 50 percent is "deeply flawed" he says. Resveratrol, believed to activate the enzyme, is also a pharmaceutical dead end, he says.

Dr. Gems and his team said they found the links between sirtuins and life extension stem from other factors, and, of the previous experiments, "... none seem to stand up to close scrutiny". The earlier experiments failed to account for other genetic differences between genetically-modified creatures and the control (normal) subjects with which they were compared. The Gems study also refutes claims that dietary restriction-induced longevity – which is not itself in dispute – depends upon sirtuins.

After steps were taken to ensure the only difference between the test animals was higher sirtuin levels, lifespan enhancing effects disappeared. Other genetic differences appear to have slipped notice. Dr. Guarante, who led the original studies, admitted in *Nature* magazine that his earlier experiments had been flawed, and the longevity enhancements attributed to sirtuins are actually due to other as-yet undetermined genetic factors.

Dr. Gems says there's no mistake: these findings "put a final nail in the coffin," for sirtuin-based life extension research. Many researchers, however, including international pharmaceutical titan GlaxoSmithKline, are betting he's mistaken.

Sirtuins And Brain Health

Sirtuins do appear to offer other clear benefits, however. In 2011, MIT's Dr. Li-Huei Tsai showed they protect neurons and boost synaptic plasticity, offering potential hope to patients suffering from Alzheimer's, Parkinson's, Huntington's, and other neurological diseases.

Sirtuins, he says, affect both learning and memory, a role which researchers found surprising, because they've long been associated with longevity, metabolism, calorie restriction, and genome stability; this is the first time sirtuins have been found to play a part in synaptic plasticity as well. Sirtuins enhance synaptic plasticity, deactivating microRNAs that suppress *CREB*, necessary for long-term potentiation.

Supplementation

Several drugs and food supplements have been shown to slow or even reverse aging in animal models; still, none of these has yet been proven to do so in humans.

In 2002, UC Berkeley Professor Bruce Ames discovered feeding elderly rats a combination of *acetyl-L-carnitine* and *alpha-lipoic acid* (both substances now sold in health food stores) had rejuvenating effects. Says Professor Ames:

> *With these two supplements together, these old rats got up and did the macarena. The brain looks better, they are full of energy – everything we looked at looks like a young animal.*

Linus Pauling Institute colleague Dr. Tory Hagen adds:

> *We significantly reversed the decline in overall activity typical of aged rats to what you see in a middle-aged to young adult rat 7 to 10 months of age. This is equivalent to making a 75- to 80-year-old person act middle-aged. We've only shown short-term effects, but the results give us the rationale for looking at these things long term.*

The team also found the combination of lipoic acid and L-carnitine improved mitochondrial function, and therefore cellular metabolism, increasing various age-declining biomolecules, including the antioxidant *ascorbic acid*.

Aged rats were fed the supplements, and the team measured memory function with a standard water maze test, and another test of temporal memory developed by Berkeley psychology professor Seth Roberts. They say the supplementation enhanced both spatial and temporal memory, and reduced oxidative RNA damage to the hippocampus. Electron microscope images clearly reveal reduced mitochondria decay among old rats which were fed the supplements.

Hagen adds:

> With aging, we see so many different things that are occurring to mitochondria that then lead to consequences in the cell. If you tune up mitochondria, you may have a means of at least delaying the onset of a number of age-related problems that we encounter, or we can in some ways, hopefully, reverse what has already taken place.

UC Berkeley patented a combination of the supplements, and has established the company *Juvenon* to market them. The jury is still out on whether these substances provide the same benefits to humans, however.

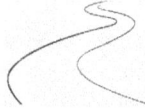

Ten-Fold Life Span Extension Reported, Carl Marziali, press release, 2008, University of Southern California; http://uscnews2.usc.edu/newstools/detail.php?recordnum=14716

Valter Longo: Groundbreaking Discovery Cancer Research, video interview, USC Davus, 2008; http://www.youtube.com/watch?v=RjABM8UmBzI

http://www.cbass.com/Strengthtraininggoodforbrain.htm

http://www.cbass.com/Aerobics&StrengthTraining&Brain.htm

An Age-Defying Quest (Red Wine Included), Jason Pontin, July 8, 2007, The New York Times; http://www.nytimes.com/2007/07/08/business/yourmoney/08stream.html

http://www.news.harvard.edu/gazette/2004/07.22/14-yeast.html

Dietary Supplements Make Old Rats Youthful, May Rejuvenate Aging Humans, 2002, press release, Bruce Ames and Tory Hagen, University of California; http://www.universityofcalifornia.edu/news/article/4001

Embryonic Anti-Aging Niche, Irina M. Conboy, Hanadie Yousef, and Michael J. Conboy, March 31, 2011, High-Impact Journal on Aging Research

Resveratrol Prevents the Wasting Disorders of Mechanical Unloading by Acting as a Physical Exercise Mimetic in the Rat, Iman Momken, Laurence Stevens, et al, 2011, Journal of the Federation of American Societies for Experimental Biology, doi: 10.1096/fj.10-177295 fj.10-177295; http://www.fasebj.org/content/early/2011/06/29/fj.10-177295

Does Grape Juice Offer the Same Heart Benefits as Red Wine? Dr. Martha Grogan, Mayo Clinic, 2011; http://www.mayoclinic.com/health/food-and-nutrition/AN00576

Resveratrol, Wikipedia, 2011; http://en.wikipedia.org/wiki/Resveratrol#Content_in_wines_and_grape_juice

The Oxidative Stress Theory of Aging: Embattled or Invincible? Insights from Non-Traditional Model Organisms, Rochelle Buffenstein, Yael H. Edrey, Ting Yang, and James Mele, Age (Dordr). 2008 Sept. 30 (2-3):99-109; Age (Dordr). 2008 Sep; 30(2-3):99-109; http://www.ncbi.nlm.nih.gov/pmc/articles/PMC2527631/?tool=pubmed

Don't Grow Old, BBC Horizon documentary, Nicola Stockley, Abigail Williams, et al, 2010; http://topdocumentaryfilms.com/dont-grow-old/

The 'Super Gene' Spotter, Amy Spiro, February 8, 2011, Jewish Week; http://www.thejewishweek.com/special_sections/healthcare/super_gene_spotter10-FldLife

N-Acylethanolamine Signalling Mediates the Effect of Diet on Lifespan in Caenorhabditis Elegans, Mark Lucanic, Jason M. Held, Maithili C. Vantipalli, Ida M. Klang, Jill B. Graham, Bradford W. Gibson, Gordon J. Lithgow, Matthew S. Gill, Nature, 2011; 473 (7346): 226 DOI: 10.1038/nature10007

Delaying the Aging Process Protects Against Alzheimer's Disease, press release, December 10, 2009, Salk Institute for Biological Studies; http://www.salk.edu/news/pressrelease_details.php?press_id=397

Hey – Wanna Live Forever? Joseph Hooper, August, 2011, *Elle* Magazine

Tests Raise Life Extension Hopes, BBC News, 2009; http://news.bbc.co.uk/2/hi/health/8139816.stm

Hungering for Longevity—Salk Scientists Identify the Confluence of Aging Signals, press release, February 17, 2011, Salk Institute for Biological Studies; http://www.salk.edu/news/pressrelease_details.php?press_id=472

When Less is More: How Mitochondrial Signals Extend Lifespan, January 06, 2011, release, Salk Institute for Biological Studies; http://www.salk.edu/news/pressrelease_details.php?press_id=458

A Novel Pathway Regulates Memory and Plasticity via SIRT1 and miR-134, Jun Gao, Wen-Yuan Wang, Ying-Wei Mao, Johannes Gräff, Ji-Song Guan, Ling Pan, Gloria Mak, Dohoon Kim, Susan C. Su & Li-Huei Tsai, 2010, Nature 466, 1105–1109, doi:10.1038/nature09271

Telomeres, Hesed Padilla-Nash and Thomas Ried, 2009, National Institutes of Health,

Progerin and Telomere Dysfunction Collaborate to Trigger Cellular Senescence in Normal Human Fibroblasts, Kan Cao, Cecilia D. Blair, Dina A. Faddah, Julia E. Kieckhaefer, Michelle Olive, Michael R. Erdos, Elizabeth G. Nabel, Francis S. Collins, Journal of Clinical Investigation, 2011; DOI: 10.1172/JCI43578

Discovery Could Lead to New Drugs to Fight Alzheimer's and Other Neurological Diseases, 2010, Anne Trafton, MIT News Office

Walnut Extract Inhibits LPS-Induced Activation of BV-2 Microglia Via Internalization of TLR4: Possible Involvement of Phospholipase D2, Lauren Willis, Donna Bielinski, Derek Fisher, Nirupa Matthan, and James Joseph, 2010, Inflammation, 33(5):325, USDA/Agricultural Research Service; http://www.ars.usda.gov/research/publications/publications.htm?seq_no_115=246811

441

Scientists Discover Clues to What Makes Human Muscle Age, Sarah Yang, 2009, press release, University of California, Berkely; http://berkeley.edu/news/media/releases/2009/09/30_muscle.shtml

New Evidence Links Sirtuins and Life Extension, 2009, Anne Trafton, MIT News Office,

Neuronal SIRT1 Regulates Endocrine and Behavioral Responses to Calorie Restriction, Dena Cohen, Leonard Guarente, et al, 2009, Genes and Development

Telomerase Reverses Ageing Process, Dramatic Rejuvenation of Prematurely Aged Mice Hints at Potential Therapy, Ewen Callaway, 2010, Nature News, doi:10.1038/news.2010.635; http://www.nature.com/news/2010/101128/full/news.2010.635.html

New Protein Linked to Alzheimer's Disease, Jamie Talan, press release, May 24, 2011, North Shore-Long Island Jewish (LIJ) Health System;

Identification of Serum Biomarkers for Aging and Anabolic Response, Camellia Banerjee, Jagadish Ulloor, Edgar L Dillon, Qusai Dahodwala, Brittani Franklin, Paola Sebastiani, Melinda Sheffield-Moore, Randall J Urban, Shalender Bhasin and Monty Montano, 2011, Immunity & Ageing; doi:10.1186/1742-4933-8-5; http://www.immunityageing.com/content/8/1/5

Restricting Calories Lowers Body Temperature, May Predict Longer Lifespan, Jim Dryden, press release, May 10, 2011, Washington State University; http://news.wustl.edu/news/Pages/22291.aspx

Long-term Calorie Restriction, But Not Endurance Exercise, Lowers Core Body Temperature in Humans, Soare A, Cangemi R, Omedei D, Holloszy JO, Fontana L. Aging, vol. 3 (3) March 2011;

The Mindfulness Chronicles: On "The Psychology Of Possibility", Cara Fienberg, September 2010, Harvard Magazine; http://harvardmagazine.com/print/28444?page=all

Mind-Set Matters: Exercise and the Placebo Effect, Alia J. Crum and Ellen J. Langer, 2007, Psychological Science, DOI: 10.1111/j.1467-9280.2007.01867.x Psychological Science February 1, 2007 vol. 18 no. 2 165-171; http://pss.sagepub.com/content/18/2/165.abstract

The Influence of Age-Related Cues on Health and Longevity, Laura M. Hsu, Jaewoo Chung and Ellen J. Langer, 2010 doi: 10.1177/1745691610388762 Perspectives on Psychological Science, vol. 5 no. 6 632-648; http://pps.sagepub.com/content/5/6/632.abstract

Researchers Find New Clues About Aging, June 13th, 2011 press release, National Institutes of Health; http://medicalxpress.com/news/2011-06-nih-clues-aging.html

Association of Marine Omega-3 Fatty Acid Levels With Telomeric Aging in Patients With Coronary Heart Disease, Ramin Farzaneh-Far, MD; Jue Lin, PhD; Elissa S. Epel, PhD; William S. Harris, PhD; Elizabeth H. Blackburn, PhD; and Mary A. Whooley, MD; JAMA. 2010; 303(3):250-257. Doi: 10.1001/jama.2009.2008; http://jama.ama-assn.org/content/303/3/250.full?sid=98bc6cf5-4ef1-4778-a8a3-fe943ddab74c

Gene Tweak Reverses Aging in Mouse Skin Cells, Ed Edelson, 2007 Health Day;

Climbing the Ladder to Longevity: Critical Enzyme Pair Identified, press release, June 24, 2009, Salk Institute for Biological Studies; http://www.salk.edu/news/pressrelease_details.php?press_id=363

'Longevity Gene' May Be Dead End: Study, Agence France-Presse, Wednesday, September 21st, 2011

442

PART IV: CONNECTING

Charisma

"Not brute force, but only persuasion and faith are the kings of this world."
– Thomas Carlyle, "Latter-Day Pamphlets", 1850

"He makes people pleased with him by making them first pleased with themselves."
– Lord Chesterfield, "The Letters of the Earl of Chesterfield to His Son", 1750

"The most important persuasion tool you have in your entire arsenal is integrity."
– Zig Ziglar, "Secrets of Closing the Sale", 2004

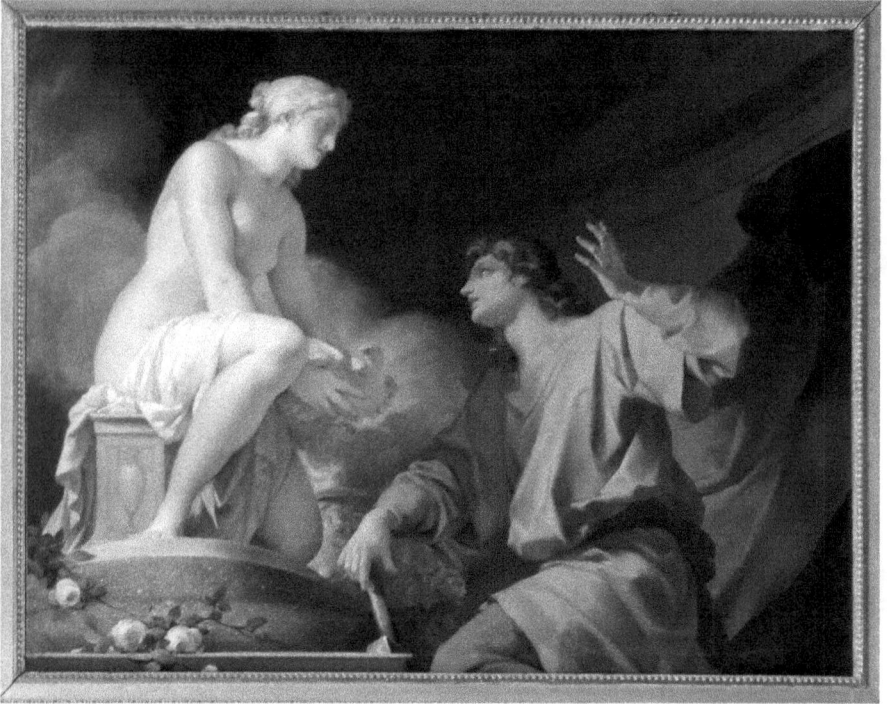

Pygmalion, Jean-Baptiste Regnault, 1786 musée national du château et des Trianons

Pygmalion was a sculptor on the Greek island of Cyprus. He had just crafted the most dazzling statue of ivory, a woman so beautiful that he fell in love with her. On the sacred festival day of Venus, Pygmalion went to the temple to offer a sacrifice to the goddess of love and a prayer to grant his deepest wish. When he returned home, he kissed the lips of his statue, and the ivory warmed as the beautiful mouth came to life. He kissed the lips again, and as he touched the ivory breasts, they softened, and everywhere he touched transformed his statue into a living, breathing woman.

The goddess had granted Pygmalion his wish. Pygmalion and *Galatea* ("she that is milk-white") were soon married and went on to build a family that would achieve great things.

Ovid's 2000-year-old myth has become a metaphor for the *Pygmalion effect* – where expectation of the good in others brings out their positive qualities. The Pygmalion effect means the greater your expectations are for others, the better they perform to live up to your expectations.

This is one type of *self-fulfilling prophecy*, where positive – or negative – judgment of others leads them to fulfill your expectations. You've already seen the deep power of the placebo effect, so you know how powerful your expectations can be upon *yourself*, but your expectations also deeply affect how you interpret everything, particularly other people, and they profoundly shape how others will respond to and interact with you.

Negative expectations are at the heart of racism, sexism, ageism, homophobia and other destructive stereotypes. Positive expectations – and an assumption of trustworthiness – encourage, uplift and motivate.

What Is Beauty?

Since the dawn of time there have been men and women whose natural features grant them a special, effortless power to attract and influence. The timeless beauty of Cleopatra, Marilyn Monroe and Angelina Jolie has captured millions of hearts and captivated generations. But what qualities do they share? From where does this mysterious power to make pulses race and thoughts wander derive?

To fully answer that question, we need to look to behavioral psychology.

Living creatures evolve in ways that best equip themselves and their progeny to survive. Human beings are no different, and the three strongest adaptive features we have evolved are *opposable thumbs* (thumbs opposite our fingers, allowing our hands to grasp and precisely manipulate objects), *bipedalism* (walking on two legs, for hunting, fighting, energy conservation and escaping predators), and, most importantly, a massive, complex brain.

The human brain evolved into a powerful tool for instantly evaluating threats and rewards. Because of this, impressions and future expectations can be formed within milliseconds of meeting someone. In other words, first impressions have tremendous importance, because they set the stage for every interaction to follow.

In stark terms of species survival, the most vital ability of that brain is *pattern recognition* – so we can, for example, instantly discern the shape of a tiger lurking in the jungle, or recognize that a piece of food is safe to eat.

Among the skills pattern recognition confers upon us are the abilities to process colors, recognize and classify shapes, words, numbers, and, lastly, faces.

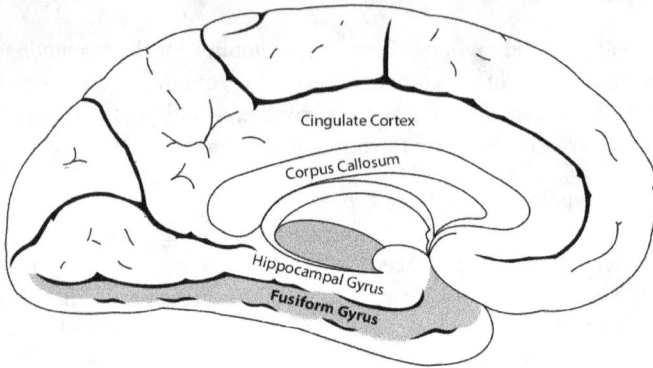

Fusiform, public domain image from Gray's Anatomy, 1858

A region of your temporal lobe called the *fusiform gyrus* seems at the center of controlling your ability to instantly and instinctively recognize faces in particular. In close conjunction with your occipital lobe and limbic system, the region allows you to instantly sense if a person is, for example:

- a stranger or acquaintance
- happy, sad, hostile, or in any other overall emotional state
- young or old
- fit or out of shape

In addition to helping you recognize people, the fusiform also participates in your instant assessment of whether or not a stranger is *a suitable gene donor* – the primary basis of "attractiveness".

> **A Dissenting View:** *Currently, the fusiform face area (FFA) is a hotly-debated issue in neuroscience. The FFA is a small section of the fusiform gyrus thought to be dedicated to face perception. It was first discovered by MIT's Dr. Nancy Kanwisher, in 1997, and is believed to handle the detection and recognition of individual faces. Becauses facial recognition is critical to survival, it's been theorized that the FFA evolved as a module specifically for dealing with faces.*
>
> *Using fMRI or PET scans to see which areas activate as subjects attempt to recognize faces, scientists determined the FFA is central to face processing, but recognition appears to derive from a larger network, with many steps and subprocesses, beginning in the retina, and including the occipital face area (OFA), and the right anterior inferotemporal cortex (aIT).*

Research has shown when the fusiform is severely damaged, you can no longer recognize friends, family members, or even someone you've just met. Additionally, you lose the ability to judge what is "beautiful" and what's not. So what, precisely, does this brain region use to judge a person as beautiful (i.e. a suitable mate)?

The latest research has nailed those principles down to an exact science – so exact that computers can now turn a facial image from "ho-hum" into "wow!" with a few simple button clicks.

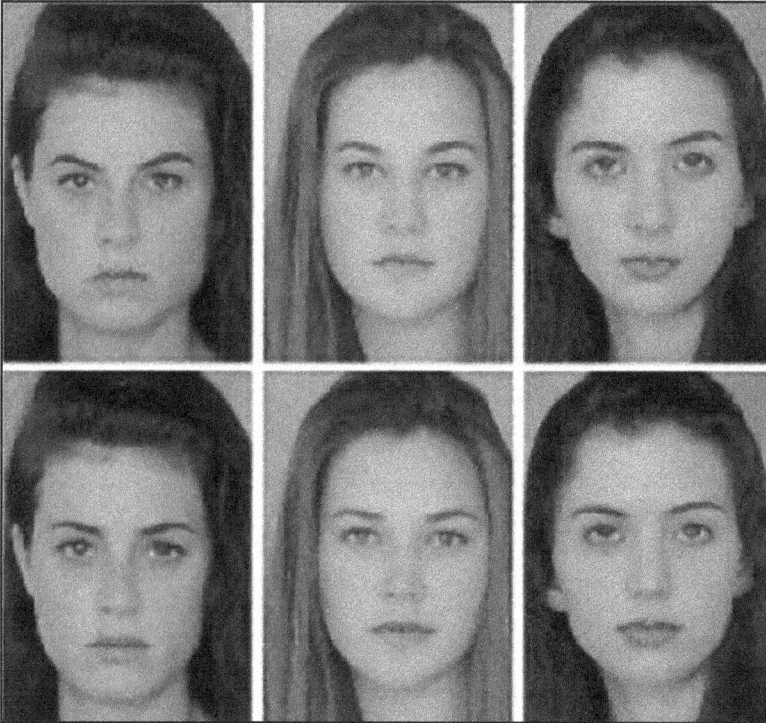

Photographs manipulated by TAU's "Beauty Machine." Top: originals; Bottom: manipulated photographs. Images courtesy of Akira Gomi and AR face database; output images courtesy of ACM SIGGRAPH.

In a 2008 study at Tel Aviv University, Professor Cohen-Or and colleagues created a database correlating to 250 different measurements and facial features, such as ratios of the nose, chin and distance from ears to eyes, and created a program that instantly applies the changes to a fresh image. A video of the presentation can be seen online: http://www.youtube.com/watch?v=lVbrUuwK-8g&feature=player_embedded

Says Prof. Cohen-Or:

Beauty can be quantified by mathematical measurements and ratios. It can be defined as average distances between features, which a majority of people agree are the most beautiful. I don't claim to know much about beauty. For us, every picture in this research project is just a collection of numbers."

I. Symmetry

The ancient Greek mathematician Pythagoras first suggested 3000 years ago that the secret of beauty lay in "harmony" or "balance" that was pleasing to the eye. He came up with a formula for the *Golden Mean* or *phi*, which dictated that if the length and the height of an object are in harmony (a mathematical ratio of 1 to 1.618), it creates a perfect sense of balance in art or design. Since that day, engineers, artists and architects have used the formula worldwide to make timeless masterpieces from the Parthenon to Leonardo da Vinci's Madonna and Child.

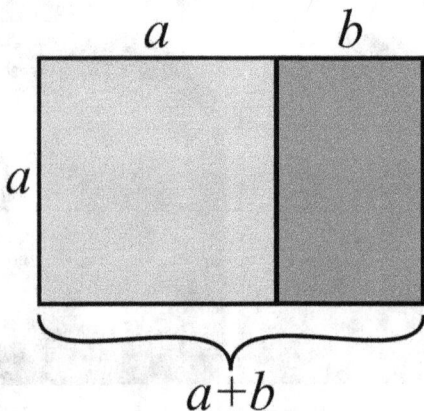

$$a \qquad b$$

$$a$$

$$a+b$$

Phi - the golden ratio or Divine Proportion - divides a line segment into two parts - a smaller portion measured against the entire length - at 1 to 1.618. This ratio has been deliberately used to create the most enduring works of art in history, including the Parthenon, Mona Lisa, Taj Mahal, Last Supper and more. It's used in modern design, and the faces of classic beauties such as Marilyn Monroe conform to it.

This formula is still a standard by which objects of beauty are created, but for human beings, a simpler standard is one of the major determinants of beauty: evenness on both sides of the face and body. That is, the more the left half of a person's face and body resembles the right half, the more attractive he or she is. This "mirror image" effect of left and right is called *symmetry*. An excellent example of someone with high symmetry in her facial features is Angelina Jolie.

Through experimentation, scientists have found that even babies prefer to look at symmetrical faces, so it's an innate, unconscious preference; it's also the same in every culture on the planet – men and women find facial features that match on the left and right to be attractive in every culture. Studies show this also affects sexual arousal and general physical attraction. What's more, this also holds true even in the animal and insect kingdoms.

The reason appears to be that living creatures naturally grow symmetrically – unless their symmetry has been misshapen by trauma such as damage from disease, or from losing a battle with a competitor. Thus, a creature that has reached adulthood with no deformative scars or signs of disease registers in our instinctive minds as a mate with high survival skills, and we are drawn to them for reproductive reasons – our subconscious mind says mating with such outwardly healthy people will give us strong, healthy babies.

II. Waist-to-Hip Ratio

From the jungles of Borneo to the boulevards of Paris, men and women find partners with a very specific *waist-to-hip ratio* to be the most attractive. When the size of the waist is compared to the size of the hips, .7 is the magic number. This means that the woman's waistline is 70% the size of her hips. Her waist and hips may both be large or small, but if they're in this ratio, we automatically find her body to be attractive.

Again, this comes down to evolutionary biology: people subconsciously choose mates with the best chance of helping them make healthy babies, and scientists have found that, all other factors being equal, a woman whose *WHR* (waist to hip ratio) is exactly .7 has up to a 1000% better chance of becoming pregnant than a woman with a less favorable ratio. Disease, injury and weight gain, all of which change WHR, impair a woman's ability to give birth. (To find your own waist to hip ratio, divide your waist size by your hip size using a calculator.

III. Average Features

By showing computer composites of facial features to human subjects, researchers have also discovered that the more typical ("average") in proportions a face is, the more beautiful people tend to think it is.

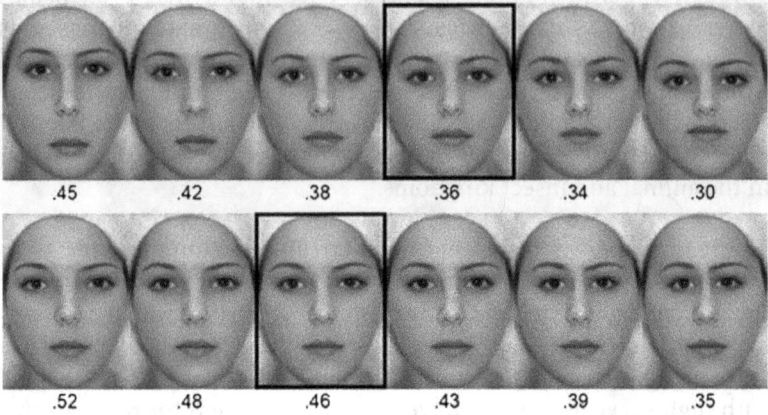

Dr. Kang Lee, University of Toronto, 2009. Used with permission

Joint research at UC San Diego and the University of Toronto has revealed the universally "ideal" arrangement of facial features for women, the mathematically optimal relation between the eyes, mouth and the edge of the face. By manipulating eye-to-mouth and eye-to-eye ratios in a series of photographs, the researchers discovered that women's faces were consistently judged more attractive by subjects when the vertical space between their eyes and mouth was approximately 36 percent of the face's length, and the horizontal space between their eyes was approximately 46 percent of the face's width.

According to Dr. Kang Lee:

> *We already know that different facial features make a female face attractive – large eyes, for example, or full lips. Our study conclusively proves that the structure of faces – the relation between our face contour and the eyes, mouth and nose – also contributes to our perception of facial attractiveness. Our finding also explains why sometimes an attractive person looks unattractive or vice versa after a haircut, because hairdos change the ratios.*

Adds colleague Dr. Pallett:

> *People have tried and failed to find these ratios since antiquity. The ancient Greeks found what they believed was a 'golden ratio' – also known as 'phi' or the 'divine proportion' – and used it in their architecture and art. Some even suggest that Leonardo Da Vinci used the golden ratio when painting his 'Mona Lisa.' But there was never any proof that the golden ratio was special. As it turns out, it isn't. Instead*

of phi, we showed that average distances between the eyes, mouth and face contour form the true golden ratios.

The team believes that in addition to symmetry, humans use a mental "averaging process" for an ideal facial width and length ratio that constitutes beauty. We are evolutionarily inclined to find such average faces beautiful.

It's their joint conclusion that, as with symmetry, we have evolved to find average facial features the most attractive. Researchers suggest this may be because it's easiest for the fusiform to quickly process average features. Aside from these three major aspects of beauty, people have always found youth, healthy vigor, and smooth, clear skin to be attractive.

Dr. Stephen Marquardt, founder of Marquardt Beauty Analysis in Huntington Beach, California is a former oral and facial surgeon at UCLA with a similar finding. He's constructed a proportional template of the ideal face used as a guide for plastic surgeons and software. His "beauty mask" template can be superimposed over pictures of people to determine how closely they conform to these ideal mathematical proportions.

Dr. Marquardt believes that each of us carries a subconscious image of what the ideal human face is supposed to look like, and the more someone's face conforms to this ideal, the greater its attractiveness:

> *Plato (427-347 BCE) discussed his "Forms", postulating that all objects have an "ideal" "form" or structure. In particular, he taught that these "Forms" were pure or perfect objects of mathematical or other conceptual knowledge. He felt that these "pure" forms existed only in the realm of knowledge and never in the reality of human everyday existence. Individual things in the realm of appearance are beautiful only insofar as they participate in, correlate with, or approach in structure these universal "Forms" of Beauty.*

> *Karl Jung (1875-1961) took the concept of Plato's "Forms" further and presented his own Theory of Archetypes. In Jungian Psychology an Archetype is "an unconscious idea, pattern of thought, image, etc., inherited from the ancestors of the race and universally present in individual psyches". In simpler terms we could basically refer to an archetype as an "instinct".*

> *We now believe that the image of the "ideal" human face is indeed an "Archetype"; a subconscious image which we are born with and carry throughout our lives. This archetype has evolved in order to help us identify members of our own species and further sort members of our species according to their relative health and ability to successfully reproduce and to provide other resources to us and those who are close to us.*

451

However, while Martquardt says his phi mask is unisex and multiracial, his detractors say it's only an ideal for Caucasian features.

Scientists do agree, however, that most men prefer women with tiny jaws and noses, large eyes and pronounced cheekbones – what is typically described as a "baby face". Conversely, woman with "mature" features, such as a large nose and small eyes, tend to receive greater respect from men. What's fascinating is that researchers have also found that women find different male facial features beautiful based on their menstrual cycles. That is, women tend to prefer heart-shaped, small-chinned, mature faces with full lips (feminine facial characteristics), but when they are having their periods, the same women prefer men with more masculine facial characteristics, such as square features, a strong brow, high forehead and broad jaw.

It's been theorized that a clandestine romp with a physically strong and aggressive man at the height of a woman's fertility would allow her to become impregnated with the sperm that carries DNA for children with the greatest chance of survival. Then bonding with a more sensitive, responsible (feminine) mate would assure protection during her vulnerable periods of pregnancy, childbirth and child rearing.

Confidence, physical strength, and a "powerful bearing" are also perceived as attractive qualities in men, with tallness universally conferring status. Research indicates women are most attracted to men at least 10% taller than themselves, with broad shoulders and a slim waist – a "v-shaped" upper body. John Barban and Brad Pilon, authors of the 2008 diet and exercise program *The Adonis Effect,* take it a step further, claiming the ideal waist to shoulder ratio is 1:1.6, citing the Golden Mean and a 1998 Archives of *Sexual Behavior* study.

Studies have also found that people are overwhelmingly more attracted to those who are friendly than those who act cold or arrogant. An exciting, warm-hearted, open personality significantly raises perceived attractiveness. Additional personality traits such as intelligence, honesty, amiability, leadership, kindness and mental stability also raise perceived attractiveness. Your individual interpretation of what is "attractive" appears to evolve over your lifetime, with superficial beauty being most important to young women, and personality traits becoming more important over time. Finally, researchers have noted that we are generally attracted to mates with facial features resembling our parents', and that the facial features of couples often tend to be similar.

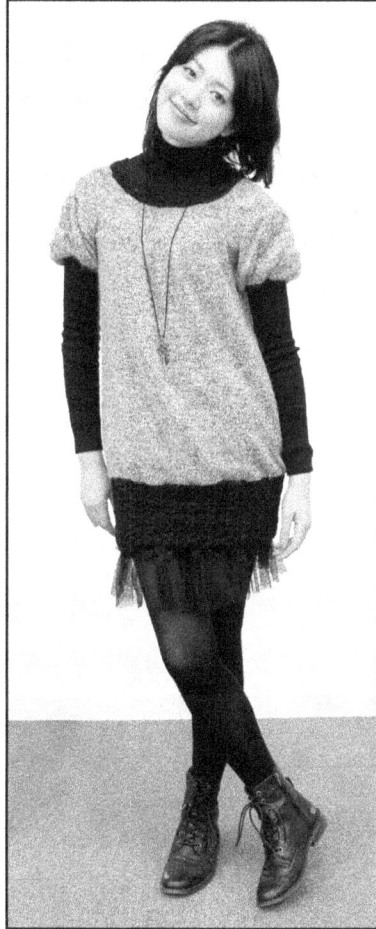

A symmetrical face, smooth skin, small chin, large eyes, full lips – traits of feminine beauty universally and instinctively recognized. Model: Yumi Takano; Photographer: Christopher Jue; copyright 2010, Polyglot Studios

The Advantages Of Beauty

Researchers have found that attractive people earn higher salaries, receive better grades in school, are favored by parents, receive lighter punishments in court, reach higher military ranks and job status, achieve more successes, have more sex, make more friends, enjoy better service and are treated better than those who are plain. Moreover, psychologists have discovered a *halo effect*: when people meet someone attractive, they often instantly assume many good things about them before a word is spoken – often automatically believing attractive people are honest, intelligent, hardworking, kind, etc. Research also shows that how you feel about your own physical attractiveness can influence the opinion of others to a great degree – confidence (and self-talk) pays real dividends.

The Disadvantages

Natural beauty is something that usually doesn't have to be earned, and some of those deemed unattractive in society can be resentful of what they see as "unfairness in life". Additionally, plain people are often worried that more beautiful people may steal their mates or have unfair advantages in the workplace. Finally, the mentally ill may project their own fantasies onto attractive people, putting them at risk of stalking or worse.

If you are lucky enough to be born naturally beautiful, think of Angelina Jolie, Brad Pitt, George Clooney and Leonardo DiCaprio as examples of standards of kindness and behavior to emulate. Being selfish or reckless (like certain notorious celebrities we all know) can sink your reputation, but if you're kind and generous, you will be regarded highly.

Why And How Cosmetics Work

Take a look at the following picture. Which of the two faces is male, and which one is female?

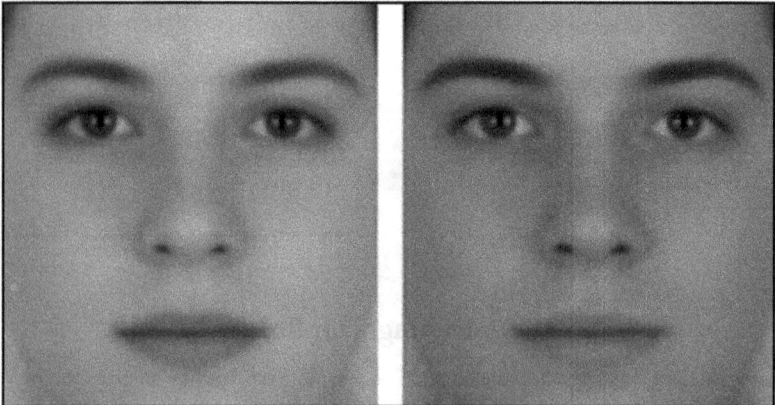

Reprinted with permission from Professor Richard Russell, Gettysburg College, 2009

It may surprise you to know that they're exactly the same image, with contrast heightened on the left to create what we perceive as more "feminine" features. According to Gettysburg College Psychology Professor Dr. Richard Russell, no matter what the race, women's skin is lighter than men's, though eyes and lips tend to be the same. This contrast in features is what our brains use to help determine facial gender recognition. Cosmetics enhance a woman's facial contrast, heightening perceived femininity and attractiveness. According to Dr. Russell:

> *Though people are not consciously aware of the sex difference in contrast, they... use the amount of contrast in a face to judge how masculine or feminine the face is, which is related to how attractive we think it is. Cosmetics are typically used in precisely the correct way to exaggerate this difference, Making the eyes and lips darker without changing the surrounding skin increases the facial contrast. Femininity and attractiveness are highly correlated, so making a face more feminine also makes it more attractive. The findings offer some clues to help unravel 'the mysteries of mateship rituals'.*

Social Status

In 2011, the National Institute of Mental Health published studies showing your social status influences your responses to others. Those of high socioeconomic status have a greater amount of brain activity in response to other high-status people, while people with lower status respond more to others of low status. The differences register in the *ventral striatum*, a region central to processing the value of rewards.

How you interact and behave around others is largely determined by their social status in relation to your own, so information related to social status is important, according to Dr. Caroline F. Zink of the National Institute of Mental Health. And the value people assign to another's status seems dependent upon their own.

While fMRI monitored their ventral striata, volunteers of varying social status looked at information about a person of relatively higher status and then about a person of relatively lower status. Their brain responses varied depending upon their own relative status. Humans, like other social species, decide what is appropriate behavior based upon assessments of social status. Socioeconomic status isn't written in stone, however; it can vary over time.

When determining appropriate emotions and behavior, you evaluate your environment, and the ventral striatum seems to be the center of activity for this evaluation. This is because people tend to view the benefits of social status mainly in terms of rewards.

A 2010 study by Dr. Martinez and a team of colleagues at Columbia University discovered that the density of dopamine receptors in the striatum correlate with social status and support. After determining the social status of healthy volunteers, Dr. Martinez and his team ran PET scans to measure their dopamine type 2 receptors. The findings indicate people of higher social status have a greater capacity to enjoy life, finding it more stimulating and rewarding, due to increased dopamine receptors within their striata.

According to Dr. John Krystal, Editor of *Biological Psychiatry*, this partly helps explain the human drive to achieve social status. People with more D2 receptors are more strongly motivated and engaged by social situations, driven by their mesolimbic reward pathways to become high achievers and have higher social support levels.

On the other hand, low levels of dopamine receptors correlate with lower social status and social support from friends, family, or partners. The work of Dr. Nora Volkow, Director of the National Institute on Drug Abuse, implies that D2 receptor-deficient individuals are vulnerable to lower social status and social supports, and these social factors heighten the risk of alcohol and substance abuse.

Developing Charisma

We all know someone who can walk into the room and immediately "own" it. So what special magnetic characteristic do they possess – this air of effortless persuasion? While you might not have been born with the magnetism of Angelina Jolie or George Clooney, you *can* refine your image and personality to make yourself more attractive and credible. Here are some pointers:

Polish your Exterior – Always pay attention to what you wear, to your posture, grooming and overall appearance.

Get an Outside Opinion – Learn how others perceive you through the advice of trusted friends, photographs and videotapes of yourself. Keep a list of what you like about your appearance and start to fix what you don't.

Speak with Conviction – If you know what's important to you in life, you can convey it more powerfully. When you're passionate about an issue, you're more persuasive, articulate, and attractive.

The Power Of A Smile

HealthTap and Wellsphere CEO Ron Gutman has long conducted research into helping people live healthier, happier lives. In *The Untapped Power of Smiling*, he describes some of the incredible facts about smiling:

A 2000 study of 30-year-old yearbook pictures found women's smiles to be a predictor of their well-being and success throughout their lives; measuring smile width, scientists could predict how long-lasting and happy their marriages were, their scores on tests measuring happiness and well-being, and how much they could inspire others later in life. Those who smiled widest were consistently in the highest ranks for all categories.

In a similar 2010 study at Wayne State University, Professors Ernest L. Abel and Michael L. Kruger used smiles of famous athletes on baseball cards to predict how long they would live:

> *Emotions affect personalities and life outcomes by influencing how people think, behave, and interact with others. People with positive emotions are happier and have more stable personalities, more stable marriages, and better cognitive and interpersonal skills than those with negative emotions, throughout the life span.*

Their startling finding was that players with the biggest smiles outlived their peers by an average of seven years.

Says Gutman, smiling is a basic fundamental instinct common to humans around the globe and throughout history. In fact, smiling is such a fundamental, natural expression, 3D ultrasound shows babies do it while in the womb, and almost continuously throughout infancy.

Apparently, we're not only hard-wired to smile, but also to respond to smiles from others; studies at Sweden's Uppsala University have proven that seeing a smile suppresses normal control over facial muscles – compelling you to break into a smile in response. It's also naturally difficult to frown in response to someone else's smile. Gutman suggests that (presumably via mirror neurons), your automatic reflex to mimic a smile allows you to physically experience the emotions of the smiler you're watching, and helps you in interpreting the emotional meaning and authenticity of the smile.

In research performed at the University of Clermont-Ferrand in France, subjects were asked to interpret real vs. fake smiles, while holding a pencil in their mouths to repress the muscles that help us smile. Without the pencils in their mouths, subjects were excellent judges, but with the pencils – *when they could not mimic the smiles they saw* – their judgment was impaired.

A 2009 study at Echnische University in Munich used Botox – weakened botulism toxin – to temporarily paralyze the smiling muscles of test subjects, and scanned their brain activity before and after. They discovered that mimicking facial expressions alters limbic system activity, showing how emotions are transferred from person to person via facial expressions – smiles or other expressions.

Smiling has also been correlated with a significant reduction in stress hormones such as cortisol and adrenaline, lower blood pressure, and an increase in health- and mood-improving endorphins. Seeing the smile of someone you love or admire smile has particularly amazing physiological effects: a 2005 study led by Dr. David Lewis, author of *The Secret Language of Success,* involved fMRI scans and heart-rate monitors, used to measure the effects of a number of pleasure-inducing stimuli.

109 test subjects were, in turn, given chocolate, money, and shown photos of smiling friends, family and loved ones. In comparing the health effects of each reward, a child's smile triggered positive stimulation equivalent to 2,000 chocolate bars or over $21,000, while the smile of a loved one triggered positive activity equivalent to 600 chocolate bars or over $11,000, and a friend's smile elicited 200 bars of chocolate or $200 worth of positivity.

Smiling also enhances your attractiveness; a 2007 study conducted at the University of Aberdeen in Scotland, found that a direct gaze with a smile enhanced both likeability and sexual attractiveness.

Quantum-Level Charisma

If you want to persuade or otherwise influence others, psychologists have outlined the most powerful techniques, based upon fundamental human motivation.

It's well-understood that sentient creatures avoid negative stimuli such as pain or discomfort, and approach positive stimuli, such as pleasant physical sensations, or emotions.

While humans, with our advanced cortices, have the capacity for much more complex experiences and motivations than insects, reptiles or other less mentally-evolved creatures, we still share the same fundamental basis of motivation, as well as common behavioral traits that have been well-studied and, within the last decade, understood quite deeply.

Said by many to be the greatest book on persuasion ever written, Professor Robert B. Cialdini's *Influence: The Psychology of Persuasion* describes what motivates people, and how this can be turned to your advantage in virtually any situation. He lists six *Weapons of Influence* used by the most effective marketers, salespeople, and canny negotiators throughout everyday life.

Dr. Cialdini followed up his "must-read" international smash hit book with a joint 2004 study entitled *Social Influence: Compliance and Conformity*. In the paper, Dr. Cialdini and co-author Dr. Noah J. Goldstein gathered and summarized the most important research on influence, compliance and conformity between 1997 and 2002. They stating that people "...are motivated to form accurate perceptions of reality and react accordingly, to develop and preserve meaningful social relationships, and to maintain a favorable self-concept." They summarized these as "three goals fundamental to rewarding human functioning":

1. *Affiliation* – the desire to be an accepted member of one or several social circles)

2. *Accuracy* – the desire to learn and use the "best" (most practical and beneficial) techniques for managing life issues and relationships

3. *Maintaining a Positive Self-Concept* – the need to be true to an inner identities, and to maintain a consistent worldview

Affiliation boils down to the simple human desire to be liked. Research has shown that positive human touch and social interaction cause the brain to release mood-enhancing endorphins, raise self-esteem and elevate mood. Conversely, rejection feels terrible, releases the stress hormone cortisol, lowers the hormone testosterone, makes self-esteem drop, and worsens mood.

Because we want to be liked and socially accepted, we act in ways we think will be please people whose approval we desire. And because it's the simplest, safest way to receive approval from a large number of people, people like to become part of a group, which often leaves them open to the influence of *opinion leaders*, who may not always be acting in the best interest of their followers.

Accuracy is our constant desire to do things in the best, most efficient and/or rewarding way possible. We want to know the "best way to get along with others" or the optimal route to and from work, or "easy time-savers in the kitchen". We also tend to look to others around us to assess whether or not we're doing things "correctly".

Maintaining a Positive Self-Concept is our need to preserve ideas about ourselves and what kind of people we are, as well as our personal world view. Out of necessity, human beings have evolved to behave consistently, generally through habit formation. This means if you think of yourself as a people person, you're going to do things to fit that label.

If a friend wanted to manipulate you into going to a party you were reluctant to attend, they could trigger this subconscious goal by saying something like, "you mean you're not going? You always go! Come on, you *love* mingling!"

A secondary part of this unconscious drive to maintain consistency is the need to maintain long-held worldviews. If you believe people are basically good at heart, you're likely to listen to messages that bolster that worldview, and tune out conflicting ones.

Six Weapons Of Influence

Professor Robert Cialdini's *Weapons of Influence* shows how successful persuaders – be they politicians, salesmen, middle managers or even spouses – capitalize upon certain human needs. You can be certain that virtually every modern advertisement you see or political speech that you hear has been written by someone who studied Professor Caldini's work – it's been updated as a university textbook, translated into 25 languages, and sold 2 million copies since its first publication in 2001. The six weapons of influence are:

1. ***Reciprocity*** – When you receive something nice from another person, you feel like you owe them something in return. A free coffee sample in the shopping mall or even a compliment on how someone is dressed are "favors" salesmen use to you feel you owe someone a kindness in return. As the Japanese proverb says, "The most expensive things are those that are offered for free".

2. ***Commitment and Consistency*** – The cliché "sticking to your guns" comes close to describing how this persuasion technique works. Once a person's made a decision or acted in a certain way, they will probably do it again and continue to do so, to maintain their idea of who they are and justify that their actions are "correct".

   Advertisers exploit this in building brand loyalty with ads suggesting you're a "Marlboro Man" or clothing that says you're "Juicy". Interestingly, a new study has found that brand identities have even come to heighten people's perceptions of themselves, so that carrying Victoria's Secret bags made mall shoppers regard themselves as better-looking, more glamorous and feminine than shoppers with non-branded bags, and using a pen with the MIT logo made people believe themselves to be more intelligent, and have greater leadership qualities.

3. ***Social Proof*** – Otherwise known as the principle of "monkey see, monkey do" – if you see others taking a certain course of action,

you subconsciously accept this as proof of its logic. You can have fun with this one: stop in the middle of the sidewalk and stare up into the sky for quick proof of how powerful this effect is.

Even just hearing "everybody's got one!" is enough to trigger an inner "Well I want one too!" impulse. My favourite personal example of this principle at work is found in *The Adventures of Tom Sawyer*, in chapter two, free for downloading online here: http://etext.lib.virginia.edu/toc/modeng/public/Twa2Tom.html

Dr. Cialdini cites the use of laugh tracks in comedy as an example of media exploitation of this principle – subconsciously we believe that if others are laughing, what we're watching must be funny....

4. *Liking* – This principle is pretty obvious – if you like someone, you'll value his or her opinion, and you're thus more open to persuasion. Particularly attractive people have an advantage here, which is why models and movie stars are used to endorse products. Finding similarities is another powerful way to build rapport quickly – we like people who we believe are similar to us.

5. *Authority* – If somebody has a title, we often automatically obey them, sometimes even against our better judgment, as in the infamous "shock experiments" conducted by Yale University psychologist Stanley Milgram.

6. *Scarcity* – Ads that shout, "Buy now! Time is running out!" illustrate this principle in action. In short, we want what we can't have. If it seems there's a limited supply of something, our impulse is to grab our own fair share. This ties in neatly with the principle of *social proof* – subconsciously we're compelled to believe "If everyone else is buying that, it *must* be good!"

It would be irresponsible to end our discussion on persuasion here. While it's certainly possible to use these techniques in selfish, manipulative ways, it's far better for many reasons to use this knowledge ethically, looking for ways to benefit others as well as oneself, the classic "win-win" stance.

Social Bulldozers

Authority figures share certain behaviours. They tend to smile less often, interrupt others more frequently, and speak in louder voices, according to 2011 studies conducted at the University of Amsterdam. By breaking proper rules of social decorum, they convey the impression of power and status.

Because people with a lot of money and influence have fewer rules constraining them, and greater access to resources, knowledge and support, they experience a much different reality than most people. Conversely, powerless people are limited in their behavior, and compelled to follow rules by threat of punishment. These rules of social behavior are called *norms*, and experiments show that those who break them appear more powerful.

Norm violators are seen as having the freedom to do whatever they like, so acting in this manner among strangers makes you appear powerful, according to Dr. Gerben Van Kleef, who led the study.

Volunteers in his study were asked to evaluate a visitor who violated norms, taking employee coffee without asking, or posing as a bookkeeper that broke accounting rules. The volunteers consistently found these rule breakers to be more "in control" and "powerful" compared with people who didn't steal coffee or break bookkeeping rules. One caveat is that this may vary by culture; such violations of unspoken rules would likely be seen as much more serious in Japan than in America, for example.

Like rule-breaking, acting rudely also conveys an air of power. Volunteers watched videos of a man in a sidewalk café acting rudely or politely and gave their impressions. When the actor put his feet up on a chair, tossed cigarette ashes on the ground and brusquely ordered his food, volunteers were much more likely to describe him as a "decision-maker", with the ability to get people to listen to him than the same actor being polite.

In a related study, Dr. Van Kleef and his team brought volunteers into the lab with actors who assumed the roles of rule breakers or rule followers. The polite actor acted normal and considerate, while the rule breaker came late, threw his bag onto a table and put his feet up. Volunteers reported that the rule breaker was more powerful and able to compel others to do what he wanted.

Seven Types Of Personal Power

Karen Burns, author of *The Amazing Adventures of Working Girl: Real-Life Career Advice You Can Actually Use* says influence comes from several different sources, and knowing about them increases your effectiveness. Consider how you can increase your personal influence in each of the following ways:

1. *Authority* – This is the most overt form of influence, bestowed with the title of "president" or "department head", etc. However, the title alone isn't enough – to ensure your influence continues, you must

have at least one of the other forms of power, or you will quickly find your influence fading.

2. **Wealth** – When you have or control access to money or material goods that someone else wants, you have significant influence. However, this is not based upon who you are – when you no longer possess or have access to them, your influence will completely dissipate. An excellent story that illustrates this kind of power and its subsequent loss is the novel *The Bonfire of the Vanities* by Tom Wolfe.

3. **Connections** – Knowing who to introduce to whom, and where to go for information makes you a "mover and a shaker" that others want to know. An excellent example of someone who exploited this influence was Enoch L. Johnson, the Prohibition-era statesman and gangster fictionalized as "Nucky" Thompson in the HBO television series *Boardwalk Empire*.

4. **Knowledge** – Being an expert at a given skill puts you in a unique place of power – people will come to you to help sort out their problems and offer them guidance. Think of Hugh Laurie's character in the television series House.

5. **Love** – Some people are born with charisma, a natural attractiveness that draws people to them and makes them feel affection. Charisma can certainly be developed (through the techniques here), but for some people, a natural charm is effortless.

    Unfortunately, this power can often lead to vanity or a sense of unearned entitlement. If you are one of the lucky ones born with strong charisma, take care to never let it blind you to the fundamental equality of people. Examples that immediately spring to mind are Marilyn Monroe, Cary Grant, Brad Pitt or Elizabeth Taylor.

6. **Respect** – Being known as reliable, ethical, honest, dependable, of upstanding character, and having a solid work ethic brings respect over time. Examples could include Eleanor Roosevelt or Mother Teresa.

7. **Fear** – If you have the ability to physically, socially, emotionally or financially punish others, it will give you influence over them. However, using this kind of power can breed deep resentment and hatred, so it's best when never used, but only implied. Of course, Adolph Hitler and Joseph Stalin are examples of this kind of power.

Ms. Burns cautions that power can become addictive and easily abused, but abuse of power is an obvious sign of insecurity and weakness. Take care to use your own influence in life for to spread happiness and growth instead of misery and discord.

Online: Virtual Charisma

In a rapidly modernizing society, face-to-face first meetings are being replaced with online introductions through social networking sites. If you're interested in creating a powerful first impression online, dating site *OKCupid.com* has some excellent advice for you. Out of over 500,000 first contact messages, OKCupid found only 32% receive one or more responses, but some people get consistently better reply rates. By looking at keywords and phrases and how they affected reply rates, the company devised a set of guidelines for online introductions. In order of importance, they suggest the following:

1. *Sound Intelligent* – Grammar and spelling mistakes as well as slang and "netspeak" were deal-breakers. Examples of what they deemed "huge turn-offs" included "ur", "u", "wat", "wont", etc. The exceptions were expressions of amusement like "haha" and "lol".

2. *Dial Back the Hornies* – Don't compliment someone's appearance during initial contact (men or women). It suggests desperation and hints the sender is unattractive. General compliments, however, seem to elicit favorable responses. The keywords "awesome", "fascinating" and "pretty good" worked well, as did messages showing interest in what the other had to say, with "you mention" ranking at the top.

3. *Novelty is Powerful* – Saying "hi" and "hello" doesn't fare well, but jumping right into what you want to say is the best approach, followed by informal, casual greetings like "how's it going?", "what's up?", and "howdy".

4. *Individuality is Attractive* – bringing up specific individual preferences in music, social activities and/or other tastes are an apparently effective way to make a connection.

5. *Humility is a Virtue (for men)* – Although confidence is king in the real world, online, being a little more humble has a much more beneficial impact. The words "kinda", "sorry", "apologize" and "probably" all made for much more successful interactions. The one exception was the word "please", which, the authors note, may smack of desperation.

6. *Avoid Religion* – Self-proclaimed atheists received the highest response rate at 56%.

7. *Brevity Attracts* – The ideal length of a first message is 200 characters from men, and only 50 characters from women.

Be More Photogenic

OKCupid.com next studied 7,000 profile photos from their database, comparing how many contacts each picture yielded. They analyzed three parameters:

- *Expression and Pose* – (smiling, looking straight ahead, pursing the lips flirtatiously, etc.

- *Context* – (environment, alone or among friends, activity, with a pet, car, etc.

- *Revelation* – (showing cleavage for women or muscles for men, face, etc.

An interesting initial finding was that profiles which didn't show the subject's face were just as successful in getting responses as those which showed the face – as long as the pictures showed "...something unusual, sexy, or mysterious enough to make people want to talk to you." So what *were* the best ways to take a profile picture?

For Women – Holding the camera overhead and tilting the head down ("the MySpace shot") while making eye contact and pouting at the camera was by far the single most effective photo type for women (cleavage or no cleavage).

Women got the worst response when seeming to flirt off-camera (presumably with someone else?).

The Cleavage Shot was also very successful, drawing 49% more contacts per month than average. As women's ages went up, they tended to get fewer responses, BUT, when they were older AND showed cleavage, their responses went up. Additionally, doing something interesting (such as playing an instrument), or posing with an animal generated a lot of contacts. Travel pictures ranked a distant third.

For Men – For men, smiling was NOT an effective approach. In fact, the most responses were generated by pictures where the man looked away from the camera with disinterest (not smiling) – the effect was about a 50% increase in responses. Presumably a shot from below would be even more effective, as we'll see shortly. Appearing to flirt away from the camera was likewise the worst thing men could do. Guys also fared poorly in formal clothes – casual clothes seemed to be more effective.

Among other types of pictures that generated interest were posing with an animal, showing off muscles (only for men aged 19 to 31, and the effect decreased significantly with age), being engaged in a fun or interesting activity, or having fun with friends – presumably because they make someone look "more normally adjusted and well balanced".

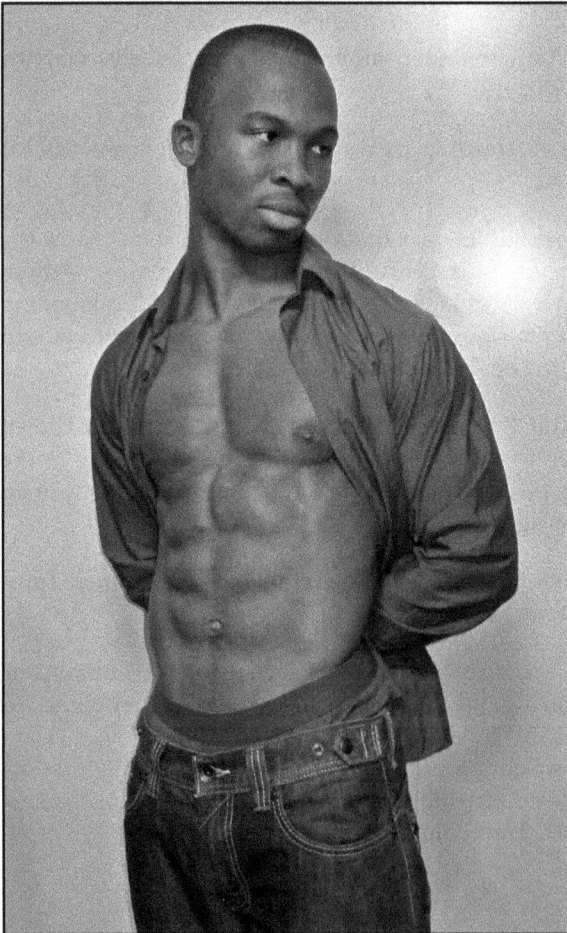

Pro kickboxer Arthur Sorsor demonstrates an optimal profile pose. Photo used with permission, photographer anonymous

Research has also shown women consistently look for cues on a man's desirability based on how other women seem to judge him. A group of women smiling at the man in the picture seems to boost judgments of his attractiveness considerably.

Use Good Equipment

In another survey of over 11 million online subscribers, OKCupid also found the more complex the camera, the more attractive pictures will be – a digital Single Lens Reflex (where you can adjust and change the lenses) gives the best results. Automatic cameras give generally baseline results, and pictures taken with phone cameras fared the worst.

Additionally, blurring out the background and sharply focusing in on just the main subject with a shallow depth of field enhances pictures tremendously, according to their findings. This is achieved by using a *wide aperture* setting – like the iris in your eye, the aperture changes the amount of light allowed to enter the camera.

The best times to take have your picture taken, they've found, were between 1 pm to 4 pm and 2 am to 7 am; 7 am to noon and 6 pm to 10 pm were the worst. Using direct flash adds seven years to your appearance, so the flash should be softened by bouncing it off of walls.

OKCupid also recently debuted a new service that allows you to upload pictures and get detailed feedback on which are your best, what category of people like them and where they're located. The service is called "MyBest-Face", and can be found here: http://www.okcupid.com/mybestface

---

Capitalize on Your Flaws Another OKCupid study examined the profiles of 11 million men and women and found the surprising fact that emphasizing one's unusual features draws more positive responses.

What's Your Angle?

According to the latest research, people appear more attractive to the opposite sex by changing the angle of their faces. Dr. Darren Burke, a senior psychology lecturer at the University of Newcastle, Australia, and his wife, Dr. Danielle Sulikowski, conducted the study as a team, using computer-generated 3D male and female faces.

As the computer images were tilted up and down among five different positions, participants rated each face for attractiveness, masculinity and femininity. Said Dr. Burke, women are more alluring when tilting their heads downwards and looking up, while men look more masculine when tilting their heads backwards and looking slightly downward.

In other words, an upwardly tilted face is judged to be more masculine and less feminine, and a downwardly tilted face is judged to be more feminine and less masculine. Drs. Burke and Sulikowski believe this mimics ideal height differences between men and women – when a woman tilts her head forward, with her chin downwards, she is recreating the way a taller man would see her.

According to Dr. Burke, "For women, a slight downward tilt of the head simulates the view from above and that is most feminine and most attractive; for men, a slight backward tilt of the head is judged as most masculine, which can make the man more attractive."

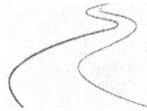

Pygmalion, Wikipedia, 2010

Intro to Psychology, Lecture 17, Professor Paul Bloom, April 16, 2007, Yale University

Discriminating Individual Faces From Neural Activation, December 29, 2007, Johan Carlin, MA, Cambridge University

Dopamine Type 2/3 Receptor Availability in the Striatum and Social Status in Human Volunteers, Martinez et al., 2010, Biological Psychiatry; 67 (3): 275 DOI: 10.1016/j.biopsych.2009.07.037; http://www.ncbi.nlm.nih.gov/pubmed/19811777

Subjective Socioeconomic Status Predicts Human Ventral Striatal Responses to Social Status Information, Martina Ly, M. Ryan Haynes, Joseph W. Barter, Daniel R. Weinberger, Caroline F. Zink, Current Science, 28 April 2011 DOI: 10.1016/j.cub.2011.03.050

Breaking the Rules to Rise to Power: How Norm Violators Gain Power in the Eyes of Others, G. A. Van Kleef, A. C. Homan, C. Finkenauer, S. Gundemir, E. Stamkou. Social Psychological and Personality Science, 2011; DOI: 10.1177/1948550611398416

A Machine Learning Predictor of Facial Attractiveness Revealing Human-like Psychophysical Biases, Amit Kagian, Gideon Dror, Tommer Leyvand, Isaac Meilijson, Daniel Cohen-Or a, Eytan Ruppin, Vision Research, 2008;

Data-Driven Enhancement of Facial Attractiveness, SIGGRAPH 2008

New "Golden" Ratios for Facial Beauty", Pamela M. Pallett; Stephen Link and Kang Lee, Vision

Research 50 (2): 149–154, 2010

Stephen R. Marquardt, Wikipedia, 2011; See also: http://www.beautyanalysis.com/

Male Physical Attractiveness in Britain and Greece: A Cross-Cultural Study, Swami Viren, et al, The Journal of Social Psychology, 2007, 147,15-26;

Physical Attractiveness: The Influence of Selected Torso Parameters, T. Horvath, Archives of Sexual Behavior, Vol. 10, No. 1, 1981;

Sex Differences in Morphological Predictors of Sexual Behavior Shoulder to Hip and Waist to Hip Ratios, Susan M. Hughes, Gordon G. Gallup, Jr., 2003, Evolution and Human Behavior, 24, 173-178;

Female Judgment of Male Attractiveness and Desirability for Relationships: Role of Waist-to-Hip Ratio and Financial Status, Devendra Singh, Journal of Personality and Social Psychology, 1995, vol. 69;

Interviewing Strategies in the Face of Beauty: A Psychophysiological Investigation into the Job Negotiation Process, Carl Senior; Michael J.R. Butler, 2007 Annals of the New York Academy of Sciences: The Social Cognitive Neuroscience of Corporate Thinking;

The Biology of Beauty, Cowley, Geoffrey, June 3, 1996, Newsweek;

Personality Goes a Long Way: The Malleability of Opposite-Sex Physical Attractiveness, Gary Lewandoski, Art Aron, Julie Gee, 2007, Personal Relationships 14

A New Viewpoint on the Evolution of Sexually Dimorphic Human Faces, Dr. Darren Burke, Danielle Sulikowski, 2010, Journal of Evolutionary Psychology, 8(4): 573-585 http://www.epjournal.net/filestore/EP08573585.pdf

Expressions Of Positive Emotion In Women's College Yearbook Pictures And Their Relationship To Personality And Life Outcomes Across Adulthood, Keltner, D. and Harker, L., 2001, Journal of Personality and Social Psychology, Vol. 80, No. 1; http://education.ucsb.edu/janeconoley/ed197/documents/Keltnerexpressionsofpositivemotion.pdf

Smile Intensity In Photographs Predicts Longevity, Ernest L. Abel, E. and Kruger, M., Psychological Science (April 2010 21: 542-544); http://pss.sagepub.com/content/early/2010/02/26/0956797610363775.extract

Scanner Shows Unborn Babies Smile, BBC News September 9, 2003;

Scans Uncover Secrets Of The Womb, BBC News (June 28, 2004); http://news.bbc.co.uk/2/hi/health/3105580.stm

Attachment, Bowlby, J., 1983, Volume 2 of Attachment and Loss, Basic Books

The Repertoire Of Nonverbal Behavior: Categories, Origins, Usage, And Coding, Ekman, P. & Friesen, W. V, 1969, Semiotica, 1, 49–98).

Facial Reactions To Emotional Stimuli: Automatically Controlled Emotional Responses, Dimberg, U., Thunberg, M., Grunedal, S., 2002, Cognition and Emotion (2002) 16:4, 449–471;

469

The Voluntary Facial Action Technique: A Method to Test the Facial Feedback Hypothesis, Dimberg, U., Söderkvist, S., 2011, Journal of Nonverbal Behavior, 35:1, 17033.

The Simulation Of Smiles (SIMS) Model: Embodied Simulation And The Meaning Of Facial Expression, Niedenthal, P. Mermillod, M., Maringer, M., Hess, U., 2010, Behavioral and Brain Sciences 33, 417–480; http://lapsco.univ-bpclermont.fr/persos/mermillod/BBS_2010.pdf

The Link Between Facial Feedback And Neural Activity Within Central Circuitries Of Emotion – New Insights From Botulinum Toxin-Induced Denervation Of Frown Muscles, Hennenlotter, A., Dresel, C., Castrop, F., et. al, 2009, Cerebral Cortex, 19 (3): 537-542; http://cercor.oxfordjournals.org/content/19/3/537.short

One Smile Can Make You Feel A Million Dollars, The Scottsman, May 4, 2005, http://news.scotsman.com/health/One-smile-can-make-you.2607641.jp

Yet Another Reason to Look After Your Teeth, Press Release, British Dental Health Organization (April 30, 2005) http://www.dentalhealth.org.uk/pressreleases/releasedetail.php?id=228/

Evidence for Adaptive Design in Human Gaze Preference, C.A Conway, B.C Jones, L.M DeBruine and A.C Little, Proceedings of the Royal Society of Biological Sciences, 2007, doi: 10.1098/rspb.2007.1073 Proc. R. Soc. B, vol. 275 no. 1630 63-69; http://rspb.royalsocietypublishing.org/content/275/1630/63.full.pdf+html

A Sex Difference in Facial Pigmentation and its Exaggeration by Cosmetics, Dr. Richard Russell, Perception, 2009, Vol. 38: 1211-1219

Seven Ways to Gain Power at Work, Karen Burns, September 8, 2010, US News,

Charisma: Seven Keys to Developing the Magnetism that Leads to Success, Tony Alessandra, 2000

Influence: The Psychology of Persuasion, Robert B. Cialdini, 2001

Yes! 50 Scientifically Proven Ways to be Persuasive, Dr. Robert B. Cialdini, Dr. Noah Goldstein and Steve J. Martin, 2009

The 4 Big Myths of Profile Pictures, Christian Rudder, 2010 http://blog.okcupid.com/index.php/the-4-big-myths-of-profile-pictures/

Don't Be Ugly By Accident! Christian Rudder, August 10th, 2010 http://blog.okcupid.com/index.php/dont-be-ugly-by-accident/)

Exactly What To Say In A First Message, Christian Rudder, September 14th, 2009 http://blog.okcupid.com/index.php/online-dating-advice-exactly-what-to-say-in-a-first-message/

The Untapped Power of Smiling, Ron Gutman, 2011; http://blog.healthtap.com/2011/05/the-untapped-power-of-smiling/

Contact

*"The Creator would indeed have been a bungling artist had he intended man for a
social animal without planting in him social dispositions."*
–Thomas Jefferson, circa 1815

"To touch can be to give life." – Michelangelo

It was a heart wrenching, baffling mystery. A century ago, orphaned American babies were dying before their seventh month, 75% of them wasting away from a mysterious affliction, even with sound food and medical care. But as soon as these babies were removed from the giant, impersonal orphanages and placed into loving homes, they quickly returned to health and began to thrive.

Orphanage workers were instructed to start holding the babies; from that point forward, these babies stopped dying. The culprit was *marasmus*, an illness caused by a lack of human touch. According to Drs. Ben Benjamin, and Ruth Werner in *The Primacy of Human Touch*, because of this finding, some modern American hospitals now have hospital volunteers massage sick and premature infants for fifteen minutes, three times a day.

Babies who receive this touch therapy grow faster, gain more weight and leave the hospital sooner than their untouched counterparts, and the "volunteer grandparents" who donate their time to take care of these babies also experience huge health benefits, and have lower levels of anxiety and depression and greater self-esteem.

They say it's because, unlike other animal species, humans emerge from the womb prematurely, unable to move or function to any great degree. Unable to see clearly or distinguish sounds, their only information from the outside world is gathered through the sense of touch. Thus, the way a baby is touched early in life has a major impact on whether it survives, and these first messages about safety and well-being that babies receive through touch affect them for the rest of their lives, impacting their adult coping skills.

Research has shown baby rats which are separated from their mothers undergo measurable brain damage, with actual cell degeneration in their central nervous systems.

Young monkeys that have received nurturing deal with stressful situations with curiosity and a kind of "tentative courage", but baby monkeys raised without touch become easily overwhelmed by new experiences, and collapse into hysterical screaming when placed in unfamiliar environments or challenging situations.

Numerous studies have shown it's the same in humans – children who receive a great deal of positive physical touch usually grow into stable, mature, loving adults, while infants deprived of nurturing touch tend to grow into aggressive and even violent adults.

Oxytocin, the brain's "trust hormone", is released in the brain during contact between humans and other animals. Recent shows this plays a vital role in human happiness and well-being, increasing cooperative social behaviours and reducing cortisol levels and other stress symptoms.

"Work in the last two decades has propelled oxytocin toward the top of a list of potentially effective stress- and anxiety-reducing agents, largely due to its positive associations with mental health," says Dr. Jason Yee of the University of Illinois "…the biological basis for social connections – oxytocin – is part of the brain mechanisms that serve to make us happy," adds Claremont Graduate University's Dr. Paul Zak.

Zak and his colleagues have found that women with the highest oxytocin levels report the most life satisfaction, least depression, and have greater resilience in response to challenges. Women who tend to share are also happier, more trusting, and have stronger attachments to others.

Extensive research has shown that positive touch can also influence performance and behavior in a number of different ways, for example, a teacher giving a student a supportive pat on the back or the arm inspires the student to become more involved in class, and athletes who hug or "high-five" their teammates play better. Touch increases likeability, trust, devotion, and influence, promotes monogamy, generosity, friendliness, enhances social skills and brings people closer together.

Birth doulas – professionals who provide supportive touch and closeness to mothers giving birth – have been shown to significantly shorten labor, and reduce complications and requests for pain medication.

According to Tiffany Field, director of the Touch Research Institute at the University of Miami, the mechanisms are very well understood: pressure on the skin from touch activates mechanoreceptors called *Pacinian corpuscles,* which send a signal to the *vagus nerve.* The vagus nerve, if you recall, is cranial nerve ten, when sends branches throughout the body, to a number of internal organs, including the heart. Parasympathetic impulses from the medulla through the vagus nerve slow the heart and decrease blood pressure.

Subjects under study performed stressful tasks like public speaking, and the Field's team found that when their partners hugged or held their hands, it reduced subjects' blood pressure and heart rate.

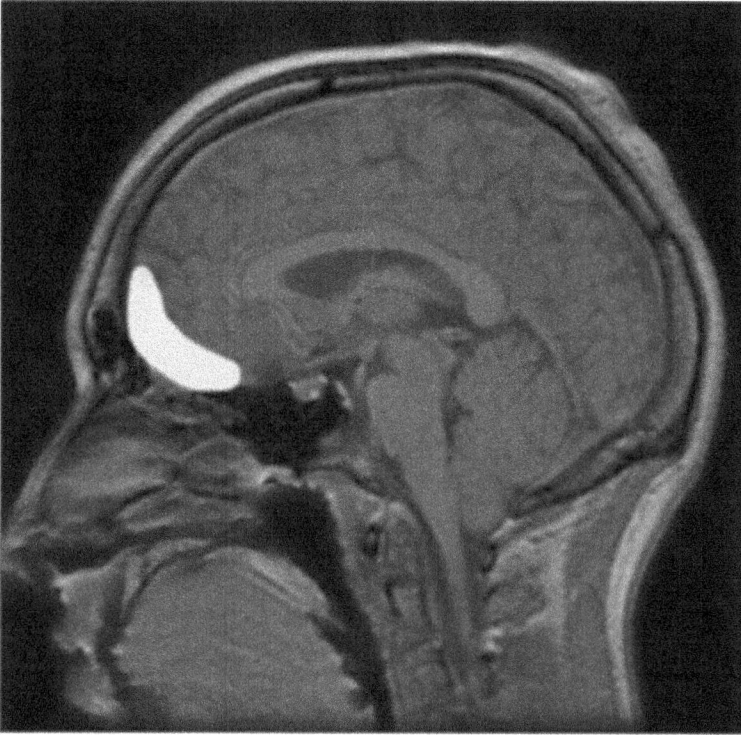

The orbitofrontal cortex, Wikipedia, public domain, 2009

In addition, the *orbitofrontal cortex* – the area above the eyes activated by dopamine and serotonin in response to pleasant fragrances or sweet tastes – "lights up", becoming highly active in response to a friendly touch.

Meanwhile, oxytocin quiets the amygdala's fight or flight response, reducing the likelihood that animals and people automatically classify others as threats, allowing them to better see faint signs of benign or friendly intent.

Once friendly contact has been initiated, the oxytocin release in both parties creates and sustains a "social loop" – a continuous positive feedback system between both parties, increasing mental and physical wellbeing.

Positive stimuli such as pleasant and friendly sights, sounds and smells can also trigger oxytocin release, and studies have shown oxytocin levels double in both humans and pets when the owners return home and meet them. Stroking an animal's fur causes an oxytocin release, and even simple eye contact with a pet can trigger the healthy chemical emission.

473

Contact with animals has even been said to inspire the mute to speak, feral children to become calm and to cure autism, as relayed in the 2009 book *Horse Boy*. In short, touch is a vital part of human life that makes us healthier, happier and lead better, more productive lives.

Compassionate Genes

The *periaqueductal grey area* in the ancient midbrain is associated with compassion in a number of mammal species, and touch activates it. This suggests compassion is an ancient, innate trait. It's activated by oxytocin (produced by the hypothalamus), and triggers nurturing, generosity and faithfulness.

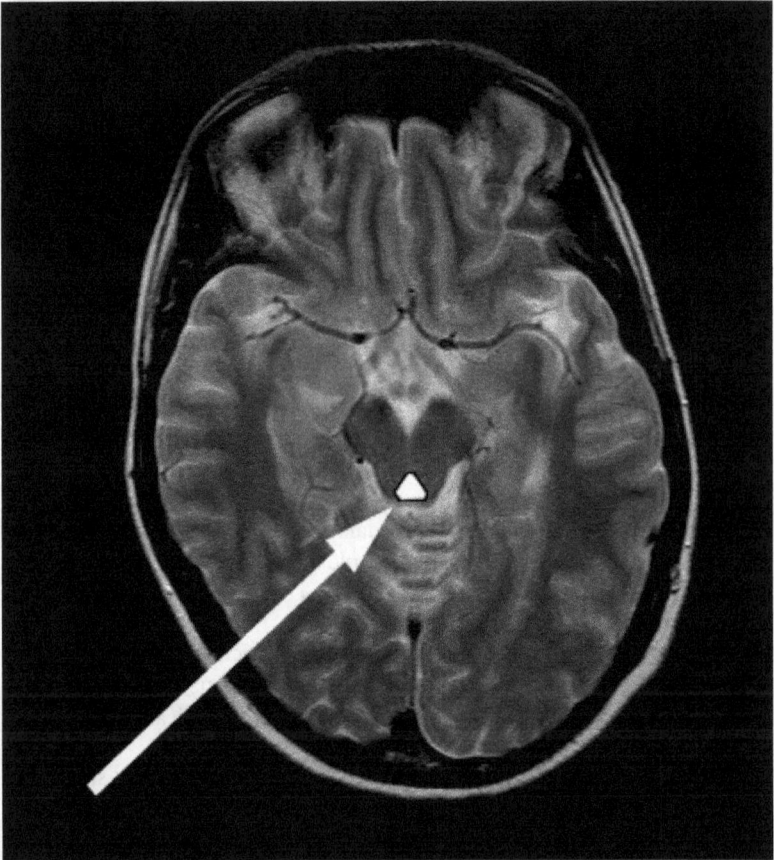

PAG, 2012 , Dr. Timothy C. Hain. Used with permission

Dr. Dacher Keltner, founder of the Greater Good Science Center at Berkeley and author of *Born to Be Good, the Science of a Meaningful Life*, says the gene most responsible for promoting altruism is *rs53576*, which governs oxytocin receptor synthesis. People born with a healthy oxytocin polymorphism are kinder, better able to read the emotions of others, and respond more compassionately to their suffering.

According to the Society for Neuroscience, multiple studies in 2010 suggest that oxytocin plays a much wider role than previously suspected. It influences an animal's sense of well-being, as well as relieving social stress and anxiety, and is strongly linked to happiness. Presumably because it enhances trust, it also increases the likelihood people will donate to public services. Its anxiety-reducing affects only appear to be powerful in the presence of friends, however, say researchers.

Most astounding of all is that oxytocin seems able to completely cancel out the addictive associations formed when taking addictive drugs among mothers in the presence of their newborns. In fact, say researchers, oxytocin seems to be just as rewarding as drugs of abuse to some animals.

The Touch-Deprived Society

According to Dr. Keltner, we're a "touch-deprived society".

Asking, "Can emotions be communicated through touch?" he separated volunteers with a barrier and had one subject touch another on the forearm through a barrier, trying to convey emotions from a list through only the sense of touch. Says Dr. Keltner, people guessed correctly about 50% of the time – five to six times the rate of chance guessing. Interestingly, men trying to read anger from women were 0% correct, while women trying to read men's compassion were 0% correct.

Unexpressive

A joint 2008 study between the University of Rome and Harvard Medical School found that people who have difficulty expressing emotion (a relatively newly-discovered disorder called *alexithymia*) have impaired data transfer across their brain hemispheres via the connective nerve tissue of the *corpus callosum*.

Keltner notes that alexithymia exists in everyone to some degree, preventing some degree of sharing and understanding of his or her own emotions, but for one in 11, the problem's severe, causing difficulties in relating, such as anxiety among others and a tendency to avoid forming relationships.

Alexithymia can often accompany post-traumatic stress disorder, and might also be linked to substance abuse, as well as eating disorders and panic disorders.

But University of Missouri assistant professor Colin Hesse says affectionate tactile communication such as hugging helps those with alexithymia. Hesse's own work has shown how such affectionate communication triggers stress-relieving hormonal releases.

Hesse and co-author Dr. Kory Floyd measured the number of close relationships and the affection and attachment levels of 921 volunteers and found that, while alexithymia made forming relationships difficult, affectionate communication markedly lessened any communication difficulties.

A Link Between Touch And Violence?

The amount of touching that occurs in different cultures varies widely. In 2009, British researchers compared the amount of physical contact between friends that could be observed in public in a number of countries. They found that, on average, during an hour, in England people touched each other 0%; in America twice, and in Puerto Rico, 180 times.

In a related study, touching behavior between couples was observed in public cafes in several countries. Couples were observed for 30-minute periods in each location, and the amount of touching between them was recorded. Among the highest touch rates was France (110 times per 30 minutes) and among the lowest was in the United States (2 times per 30 minutes).

High touch cultures also had relatively low rates of violence, while low touch cultures, had extremely high rates of both youth and adult violence – for example, in a 1994 report by the Centers for Disease Control and Prevention, the homicide rate per 100,000 was 1 in France and 22 in the United States.

Studies also suggest that French families are also likely to provide their children with more touch stimulation, and American families provide less. Dr. Keltner's team observed parents and children in Paris and Miami playgrounds, and found evidence that these cultures differed in parent touching of preschoolers, peer touching in preschoolers and peer touching among young adolescents.

Among Parisian parents, touching occurred 43% of the time, compared with 11% of the time among Miami parents. Additionally, affectionate touch between preschool children occurred 23% of the time in Paris, and only 3% of the time in Miami. However, aggressive touching occurred 37% of the time on Miami playgrounds and only 1% of the time on Paris playgrounds, says Dr. Keltner.

Dramatic, Life-Changing Effects

Touch inspires, instills courage, builds bonds, and alleviates pain.

Dr. Tiffany Field, PhD. is the Director of The Touch Research Institute at the University of Miami Medical School. She says that her experiments show prematurely-born babies who received only three daily 15-minute sessions of touch therapy for 5-10 days gained 47 percent more weight than those who only received standard medical treatment. Touch therapy is also said to reduce Alzheimer's disease "precipitously", and that doctors who initiate touch with patients appear to increase survival rates.

Touch also triggers, says Dr. Keltner, the immune response, which is probably why a lot of touching seems to extend lives. It also activates the orbitofrontal cortex, builds cooperative relationships, signals safety and trust, soothes, and activates the vagus nerve to calm cardiovascular stress.

In *prisoner's dilemma* experiments, researchers have found a simple pat on the back increases cooperation by 200%, producing the same neurochemical rewards as eating chocolate, according to Keltner. He also says NBA basketball teams whose players touch each other more tend to win more games. Similarly, research by Darlene Francis and Michael Meaney at McGill University has shown that rats whose mothers groom them frequently when they are infants grow up to be calmer and more resilient to stress, with stronger immune systems.

Keltner notes that Charles Darwin said sympathy proliferates through natural selection – that is, communities with the highest numbers of compassionate members tend to survive and pass the trait on to their offspring. In fact, says Keltner, among humans, in every culture studied, kindness was the single most important factor in mate selection, and "… cultures in which there was more physical affection toward infants had lower rates of adult physical violence and vice versa."

The Master Relationship Secret

"The most important single ingredient in the formula of success is knowing how to get along with people." – President Theodore Roosevelt, "The Winning of the West", 1894

"Pretend that every single person you meet has a sign around his or her neck that says, 'Make me feel important.'
Not only will you succeed in sales, you will succeed in life."
– Mary Kay Ash, "Miracles Happen: The Life and Timeless Principles of the Founder of Mary Kay Inc.", 1994

"People will do anything for those who encourage their dreams, justify their failures, allay their fears, confirm their suspicions and help them throw rocks at their enemies."
– Blair Warren, "The Forbidden Keys to Persuasion", 2003

"If you judge people, you have no time to love them."
– Mother Teresa, "Essential Writings", 2001

The single most important trait you need to succeed, says motivational psychologist Dr. Heidi Grant Halvorson, is trustworthiness. Author of *Succeed: How We Can Reach Our Goals*, she says that, no matter how honest you may truly be, trustworthiness can easily be undermined by how others perceive you: If you look like you have little willpower, people won't trust you. This means your boss won't give you key assignments, promotions, or the freedom to do things your way or to take risks. And your coworkers or employees won't give you their best, or relay all the information you need to make the best decisions. This, she says, is logical;

> *If you think about it, this makes a lot of intuitive sense. We trust people because we know that when things get hard, or when it might be tempting for them to put their own interests first, they'll resist temptation and do what's right.*

Studies show that when you engage in behaviours that are indicative of low self-control, your trustworthiness is diminished. In other words, all those things you know you shouldn't do – smoking, overeating, impulsive spending, being lazy, late, disorganized, excessively emotional or having a quick temper – may be even worse for you than you ever realized, because of the collateral damage they are doing to your reputation. So if you want to be trusted, you're going to have to conquer these trust saboteurs.

As we saw in previous chapters, your willpower can be strengthened through use, just like your body's muscles. And just as even the strongest muscles can be worn out by overwork, your willpower can become taxed; everyday activities such as making decisions or trying to convey a good impression sap this resource. When you put too much strain upon it at once, or for too long, your "self-control supply" runs out, no matter who you are. This is when the chocolate cake, the beer, or the impulse to lash out in anger wins – and you lose.

Thus, if you're serious about wanting to resist your impulses, you need to recognize the limits of your willpower. When you're drained and exhausted from a stressful day, your "willpower well" will have run dry. Because of this, you need to plan ahead, to avoid the environmental cues that pull you in, driving you toward your unhealthy impulses. Plan ahead for what to do as an alternative to giving in to your cravings when they emerge.

Fortunately, your capacity for willpower returns, if you allow yourself some rest, eat properly and remove yourself from stress. Says Dr. Halvorson:

> When rest is not an option, recent research shows that you can actually speed up your self-control recovery, or give it a boost when reserves are low, simply by thinking about people you know who have lot of self-control. (Thinking about my impossibly self-possessed mother does wonders for me when I'm about to fall off the no-cheesecake wagon. Or, you can try giving yourself a pick-me-up. I don't mean a cocktail – I mean something that puts you in a good mood. (Again, not a cocktail – it may be mood-enhancing, but alcohol is definitely not willpower-enhancing, nor trust-enhancing). Anything that lifts your spirits should also help restore your self-control strength when you're looking for a quick fix.

Dr. Halvorson says research shows your willpower can be developed and strengthened over time with daily activities such as exercising, keeping track of your finances or eating habits, and even just sitting up straight every time you remember. Each of these, she says, will help strengthen your capacity for self-control.

Studies show that people given free gym memberships who kept up a regular exercise program for two months got physically healthier, smoked fewer cigarettes, drank less alcohol, and ate less junk food. They had greater control over their anger, spent less money impulsively, didn't leave dishes in the sink or otherwise procrastinate, and they missed fewer appointments.

"In fact," she says, "every aspect of their lives that required the use of willpower improved dramatically."

> So if you want to build more willpower, start by picking an activity (or avoiding one) that fits with your life and your goals – anything that requires you to override an impulse or desire again and again, and add

479

this activity to your daily routine. It will be hard in the beginning, but it will get easier over time if you hang in there, because your capacity for self-control will grow. Other people will notice the change, and trust you more. Armed with more willpower and the trust of those around you, you'll be more successful than ever before.

Valuing Others

Similarly, the single most fundamentally powerful step you can take to strengthen your relationships in every aspect of your life is to simply change your focus. Stop thinking about yourself and focus entirely upon the person with whom you are interacting, with full eye contact and attention.

The person in front of you needs to be the most important person in the world to you at the moment she's speaking; let her know she is. Consider how she benefits from this communication – What's in it for her? Then show her she matters to you by verbally acknowledging that you recognize and care about her need.

One of the easiest and most important ways you can show people they matter is by remembering details about them. In the business success book *Swim With the Sharks Without Being Eaten Alive*, consultant Harvey MacKay suggests keeping note cards of contacts you make – their names, any personal details you learn about them – anniversaries, hobbies, upcoming important events, etc. When you ask an acquaintance "how was your trip to the mountains?" or talk about golf with him (if that's his hobby), it opens doors and wins you a friend. At a minimum, you need to always remember names – it's a sign of simple respect. Use someone's name the first time you meet them – it will help you remember.

The easiest way to begin valuing and increasing awareness of others is through simple curiosity. Ask yourself questions about the strangers you see around you – where they're from, their backgrounds, their hobbies, hopes and dreams. Look for things you might have in common with them.

An excellent game for learning about people is to simply sit at a café and watch the crowds walk by. As people pass, ask yourself detailed questions about them.

Gloating – *The Germans have a special term for the nasty emotion* **schadenfreude** – *taking pleasure in the misfortune of others. This is a quality you want to completely remove from within yourself – learn to genuinely enjoy the success of others and share in their disappointments. Empathy is a powerful bonding agent, and is common among those who have evolved beyond their own personal insecurities.*

Power Listening

Communications experts train their students with the following, incredibly powerful formula: when someone's speaking to you, face them directly, make full eye contact, and give them 100 percent of your focused attention. Clear your mind – don't think about how you're going to answer them. Stop and FULLY concentrate on what they're telling you. Pause a moment before replying. Repeat their words back to them to be sure you understood what they meant, for example, "So you're saying that you believe A and B, but not C?"

The combined effect of these steps makes an unforgettable positive impression on those you talk with. Please experiment with this technique today with the people around you.

Truly Connecting

Dr. Brené Brown of the University of Houston says she is a "vulnerability specialist". She describes a rare type of people she calls "whole-hearted", who are fully engaged in life and deeply connected to others in meaningful, deep ways. This connection is vital to humans. She says her years of research have taught her three keys to connecting – and happiness – in life:

1. *Courage* – Allowing yourself to be seen for who you truly are. Wearing your heart on your sleeve endears you to others and opens you up for deep connections. Courage is Latin for telling your story from your heart. The courage to be authentic, willing to let go of who you think you "should" be, and being who you really are is critical for true connection.

    Shame is when people hate pieces of themselves and fear revealing them, because they believe it will drive others away or they won't "fit in". But this shuts out deep communication. Communicating honestly who you are – your strengths and weakness – is what opens and strengthens deep connections with others. This also entails being willing to risk having your heart broken or be disappointed, however. "...vulnerability is the core of shame and fear and our struggle for worthiness, but it appears that it's also the birthplace of joy, of creativity, of belonging, of love." You have to be willing to take pain and unhappiness to win joy and love. You also have to be willing to let go and fully experience joy – be willing to love someone completely, for example, even if it leaves you open to pain.

2. *Compassion* – This is the willingness to be open and kind to others - empathy. Courageous people, what she calls "whole hearted" are

initially kind to themselves. This is necessary at the outset. You can't be compassionate towards another if you're unkind toward yourself. Whole hearted people say inwardly, "I'm enough", and have a full self-acceptance. People who are whole hearted also carry a sense of worthiness – believing they're good enough to deserve love, and this very openness brings it into their lives.

3. **Connecting** – We typically numb vulnerability and close ourselves off to deep-level connections. But in shutting down negative feelings through addictions or distractions, we also numb good feelings like happiness and joy. This starts a cycle of unhappiness.

When others express shame, it can trigger our own, but we need to stay open in the midst of it to grow. We also try to create certainty, out of fear, blaming others when things don't go the way we want. Blame is a way of discharging pain and fear.

The Magic Word – *The best boss I ever had was a master communicator. The office manager of the biggest real estate agency in Vancouver at the time, she knew how to bring out the best in everybody. Aside from being a master at power listening, and from genuinely caring about the welfare of her employees, she knew how to make people feel really valued, happy and motivated.*

I used to watch how she worked, hoping to learn as much as I could from her management style. One habit she had, that I have since learned has the most amazing effects, is a single-word response. When somebody has done something for you, rather than "thank you", try "perfect". People will light up. You will instantly make them feel great. They have done something not just well, but perfectly. Try it and see.

Loving Communication

In *Feeling Good Together: The Secret to Making Troubled Relationships Work*, Dr. David Burns says there are some simple guidelines you can remember and follow to enhance communications with your significant others:

He suggests remembering the acronym *EAR* – *Empathy* (listening carefully), *Assertiveness* (honestly and fully expressing yourself), and *Respect* (caring for and about your partner). The first step, *Empathy*, means trying to understand your partner's point of view, listening attentively, and carefully considering what you hear, even when you are hearing things you find unpleasant.

The second step, *Assertiveness*, means expressing your feelings openly, using "I feel" statements, such as "I feel unhappy when you...". It's import to express yourself considerately to avoid hurting your partner's feelings. If you act aggressively by shouting, finger-pointing or blaming your partner, the situation will only worsen.

Treating your partner with *Respect* and a considerate, caring attitude even when you're irritated or exasperated will help solve problems more effectively. Acting competitive, superior or adversarial, on the other hand, will only worsen a situation. Here are some communications behaviours Dr. Burns says should be "red flags". If you or your partner start to follow one of these patterns, you should take a time out and restart the discussion in a healthier manner:

- *Defensiveness* – Insisting you're in the right, refusing to admit your own shortcomings, or somehow implying a problem is entirely your partner's fault

- *Aggression* – Name-calling, acting patronizing or derisive, implying your partner is defective or otherwise putting them down. Listing problems in the past and/or responding to criticism with counterattacks

- *Intellectualization* – Pretending you're not part of the problem, that you're not upset or disengaging yourself from the problem by offering "helpful" advice instead of listening

- *Passivity* – Acting helpless, or saying you've tried everything, but nothing ever works. Acting like the victim of your partner's tyranny, or putting on an "I'm so horrible" act to duck the issues

- *Passive aggression* – "clamming up", leaving messes for your partner to clean, pouting, procrastinating or slamming doors.

- *Magical thinking* – Expecting your partner to be able to automatically read your mind and/or feelings

Additionally, phrases that begin with "you always" and "you never" should send up an immediate red flag in your mind. If you find yourself saying "you always" or "you never", immediately stop and think of a less judgmental way of expressing what you want to say; it's always better to express yourself in terms of how *you feel*, rather than labelling your partner. For example, "I feel like we don't talk enough" is much more productive than "You never tell me what's going on!"

Fighting Fair

Destructive criticism in the form of insults, blaming and labelling are a danger sign to watch out for, and a hot button during arguments. When it comes to issues of contention, such as money management, sex, disciplining children, etc., it's vital to focus on the issue, rather than laying blame.

"You always", *"you're so..."* or, *"you're such a..."* are sure signs that a label is about to follow. It also indicates that your partner's been carrying feelings of resentment for a long time, rather than communicating complaints (and dealing with them) when they arise.

In the heat of anger, it becomes easy to lose control and start character assassination. This is the point at which learning to make your prefrontal cortex resume control over your limbic system is both hardest to do, and when it's most important – after all, what could possibly be more important in life than the person you care about the most?

If you let something bother you again and again, and feel like your appeals to your partner are having little or no effect, the natural tendency is to become frustrated, but it's important to focus on the issue rather than accusing your loved ones of having character faults.

Contempt in particular is deadly to a relationship. When anger turns into contempt, it means you've been dismissed, and is a stance of moral superiority. The smirk of derision or sneer of contempt, with a label like "wimp", "slut", "asshole" or "bitch" is pure poison, guaranteed to have destructive, likely permanent effects.

Relationship expert Dr. John Gottman says contempt is the single most definite predictor that a couple would separate within a matter of a few short years. The recipient of that contempt (or its close relative emotion disgust) would also suffer health problems, from colds and flus to bladder and yeast infections and gastrointestinal ailments.

The facial expressions of contempt (the eyes rolling upward or the lip curling into a sneer) are easily recognizable and should serve as a warning signal that a toxic emotional exchange has begun.

Contempt, disgust and criticism on a habitual basis mean that one or both partners has come to silently judge his or her partner for the worse. From the point this negative assessment has formed, a habitual undercurrent of negative judgment will color the perceptions and mutual communication of partners in the worst possible way. In other words, the labels you attach to others raise the possibility that you're setting yourself up to permanently treat them with a negative bias.

484

In defending herself against your negative labelling, your spouse or partner may well lose control of the limbo-cortical mental battle, lashing out in anger, or *stonewalling*, shutting down channels of communication in a tremendously frustrating and counterproductive attempt to withdraw from the anxiety of the exchange.

This strategy is usually employed by men. What women may not realize is it's because marital arguments result in much higher releases of stress hormones in men, creating extreme physical discomfort. Stonewalling is a coping strategy which allows men to physically recover – heartbeat has been shown to drop significantly as a result of this form of disengaging from an argument.

Remember that your thoughts and actions are colored by your inner environment – your "schemata" – the total unconscious-level feelings, assumptions, thoughts and beliefs you carry about yourself and those you interact with. Do you feel like a victim? Do you feel powerless? Do you believe your partner is unfair, dishonest, a tyrant? Do you feel you're being treated with dignity and fairness?

Also remember that once we build our schemata, we tend to find (pay attention to) things that support our beliefs, feelings and ideas, and tend to act in ways that make our predictions come true. If you think you're a victim, you'll be constantly analyzing your partner's words and actions for clues that confirm that you're being treated unfairly. Even innocent or kind remarks and gestures can easily be misread when you're carrying this kind of preconceived negativity.

And if you've built up this neural circuitry by thinking the same things over and over again, they are most easily repeated, harder to break away from, and can easily and progressively lead to ever more quickly- and deeply-triggered emotional hijackings – despair or anger at a situation that "will never change" – almost certainly because you've decided consciously or unconsciously that's the way it will be.

Eventually, as a result of this way of thinking, both you and your partner can reach a state of *hypervigilance*, always on guard and expecting an insult, attack or slight. Communication will become an exercise in futility – one or both of you will habitually give up with an "it's useless" mental shrug of the shoulders.

At this stage in a relationship's breakdown, both of you have withdrawn in mutual surrender, and will begin to live separate lives. This, of course, is the beginning of the end for most marriages.

Fortunately, the strategies for rescuing such a relationship are quite clearly defined in psychotherapy:

1. Be willing to offer – and accept – conciliations. These verbal "olive branches" or "piece offerings" are aimed at cooling down rising emotions, and require humility to offer.

2. Care enough about your partner to listen carefully (and actually consider) her point of view

3. Stick to talking about the issues bothering one or both of you – don't get sidetracked by irrelevancies or engage in blaming, criticizing or name-calling. Let your partner know how the issue makes you feel. For example: "When you say 'I just want to watch the game and relax after work without being bothered', it makes me feel like I'm not important to you". Your partner may genuinely have no idea how you feel.

4. Be specific – talk about specific incidents and how they made you feel

5. Don't assume the other person knows what you're thinking or feeling.

6. Try to understand the situation from your partner's point of view (for example, perhaps your partner's money worries come from having been very poor in childhood)

7. Be willing to trust and believe – if you assume the best (or the worst) of people, they will intuitively pick up on this and usually live up to your expectations

8. Think about why you're upset – is this due to experiences in your childhood that may be coloring your perception of what's happening now?

9. Some incredibly powerful phrases that have an immediate effect on others are, "I'm sorry", "you're right" and, of course, "I love you"

10. Remember that one of the reasons you're feeling such overwhelming emotions is because you care *so* much – you're very invested emotionally, having given so much of your time and energy to build the relationship. And your romantic relationships are grounded upon the social lessons you learned in childhood and infancy. We all fight fiercely to protect ourselves against abandonment and emotional deprivation, and to ensure we get the nurtur-

ing, love, respect and feelings of being needed that every human being thrives upon. If you can start to listen for your partners' and your own needs *behind* the emotions you're hearing, you can start to understand and work towards repairing the relationship.

11. Watch for your own negative inner statements. Red flags should go up if you mentally tell yourself, "I'm not putting up with *this* anymore!" or "I don't deserve to be treated like *this*!" or "How *dare* he!" or "She's always such a *bitch*!"

12. If you find yourself getting angry, listen to the words you're telling yourself, and then think about them – where they come from, why they have power, and if they're based upon a realistic assessment of the current situation. Are these things fair? Are they really always true?

13. Remember that the best way to have these cognitive tools for relationship and emotional management at hand when you need them most is by using them – the more you use the same neural pathways, the stronger and more easily accessed they become. And then, in the heat of the moment, you can avoid being overtaken by the dragon.

14. Additionally, if you're going to hash out emotional issues with someone important to you, be sure to do it in person and only between the two of you. (Unless of course you're both at a counsellor's office together.)

Wired Differently – Motivations Of Men And Women

Georgetown University linguistics Professor Deborah Tannen opened up an entirely new field of communications study when she began to notice that men and women consistently communicated differently.

She went on to publish her observations and advice in the 1990 book, *You Just Don't Understand: Women and Men in Conversation*. Among conclusions she reached are that our social strategies differ: women tend to seek consensus, agreement, and bonding to build social networks, while men seek to compete and dominate in social hierarchies.

So a man's typical impulse is to use status, physical stature, wealth, intelligence or some other personal trait to his advantage, to either establish his dominance or to deflate another's relative social standing, in a constant game of what we call *one-upmanship*. Men also tend to be *solution-oriented* – we like to solve problems and tend to think in a more linear, analytical fashion.

Conversely, a woman will usually try to equalize social standing within her circles, often speaking in self-deprecatory ways or apologizing, in anticipation that the other women in the group will say or do something to bring her status back to the "group" level.

Because of their emphasis on connecting, over time, women tend to develop higher levels of communication skills and are significantly more adept at collaboration and reading people than most men. Men, on the other hand, tend to want to organize, build and control, and can excel in strategy.

These traits are likely from social conditioning for the most part (feminists say it's the influence of a patriarchal society).

Then Again...

On the other hand, there are marked differences in brain and endocrine structures which may be the cause of cognitive and behavioral differences between men and women. Dr. Louann Brizendine, author of *The Female Brain* and *The Male Brain*, says there are very clear, measurable differences between the male and female brain, and that these physical differences make women better at reading the meaning of facial expressions and vocal tones, and men better at using analysis to solve logical problems.

She says that research has shown every developing baby's brain begins with a "female" structure, but eight weeks after conception, testosterone levels convert some babies into men, altering development of their brains and bodies.

According to Brizendine, men have slightly larger (4% on average) brains, but women have a greater number of neural connections within their brains.

Additionally, she says, women have larger areas of the brain dedicated to communication on average, while men's brains have areas 2.5 times the size of women's which are dedicated to sexual pursuit, causing men to think about sex with much greater frequency throughout the average day.

Women also have a larger corpus callosum, the sheet of hard neural tissue that transfers data between the right and left halves of the brain more efficiently, while men tend to be more left-brain oriented – using logic instead of the right brain functions, generally associated with creativity, she adds. The deep limbic system is also larger in women, making them more in touch with their emotions, better able at expressing them and more skilful at bonding with others. She notes that this is why in every society across the world women are the primary caregivers for children. According to Dr. Brizendine,

In general, women are:

- better able to connect with others and maintain those connections

- better at reading and understanding emotions based upon facial expressions, body language, and vocal tones.

- better at caregiving

- more subject to depression, particularly during periods of strong hormonal change.

In general, men are:

- better at analyzing, problem-solving, building and creating systems

- strongest in competitive situations

- more aggressive and direct

- obsessed with rank and hierarchy

Cambridge university professor Simon Baron-Cohen has suggested that there is in fact a varying spectrum of modes of cognition and interpreting the world, a spectrum that ranges between *empathizing* and *systemizing*. He says that, due to measurable influences of prenatal testosterone on the brains of developing fetuses, in general men tend to be *systemizers*, while women tend to be *empathizers*, although there are exceptions, and people can also fall anywhere within the middle range of this scale.

> *Empathizing is the drive to identify another person's emotions and thoughts, and to respond to these with an appropriate emotion. The empathizer intuitively figures out how people are feeling, and how to treat people with care and sensitivity.*

> *Systemizing is the drive to analyze and explore a system, to extract underlying rules that govern the behavior of a system; and the drive to construct systems. The systemizer intuitively figures out how things work, or what the underlying rules are controlling a system. Systems can be as varied as a pond, a vehicle, a computer, a math equation, or even an army unit. They all operate on inputs and deliver outputs, using rules.*

He suggests that logical thinking was a skill that gave a survival advantage to hunter-gatherers (usually men), while empathizing was a skill evolved for caregivers (women). He also adds that, when it comes to aggression, males tend to engage in more direct physical aggression, hitting and punching, while females are more indirect, using gossip, ostracism, and catty remarks.

An interesting finding of his research was the tendency for newborn girls to gaze for longer periods at a person's face, while newborn boys gaze at mechanical mobiles hanging over their cribs. He says the amount of eye contact newborns make is partly dependent upon the amount of testosterone present as the fetus develops.

> *We, of course, know that with time, culture and socialization do play a role in determining a male brain (stronger interest in systems) or female brain (stronger interest in empathy). But these studies strongly suggest that biology also partly determines this.*

If you're curious about where you fall in the E-S spectrum, you can take the free online test here: http://eqsq.com/eq-sq-tests/

Thinkers Vs. Feelers

Three joint studies at the University of Illinois and Stanford University in 2010 showed another fundamental difference in cognitive strategies: people tend to evaluate and describe the world in terms of either thinking or feeling.

The studies found that "thinkers" were persuaded effectively by logical language and messages, while "feelers" responded best to emotional language and messages. Professor Baron-Cohen says they also fall along a continuum, between the *Romanticizing Quotient* and the *Pragmatizing Quotient*.

Thinkers make decisions based upon practicalities and logic, and prefer to find the solutions to problems, while *feelers* make decisions based on values, emotion, and gut instinct, and care about how their actions affect their feelings and those around them.

The researchers found gender stereotypes actually generally held true, in that women are usually "feelers" and men are usually "thinkers". For example, in their studies, women responded more favorably in response to movie reviews beginning with the phrase "I feel", while and men responded more favorably to reviews beginning with "I think".

Knowing these differences can help you communicate more effectively: to get through to a *thinker* vs. a *feeler*, you needn't change the actual *content* of what you want to say – you just need to reframe the *terms* you use. This is a small and subtle shift your listeners will definitely respond to – when you use *think* or *feel*, you show you're speaking their language.

The point is that we often communicate in radically different ways, and being aware of these differences helps in understanding why. To further bridge the gap, it's helpful for women to learn more assertive communication styles, and for men to learn more empathic listening.

Homework: Watch the movies *Pay it Forward* and *Six Degrees of Separation*. Read *Manwatching: A Field Guide to Human Behavior*, by Desmond Morris and *How to Win Friends and Influence People*, by Dale Carnegie.

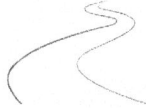

The Key Trait Successful People Share, Dr. Heidi Grant Halvorson, October 26, 2011, The Huffington Post; http://www.huffingtonpost.com/Heidi-Grant-Halvorson-phd/success-and-willpower-_b_1030250.html

Affection Mediates the Impact of Alexithymia on Relationships, 2011, Colin Hesse and Kory Floyd, 2011, Personality and Individual Differences, Volume 50, Issue 4; doi:10.1016/j.paid.2010.11.004; http://www.sciencedirect.com/

Transfer Deficit in Alexithymia: A Transcranial Magnetic Stimulation Study, Vincenzo Romeia, Luigi De Gennaroa, Fabiana Fratelloa, Giuseppe Curcioa, Michele Ferrarab, Alvaro Pascual-Leonec, Mario Bertinia, 2008, Psychotherapy and Psychosomatics, DOI: 10.1159/000119737; http://content.karger.com/ProdukteDB/produkte.asp?doi=119737

Born to Be Good: The Science of a Meaningful Life, Dr. Dacher Keltner, 2009, New York: W. W. Norton & Company;

Affectional Bonding For The Prevention Of Violent Behaviours: Neurobiological, Psychological And Religious/Spiritual Determinants, Hertzberg LJ, Ostrum GF, Field JR, eds. Violent Behavior, 1990; PMA Publishing; 1990:95-124.

An Exploratory Study Of Body Accessibility, Jourard SM. 1996, British Journal of Social and Clinical Psychology; 5:221-231

National Center for Injury Prevention and Control International Comparisons of Homocide Rates in Males 15-24 Years of Age, 1988-1991. Atlanta, GA: Centers for Disease Control and Prevention; 1994.

Preschoolers in America Are Touched Less And Are More Aggressive Than Preschoolers In France. Dr. Tiffany Field, 1999, Early Child Development and Care; 151:11-17

American Adolescents Touch Each Other Less And Are More Aggressive Toward Their Peers As Compared With French Adolescents, Dr. Tiffany Field, 1999, Adolescence ;34:753-758

Touch and Massage in Early Child Development, Dr. Tiffany Field, et al 2004, Johnson & Johnson Pediatric Institute, L.L.C. ISBN 0-931562-30-9

The Primacy of Human Touch, Ben Benjamin, PhD and Ruth Werner, LMT, http://www.benbenjamin.net/pdfs/Issue2.pdf

Human Connections Start With A Friendly Touch, Michelle Trudeau, National Public Radio, September 20, 2010;

The Effect of a Supportive Companion on Perinatal Problems, Length of Labor, and Mother-Infant Interaction, Sosa, R, , et al, 1980, The New England Journal of Medicine, 303(11):597-600

Labor Support by a Doula for Middle-Income Couples: the Effect on Cesarean Rates, Dr. John H. Kennell, and Susan K.McGrath, 1993, Pediatric Research, vol. 33, no. 12A

The Biology of the Horse Boy – Can Children Ride Horses Out of the Depths of Autism? Meg Daley Olmert, April 2, 2009, Psychology Today, http://www.psychologytoday.com/blog/made-each-other/200904/the-biology-the-horse-boy

Studies Expand Oxytocin's Role Beyond "Cuddle Hormone, News Release, Kat Snodgrass and Todd Bentsen, 2010, Society for Neuroscience; http://www.sfn.org/index.aspx?pagename=news_111410a

Intranasal Oxytocin Increases Positive Communication and Reduces Cortisol Levels During Couple Conflict, Dr. Beate Ditzen, et al.2008, Journal of Biological Psychiatry

Feeling Good Together: The Secret to Making Troubled Relationships Work, David Burns, 2008

They Just Can't Help It, Simon Baron-Cohen, April 17, 2003, The UK Guardian

The Male Brain, The Female Brain, Dr. Louann Brizendine, 2008, 2011

Think' Versus 'Feel' Framing Effects in Persuasion, Nicole D. Mayer and Zakary L. Tormala, 2010, Personality and Social Psychology Bulletin, 36 (4), 443-54

Sex

"I'll have what she's having" – Estelle Reiner, "When Harry Met Sally", 1989

*"There's very little advice in men's magazines, because men think,
'I know what I'm doing. Just show me somebody naked.'"*
– Jerry Seinfeld, Live on Broadway: I'm Telling You for the Last Time, 1998

"Tell him I've been too fucking busy – and vice versa."
*– American writer Dorothy Parker, while honeymooning, in response to a request by
New Yorker editor Harold Ross, who was asking why her book review was late, 1934*

"It's so long since I've had sex I've forgotten who ties up whom."
– Joan Rivers, "Enter Talking", 1986

Surprise! Sex Is Good For You

Research still has a fair distance to go before we fully understand all the mysteries of human sexuality, but one could say we're getting to third base.

One of the perhaps less surprising fruits of sex research is just how darned healthy bonking happens to be. For example, middle-aged men who have two or more orgasms a week are 200% less likely to die than those having fewer, according to a ten-year study published in the 1997 British Medical Journal. In 2001, another study focused on cardiovascular health, showing those who had sex three or more times weekly were 50% less likely to suffer heart attacks or strokes.

But for all the health and mood-boosting benefits of a rousing game of rugby-on-the-couch, according to Dr. Julia Heiman, current director of the Kinsey Institute, remarkably little is known about the actual biological processes underlying the orgasm. All that's rapidly changing.

Taking One For The Team

In March, 2011, *New Scientist* reporter Kayt Sukel agreed to a novel experiment: she was about to stimulate herself to orgasm for the betterment of mankind, as Dr. Barry Komisaruk of Rutgers University scanned her brain with an fMRI machine. Sukel was one of a number of volunteers participating in a study of the neurological processes underlying sexual arousal and orgasm.

As Sukel stimulated herself to orgasm, fMRI scans revealed that over 30 of her brain regions activated throughout the sequence, including regions involved in processing touch, memory, reward and pain.

493

Imagined stimulation without manual stimulation activated the same brain regions as actual stimulation, to a lesser degree, though the PFC showed greater activation during the imaginary segment than during actual stimulation.

Dr. Komisaruk believes this heightened PFC activity is due either to the generation of fantasy, or to direct cognitive control ("top-down" control) of physiological functions – of our own pleasure. Eventually, he hopes to use neurofeedback to help women with anorgasmia achieve climax.

His fMRI scan sequences have since been used to create the world's first movie of the female brain as it approaches, experiences and recovers from an orgasm. As the animation plays, activity first builds up in the genital-responsive region of the sensory cortex, a response to being touched. Activity then spreads to the limbic system.

As orgasm arrives, activity accelerates in the cerebellum and frontal cortex, perhaps because of greater muscle tension. During orgasm, activity reaches a peak in the hypothalamus, which releases oxytocin, causing pleasurable sensations and stimulating uterus contraction. Activity also peaks in the nucleus accumbens, the brain's primary limbic dopamine target for reward and training. You can see the online animation here: http://www.thevisuald.com/read_videoguide.php?id_url=1033607627

Orgasm Science

The state of orgasm is a previously unseen level of consciousness that Dr. Komisaruk hopes may help in devising new kinds of pain killers, which make use of the PFC's role in controlling physical sensations like pain. He and his team also hope to uncover what goes wrong in both men and women who cannot reach sexual climax; an estimated 25% of American women have difficulty in achieving orgasm, while 5 to 10% are anorgasmic – completely incapable of climaxing.

His studies have revealed what many have long maintained – that there are multiple routes to orgasm. He's currently focusing upon the sequences, particularly the heightened PFC activity when women climax.

The PFC is involved in such aspects of consciousness as self-evaluation and considering things from another's perspective. This heightened activity is also present among women who can climax through fantasy alone. Because fantasy and self-referential imagery are often described as key to the sexual experience, Komisaruk and his team hypothesized that the PFC plays a key role in creating physical responses to imagination without tactile stimulation.

Different Roads To Bliss

Interestingly, Dr. Janniko Georgiadis of the University of Groningen in the Netherlands found contradictory results – that the PFC shuts down during orgasm. He believes the orbitofrontal cortex may be the center of sexual control, and that orgasm is a function of letting go of this control. This deactivation is, he contends, a previously undiscovered, altered state of consciousness. Georgiadis believes the inability to let go and achieve this altered state may underlie the inability of some women to climax. A willful release of fear and anxiety may be central to the process of achieving orgasm.

It's possible that the discrepancies between Georgiadis' and Komisaruk's findings may be due to separate methods for reaching orgasm – volunteers in Komisaruk's studies stimulated themselves to orgasm, while those in Georgiadis's were stimulated by their lovers.

Not Getting There – While healthy men have no difficulties in reaching orgasm, in various studies, about 25 percent of women report difficulties, and perhaps 10 percent of American women have never experienced orgasm. Among those women who do regularly, orgasm is only achieved from 50 to 70 percent of the time.

This may be due to an inability to "let go of inhibitions.", and seems closely related to both performance anxiety (sexual stage fright) and an unwillingness to pursue one's own physical satisfaction independently of one's partner's. Some women become so worried about pleasing their partners that it causes ongoing anxiety, which can worsen the problem.

But a 2005 study of 2,000 twin women by Dr. Tim Spector in London found the causes to be genetic in 34% to 45% of reported cases – some women are genetically predisposed to have trouble in reaching orgasm, a condition called *anorgasmia*.

Come Again?

At the peak of sexual pleasure, orgasm is controlled by the autonomic system, and generally culminates in a 15- to 20-second cycle of rapid muscle contractions in the pelvic muscles surrounding the genitals and anus. In men, these contractions propel sperm out of the penis, in women, uterine contractions are thought to pull sperm cells in to promote fertilization.

Orgasm is typically achieved by genital stimulation – in women, stimulating the clitoris, although some women can also achieve orgasm through nipple and/or G-spot stimulation; in men, stimulating the penis results in orgasm and (usually) ejaculation. Both the clitoris and penis are structurally analogous, and are developed from the same structure in the embryo.

Women generally take about 20 minutes of stimulation to reach orgasm, but men can climax in as little as two minutes or less. As the genitals (or other erogenous areas) are stimulated, activity gradually begins to decline in brain regions responsible for fear, anxiety and behavioral control. This switching off eventually reaches its height during orgasm, when parts of the brain essentially shut down, resulting in a trance-like state.

Exceptionally rare cases of women able to reach orgasm simply through thought alone have also been recorded in Dr. Komisaruk's lab, where he also found several of his female volunteers were able to reach multiple or even constant states of orgasm.

In 1995, it was even demonstrated that some men can achieve multiple orgasms as well – an ability taught by tantric meditation. Sensations for orgasm are relayed by the spinal cord, from the *sacral nerve root*. Direct stimulation triggers orgasm. In theory, it's even possible to trigger this orgasm reflex in a dead person, if there is an oxygen supply to the sacral nerve, according to brain death expert Dr. Stephanie Mann.

Dr. Komisaruk and partner Beverly Whipple discovered in 1997 that orgasms could also be induced by the injecting *vasoactive intestinal peptide* into the spine. Their interest was first piqued after discovering this neurotransmitter nearly doubles pain tolerance in women.

The Sweet Spot

Erogenous zones (sexually stimulating regions) vary widely from person to person, and even changing with age, but in the genitals, relative sensitivity is more generally consistent, with the exception of the Gräfenberg Spot, named after Ernest Gräfenberg. In women, the G-Spot (Gräfenberg Spot) is still an area of contention among researchers. However, if you explore a little yourself, I think you'll find the debate can be quickly settled.

The region varies in size, surrounding the urethra behind the pubic bone in women; it can be touched on the anterior (frontal) wall inside the vagina. Some laboratory experiments have shown that the vagina's anterior wall in the 12 o'clock position, while a woman lies upon her back, is most sensitive to physical stimulation. Stimulating the deep-lying tissue surrounding the urethra by pressing up against the internal surface in a "come here" finger motion has been found most likely to produce orgasms. Stimulation of the posterior wall, at the 6 o'clock position, was least likely to produce orgasms.

To reach the area, place your fingers one or two inches into the vaginal canal and hook them inward and downward toward the belly button. You will eventually find an area that feels different from the surrounding tissue, a wet, spongy region. Gentle stimulation to the area, particularly combined with stimulation of the clitoris, can yield some dramatic results. The latest metastudies indicate a G-spot per se doesn't exist, but that this region is usually a nexus of dense nerve centers that exits in some but not all women.

The Mountain That Took 2000 Years to Find

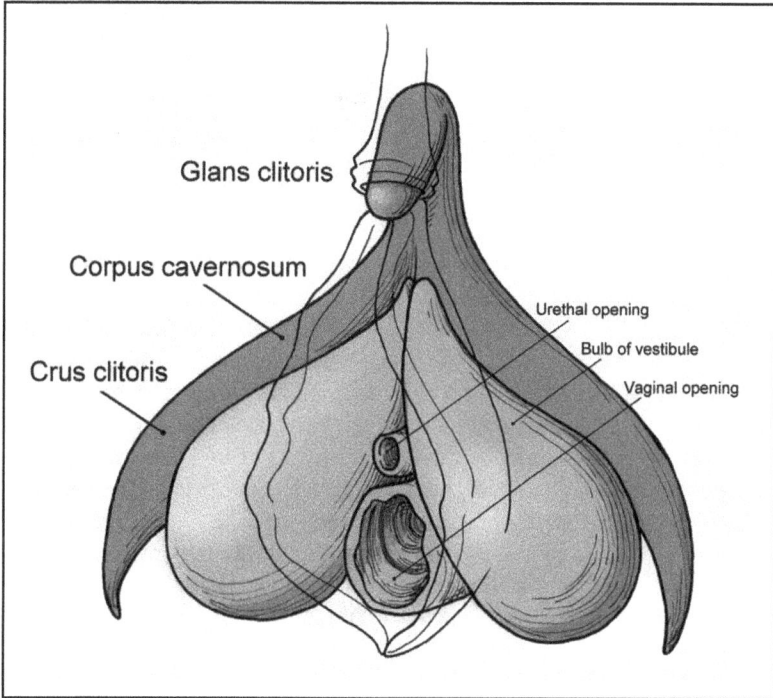

In 2006, urological surgeon Dr. Helen O'Connell of Australia's Royal Melbourne Hospital said it was finally time to nip female sexual anatomy misconceptions in the bud. Her decades of work as a surgeon specializing in the region in question, combined with magnetic resonance imaging (MRI), led to her announcement that surprise! we've had it all wrong from the outset. Her discovery has since led to a rewriting of all the classic textbooks on human anatomy.

Dr O'Connell first discovered the mistake 17 years ago. After repeatedly failing a medical exam, in frustration, she turned to her anatomy texts, only to discover they had it completely wrong. The clitoris, derived from the Greek word for "little hill" turns out to be more of a mountain than a molehill. Says Dr. O' Connell, it's at least as large as the penis, perhaps larger:

"The vaginal wall is, in fact, the clitoris. If you lift the skin off the vagina on the side walls, you get the bulbs of the clitoris - triangular, crescental masses of erectile tissue. During arousal, the entire structure becomes engorged." Image: Wikipedia, 2009, public domain

Your Brain On Sex

EEG readouts and PET scans show orgasmic brain activity patterns are similar between men and women. fMRI and PET studies show the brain lights up like a Christmas tree during sexual stimulation, with heightened activation of the interconnected *limbic regions* (amygdala, hippocampus, hypothalamus) as well as the thalamus, cingulate cortex, striatum, insula, septum, reticular formation, central gray, neocortex and cerebellum. Together, these systems provide communicative links between the cognitive and emotional regions of the brain, integrating sensory, cognitive, emotional, visceral, and motor processes, all of which make up the experience of an orgasm. Specific genital regions transmit signals to the brain via specific nerves, explaining why orgasms vary in quality, depending on whether they are induced from the clitoris, vagina, cervix, anus, penis or testicles.

Additionally, there is a demonstrable link between brain regions that process pain and those which process sexual response; during sexual activity, the *O face* or (more coarsely), the *fuck face* looks remarkably like someone is suffering or in pain. The common link in the chain appears to be the anterior cingulate cortex, which activates in response to painful stimulation as well as genital stimulation. This brain center has been suggested as the sole region where the "suffering" part of pain is represented to consciousness.

Researchers at the University of Groningen in the Netherlands have been taking PET scans of volunteers' brains during sex, and say that both men and women respond in generally the same way to sex. In both, activity in the lateral orbitofrontal cortex, a region behind the left eye thought to be involved in decision-making and behavioral control, switches off during orgasm. According to researcher Janniko R. Georgiadis, this means having an orgasm is a surrender of control, similar to the brain activity seen when someone shoots heroin.

According to head researcher Dr. Gert Holstege, deactivation of large parts of the brain in women is particularly pronounced, primarily in the "fear centers". The amygdala and hippocampus quieten markedly in women, leading Dr. Holstege's team to surmise that a need for safety – a reduction in fear and anxiety – is a key component for women to achieve orgasm.

In women, the periaqueductal gray (PAG) in the brain stem also activates. This region is responsible for pain reduction, activating the raphe nuclei to trigger endorphin (painkiller) release along the spine. In men, the insular cortex activates. This region reports the physical sense of self, integrating body sensations including heartbeat, pain, the sense of smell, heat and cold, and is thought to play a major role in emotion recognition, by reporting the body's emotion-related states (such as an elevated heartbeat) to the brain.

Dopamine and Oxytocin in Balance *The main neurochemical agent driving romantic love (and its decline) is dopamine. This is the "juice" powering the reward circuitry of the mesocorticolimbic reward pathway, giving us the capability to assess things in our environment as "good, bad, or indifferent."*

This is the basis of cravings – your brain's neurochemical response to needs for homeostasis. The greater the dopamine release, the stronger the activation of the mesocorticolimbic reward pathway, and the greater the desire becomes. High-calorie foods trigger a larger dopamine release than low-calorie foods, which is why we crave doughnuts instead of salad – this reward pathway has been programmed from an ancient, evolutionary perspective in which calories mean survival.

Ultimately, what this means is that you're not actually craving a chocolate fudge sundae, the admiration of your co-workers, or a night of hot passion with your fantasy girl (boy) – it's the squirt of brain-function-enhancing dopamine into your nucleus accumbens that has you all worked up.

Dopamine facilitates brain function – it feels good, because it enhances thought and energizes you. And it's driven by novelty and the unexpected most of all. Because of its role as a neuromodulator (adjusting the effectiveness of other neurotransmitters), it is involved in a number of aspects of mood, behavior, and perception, and minute shifts in dopamine levels or receptiveness can have profoundly affect how you perceive your world and everyone in your life.

Dopamine is the basis of motivating you to seek rewards, but there are additional neurotransmitters involved in the mesocorticolimbic pathway. The actual sensations of pleasure may derive instead from opioids – your brain's natural morphine. So, while dopamine drives you toward the plate of chocolate cake or the rousing sex romp, the actual pleasurable sensations seem to arise from opioids.

Amygdala-Hippocampus – These connected regions participate in recognizing and integrating sexual stimuli, as part of their role in activating emotional responses to external sensory stimuli. The hippocampus activates during orgasm even if the orgasm has been generated by thought alone, so the hippocampus may play a large role in the cognitive parts of experiencing orgasm, as does the amygdala , which projects into the temporal and frontal lobes, appearing to screen the final stages of sensory data before it is output to the neocortex.

Cingulate Cortex – During orgasm, heart rate, blood pressure, and pupil diameter double, indicating intense sympathetic nervous system activation. This appears to activate the cingulate cortex, which activates during orgasm as well as in response to pain. Stimulating the cingulate cortex directly increases breathing and heart rate, demonstrating its connection to the sympathetic nervous system. PET studies have also shown that the cingulate cortex responds to both painful and pleasurable stimulation.

The ACC in particular is known to be involved in responding with sympathetic nervous system activation to physiological stimulation like pain and orgasm, as well as to cognitive-generated stress like worry and guilt. In terms of orgasm, the ACC appears to mediate both the intense sensations of orgasm as well as the autonomic nervous system responses during orgasm. Thus, the cingulate cortex is thought to play a central role in generating orgasms.

Hypothalamus – A cluster of neurons in the hypothalamus called the *paraventricular nucleus* triggers the secretion of oxytocin into the bloodstream, brain, and nervous system in response to sexual stimulation.

Breast, nipple, cervical, and genital sensations all converge on the PVN region, and it plays a central role in ejaculation, resulting in a significant oxytocin release within a minute of orgasm. This oxytocin release can trigger contractions during both orgasm and childbirth.

This cluster of neurons contains several specialized subgroups activated by a range of stressful or physiological changes. Many PVN neurons project to the pituitary grand, triggering the release of oxytocin or vasopressin into the bloodstream. Others regulate appetite, and autonomic brain stem and spinal cord functions.

The PVN neurons which direct sexual responses are excited by dopamine and inhibited by opioids, and the axons project to the pituitary gland, triggering oxytocin release into the bloodstream. Additional oxytocin neurons project down the spinal cord to connect with neurons in the *sacral region*, which controls erection and ejaculation.

Insula – During orgasm, the *insula* mediates *visceral* (internal) feelings of pain and pleasure. Stimulating the region electrically produces mainly visceral sensations. Additionally, PET studies have shown that as people eat chocolate while in states of high motivation and rating their chocolate as very pleasing, the insula is one of the regions activated, suggesting it is one of the areas in the brain where *salience* (reward value) is represented.

Nucleus Accumbens – In both sexes, the mesolimbic pathway activates during orgasm. Blocking dopamine function *attenuates* (weakens) the intensity of orgasms, while stimulating dopaminergic neurons intensifies them.

Your Body on Sex

Particularly sensitive nerve endings on the genitalia, nipples and other erogenous zones – which vary widely in location and sensitivity from person to person – elsewhere relay information to the brain about sensations being experienced. The clitoris in particular is extremely sensitive, with over 8,000 nerves that eventually connect to the spinal cord.

Among the nerves activated during sex:

- *hypogastric nerve* – transmits sensations from the uterus and cervix (women) or prostate (men)

- *pelvic nerve* – transmits sensations from the vagina, cervix (women) and rectum (both men and women)

- *pudendal nerve* – transmits sensations from the clitoris (women), scrotum and penis (men)

- *vagus nerve* – transmits sensations from cervix, uterus and vagina

The vagus nerve's role in orgasm is a relatively recent discovery. Among its other functions, however, is parasympathetic control of the heart – slowing heartbeat. In fact, the vagus nerve sends parasympathetic messages to every organ save the adrenal glands, and controls a few throat muscles, including the larynx, which may help explain the vocalizations emitted during the throes of orgasm.

The pelvic nerves function as a bundle, with both sympathetic (arousal) and parasympathetic (calming) effects, working together to provide sensory messages from the pelvis to the brain, and motor control from the brain to the pelvis. In the pelvis, the parasympathetic nervous system also helps with waste elimination, controlling muscles which transport urine from the kidneys to the bladder and feces through the intestines.

The process seems to be primarily controlled by dopamine and oxytocin, produced during sexual arousal, although several other excitatory and inhibitory neurotransmitters also play a role, including serotonin and noradrenaline.

During ejaculation, the ventral tegmental area produces a substantial release of dopamine. After orgasm subsides, there is a period of time called the refractory period, in which the body eases into relaxation, prompted by release of the hormones oxytocin and prolactin.

Hypogastric Nerve – Along with the pelvic nerve, the hypogastric nerve also relays sensations from the uterus and cervix to the brain in women, and from the prostate and testes to the brain in men. Pressure on the prostate (the area between the anus and testicles in men) also heightens male orgasm.

Pudendal Nerve – The clitoris transmits sensations via this nerve in women, and the penis and scrotum in men.

Pelvic Nerve – The pelvic nerve provides sensory impulses to the brain from the vagina, cervix, rectum, and urinary bladder. The pelvic nerve can reportedly lead to orgasm in both women and men if stimulated genitally or via the rectum. Breast or nipple stimulation is also thought to activate the same afferent nerves that read genital stimulation. For some women, simultaneously stimulating the rectum along with the clitoris, vagina, and/or cervix can heighten the complexity and intensity of orgasm.

"Cross-talk" can exist between sensations derived from vaginal and rectal stimulation, probably because the same nerve (the pelvic nerve) relays sensory information from both organs. In other words, stimulation of vaginal, clitoral or cervical nerves can in some circumstances lead to a feeling of the need to defecate, and stimulation of the rectum can also relay sexual pleasure. The pelvic nerve also appears to be sometimes activated by stimulation of the G spot, and can result in "female ejaculation" from the urethra among some women. Personal field studies have verified this.

Vagus Nerve – The most recent research suggests vagus nerves also convey pleasurable sensations from the cervix. In women, the clitoris, vagina, and cervix all send sensory messages to the brain along different nerve pathways (the clitoris from the pudendal nerve, the vagina primarily by the pelvic nerve and the cervix primarily by the hypogastric, pelvic, and vagus nerves). Stimulating each in isolation can result in orgasms of varying sensations, but combining stimulation of all three heightens and intensifies the overall effect.

Evolutionary Functions

Evolutionary psychology often allows us to provide excellent "best guesses" as to why a behavior or feature has evolved. In the case of orgasm, it's pretty obvious – intense pleasure drives us to frequently seek out sex, which in turn promotes reproduction. And in women, some studies seem to indicate that oxytocin increases uterine contractions that aid fertilization, helping suck sperm into the fallopian tubes.

Female Orgasm And Reproduction

Female sexual excitement includes erection of the clitoris and swelling of the labia (lips) with blood as excitement builds, culminating in a series of orgasmic muscle contractions. Masters and Johnson first mapped the female sexual response in 1966, noting it follows four phases:

- *Excitement:* image, fantasy, memory, sensory stimulus

- *Plateau:* increased blood flow to vagina, vaginal dilation, vaginal lubrication

- *Response or orgasm:* muscle contraction of lower anus and lower pelvic muscles, uterine contractions, vaginal contractions (orgasm)

- *Resolution:* satisfaction, relaxation (decreased blood flow to sex organs, relaxation of muscle tone), euphoria

In women, erectile tissue similar to men's plays a similar role in sexual excitement, increasing blood flow and swelling in the region as excitement builds. Meanwhile, the parasympathetic nervous system triggers a release of vaginal secretions to decrease friction and help semen migration.

During orgasm, a woman's blood pressure and heart rate nearly double their resting rate, increasing blood flow throughout the body. Pain sensitivity also halves, although other kinds of touch sensitivity are not decreased. The uterus contracts rhythmically, leading to the suggestion that these contractions have an "upsuck" effect which draws semen into the uterus and eventually up the fallopian tubes to meet an ovulated egg.

Evidence for this theory has been demonstrated in the animal kingdom; the Danish National Committee for Pig Production discovered that sexually stimulating sows during artificial insemination produces a six-percent increase in the number of young produced.

Male Orgasm And Reproduction

In men, plexus nerves stimulate muscles in coiled *helicene arteries* to relax and allow blood to fill the penis, making it *tumescent* (swollen and rigid) for sexual activity. Physical stimulation or *psychogenic* (fantasy-induced) arousal activates nerves extending from the sacral region of the spinal cord which terminate in *corpora cavernosa* – tissues which swell with blood, resulting in erections. This is followed by ejaculation, a wave of cycling muscle contractions generated by the sympathetic nervous system that ejects sperm. During *remission,* the penis once again returns to a *flaccid* (limp) state.

Physical stimulation of penile skin transmits signals to the spinal cord and related nerves release nitric oxide and acetylcholine, which stimulate *second messenger* chemicals.

Phosphate molecules combine with protein in the smooth muscle, expanding the proteins to relax the muscles, "like fingers loosening their grip on a hose". A dilation of sinusoids (gates) and expansion of arteries increases blood flow into spaces within the penis, filling them with blood to produce an erection.

During orgasm, pelvic muscles contract to ejaculate semen. This emission is produced by contractions of smooth muscle in the testes, the paired glands called the seminal vesicles, and the prostate gland.

Stimulated by the hypogastric nerve, the seminal vesicles contract by a travelling wave of muscle contraction and relaxation to propel semen outward. Erections usually subside after ejaculation, as sympathetic hypogastric nerves stimulate muscles to reopen the veins, so trapped blood is expelled and the penis once again becomes flaccid.

Sex Hormones And Development

Testosterone and additional sex hormones help develop and maintain functionality of the neural circuitry of sexual behaviours, modulating brain activity like pituitary secretion and PVN neurotransmission. Hormones appear to govern human sexuality via two brain processes – the *organizational* (causing the brain and body to develop typically feminine or masculine characteristics), and the *activational*, (causing typically feminine or masculine behaviours).

Organizational processes occur during *perinatal* (in the womb) development, resulting in sexual differentiation of the brain, which will develop either female or male neural components.

Development of the neural circuitry necessary for male sexual behavior results from testosterone secretion by the testis during prenatal organization. Testosterone and similar steroid hormones trigger structural changes throughout several CNS regions, even determining the connection patterns and number of neurons in brain *nuclei* (neural clusters).

In addition to organizing brain development, testosterone also initiates male sexual response during puberty, and regulates libido; testosterone levels in the blood have been shown to correlate with the frequency of sexual fantasies. Testosterone appears to activate sexual desire, although it's not involved in the neural activity of sexual arousal or orgasm.

It does, however, maintain the ability of neural circuits to respond to the complex sensations generated by genital stimulation. Most *androgenergic* neurons (nerves with androgen receptors) are found in the hypothalamus and preoptic area, although primates have been found to also possess them in the amygdala and bed nucleus of the stria terminalis. These regions are known to be at the heart of libido.

Interestingly, in women, even high-dose estrogen treatment fails to stimulate libido, sexual arousal, or orgasm, but testosterone and possibly other androgens like DHEA act as aphrodisiacs for them; long-term testosterone administration with skin patches has been shown to significantly improve all aspects of female sexual activity, including orgasm. Estrogen, while ineffective on its own, appears to act *synergistically* (in concert) with androgens to boost female libido.

In fact, it's believed that both men and women use a combination of androgen and estrogen, naturally metabolized from testosterone, for normal sexual response.

Surprisingly, even paraplegics are capable of orgasm: in 2004, Drs. Barry Komisaruk and Beverly Whipple of Rutgers University discovered that women with severed spinal cords could feel cervical stimulation and even reach orgasm, although, since their spinal cords were severed, their brains could not receive signals from their hypogastric or pelvic nerves. MRI scans showed that signals from the vagus nerve, which bypasses the spinal cord, was relaying the signals. Read the study online: http://www.scribd.com/doc/302148/Functional-MRI-of-the-Brain-During-Orgasm-In-Women)

Homework: ...

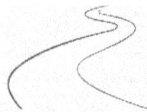

Sex on the Brain: Orgasms Unlock Altered Consciousness, Kayt Sukel, 11 May 2011, New Scientist; http://www.newscientist.com/article/mg21028124.600-sex-on-the-brain-orgasms-unlock-altered-consciousness.html?full=true&print=true

Human Sexual Response, William H. Masters, Virginia E. Johnson, 1966

The Kinsey Institute New Report On Sex, June M. Reinisch and Ruth Beasley, 1991

The Complete Illustrated Kama Sutra, Lance Dane, 2003

The Happy Hooker, Xaviera Hollander, 1972

Double Your Dating, David DeAngelo, 2001

Fear of Flying, Eric Jong, 1973

Female Orgasm Black Book, Lee Jenkins, 2007

Anatomy of the Clitoris, Helen O'Connell, Kalavampara Sanjeevan, John M. Hutson, October 2005, The Journal of Urology 174 (4 Pt 1): 1189–95 http://www.jurology.com/article/S0022-5347%2801%2968572-0/abstract

Sexual Secrets: The Alchemy of Ecstasy, Nik Douglas and Penny Slinger, 1979

Raw Talent: The Adult Film Industry As Seen by Its Most Popular Male Star, Jerry Butler, Robert Rimmer and Catherine Tavel, 1999

Time For Rethink On The Clitoris, Sharon Mascall, BBC News, 11 June 2006

Functional MRI of the Brain During Orgasm In Women, Barry R. Komisaruk and Beverly Whipple, 2005, Annual Review of Sex Research 16:62-86

The Science of Orgasm, Barry R. Komisarak, Carlos Beyer-Flores and Beverly Whipple; "The Joy of Sex: The Ultimate Revised Edition", Alex Comfort, 2009; "How Sex Works", Dr. Sharon Moalem, 2009)

Tulane: The Emergence of a Modern University, 1945 – 1980, Clarence L. Mohr and Joseph E. Gordon, 2001, Louisiana State University Press

The Three-Pound Universe, Judith Hooper and Dick Teresi, 1986; 1991 ISBN: 0-874-77650-3

The Brain from Top to Bottom, McGill University; http://thebrain.mcgill.ca/flash/i/i_03/i_03_cr/i_03_cr_que/i_03_cr_que.html

The Orgasmic Mind: The Neurological Roots of Sexual Pleasure, Martin Portner, 2008, Scientific American Mind, http://www.scientificamerican.com/article.cfm?id=the-orgasmic-mind

Bremelanotide Fact Sheet, Palatin Technologies, 2009; http://www.palatin.com/pdfs/bremelanotide.pdf

What Happens in the Brain During an Orgasm? Shanna Freeman, 2008, Discovery Fit & Health http://health.howstuffworks.com/sexual-health/sexuality/brain-during-orgasm.htm

Cupid's Poisoned Arrow: From Habit to Harmony in Sexual Relationships, Marnia Robinson; ISBN: 978-1-55643-809-7, North Atlantic Books; http://www.amazon.com/Cupids-Poisoned-Arrow-Harmony-Relationships/dp/1556438095

Parasympathetic nervous System, Wikipedia, 2011

The Science of Orgasm, Barry R. Komisaruk, Carlos Beyer-Flores, Beverly Whipple, 2006, Johns Hopkins University Press, ISBN-10: 080188490X; http://www.amazon.com/Science-Orgasm-Barry-R-Komisaruk/dp/080188490X

Orgasm Pill no Pleasure for Rutgers Professors, Josh Funk, Friday, June 16, 2006, Daily Nebraskan; http://www.dailynebraskan.com/news/orgasm-pill-no-pleasure-for-rutgers-professors-1.301849

Mary Roach: 10 Things You Didn't Know About Orgasm, February 2009, TED Talks; http://www.ted.com/talks/lang/eng/mary_roach_10_things_you_didn_t_know_about_orgasm.html

Strange Sex: The Mental Orgasm, 2010 Discovery Communications, LLC; http://tlc.discovery.com/videos/strange-sex-videos/

Sex and the Secret Nerve, R. Douglas Fields, 2009, Scientific American, Inc.

508

Love

"She walks in Beauty, like the night
Of cloudless climes and starry skies,
And all that's best of dark and bright
Meet in her aspect and her eyes."
– *"She Walks in Beauty", Lord Byron, 1814*

"There's this place in me where your fingerprints still rest,
your kisses still linger, and your whispers softly echo.
It's the place where a part of you will forever be a part of me."
– *attributed to Indiana University Professor Gretchen A. Kemp, circa 1975*

"Sometimes your nearness takes my breath away;
and all the things I want to say can find no voice.
Then, in silence, I can only hope my eyes will speak my heart."

"I will ask no more of life than this:
that I might love you through all my days,
and that you may find both peace and joy
in the constancy of my heart."

"...And when we grow old
I will find two chairs
and set them close each sunlit day,
that you and I - in quiet joy -
may rock the world away."
– *Robert Sexton, American artist, from his original prints, 2004*

Love is one of the most fundamental of all human emotions, compelling some of the most heroic acts of courage, self-sacrifice and nobility in human history – and some of the blackest acts of cold-hearted brutality. So what's it doing in us – how does it "work"?

Studies on both animals and humans have uncovered the biochemistry underlying love. Researchers have begun to understand love as part of the highly-evolved, naturally-wired motivation and reward system in the animal brain; the neurochemical processes are the result of billions of years of evolutionary adaptation in both animals and people, maximizing the opportunities for procreation and the continued survival of a given species.

When looking at potential mates, animals like you and I are subconsciously assessing their genes for the potential to help us create healthy children – to pass on these genes to future generations.

509

So attractiveness, as we've seen in our previous chapter on beauty, is largely dependent upon subconscious judgments of how genetically suitable a potential partner is for creating healthy offspring, although subjective factors such as your phenotype, hormonal programming, and childhood environment also play a large role in your selection of a mate.

Chemistry

In humans, when we see a potential mate, in about two-tenths of a second, our brains engage in complex simultaneous biochemical processes across several brain regions, launching a variety of hormones, proteins and neurotransmitters.

As for love, extensive studies have shown the same processes at work in the brains of the moonstruck as in drug addicts – love seems to be every bit as addictive as cocaine, and for exactly the same neurological reasons. And, just as with addictive drugs, love's addiction can create *tolerance* (a weakened response requiring ever stronger doses of the "drug" – in this case, the object of one's affections); *withdrawal* (pain experienced in the absence of the drug); and *relapse* (a tendency to fall back into the addiction cycle long after recovery). Obsessive love in particular also has many neurological similarities to mental illness.

Initial pangs of love are generated in the *caudate*, the apostrophe-shaped central brain region that plays a central role in arousal and experiencing sensations of pleasure. When the caudate is activated, your brain is flooded with a pleasurable rush of dopamine, and you want to continue the euphoric state, so you're motivated to try to please the object of your affection in various ways.

fMRI scans show that volunteers who describe themselves as madly in love have heightened caudate activity, coupled with reduced prefrontal cortex activity, showing a lack of judgment and impulse control over their feelings. This is why, as the BBC reports, "When it comes to love, it seems we are at the mercy of our biochemistry."

Rutgers University Biological Anthropologist Dr. Helen Fisher says there are three distinct phases of love, each marked by a different combination of neurochemical activity:

1. In phase one – **lust** – the sex drive spurs the hypothalamus to trigger hormone synthesis in the pituitary gland. This makes gonads release testosterone and estrogen, heightening libido.

2. Phase two, **attraction**, includes obsessive thinking about the object of affection. People may have no appetite and lose the ability to sleep, spending hours in daydreaming about the object of their affections. In this phase, dopamine release is accompanied by nor-epinephrine, cortisol and nerve growth factor (NGF), all of which lead to racing heartbeat, flushed cheeks, distractedness, and a ten-dency to see the positive characteristics and to attach great weight to even the smallest of interactions with the loved one.

3. *Attachment* is the third phase of love, in which a couple bonds and usually bears children. In this stage, the hypothalamus and pi-tuitary release oxytocin and vasopressin, hormones that build trust and feelings of mutual closeness. Sexual intercourse is responsible for additional oxytocin and vasopressin releases, as well as signifi-cant dopamine release, leading us to seek to repeat the behavior, and to draw ever closer to our sexual partners.

Dr. Lucy Brown, a professor at New York's Albert Einstein College per-formed fMRI scans on college students experiencing new romantic love. While they were scanned, the volunteers looked at photos of the ones they loved. Brown's team discovered that the caudate – involved in habit-forming and craving – became highly activated. Within the region, the ventral teg-mental area became highly active, producing high levels of dopamine, the powerful neuromodulator at the heart of all motivation.

According to Dr. Brown, when you fall in love, the ventral tegmental area appears to flood the brain with dopamine; the caudate, in turn, then sends signals for more dopamine. And the greater the dopamine release, the greater the "high". In other words, falling in love activates precisely the same system as snorting cocaine.

Lust, however, appears to activate entirely different regions – primarily the hypothalamus and amygdala – centers involved in creating hunger and arousal, among other motivational instincts.

In the year 2000 at London's University College, neurobiologists Andreas Bartels and Semir Zeki tested which brain regions activate at the sight of one's beloved.

17 subjects said to be "deeply and madly in love" were examined with fMRI scans while observing first photographs of loved ones and later those of friends, and these scans were compared. The insula, anterior cingulate cortex, and striatum activated; the insula and cingulate cortex are related to a number of emotions, so this was unsurprising, but activation of the striatum – an area believed to be responsible for motor planning – was surprising.

Sometimes, however, relationships are broken, and there is grief, especially when there is separation from the beloved. Najib et al., (2004) studied the brain of 17 women experiencing grief, who were turning their situation over and over in their mind (i.e. *ruminating*).

The team used fMRI to show that acute grief increases the activity in several posterior brain regions, and decreased activity in the thalamus, striatum, and cingulate cortex. For women that experience a larger grief, the decrease in activity in these regions was larger.

A study four years later at Rutgers NYSU and the Albert Einstein College of Medicine studied the neural basis of love in its earliest stages, from 1 to 17 months, and found activation concentrated in the ventral tegmental area and caudate, and the more passionate the love was reported to be, the greater was the response in the caudate.

Beauty Is in the Medial OFC of the Beholder

According to Dr. Semir Zeki of University College London, beauty is indeed subjective – it depends entirely upon who's looking at the object in question.

When we enjoy a work of art or music, a region of the frontal lobe called the medial orbitofrontal cortex activates. This same region takes part in consciously recognizing rewards of stimuli in the environment (salience). This innate appreciation of beauty applies to a variety of media – visual, auditory, even physical attractiveness.

Twenty-one study participants from a variety of cultures and ethnicities was asked to rate either a series of paintings or musical excerpts as beautiful, indifferent or ugly. They next viewed the pictures or listened to the musical excerpts within an fMRI scanner.

Drs. Zeki and Tomohiro Ishizu discovered that the medial orbitofrontal cortex, part of the mesocortical pleasure pathway, becomes more active while people listen to music or watch pictures they find to be aesthetically pleasing (beautiful). However, no single region consistently activated in response to works of art the volunteers had rated as "ugly".

Studies have previously shown that this same region is activated by an attractive face, and even more so when that face smiles at the viewer. As one might suspect, the visual cortex (occipital lobe) also activated while subjects viewed paintings, and the auditory cortex (temporal lobe) as they listened to music.

Interestingly, the caudate also increased in activity with the viewer's perception of beauty – the more pleasing the artwork, the greater the caudal activation. The caudate has previously been found to activate strongly during romantic love, which indicates a biological link between beauty and love.

Says Dr. Zeki, the degree of activation is entirely subjective – it's based upon personal preferences: while some find pleasure in a Tchaikovsky concerto, others will respond more strongly to a Led Zeppelin anthem.

Picky, Picky: How We Select Our Mate(s)

According to Yale University's Dr. Paul Bloom, the psychological component of human attraction is based upon *similarity, familiarity* and *proximity*. If you think someone is like you, they're nearby, and you frequently interact, the likelihood of your mutual attraction increases.

According to dating guru David DeAngelo, another major part of the puzzle is *social value*. We want someone we perceive as having high status. For heterosexual men, this means a physically attractive and socially adept woman; for heterosexual women, it means a self-assured, economically competent, physically healthy and socially dominant man.

Physically, however, all of our sensory organs are engaged in helping us choose a partner.

Pheromones are chemical molecules that trigger hormonal changes and provide clues about the genetic "fitness" of a prospective mate. These *odorants* bind to receptors in the mucus membrane of the nose, where their chemical properties can be broken down and analyzed by the *rhinoencephalis* (nose brain).

Dr. Elisabeth Oberzaucher of the University of Vienna ran a series of experiments in which she had females rate the "pleasantness" of t-shirts worn by various men during exercise.

Testosterone and androstenone are secreted at higher levels by more physically attractive men, in the sense that they are more genetically appealing, i.e. younger, fitter and more symmetric in appearance). Women find the direct scent repellant – except when they're ovulating, and therefore most fertile.

Then there is androstadienone, said to be the first true pheromone identified in humans. A *metabolite* (chemical product) of testosterone, androstadienone subtly alters the mood of heterosexual women and homosexual men. While it reputedly doesn't specifically alter overt behavior, it appears to increase attentiveness to emotional cues and to improve mood through raising cortisol levels.

The validity of pheromone studies are still very much under dispute, and the claim that humans – like other animals – have a functional *Vomeronasal Organ (VNO)* detection system for them is also widely regarded with skepticism by the scientific community. (See book one - "Cranial Nerve Zero").

The first kiss, however, is the ultimate test of compatibility – in the exchange, five of the 12 cranial nerves are activated, engaging taste, touch and scent, and hormonal and health cues are exchanged, signalling subconsciously how appropriate someone is as a partner.

Voice also appears to subconsciously transmit information about sexual promiscuity, and, it's been claimed, physical attractiveness – "nice voices" correlate with attractive physical characteristics. Because of this, Dr. Gordon Gallup of State University of New York, Albany suggests having a phone conversation before ever accepting a blind date.

The BBC has an interesting online test to measure what kind of partner you're attracted to:

http://www.bbc.co.uk/science/humanbody/mind/surveys/faceperception1/

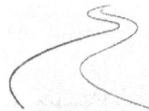

The Sex Researchers, season one, episode two, BBC One, 2011

Smelling a Single Component of Male Sweat Alters Levels of Cortisol in Women, Wyart C, Webster WW, Chen JH, Wilson SR, McClary A, Khan RM, Sobel N (February 2007) Journal of Neuroscience 27 (6): 1261–5. doi:10.1523/JNEUROSCI.4430-06.2007. PMID 17287500; http://www.ncbi.nlm.nih.gov/pubmed/17287500

Subthreshold Amounts of Social Odorant Affect Mood, but not Behavior, in Heterosexual Women When Tested by a Male, but not a Female, Experimenter, Johan N. Lundström and Mats J. Olsson, 2005, Biological Psychology, doi:10.1016/j.biopsycho.2005.01.008; http://www.sciencedirect.com/science/article/pii/S0301051105000396

Cognitive and Physiological Responses of Men to Female Pheromones, Astrid Jütte, 1997, New Aspects of Human Ethology, New York, Plenum Press, pp. 206; http://www.amazon.com/Aspects-Ethology-Recent-Advances-Phytochemistry/dp/0306456958

Putative Human Pheromone Androstadienone Attunes the Mind Specifically to Emotional Information, Tom A. Hummera, and Martha K. McClintock, 2009, Hormones and Behav-

ior, doi:10.1016/j.yhbeh.2009.01.002; http://www.sciencedirect.com/science/article/pii/
S0018506X09000051

*Human Pheromones: A Critical Review of the Evidence for the Existence (1) Human Phero-
mones and (2) a Functional Vomeronasal Organ (VNO) in Humans,* Tim Jacob, 1999-2005,
Cardiff University; http://www.cf.ac.uk/biosi/staffinfo/jacob/teaching/sensory/pherom.html

The Biochemistry of Love's Ecstasy and Agony, Dr. Glenn D. Braunstein, 2011 The Huffington Post

Human Body & Mind: The Science of Love, author unattributed, 2011 BBC Science

Lullabyes for Getting Laid, Julia Smith-Eppsteiner, 2011, The Michigan Daily

Loving With All Your ... Brain, Elizabeth Cohen, February 14, 2007, CNN; http://articles.cnn.
com/2007-02-14/health/love.science_1_scans-caudate-amygdala?_s=PM:HEALTH

The Neural Basis of Romantic Love, Bartels A, Zeki S, 2000 Nov 27, Neuroreport; 11(17):3829-
34.; http://www.vislab.ucl.ac.uk/pdf/NeuralBasisOfLove.pdf

*Reward, Motivation, and Emotion Systems Associated With Early-Stage Intense Romantic
Love,* Arthur Aron, Helen Fisher, Debra J. Mashek, Greg Strong, Haifang Li and Lucy L.
Brown, Journal of Neurophysiology, 94:327-337, 2005. doi:10.1152/jn.00838.2004; http://
jn.physiology.org/content/94/1/327.full.pdf

Toward A Brain-Based Theory of Beauty, Tomohiro Ishizu, Semir Zeki, PLoS ONE, 2011;
6 (7): e21852 DOI: 10.1371/journal.pone.0021852; http://www.plosone.org/article/
info%3Adoi%2F10.1371%2Fjournal.pone.0021852

Beauty in a Smile: the Role of Medial Orbitofrontal Cortex in Facial Attractiveness, J.
O'Doherty, J. Winston, H. Critchley, D. Perrett, D. M. Burt and R. J. Dolan, 2003, Neuropsy-
chologia;41(2):147-55. http://www.sciencedirect.com/science/article/pii/S0028393202001458

Happiness

If you observe a really happy man you will find him building a boat, writing a symphony, educating his son, growing double dahlias in his garden. He will not be searching for happiness as if it were a collar button that has rolled under the radiator."
– W. Beran Wolfe, "How to be Happy Though Human", 1931

"Happiness is an inside job." – William Arthur Ward, "Fountains of Faith", 1970

"One of the main aspects of spiritual maturity is having a connectedness with others. This is defined as having an appreciation of a common bond with all of humanity and, in particular, relationships with others. Relationships can be stifled by self-absorption, selfishness, meanness, greed, narcissism, pride, and so on. On the other hand, relationships are fostered by moving beyond individual ego worlds and participating in daily acts of self-transcendence, mindfulness of others, self-forgetfulness, generosity, compassion, listening, helping, patience, humility, and so on."

– Pamela Waters, "Spirituality in Addiction Treatment and Recovery", 2005

"Since you get more joy out of giving joy to others, you should put a good deal of thought into the happiness that you are able to give."
—Eleanor Roosevelt, "You Learn By Living", 1960.

"Each morning when I open my eyes I say to myself: I, not events, have the power to make me happy or unhappy today. I can choose which it shall be. Yesterday is dead, tomorrow hasn't arrived yet. I have just one day, today, and I'm going to be happy in it."
– Groucho Marx, "The Essential Groucho", 2003

" "People say that money is not the key to happiness, but I always figured if you have enough money, you can have a key made."
– Joan Rivers, "Bouncing Back: I've Survived Everything..." 1997

Happiness. What exactly is it?

Merriam Webster dictionary describes it as "a state of well-being and contentment: joy". That's simple enough, but the REAL question is: how do you get it?

Modern research has found a number of attributes happy people share: strong relationships and an active social life, extroversion, satisfaction from long-term marriage, employment, good health, political freedom, an optimistic personality, regular physical exercise, religious involvement, a solid income and proximity to other happy people.

Whereas westerners have long sought happiness through external events, objects or circumstances, easterners have focused for thousands of years on developing inner abilities, studying methods for achieving optimal mental states. Says happiness expert Dr. Lance P. Hickey, this is why modern Americans have trouble in achieving happiness: in pursuing it, we look outwardly, believing it to be somehow distant from us, when in fact the keys lies in inner development.

Harvard psychologist Dan Gilbert, author of *Stumbling on Happiness* points out, "We have within us the capacity to manufacture the very commodities we are constantly chasing": it's not the external things that you strive for which give you satisfaction in and of themselves, but your own thoughts and the neurotransmitters and hormones they generate which affect your moods.

That's all well and good – we've looked at the brain chemistry and mechanisms underlying happiness, so what are the sources?

It turns out that the number one factor in happiness, according to decades of research, is found in human relationships. Mihaly Csikszentmihalyi, said to be the world's best authority on positive psychology says:

> *Almost every person feels happier when they're with other people.... It's paradoxical because many of us think we can hardly wait to get home and be alone with nothing to do, but that's a worst-case scenario. If you're alone with nothing to do, the quality of your experience really plummets.*

There are, of course, a number of other life circumstances that can contribute to happiness. Former president of the American Psychological Association Dr. Martin E. P. Seligman teaches psychology at the University of Pennsylvania. He spoke at the Feb. 2004 TED seminar in Monterrey, California on the state of psychology, saying it has, until now, focused generally on fixing what's gone wrong. This, he says, is the wrong approach.

In his 25 years of clinical experience, he says the most that can ever be achieved is to bring a formerly depressed, anxious or mentally ill patient to a "zero" level – basically a null state, emotional emptiness.

Now Dr. Seligman leads the University of Pennsylvania's Positive Psychological Center, where they have examined thousands of studies around the world to derive at what happiness means and how to achieve it. Says Dr. Seligman, there are three paths to happiness:

Hedonism – living a life of pleasure

Engagement – absorption in the pleasure of using your true skills at high levels of mastery

Altruism – finding a "higher purpose" to serve with your strengths

He says that thousands of studies show that a life of pleasure-seeking can bring happiness, but this happiness appears to be transitory and shallow.

The other two paths to happiness require knowing your signature strengths and then recrafting your life to use them as much as possible, in work, friendship, family and play. To find your own "signature strengths" and learn more effective ways of maximizing joy in your life, please visit: http://www.authentichappiness.org

For example, if you're particularly skilled at analytical thinking, a job in sales is likely to lead to misery, unless, for example, you move into customer satisfaction, motivation research, market analysis and the like. Conversely, if you love to talk and meet new people, perhaps recruitment or sales is the perfect fit.

The third path to happiness – altruism – has been shown time and again to be the most effective means of achieving happiness and fulfillment in life, leading to significant and statistically proven increases in productivity, longevity and health.

Hedonism – The most fleeting and superficial form of happiness is pleasure, says Seligman, although the majority of westerners build our lives around pursuing it obsessively, usually through *materialism* – acquiring money or objects. But *can* money buy happiness?

Well, yes and no, say scientists. It all depends on how it's used: a 2009 San Francisco State University study found that purchasing *life experiences* instead of material possessions leads to greater happiness: while a shiny new toy may provide fleeting pleasure, eventually you'll grow bored of it and go off in search of a new novelty.

"Purchased experiences provide *memory capital*," says assistant psychology professor Ryan Howell. "We don't tend to get bored of happy memories like we do with a material object." What's more, materialistic people are less liked among their peers than people seeking pleasure through experiences, according to University of Colorado psychology Professor Leaf Van Boven.

Engagement – Many psychologists believe the highest state of human happiness is achieved during *peak* or *flow experiences*, where your mind becomes completely engaged in an activity, and your body just "flows" with effortless skill and competency; you "let go" and forget yourself, acting without conscious effort, but with a heightened awareness of the moment (athletes often describe this as *being in the zone*). During the flow experience, you lose all sense of self – physical needs and sensations, emotions, the passage of time, and self-awareness.

To bring about flow states, the activity has to be something voluntary, enjoyable, and one that is challenging and requires skill. *Focused attention* is apparently the key, and this can be learned and improved through mastering activities such as meditation, yoga, and martial arts training. Simple, regular exercise such as running is another means of learning to engage in the present moment and improve focused attention. People who experience flow in daily life have been shown to have better concentration, self-esteem, and health.

Altruism – Religious faith or belief that life has meaning also makes people happier, according to statistics. In fact, it also helps people survive the worst of circumstances. According to Dr. Seligman, learning your life purpose comes from discovering your strengths and finding new ways to use them, particularly in helping others. Helping others adds meaning to your life – giving you a sense of purpose, because you matter to someone else.

Along these lines, University of California psychologist Sonja Lyubomirsky recommends that performing at least five "good deeds" a week, especially all in a single day, gives a measurable boost in mood and health.

Psychologist Viktor Frankl's amazing *Man's Search for Meaning* recounts his harrowing story of survival in the Auschwitz and other Nazi concentration camps for five years. Frankl observed that only those with deep faith of one sort or another had the spiritual stamina to survive. Like Abraham Maslow, it's Frankl's contention that finding such meaning in life is humanity's highest purpose.

Your Happiness Setpoint

Life's triumphs and tragedies – the "slings and arrows of outrageous fortune" – can bring joy or disappointment, but psychologists have discovered that each of us tends to eventually return to an emotional *set point*, an individual baseline of satisfaction or anxiety.

In 2008, an international team of scientists at Edinburgh University and the Queensland Institute for Medical Research found support for the premise that each of us is born with a happiness setpoint, a base level of personal happiness to which we bounce back – or plummet – depending on our genetics.

Using the *Five-Factor Personality Model* (see The Path Book I) to study 973 pairs of genetic twins, the researchers discovered that subjects who are sociable, conscientious, and don't worry excessively are generally happier. They believe this mixture of personality traits acts as an "emotional buffer" in the face of adversity. These traits appear to come from genes which predispose an individual to happiness in life – providing a reserve of happiness to be called upon during difficulty.

Still, they note that, while these inherited traits may increase the likelihood of life happiness, about 50 to 66 percent of the "happiness equation" is still derived from environmental factors such as health, major life events, socio-economic status, relationships and careers.

Happy Genes

Behavioral economist Jan-Emmanuel De Neve of the London School of Economics and Political Science (LSE) found a direct link between a specific gene and individual happiness, as measured by life satisfaction. The gene is an *allele* (variant) of 5-HTT, which encodes mRNA and proteins used to make serotonin reuptake transporters. The 5-HTT gene can be long or short, and the longer allele manufactures more serotonin transporters. Each half of a chromosome pair is inherited from one parent, so one can have a combination of long+long, short+short, or both alleles.

Matching 5-HTT alleles to happiness surveys, De Neve's team studied 2,500 volunteers. Those with efficient (long-long) 5-HHT alleles consistently reported much greater life satisfaction, either "very satisfied" (35 per cent) or "satisfied" (34 per cent) – compared with 19 percent in both categories for those with the less efficient (short-short) form.

Naturally, De Neve notes, this single gene isn't the sole determinant of human happiness; other genes and life experiences significantly help shape individual happiness, but it appears the theory that each of us is born with a basic set point of happiness is true, primarily due to the influence of genetics in serotonin circulation.

A related study prepared by De Neve, Harvard Medical School's Nicholas Christakis, UCal's James H. Fowler and Bruno Frey (University of Zurich) further developed the research to show that genetics comprise about one-third of the variation in human happiness.

These genetic set points have been shown through research to be stable over the years. However, according to Virginia Commonwealth University psychiatrist Kenneth S. Kendler, extreme adversity – on the order of severe childhood abuse or war trauma – can have lasting effects as well. Kendler's research demonstrates that life experiences can influence set points for anxiety and depression, possibly even more than genes.

With an international team of researchers from Amsterdam, America, and Sweden, Dr. Kendler studied data from over 12,000 identical twins (those who share the same genes), ranging in age from 10 to 66. Because their lives unfold along different paths, it's possible to study the specific impact of environmental factors on personality. The twins in the study had filled out surveys describing their levels of anxiety and depression three times over the course of five to six years.

Building a composite of life segments ranging from prepubescence through adulthood and retirement, VCU's Dr. Charles Gardner discovered a distinct statistical curve. Set points among 10-year-old twins were identical or nearly so, but as twins grew into adolescence and beyond, these set points increasingly diverged, until levelling out at about 60 years of age. This massive study proves that while set points are individually stable, not changing willy-nilly, they aren't immutable, but are subject to change over time.

By studying the difference between these set points among genetically identical twins, the scientists found that, although genes may help determine emotional predilections, life experiences can shift temperaments. According to Dr. Kendler, the effects of life experiences are lasting, so what determines an adult's emotional set point is a mixture of both genetic factors and the sum total of life experiences.

Self-Esteem And Your Health

High self-esteem is more than just a matter of feeling good – it also has a marked effect on your body as well. Regarding yourself with respect translates into boosts to your cardiovascular and immune system health. First, in the face of threats, high self-esteem grants greater feelings of security. This translates directly into reduced cortisol levels in response to stress – stress which, in modern society, is usually more about social status than physical danger.

Psychologist Andy Martens of the University of Canterbury, New Zealand, led a study to measure the effects of self-esteem upon the parasympathetic nervous system, which calms the body – the physiological opposite effect of the "fight or flight" response. The team asked 184 subjects to rate their levels of self-esteem every day for two weeks. Next, the researchers gave these volunteers bogus feedback regarding their intelligence or personality, aimed at raising or lowering their self-esteem.

The researchers then analyzed *cardiac vagal tone* – the effects on the heart when only parasympathetic nervous system fibers (in the vagus nerve) are in control of heart rate. These parasympathetic nerve fibers slow heart rate from about 70 bpm to 60.

The PNS slows and calms the heart, counteracting the sympathetic nervous system's triggering of the "fight or flight" state. Over prolonged periods of time, in this way, the PNS reduces the physiological effects of stress such as inflammation. An underactive PNS can eventually result in cardiovascular problems and autoimmune disease.

Dr. Martins consistently found a correlation between high self-esteem and healthy vagal tone. While the effect was small, Martens says it is an important first step in establishing the self-esteem/health connection. His advice for boosting self-esteem is to surround yourself with caring family and friends, which he believes to be much more effective than simple positive thinking. He says that low self-esteem isn't just a matter of foul moods; it means the body is malfunctioning, raising the possibility of future health problems.

Be Good To Yourself

Duke University psychologists have likewise reported that people who use kinder self-talk are better able to deal with troubles in life. Self-compassion, the ability to be kind to yourself when things take a turn for the worse, helps decrease disappointment, anger and depression, according to Professor Mark R. Leary, who lead the 2007 study. Self-compassion is said to involve three elements:

- *self-kindness* (rather than self-criticism)

- *common humanity* (viewing negative experiences as part of everyone's life)

- *mindful acceptance* (being tolerant, composed and accepting of stress instead of surrendering to despair, painful feelings and thoughts)

The difference between those who exercise self-compassion and those who don't is that when someone is kind to herself, she doesn't add an extra layer of negativity. Those who beat themselves up over mistakes or failure can become overwhelmed by the added distress in an already unpleasant situation. Self-compassionate people judge themselves less based upon the events, presumably because they're kind to and accepting of themselves, whether things go well or not. The authors believe the greatest benefits of high self-esteem come from self-compassion.

Do you treat yourself as well as you treat your friends and family? People who are supportive and understanding of others may all too often be very critical of and unkind to themselves for what they see as shortcomings in personality, behavior or appearance. But being kind to yourself and accepting your imperfections is, believe the researchers, critical to health and longevity, resulting in reduced anxiety and depression, and greater happiness and fulfillment. Self-compassion appears to even have a marked effect on diet and weight.

University of Texas Professor Kristin Neff says it's important to distinguish between self-compassion and self-indulgence. The main reason people aren't kinder to themselves, she says, is a worry that they may become overly self-indulgent, and so they accept the cultural beliefs that being hard on themselves is constructive and "keeps them in line".

But imagine enforcing such cold behavior on a small child you love. Hopefully, it's unthinkable – we don't like to be cruel to those we care about. especially if they're vulnerable. Adopt the same nurturing standard for yourself – avoiding self-criticism and negativity – and your life will improve dramatically.

Self-Compassion And Health

The reason you don't let your children eat five big tubs of ice cream is because you care about them. With self-compassion, if you care about yourself, you do what's healthy for you rather than what's harmful to you.

In her new book *Self-Compassion: Stop Beating Yourself Up and Leave Insecurity Behind*, Dr. Neff suggests some helpful self-compassion exercises, such as meditation or writing yourself a letter of support, as if to a friend for whom you feel concern. Additionally, she suggests listing your strengths and weaknesses (which you should rephrase as "areas I am improving"), thinking about positive courses of action you can take for improvement, and reminding yourself that nobody's perfect.

A related 2007 Wake Forest University study found that just a single session in practicing self-compassion led to improved self-control over junk food. Says Harvard Medical School psychotherapist Jean Fain, author of *The Self-Compassion Diet*, self-compassion is the critical missing component of every weight-loss plan; most plans involve being unkind to yourself, engaging in deprivation and being hard on yourself. But being kind to yourself is a far more productive habit you can acquire through regular practice.

It Ain't Easy Being Green

Human beings seem driven by the impulse to impose order upon the environment: building houses, cities, paving sidewalks, pouring concrete everywhere, until everything is one massive, lifeless grey grid. It seems we have an instinctual drive toward order, predictability, even (illusory) control over nature.

But I've always thought it's unhealthy. Though I've never read studies to support it, I've always held the theory that the human brain, while seeking to find or impose logical patterns and rules upon the natural chaos of the world, paradoxically needs this natural disorder for healthy function. I believe cognitive "white noise" – randomness – is essential for mental health, whether it's the random sprawl of twisting roots, moss, branches and leaves, or the chaotic flow of rivers and lakes.

Of course, people have always known that nature is good for physical health, but recent research has revealed for the first time the specific benefits. Says University of Illinois researcher Dr. Frances Kuo, the healing powers of nature have been cited throughout history, but without any real scientific basis in fact. However, rigorous worldwide scientific studies over the last decade, using crime reports, immune system, blood pressure, and neurocognitive tests, have shown significant, measurable mental and physical health benefits. Says Dr. Kuo, "Rarely do the scientific findings on any question align so clearly.... The strength, consistency and convergence of the findings are remarkable."

Access to natural environments, even in the form of parks and gardens, results in better cognitive function and improved mental health, including higher levels of self-discipline and impulse control. Greenery enables greater amounts of physical activity, improves immune system function and blood glucose levels, and even enhances surgery recovery. And people with access to natural greenery have been found to be more generous, altruistic, sociable, and have a greater sense of community and mutual trust.

Conversely, people in sterile city environments have been shown to undergo breakdowns in healthy social functions, resulting in higher rates of aggression, violence, crime and loneliness. A lack of access to nature has also been linked to higher incidences of 15 out of 24 categories of diseases, heightened levels of ADHD, anxiety and depression, and even higher rates of childhood obesity and adult mortality.

Because of the strong correlation that has been demonstrated between nature and health, Dr. Kuo urges city planners to include more public green spaces, not as mere decoration, but as a vital source of health, resulting in smarter, kinder, better-adjusted, more sociable, law-abiding, cooperative and resilient citizens.

Neurochemical Benefits Of Yoga

A 2010 report, published in the *Journal of Alternative and Complementary Medicine*, says that yoga is even better than walking and other exercise for boosting mood and reducing anxiety. Dr. Chris Streeter of the Boston University School of Medicine believes this is due to yoga triggering an increase in endogenous mood stabilizers such as GABA, which helps regulate neurotransmission.

GABA production is suppressed in sufferers of mood and anxiety disorders, so psychiatrists commonly prescribe GABA-boosting drugs to reduce anxiety and improve moods.

Dr. Streeter and colleagues demonstrated that increased GABA in the thalamus after a session of yoga leads to a similar drop in anxiety and improved mood, suggesting yoga may someday be an accepted alternative or complement to antidepressant drugs.

Don't Fake it; Make it

Trying to fake a smile can actually worsen your mood, but using positive thinking (for example, remembering a favourite vacation) can bring out a sincere smile, to not only boost your own productivity and energy, but also improve the morale of all those you meet throughout your day.

Brent Scott, assistant professor of management at Michigan State University says that "putting on a happy face" in spite of your moods leads to emotional fatigue and withdrawal. Scott and doctoral student Christopher Barnes studied Michigan bus drivers over two weeks to examine the effects of fake smiles versus genuine smiles induced by pleasant memories or thinking positively.

One interesting finding was that the results were stronger among female bus drivers – women suffered greater stress by pretending to be in good moods, and had stronger effects from positive memories or *reframing* – thinking about situations in a more positive manner.

Cultivating Kindness

Start to learn situational awareness. If you don't already, you need to start noticing the old lady with the cane, who may need your seat because of her arthritis. Be willing to help the pregnant mother loaded down with shopping bags on the staircase. Be aware that your actions always have consequences – the simplest kindness may change a person's life. Conversely, rudeness may bring deep distress – or close a door to you forever.

Develop kindness and respect for everyone and everything you meet (including your waitress at the family restaurant, the clerk at the 7-11, even [perhaps especially!] the dirty, homeless man in the gutter), for a number of reasons, both selfish and altruistic:

- Kindness makes you happier, more attractive, more fulfilled, healthier and longer-lived. According to 2008 research at the University of Miami, the feel-good hormone oxytocin, produced by acts of kindness or positive physical contact such as hugging, reduces potential damage to blood vessels and the chance of heart attacks by an astounding 24 to 26 percent. So by bonding with others or showing simple acts of kindness you're producing oxytocin, and hugely reducing your heart disease risks.

- Happiness and goodwill are contagious. Making somebody happy uplifts both your spirits, and will be carried around by both of you throughout the day. And, let's face it, there's already enough misery and suffering in the world. Be one of the "good guys".

- You don't know the other person's story. You might be surprised at their life stories.

- You never know who else might be watching and judging you (a boss, the boy you're trying to impress, etc. If you believe in an afterlife, it may even be your grandfather and grandmother watching you when you're rude to that coworker or stranger.

- You never know where fate will bring the two of you in the future. As the American actor Jimmy Durante once said, "Be nice to people on your way up because you meet them on your way down."

Let me give you a powerful personal example of how fate can work:

At one point, I went to work in a small print shop run by a young family man named Mickey. He was smart, hardworking, had integrity, and was good at his job and a nice enough fellow, but while he was away, his assistant Christina would be incredibly rude and domineering, running the office like a Nazi camp commandant, shouting at and insulting coworkers and even customers. The day came when I reached my limit of tolerance, and I lost control of my emotions. When she loudly *slammed* a pile of books down behind me and snidely added "*These* don't belong *there!*" then stomped away, I decided I'd had enough.

I lost my temper. Pointing my finger at her like a weapon, I shouted, "Listen! I've had *enough*! *This* is *my* department, and *that* is yours! From now on, *stay* the *Hell* away from *my area!*" and stormed off, leaving her blinking in surprise. The next day, the company owner called me in and fired me. It was unpleasant, but an important life lesson. I learned from it and moved on.

As fate would have it, three months later, I found myself shopping in the supermarket, and, to my surprise, ran into Christina. She was like a different person; quieter, polite, chastised. I couldn't help but feel sorry for her as she told me she'd been fired for acting like a petty tyrant. It seemed like karma – the universe serving up justice.

But the story doesn't end there. One of the customers, for whom I had always worked extra hard, was married to the office manager of a major real estate agency. He gave me his wife's business card and urged me to call her.

I got hired and began to work for the agency. Over the course of two years, as I got better at my job, I was given more and more responsibility, until I was in charge of the department. I began to realize that the company was spending tens of thousands every year and wasting thousands of hours sending work out to suppliers – work that could be done within the company for a fraction of the cost and in a fraction of the time. I wrote up an analysis of the situation and gave it to the corporate president. He agreed with my assessment, and a digital printing press was installed so we could begin production in-house.

As fate would have it, one of our biggest suppliers was my former boss Mickey and his shop. I didn't know in advance, but the real estate company where I now worked had been providing 75% of his income. When he lost us as a client, it hit his store so hard that it drove him completely out of business within three months. I felt very sorry for the way things happened, but learned another unforgettable lesson from the experience: Fate can instantly change the power dynamics of every relationship.

The Hell Of the Hungry Ghosts
and the Religion Of Consumerism

"That's all your house is – a place to keep your stuff while you go out and get more stuff" – George Carlin, Comic Relief, 1986

"Be on your guard against all kinds of greed; life does not consist in an abundance of possessions." – Jesus Christ, Luke 12:15, King James Bible

"Only after the last tree has been cut down, only after the last river has been poisoned, only after the last fish has been caught, only then will you find money cannot be eaten." – Cree Indian Prophecy, original date and author unknown

In the Buddhist religion, one of the kingdoms of Hell is known as The *Realm of Hungry Ghosts*. In this place of torment, the living dead are cursed to wander endlessly, craving, full of desires which can never be fulfilled.

The Hungry Ghosts have huge, empty bellies, but thin necks which don't allow nourishment through, and in their mouths, food turns to fire and ash. Constantly hungry, these creatures are doomed to remain perpetually unfulfilled, and can never leave Hell because they cannot conquer their cravings. Here, Hell is a metaphor for the misery of constant unfulfillment. This is an apt metaphor for modern consumerism, where believing happiness can be achieved through endless consumption leaves you doomed to be spiritually unfulfilled.

Consumerism has become something of a religion in modern society. Compare Buddhism's Four Noble Truths:

1. Life is suffering

2. Suffering arises from desire

3. Suffering ceases when attachment to desire ceases

4. Detachment comes through walking the Path of kindness, morality, self-mastery and the search for truth and clarity

Consumerism teaches essentially the opposite. Its equivalent wisdom says:

1. Life is suffering

2. Suffering arises from unfulfilled desire

3. Suffering ceases when desires are fulfilled

4.   The fulfillment of desire comes through acquiring material goods

But as a country singer once said, using things and loving people, not vice versa, is always the best advice. If you're feeling unhappy, perhaps you're looking for happiness in the wrong places. It's something worth considering.

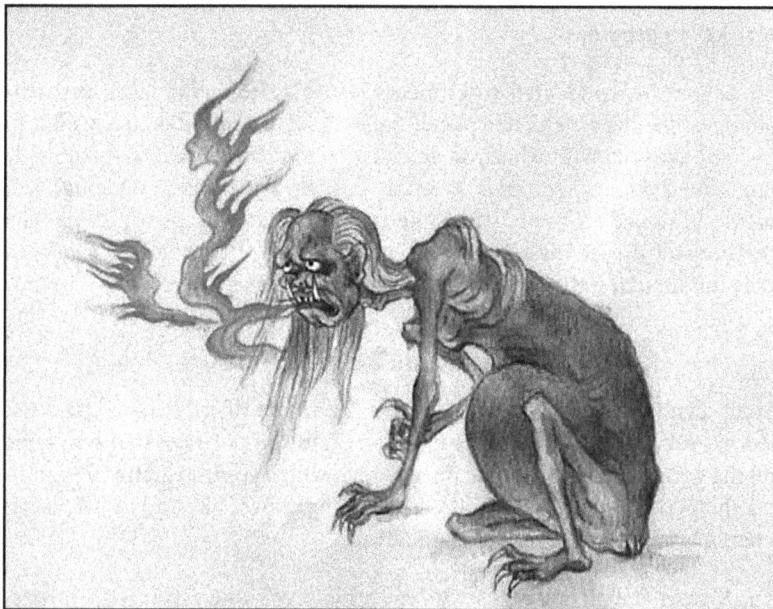

Hungry Ghosts (gaki) are demi humans with big, perpetually empty stomachs, tiny mouths, and necks so thin they cannot swallow. They experience constant hunger, unable to attain satisfaction or fill their bellies. Perpetually empty, they always seek fulfillment from outside of themselves. No matter how much they have, they are never satisfied. "Gaki-zoshi", Late-12th Century, Kyoto National Museum, Japan.

Your Experience Simulator

Harvard psychologist Dr. Dan Gilbert, author of *Stumbling on Happiness*, says your prefrontal cortex is an *experience simulator*. Its evolutionary purpose, he says, is to allow you to try things out in your head before you do them in real life. This, he says, is something no other animal can do. However, your personal experience simulator is usually off base. *Impact bias* is its tendency to predict events will have a much greater impact than they do, while in reality events tend to be shorter and much less significant than your brain predicts.

His point is that when you predict, you vastly overestimate how happy you'll be if you obtain the things you're chasing. He says we seek happiness outside ourselves, but in fact, you can synthesize it in your head. It's all within you. He cites the example of 78-year-old Moreese Bickham, who was released after 37 years of incarceration in a Louisiana State Prison, for a crime of which he was eventually proven innocent. When asked if he had any regrets, Bickham responded, "I don't have one minutes' regret. It was a glorious experience!" Moreese Bickham had learned to relish life for its own sake, the true key to happiness.

Dr. Gilbert has conducted experiments that show how abundance can actually *frustrate* happiness; one of the greatest secrets in life is in learning to become satisfied with what you actually have, and with where you already are – the *attitude of gratitude*, as some self-help gurus call it. Although you are conditioned to want "stuff", the greatest minds in history have been teaching for thousands of years that you have everything you really need for true fulfillment, right now, right here, inside of you.

The Attitude of Gratitude

Sonja Lyubomirsky suggests keeping a "gratitude diary", where you write down everything you're thankful for. She says studies show that reviewing all the good things in your life once a week with a spirit of gratitude significantly increases overall life satisfaction and improves physical health, raises energy levels and relieves pain and fatigue.

Dr. Martin Seligman proposes a "gratitude visit", where you write a letter thanking a teacher, pastor or grandparent – anyone who has helped you and for whom you're thankful – and then visiting them to read your letter of appreciation in person. This significantly boosts the endocrine effects of happiness up to a month later. A longer-lasting exercise he recommends is "three blessings" – writing down three things that went well, along with the reasons why, every day.

In the end, psychologists agree that the root of true happiness isn't money, fame, recognition, or career success, but having meaningful social relationships – suggesting that the single best way to immediately begin cultivating happiness is to invest your energy in building your social ties. Happiness, it seems, is deeply rooted in love and kindness.

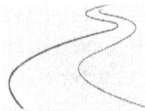

Oxytocin Attenuates NADPH-Dependent Superoxide Activity And IL-6 Secretion In Macrophages And Vascular Cells, Angela Szeto, Daniel A. Nation, Armando J. Mendez, Juan

Dominguez-Bendala, Larry G. Brooks, Neil Schneiderman, and Philip M. McCabe, 2008; 2008, The American Journal of Physiology - Endocrinology and Metabolism; doi: 10.1152/ajpendo.90718.2008; http://ajpendo.physiology.org/content/295/6/E1495.full.pdf+html

Dr. Martin Seligman, TED, February, 2004; http://www.ted.com

A Multilevel Field Investigation of Emotional Labor, Affect, Work Withdrawal, and Gender, Brent A. Scott, Christopher M. Barnes, Academy of Management Journal, Volume 54, Number 1 February 2011

For A Better Workday, Smile Like You Mean It, press release, author unattributed, 2011, Michigan State University;

Better Mood and Better Performance: Learning Rule Described Categories Is Enhanced by Positive Mood, Ruby T. Nadler, Rahel Rabi, John Paul Minda, 2010, Psychological Science; 21: 1770-1776 DOI: 10.1177/0956797610387441

Causal Impact of Employee Work Perceptions on the Bottom Line of Organizations, J. K. Harter, F. L. Schmidt, J. W. Asplund, E. A. Killham, S. Agrawal. Perspectives on Psychological Science, 2010; 5 (4): 378 DOI: 10.1177/1745691610374589

Status and the Evaluation of Workplace Deviance, H. R. Bowles, M. Gelfand, Psychological Science, 2009; 21 (1): 49 DOI: 10.1177/0956797609356509

Workplace Aggression, Manon Mireille LeBlanc, Julian Barling, 2004, Current Directions in Psychological Science; 13 (1): 9 DOI: 10.1111/j.0963-7214.2004.01301003.x

Employee Control and Occupational Stress, Paul E. Spector, Current Directions in Psychological Science, 2002; 11 (4): 133 DOI: 10.1111/1467-8721.00185

Effects of Yoga Versus Walking on Mood, Anxiety, and Brain GABA Levels: A Randomized Controlled MRS Study, Chris C. Streeter, Theodore H. Whitfield, Liz Owen, Tasha Rein, Surya K. Karri, Aleksandra Yakhkind, Ruth Perlmutter, Andrew Prescot, Perry F. Renshaw, Domenic A. Ciraulo, J. Eric Jensen, 2010, The Journal of Alternative and Complementary Medicine; 16 (11): 1145 DOI: 10.1089/acm.2010.0007

Nine Things Successful People Do Differently, Heidi Grant Halvorson, February 25, 2011, Harvard Business Review

Happiness Has A Dark Side, Association for Psychological Science, 2011, ScienceDaily; http://www.sciencedaily.com /releases/2011/05/110516162219.htm

Functional Polymorphism (5-HTTLPR) in the Serotonin Transporter Gene is Associated with Subjective Well-Being: Evidence from a US Nationally Representative Sample, Jan-Emmanuel De Neve, 2011, Journal of Human Genetics, doi:10.1038/jhg.2011.39; http://www.stat.columbia.edu/~cook/movabletype/mlm/deneve1.pdf

Genes, Economics, and Happiness, Jan-Emmanuel De Neve, Nicholas A. Christakis, James H. Fowler, and Bruno S. Frey, 2010, Social Science Research Network; http://papers.ssrn.com/sol3/papers.cfm?abstract_id=1553633

London School of Economics and Political Science, press release; http://www2.lse.ac.uk/

531

newsAndMedia/news/archives/2011/05/happiness_gene.aspx

Happiness Is a Personal(ity) Thing: The Genetics of Personality and Well-Being in a Representative Sample, Alexander Weiss, Timothy C. Bates and Michelle Luciano, 2008, Psychological Science doi: 10.1111/j.1467-9280.2008.02068.x Psychological Science March 1, 2008 vol. 19 no. 3 205-210 http://pss.sagepub.com/content/19/3/205.full.pdf+html

Mood and Experience: Life Comes At You, press release, Divya Menon, June 24, 2011, Association for Psychological Science; http://www.psychologicalscience.org/index.php/news/releases/mood-and-experience-life-comes-at-you.html

The New Science of Happiness, Claudia Wallis, Jan. 09, 2005, Time Magazine;

A Wandering Mind Is an Unhappy Mind, Jason Castro, November 24, 2010, Scientific American;

When the Mind Wanders, Happiness Also Strays, John Tierney, November 15, 2010, The New York Times

The Power to Uplift, Pamela Paul, Jan. 09, 2005, Time Magazine

'Flow' Experiences: The Secret to Ultimate Happiness? Dr. Lance P. Hickey, January 22, 2011, The Huffington Post

Self-Compassion May be More Important Than Self-Esteem in Dealing With Negative Events, New Studies Show, press release, Duke University. Monday, May 14, 2007; http://news.duke.edu/2007/05/selfcompassion.html

Go Easy on Yourself, a New Wave of Research Urges, Tara Parker-Pope, February 28, 2011, NY TImes; http://well.blogs.nytimes.com/2011/02/28/go-easy-on-yourself-a-new-wave-of-research-urges/

Consumerism as Religion, essay, Randall Rauser, June 14, 2011

Love Yourself To Stay Healthy, 12 October 2010 by Jo Marchant

Your Critical Inner Voice: Are You Letting It Sabotage Your Relationships? Dr. Lisa Firestone, May 14, 2011, The Huffington Post; http://www.huffingtonpost.com/lisa-firestone/critical-inner-voice_b_861937.html?view=print

Parks and Other Green Environments: Essential Components of a Healthy Human, Debra Levey Larson, 2011, National Park and Recreation Assocaition; http://www.nrpa.org/uploadedFiles/Explore_Parks_and_Recreation/Research/Ming%20%28Kuo%29%20Reserach%20Paper-Final-150dpi.pdf

Afterword

"The time to be happy is now. The place to be happy is here. The way to be happy is to make others so." – Robert Green Ingersoll, The Gods and Other Lectures, 1876

"When we feel love and kindness toward others, it not only makes others feel loved and cared for, but it helps us also to develop inner happiness and peace."
– Tenzin Gyatso, (Dalai Lama), Human Rights, Democracy and Freedom, 2008

"All I'm saying is simply this, that all life is interrelated, that somehow we're caught in an inescapable network of mutuality tied in a single garment of destiny. Whatever affects one directly affects all indirectly. For some strange reason, I can never be what I ought to be until you are what you ought to be. You can never be what you ought to be until I am what I ought to be. This is the interrelated structure of reality."
—Dr. Martin Luther King Jr.

Spreading Happiness, Spreading Misery

The Pollyannaish childhood rhyme "Sticks and Stones may break my bones, but words will never hurt me", it turns out, couldn't be more wrong.

The very latest research at Harvard Medical School shows that parental and peer verbal abuse in the first 20 years of life causes significant physical damage to the brain, specifically in the corpus callosum, a large bundle of nerves which carries almost all neural traffic between hemispheres of the cerebral cortex, affecting memory, attention, perceptual awareness, thought, language, and consciousness. When it's damaged, sufferers have a weakened capacity for moral judgment, and are at a greater risk of cravings, drug abuse and dependencies, as well as a number of psychiatric disorders.

Through a new invention called *Diffusion Tensor Imaging* (DTI), which measures neural flow patterns, Harvard Medical School's Dr. Martin Teicher and his colleagues were able to pinpoint the precise areas damaged by exposure to criticism, humiliation, blaming, or other verbal abuse.

Teicher says the causes include an excess of stress hormones, impaired growth of the neural electrical insulation and changes in neurotransmitters. The damage, says by Dr. R. Douglas Fields, senior investigator at the National Institutes of Health, "can be seen as clearly as a bone fracture on an X-ray."

Similar damage occurs in the brains of people subjected to violent or sexual abuse in their formative years, but verbal abuse seems to cause greater damage to the brain than physical abuse, and it increases the likelihood that victims will later suffer from addictions or psychiatric disorders such as depression, anxiety, hostility and loneliness. The longer the abuse continues, and the greater its severity, the greater the damage and subsequent risk become.

It has long been known that this kind of abusive behavior continues to be "passed down" through generations within families, but we now know that misery also spreads outwardly, just like a biological disease. Another 2010 Harvard study, conducted by biophysicist Alison Hill, used data collected over the past 62 years to show that emotions are "contagious".

In other words, you can "catch" hostility, loneliness, selfishness, cynicism and sadness just like a cold. However, this doesn't mean you should dump your negative friends if you truly love them; research says you're likely consigning them to a sad life of health problems from heart disease to Alzheimer's.

As damaged people become more defensive and alert to social threats, they become more self-protective, less social, and alienate the very people around them they need most for their own well-being, transmitting their loneliness to those around them. A far healthier life strategy than abandonment for both of you is to offer a helping hand, because the good news is that helping others is very, very good for you, and happiness is also contagious. In fact, researchers have been able to calculate that the chance of being happy increases 11% for every happy friend in a person's life.

In fact, a 20-year British study published in 2008 found that the single most important criterion for happiness is connections to other happy people. A similar 2010 study found that good deeds "spread like a domino effect".

Based upon these findings, University of California Political Scientist James Fowler and Harvard Sociologist Nicholas Christakis devised a "be kind to a stranger" game, showing that one act of random kindness spurred dozens in response. Perhaps we can start a movement for an international "Be Kind to a Stranger" Day.

The basis is apparently mimicry, the effects of "social proof" instead of selfish calculation of subsequent rewards. So when people are irrationally kind, others are compelled to copy the behavior. And what's even better is that the effects are lasting. "You don't go back to being your "old selfish self", says Dr. Fowler. Kindness is not only catching, it's habit-forming.

Polite behavior is another contagious facet of human kindness with mutual benefits. As Dr. R. Douglas Fields writes in *The Other Brain*, politeness is a set of behaviours designed to promote structure and predictable order in societies, reducing what he calls the *neurotoxin* of stress, particularly the

534

stress of interacting with strangers. The more crowded the environment, the greater the stress and the need for these formalities. In other words, being polite is actually physically healthy for you and for others.

Even the simple act of smiling makes positive, healthy chemical changes in your mind and body, and has a similar effect on the people around you (not to mention making you appear more attractive, poised, in control and likeable).

Helping others has also been shown to have enormous positive psychological and health benefits, even when the act itself is demanding and stressful. Volunteer work in particular helps not just the recipients, but the volunteers to satisfy emotional needs, master new skills and have a greater sense of purpose, accomplishment and general well-being. Extensive research shows this confers "significant health benefits", including alleviating pain, stress and depression, reducing heart disease and even extending lifespan.

Allan Luks, author of *The Healing Power of Doing Good: The Health and Spiritual Benefits of Helping Others*, says that after performing an act of volunteerism, the body releases a rush of endorphins – natural pain killers released during moments of extreme pleasure, such as winning a lottery. He calls this the "helper's high", and adds that once these are released into the body, it creates a lasting sense of well-being that boosts health.

"...it miraculously improves both your health AND the community's through the work performed and the social ties built," says Dr. Thomas H. Sander, executive director of the Saguaro Seminar: Civic Engagement in America at the Harvard Kennedy School of Government. "Civic Engagement and volunteering is the new hybrid health club for the 21st century that's free to join."

A 2004 study at the Center on Aging and Health at Johns Hopkins Medicine also found that volunteering for those between the ages of 60 and 86 "... significantly increased physical, cognitive and social activity". The conclusion was that helping others on a regular basis actually slows the aging process.

Stephen Post, director of the Institute for Research on Unlimited Love, which studies altruism, compassion, and service, says, "The helping impulse is very fundamental. When it is locked off we do not flourish. It starts with a shift from thinking, 'I am the center of the world,' to a willingness to act toward others in helpful ways." Approximately two hours a week of volunteering is all that's required to experience the health benefits, he adds.

So in the end, it seems your parents really were onto something when they told you "It's better to give than to receive".

Consider Your Impact On The World

David Nichtern, a Buddhist instructor, likes to talk about the ripple effect that your treatment of others can have. Common courtesy, respect and thoughtfulness towards others in even the smallest of ways have a rippling effect like a pebble tossed into a pond.

Metaphorically, he describes how we interact with the world as planting spiritual seeds that will eventually ripen, some sooner than others. Like the tiny acorn which, under the right conditions, can grow into a mighty oak, human interaction plants small seeds that can result in major real-world events.

Every encounter with another gives you a choice as to how you'll interact with them. Buddhist mindfulness training aims to teach a greater awareness of moments that usually barely register as we go through our days on autopilot.

Do you actually ever meet the eyes of the waitress serving you at the local cafe? Smile at her? Consider how tough her job might be – eight to ten hours of standing, rushing back and forth, carrying heavy objects, listening to constant complaints and noise, cleaning up dirty leftovers?

What about the bus driver, parking attendant, cashier?

You can be sure that when you smile at someone else, or say a kind word, it has an effect and, depending on the circumstances, sometimes that effect can be profound. Say Nichtern, "...everything we want to build up from there – like compassion, decorum, elegance, well-being, peace, harmony – has these small gestures as its basis."

Conversely, he says, "...if we manifest grasping, aggression and ignorance in the smallest details of our interaction with others, these energies gather power and strength like an avalanche." The effects aren't just theoretical or metaphysical. Studies show there are demonstrable, real-world effects.

Every living person wants to feel he has value and is understood. By recognizing the unique qualities he holds dear – the personal aspects by which he identifies himself – you'll make him come alive. So the next time you meet someone new, ask yourself, "What's the one thing would she like others to recognize about her?" Knowing the answer to that single question will work unbelievably powerful magic in your life.

In the end, *The Path* to self-actualization, to fulfillment, to enlightenment, is followed by being true to your nature and accepting of the truth in world around you. Some ancient wisdom can help you navigate the way:

- Speak the truth, avoiding slander, gossip and abusive speech.

- Behave peacefully and harmoniously, refraining from theft, murder and overindulgence in physical indulgence.

- Avoiding earning a living in ways that cause harm, that exploit people or kill animals, or involve selling intoxicants or weapons.

- Cultivate a positive frame of mind, freeing yourself from evil and unwholesome states, and preventing their future emergence.

- Develop awareness of your body, its sensations, your feelings and your states of mind, and the mental focus that allows this awareness.

My final wish for you is that my work has shone a little light upon your Path, one that will bring you the greatest of happiness, love and light.

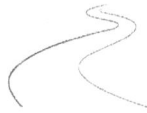

White Matter Tract Abnormalities in Young Adults Exposed to Parental Verbal Abuse, Jeewook Choiabd, Bumseok Jeongae, Michael L. Rohanac, Ann M. Polcariab, Martin H. Teicher, Harvard Medical School, Biological Psychiatry, February, 2009, Volume 65, Issue 3, Pages 227-234;

Hurtful Words: Association of Exposure to Peer Verbal Abuse With Elevated Psychiatric Symptom Scores and Corpus Callosum Abnormalities, Martin H Teicher, Jacqueline A Samson, Yi-Shin Sheu, Ann Polcari, Cynthia E McGreenery, The American Journal of Psychiatry, December, 2010; 167: 1464 – 1471;

The Other Brain, R. Douglas Fields Ph.D., 2009;

Emotions as Infectious Diseases in a Large Social Network: the SISa Model, Alison L. Hill, David G. Rand, Martin A. Nowak and Nicholas A. Christakis, 2010, Proceedings for the Royal Society;

Dynamic Spread of Happiness in a Large Social Network: Longitudinal Analysis Over 20 Years in the Framingham Heart Study, James H. Fowler and Nicholas A. Christakis, 2009, British Medical Journal 338;

Cooperative Behavior Cascades in Human Social Networks, James H. Fowler and Nicholas A. Christakis, 2010, Proceedings of the National Academy of Sciences, Vol. 107 No. 10;

Loneliness: human nature and the need for social connection, John T. Cacioppo and William Patrick, 2008;

The Therapeutic Effects of Smiling, Millicent H. Abel and Rebecca Hester, 2002, An Empirical Reflection on the Smile;

Volunteer Work as a Valuable Leisure Time Activity: A Day-Level Study on Volunteer Work, Non-Work Experiences, and Well-Being at Work, Dr. Eva J. Mojza et al, 2010, Journal of Occupational and Organizational Psychology;

The Healing Power of Doing Good: The Health and Spiritual Benefits of Helping Others, Allan Luks, 2001

The Ripple Effect of Common Courtesy, David Nichtern, 2011, The Huffington Post; http://www.huffingtonpost.com/david-nichtern/the-ripple-effect-of-comm_b_853232.html

About the Author

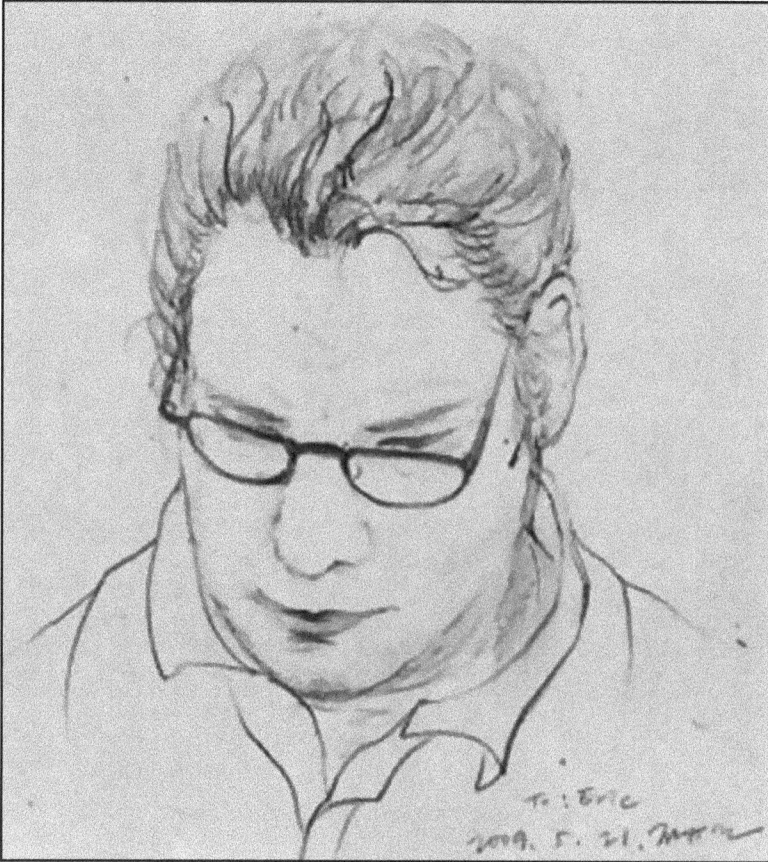

Pencil sketch, Yu Sun, 2010

Eric A. Smith is a freelance journalist, instructor and musician in Tokyo, Japan. A graduate of the University of North Carolina, he was a science reporter and photographer for The Beacon newspaper in Research Triangle Park before moving to Canada and opening his first company Hot Damn! Design.

Smith has taught IT and graphics at La Salle, Capilano and Dorsett Colleges, and trained the design staff of Pacific Press, the largest newspaper publisher in western Canada. He was also a volunteer associate editor of world-acclaimed Adbusters magazine.

Since arriving in Tokyo, he has earned JLPT certification in Japanese and established the design company Polyglot Studios, KK. In his spare time, he sings and writes original rock and folk songs, plays guitar and drums, and trains in weightlifting and Brazilian jiu jitsu. His cats are named Onion and Beebee.

www.ingramcontent.com/pod-product-compliance
Lightning Source LLC
Chambersburg PA
CBHW050447270326
41927CB00009B/1643